MALIGNANT HYPERTHERMIA

D1733149

EARLY SIGNS:

(not all need be present for a confirmed diagnosis)
- ☐ tachycardia (sudden, unexplained)
- ☐ tachypnea, spontaneous ventilation
- ☐ unstable blood pressure
- ☐ arrhythmias
- ☐ dark blood in surgical field despite adequate inspired oxygen
- ☐ cyanotic mottling of skin
- ☐ profuse sweating
- ☐ fever: rapid rise in temperature (1°F/15 min), sustained rise (to as high as 108°F [42.2°C] or more)
- ☐ fasciculations and/or rigidity (sometimes involving total body); trismus is an early sign
- ☐ discolored urine
- ☐ central venous desaturation
- ☐ central venous and arterial hypercarbia
- ☐ metabolic acidosis
- ☐ respiratory acidosis
- ☐ hyperkalemia
- ☐ myoglobinuria/myoglobinemia
- ☐ elevated CPK (late)

MH HOTLINE (209) 634-4917

For the name and telephone number of the MH consultant physician on call, dial the MH hotline number and ask for "index zero". MALIGNANT HYPERTHERMIA ASSOCIATION OF THE UNITED STATES

SUGGESTED STANDARD TREATMENT REGIMEN:

1. Stop anesthesia and surgery immediately. Change rubber goods and anesthesia machine.
2. Hyperventilate with 100% oxygen (flow: 8-10 liters).
3. As soon as possible, administer: dantrolene sodium I.V. (starting dose of 1 mg/kg up to maximum cumulative dose of 10 mg/kg) by rapid infusion; and procainamide I.V. (15 mg/kg over 10 minutes) if required for arrhythmias.
4. Initiate cooling:
   a) I.V. iced saline solution (not Ringer's lactate): 15 ml/Kg/10 min for 30 min.
   b) Surface cooling with ice and hypothermia blanket.
   c) Lavage of stomach, bladder, rectum, peritoneal and thoracic cavities with iced saline.
   d) If necessary, extracorporeal circulation and heat exchanger (femoral to femoral).
5. Correct acidosis and hyperkalemia (1–2mEq/Kg sodium bicarbonate stat guided by pH and P_aCO_2).
6. Secure monitoring lines: ECG, temperature, Foley catheter, arterial pressure, central venous pressure. Monitor: ECG, temperature, urinary output, arterial pressure and blood gases (P_aCO_2, P_aO_2), and pH, central venous pressure, electrolytes (K,Na).
7. Maintain urine output of at least 2 ml/kg/hr: administer mannitol 0.125 g/Kg I.V. and furosemide 1.0 mg/Kg I.V. (up to 4 doses each).
8. If desirable, administer 0.2 units/Kg of insulin in 50% D/W (1 ml/Kg) as an I.V. bolus to provide energy to cells.
9. Monitor patient until danger of subsequent episodes is past.
10. Post crisis follow-up therapy: administer oral dantrolene sodium 1-2 mg/kg q.i.d. (for 1 to 3 days).

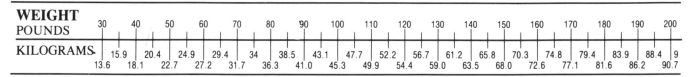

WEIGHT POUNDS	30	40	50	60	70	80	90	100	110	120	130	140	150	160	170	180	190	200
KILOGRAMS	15.9	20.4	24.9	29.4	34	38.5	43.1	47.7	52.2	56.7	61.2	65.8	70.3	74.8	79.4	83.9	88.4	9
	13.6	18.1	22.7	27.2	31.7	36.3	41.0	45.3	49.9	54.4	59.0	63.5	68.0	72.6	77.1	81.6	86.2	90.7

A PRACTICE OF ANESTHESIA
FOR INFANTS AND CHILDREN

THE SCIENTIFIC BASIS OF CLINICAL ANESTHESIA

Series Editors
Richard J. Kitz, M.D. and Myron B. Laver, M.D. (deceased)

A PRACTICE OF ANESTHESIA FOR INFANTS AND CHILDREN

Edited by

JOHN F. RYAN, M.D.
Associate Professor of Anaesthesia,
Harvard Medical School
Anesthetist, Massachusetts General Hospital

I. DAVID TODRES, M.D.
Associate Professor of Anaesthesia (Paediatrics)
Harvard Medical School
Anesthetist and Pediatrician, Massachusetts General Hospital

CHARLES J. COTÉ, M.D.
Associate Professor of Anaesthesia
Harvard Medical School
Associate Anesthetist, Massachusetts General Hospital

NISHAN G. GOUDSOUZIAN, M.D.
Associate Professor of Anaesthesia
Harvard Medical School
Anesthetist, Massachusetts General Hospital

W.B. SAUNDERS COMPANY
Harcourt Brace Jovanovich, Inc.
Philadelphia London Toronto Montreal Sydney Tokyo

W. B. SAUNDERS COMPANY
Harcourt Brace Jovanovich, Inc.

The Curtis Center
Independence Square West
Philadelphia, PA 19106

Library of Congress Cataloging in Publication Data
Main entry under title:

A Practice of anesthesia for infants and children.

(The Scientific basis of clinical anesthesia)
Includes index.
1. Pediatric anesthesia. I. Ryan, John F.,
1935-   . II. Series. [DNLM: 1. Anesthesia—in
infancy and childhood. WO 440 P895]
RD139.P73   1985   617'.96   85-12700
ISBN 0-8089-1732-3

Library of Congress Catalog Number 85-12700
International Standard Book Number 0-8089-1732-3
Printed in the United States of America
88 89 90 10 9 8 7 6 5

Dedication

To our parents, spouses, and children, who supported our efforts to pursue the goal of excellence in pediatric anesthesia.

Contents

Preface

Good ideas like good grapes need to ferment, then rest comfortably, perhaps for years before emerging as a school of thought and practice or as a vintage wine which is savored and consumed. Both enrich the quality of life.

The genesis of *A Practice of Anesthesia for Infants and Children* was more than a decade ago. It would be designed to describe a school of anesthesia concepts and procedures practiced by the pediatric anesthesia team at the Massachusetts General Hospital and selected students of the group now on the faculty of other Boston hospitals.

A school evolves over time when a number of faculty with different educational backgrounds, experiences, and practices, begin to develop common goals, philosophies, and patterns of care that transcend the individual contributions, representing a distillation and blending that results in a truly superior educational, scientific, and practice environment. The contributors are individuals who have trained and taught both in and outside the United States. Thus very diverse philosophies and experiences have contributed to the development of the school. Several are Diplomates of the American Board of Pediatrics, with one certified in Neonatal medicine; some have recently been awarded Certificates of Special Competence in Critical Care Medicine.

It is uncommon for a group of individually recognized authorities with such an eclectic background of education and research to agree on common goals, concepts and patterns of care. *A Practice of Anesthesia for Infants and Children*, represents a different approach to pediatric anesthesia texts because it isn't an individual author's experience nor catalogue of contributions from different unassociated chapter editors, but is in effect a chimera of this team's personal attitudes, experiences, and practices—verily, a school of thought, teachings, researches, and caretaking patterns. Like the vintage wine, it too is meant to be savored and enjoyed with the expectation that the anesthetic care of infants and children will improve their quality of life.

Richard J. Kitz, M.D.

Acknowledgment

This book has evolved out of the experiences of the Pediatric Anesthesia Group at the Massachusetts General Hospital and co-workers who have trained and are closely associated with us. Our aim is to share our experiences and philosophy and provide a balanced update on the current state of the art of pediatric anesthesia. We hope that this book will fulfill the need expressed by many of our co-workers for a text which is intermediate between a didactic manual and the encyclopedic text.

Many individuals have helped with this project. Our Chairman of Anesthesia, Dr. Richard J. Kitz, has contributed significantly with his stimulus and constant encouragement. Our pediatric surgeons have been an integral part of the development of pediatric anesthesia at the Massachusetts General Hospital. Our secretarial staff, Virginia Clark, Ruth Glazier, Diane Ross, and Jeanne McAdam, worked tirelessly to bring this work to fruition. We also thank Marjorie A. Coté for her meticulous review of each chapter. The excellent drawings and illustrations were supplied by Paul Andriesse.

Contributors

Charles B. Berde, M.D., Ph.D.
Assistant Professor of Anaesthesia, Harvard Medical School;
Assistant in Anesthesia, Children's Hospital Medical
    Center, Boston, Massachusetts

Charles J. Coté, M.D.
Associate Professor of Anaesthesia, Harvard Medical
    School;
Associate Anesthetist, Massachusetts General Hospital
    and the Shriners Burns Institute, Boston Massachusetts

Robert K. Crone, M.D.
Associate Professor of Anaesthesia (Paediatrics),
    Harvard Medical School;
Senior Associate in Anesthesia, Pediatrics, and
    Cardiology, Children's Hospital Medical Center,
    Boston, Massachusetts

Daniel F. Dedrick, M.D.
Assistant Professor of Anaesthesia, Harvard Medical
    School;
Anesthesiologist, Brigham and Women's Hospital,
    Boston, Massachusetts

Susan Firestone, M.D.
Instructor in Anaesthesia, Harvard Medical School;
Assistant Anesthetist, Massachusetts General Hospital,
    Boston, Massachusetts

Nishan G. Goudsouzian, M.D.
Associate Professor of Anaesthesia, Harvard Medical
    School;
Anesthetist, Massachusetts General Hospital, Boston
    Massachusetts

Paul R. Hickey, M.D.
Associate Professor of Anaesthesia, Harvard Medical
    School;
Senior Associate in Anesthesia, Children's Hospital
    Medical Center, Boston, Massachusetts

Letty M. P. Liu, M.D.
Associate Professor of Anaesthesia, Harvard Medical
    School;
Associate Anesthetist, Massachusetts General Hospital,
    Boston, Massachusetts

J. A. Jeevendra Martyn, M.D.
Associate Professor of Anaesthesia, Harvard Medical
    School;
Associate Anesthetist, Massachusetts General Hospital
    and the Shriners Burns Institute; Boston Massachusetts

Mark A. Rockoff, M.D.
Assistant Professor of Anaesthesia (Paediatrics),
    Harvard Medical School;
Associate in Anesthesia, Children's Hospital Medical
    Center, Boston, Massachusetts

John F. Ryan, M.D.
Associate Professor of Anaesthesia, Harvard Medical
    School;
Anesthetist, Massachusetts General Hospital, Boston,
    Massachusetts

S.K. Szyfelbein, M.D.
Associate Professor of Anaesthesia, Harvard Medical
    School;
Anesthetist, Massachusetts General Hospital and the
    Shriners Burns Institute; Boston, Massachusetts

I. David Todres, M.D.
Associate Professor of Anaesthesia (Paediatrics),
    Harvard Medical School;
Anesthetist and Pediatrician, Massachusetts General
    Hospital, Boston, Massachusetts

Francis X. Vacanti, M.D.
Instructor in Anaesthesia, Harvard Medical School;
Assistant in Anesthesia, Massachusetts General
    Hospital, Boston, Massachusetts

A PRACTICE OF ANESTHESIA
FOR INFANTS AND CHILDREN

1

The Practice of Pediatric Anesthesia

John F. Ryan, I. David Todres
Charles J. Coté, and Nishan G. Goudsouzian

This chapter will outline the basis of our practice of pediatric anesthesia. While general principles of safe practice are given here, individual practice is determined by the particular situation. These basic principles of practice, however, can be applied regardless of the circumstances; they provide the foundation for safe anesthesia.

PREOPERATIVE EVALUATION AND MANAGEMENT

The anesthesiologist must assume an active role in the preoperative assessment of the child. Ideally, the anesthesiologist performing the preoperative evaluation will also anesthetize the patient. A complete medical history, family history, physical examination, and chart review is performed on every patient to be anesthetized (see Chapter 4). When appropriate, the child should receive preoperative medical therapy to optimize his or her condition prior to receiving anesthesia. In addition, the emotional state of the child and family must be considered and appropriate support provided.

Familiarity with the child's clinical and psychological status is essential. Seeing the child for the first time in the operating room and then proceeding impersonally with the anesthetic procedure is both potentially hazardous to the child and unfair to the family. The anesthetic experience itself is unique for the child, and proper rapport between child, anesthesiologist, and family is crucial for success. This relationship must carry through to the postoperative phase, and special attention should be given to the relief of pain and anxiety. The anesthesiologist, with an understanding of the pharmacology of sedative and narcotic drugs, as well as the ability to perform nerve blocks, can provide valuable assistance in this respect.

The anesthesiologist must always understand the proposed surgical or investigative procedure. This facilitates the planning of an appropriate level of monitoring, as well as the selection of anesthetic drugs and technique. The anesthesiologist must anticipate the surgeon's needs regarding patient positioning and muscle relaxation, as well as the patient's need for fluid, blood and narcotics. Thus, for complex cases the anesthesiologist and surgeon should formulate a plan preoperatively, and should also completely explain that plan to the parents and child. If there are any important medical issues that require further clarification, this consultation should be a part of the preoperative evaluating and planning process. Notes on the planned surgical procedure by specialists or consultants must be carefully reviewed.

Appropriate preoperative abstinence from food and fluid should always be ordered. Special consideration must be given to the infant, where prolonged abstinence may lead to serious hypoglycemia and dehydration (see Chapter 10). It should be kept in mind that children may surreptitiously circumvent the preoperative fasting order. Thus, one must always be on guard for the possibility of a full stomach and its sequelae.

Preoperative consideration must be given to proper psychological support, any appropriate premedication, and the timing of the premedication (see Chapter 8). Premedication may be omitted because of the critical nature of the child's illness, or because the child is especially cooperative. No matter how calm they might appear, psychological support of the child and parents must never be neglected. Premedication may be administered on the ward or in the room adjacent to the operating room. Once any medication is administered, the child must always be adequately monitored for changes in cardiopulmonary function. The movement of the medicated child to the operating room must always be undertaken with safety in mind; the critically ill must be accompanied by skilled staff equipped to deal with any emergency enroute.

The possible need for postoperative intensive care, including assisted ventilation, should be anticipated and fully discussed with the parents and child (if of an appropriate age). Unnecessary concern and anxiety may then be avoided should this form of therapy be instituted.

INFORMED CONSENT

It is necessary that the risks and benefits of the anesthetic procedure be presented in clear, easily understood terms. A simple explanation to the parents of what the anesthesiologist will be doing to assure good care and safety for their child should provide the information necessary to relieve preoperative anxiety. During this explanation, reference should be made to the anesthesiologist's careful monitoring of parameters such as temperature (e.g., use of special heating blankets), heart rate and breath sounds (e.g., electrocardiogram and stethoscope), and special techniques of blood pressure measurement (e.g., intra-arterial cannulation, central venous pressure), urine output (e.g., Foley catheters), etc. An explanation of the information obtained by these monitors, and how they help to improve the safety of anesthesia, will also help to relieve anxiety. Details should not be recited in a cold and technical manner but with dialogue that responds to the parent's and child's questions and concerns. Frequently this dialogue is given too little time, leaving the parents and child insecure and unnecessarily apprehensive. Whenever invasive monitoring devices will be applied, the parents and child should be assured that in most cases these will be placed after induction of anesthesia so as to avoid patient discomfort, and that they will be removed as soon as the child's postoperative condition permits.

It is important to reassure the parents and child that the anesthesiologist is in constant attendance and is responsible for the medical well-being of the child while the surgeon undertakes the necessary operation. This not only provides reassurance, but emphasizes our role as physicians in the operating room. A high profile postoperatively, and in the intensive care unit, may contribute significantly to this phase of the patient's care, because of our special training in coping with rapid changes in physiologic status.

In discussing the procedure with the child, the child's age and level of understanding will determine how to present the concept of anesthesia, surgery, and postoperative care. Small children require reassurance that *they will not wake up during the procedure, and that they will awaken at the conclusion.* Fear of not waking is a serious concern for many children. The possibility of postoperative pain and the relief the child will receive in the form of nerve blocks and analgesics must be clearly presented to the parents and child.

THE OPERATING ROOM AND MONITORING

In order for the anesthesiologist to successfully carry out the proposed anesthetic plan, the patient's chart must be reexamined just prior to induction of anesthesia for pertinent information that may have been added at the last moment. It is most important that the patient's identification bracelet be checked, especially if the anesthetizing team is different from the preoperative evaluation team. All equipment for induction and maintenance of anesthesia, including suction and all necessary monitoring devices, must be functioning and reliable (see Chapter 23). *This must be checked personally by the anesthesiologist taking care of the child.* Too often it is presumed that certain equipment is functioning because other personnel have checked it.

The degree of monitoring must be adjusted according to the child's underlying clinical condition and the planned surgical procedure. In every situation, basic monitoring is essential; to this are added special monitoring devices as they become necessary. The basic monitors are the anesthesiologist's eyes, ears, and hands, which means the ability to observe the patient's color and chest movements, to listen for heart tones and breath sounds, and to palpate the arterial pulse. We believe that a precordial or esophageal stethoscope should be placed on every child as part of basic monitoring. All children, except those undergoing the briefest noninvasive procedures, should have an intravenous line inserted. This allows for fluid replacement and a route for the rapid and predictable administration of drugs. This is particularly important in children who have undergone prolonged fasting. Continuous electrocardiographic, temperature, inspired or expired oxygen with alarms, and intermittent blood pressure monitoring are considered routine. Expired carbon dioxide monitors, as well as those for pulse oximetry, have recently become extremely important in the early detection of "near miss" anesthetic-related problems, i.e., events which, if undetected, could result in serious morbidity or mortality.

Invasive monitoring techniques, such as arterial cannulation, central venous pressure, or pulmonary artery occlusion pressure monitoring, are required for major surgery on a stable patient where one anticipates extensive blood loss or fluid shifts, or in any medically unstable patient. The urinary catheter provides data regarding intravascular volume status and organ perfusion; it is particularly useful for long operations, procedures involving significant blood loss, or those in which wide swings in blood pressure and fluid balance can be anticipated.

If a particular variable would be monitored in the adult, then the child deserves the same treatment. Not infrequently invasive monitoring procedures are forsaken in the child because of the inexperience of the anesthesiologist with pediatric techniques; the need for invasive monitoring is thus rationalized away as being excessive. These monitors, however, allow the accurate measurement of blood pressure, cardiac output, filling pressures, and cardiac and pulmonary function. In turn they provide a safe mechanism for assessing the response to pharmacologic interventions, as well as the responses to blood product and fluid administration.

A cautionary note: with increased sophistication in monitoring, the anesthesiologist has become more distanced than ever from the patient; relying totally on mechanical monitoring devices to detect clinical abnormalities is dangerous. *The focus must always be on the child. Monitors may fail, and if, the anesthesiologist's attention is focused on the monitor in an effort to interpret it, rather than attending directly to the patient, the patient will suffer.*

INDUCTION AND MAINTENANCE OF ANESTHESIA

Significant differences in the physiology and behavior of the child, especially the newborn, in comparison to the adult, mandate that the anesthesiologist not consider the child merely a small adult.

For example, in the infant the rate of uptake of anesthetic agents is more rapid than in the adult, and the child's response to most medications is also different, indicating that changes made in inspired inhalation agents should be more gradual, and the doses of medication diluted and titrated more carefully.

The approach to the anesthetic procedure in the child is in principle similar to the adult. In practice, however, it is often advisable to modify the sequence of anesthetic induction. In the relatively stable child, after anesthesia is induced monitors may be applied without traumatic upset. In the critically ill child, however, while attempting always to approach the child in the least threatening way, establishing monitoring must not be compromised. Thus, therapeutic interventions in the very sick child and adult proceed along similar pathways.

In the child, as with the adult, monitoring begins with the basic observations of heart rate, blood pressure, respiration and temperature. The most important aspect of basic monitoring consists of using the senses of sight, hearing and touch.

CLINICAL MONITORS

Sight

Constantly observing the patient's chest excursion (depth and symmetry), the color of the nail beds, oral mucosa, and capillary refill will provide vital information regarding ventilation and perfusion.

Hearing

Constantly listening to the quality of the heart tones and breath sounds through a precordial or esophageal stethoscope will give instant feedback regarding heart rate and rhythm, cardiac output (changes in intensity of heart sounds), and ventilation. This is particularly helpful in diagnosing arrhythmias, hypovolemia, anesthetic overdose, and airway obstruction.

Touch

Intermittently examining the patient, especially palpating peripheral pulses and feeling the skin, will provide information confirming the auditory input regarding heart rate, cardiac output, blood pressure and temperature.

AIRWAY AND VENTILATION

The most important consideration in the safe practice of pediatric anesthesia is attention to the airway. Because of the unique characteristics of the infant's and child's airway, obstruction occurs readily (see Chapter 5). Thus, the anesthesiologist must maintain constant vigilance of the airway to ensure that it remains clear at all times. Airway obstruction leads to hypoventilation, but the causes of hypoventilation may also be central (e.g., drug depression) or peripheral (e.g., muscle relaxation) in origin. Thus, emphasis and attention must always be placed on the anesthesiologist constantly monitoring the adequacy of ventilation. While it is desirable to ventilate optimally and maintain a $PaCO_2$ of approximately 40 torr, rarely at the operating table is an infant or child harmed by mild to moderate overventilation; underventilation has far more serious consequences.

Constant monitoring of inspired and expired oxygen concentrations, expired carbon dioxide concentrations, and oxygen saturation (pulse oximetry) are valuable adjuncts to the senses of sight, hearing, and touch. Failure to ventilate adequately is probably the most important factor in the morbidity and mortality of children undergoing anesthesia.

FLUIDS

Intraoperative fluid management is especially important in the infant and child (see Chapter 10). The relatively small blood volume of the infant leads to rapid development of hypovolemia. Both the replacement of lost blood and basic fluid administration must be carefully titrated (using rate-limiting devices), since overhydration is easily produced. The anesthesiologist should, therefore, have a clear plan of fluid administration, and this plan should be written out on the anesthetic record. A well planned outline results in a rational and safe approach to correction of fluid deficit, maintenance, and loss.

CONDUCT OF THE ANESTHESIA TEAM

The anesthesiologist must maintain full concentration throughout the procedure; the child's safety is in his or her hands, and any inattention may place the child's life in jeopardy. Should members of the anesthesia team need to replace each other during the anesthetic procedure, it is essential that the "baton" of responsibility is passed in a smooth and coordinated manner. A clear dialogue between team members must be established regarding the nature of the surgery, the child's underlying condition, anesthetic agents, fluid and blood management, as well as any special problems. Drugs on the anesthesia machine must be clearly labelled by name and dosage, so that the child is not exposed to needless risk.

Ongoing communication between the anesthesiologist and surgeon is always important; this allows the anesthesiologist to anticipate potential changes in the child's physiological status due to surgical manipulations, and thus to deal with them immediately, appropriately, and more effectively.

The conclusion of the anesthetic procedure is fraught with potential problems. Therefore, the anesthesiologist should not be alone or relax vigilance during awakening and transferring the patient to the recovery room or intensive care unit. It is during this stage that the patient is most likely to have problems with postanesthetic excitement, vomiting, or airway obstruction (see Chapter 22).

Records of the anesthetic procedure must be accurate and complete. The anesthesiologist must avoid the compulsion, however, to complete these during the procedure if the child's condition warrants special attention.

RECOVERY ROOM

The anesthesiologist has a responsibility to the child that continues into the recovery room. Transport to the recovery room must be carried out with appropriate monitoring, attention to a clear airway, adequate ventilation, and perfusion.

In the recovery room, a clear summary of the medical and surgical problems of the child and of the anesthetic procedure is given to the nurse who will continue to monitor the child. Appropriate resuscitation equipment must be at hand. Vital signs, (temperature, heart rate, blood pressure, respiratory rate) are recorded. Special instructions are given relating to fluid management, oxygen administration, drug therapy, blood tests (hematocrit, blood gases, electrolytes, coagulation profile, etc.), and x-rays.

POSTOPERATIVE VISIT

The anesthesiologist should visit the child and family postoperatively to assess the post-anesthetic clinical course and discuss their reaction to the anesthetic procedure. A note should be placed in the child's record. All too often the anesthesiologist is a "nonperson" in the eyes of the family. If the public is to understand and respect the profession of anesthesiology, close interaction between parents, child, and anesthesiologist is necessary.

CONCLUSION

This introductory chapter outlines the fundamentals of pediatric anesthesia practice. The chapters which follow expand these fundamentals in areas which we feel from our experience will help the practicing anesthesiologist. We have reiterated specific points throughout in order to stress their importance.

2

Growth and Development

I. David Todres

As the infant matures, vital changes occur which affect the child's response to disease, drugs, and the environment. Growth is an increase in physical size, while development is an increase in complexity and function. An overview of this subject is presented so that the anesthesiologist may better appreciate the uniqueness of the child at different developmental stages. With this understanding the application of anesthetic practice to the child is built on sound scientific foundations.

Prenatal growth is the most important phase, comprising organogenesis in the first eight weeks (embryonic growth), followed by development of organ systems function, and maturation of the fetus to full-term (fetal growth). Rapid growth occurs particularly in the second trimester, and increase in weight from laying down of subcutaneous tissue and muscle mass occurs in the third trimester. The duration of gestation and the weight of the infant have an important relationship (Table 2-1); deviations from this relationship may be associated with serious effects in the infant. These effects may be the result of inadequate nutrition (maternal malnutrition or placental insufficiency), congenital viral infection, or developmental malformation.

Table 2-1

The Relationship of Gestational Age To Weight

Gestation (wk)	Mean Weight (gm)
28	1050
32	1700
36	2500
40 (full-term)	3400

Clarification of the terms used to describe the newborn infant is necessary. The term prematurity has conventionally been applied to infants who weigh less than 2500 gm at birth, and who were usually born prematurely. Some infants, however, are born at term and weigh less than 2500 gm. For this reason the designation preterm infant is preferred. A preterm infant by definition is one born before 37 weeks gestation; post-term refers to an infant born after 42 weeks. Irrespective of the time of birth, an infant may be small for gestational age (SGA), large for gestational age (LGA), or appropriate for gestational age (AGA) (Table 2-2).

A low birth weight (LBW) infant is one weighing less than 2500 gm irrespective of the duration of pregnancy. A very low birth weight infant (VLBW) weighs less than 1500 gm. Low birth weight is associated with maternal malnutrition, toxemia, placental insufficiency, genetic factors, excessive smoking, and alcohol.

The SGA infant is usually the result of intrapartum factors which lead to intrauterine undernutrition, e.g., toxemia and placental insufficiency. Other causes include intrauterine infections (rubella, cytomegalovirus), chromosomal abnormalities, and congenital malformations.[1] The SGA infant is particularly prone to hypoglycemia, poor temperature control, and mental and/or physical handicap. Problems associated with gestation and body habitus are summarized in Table 2-2.

Diabetes or prediabetes in the mother is often associated with LGA infants. This is the result of excessive amounts of subcutaneous fat laid down from increased fetal insulin in response to maternal hyperglycemia. With improved control of maternal diabetes these infants do not grow as large as with poor control; although large, the infants are often less mature.[2-4]

Gestational age estimation is an important assessment.

Table 2-2

Common Neonatal Problems Associated with Weight and Gestation

Gestation	Body Habitus	Neonatal Problems at Increased Incidence	
Premature: less than 37 wk gestation	SGA	Respiratory distress syndrome Apnea Hypoglycemia Hypomagnesemia Hypocalcemia Hyperbilirubinemia	Viral infection Thrombocytopenia Congenital anomalies Maternal drug addiction Neonatal asphyxia Aspiration pneumonia
	AGA	Respiratory distress syndrome Apnea Hypoglycemia Hypomagnesemia Hypocalcemia Hyperbilirubinemia	
	LGA	Respiratory distress syndrome Hypoglycemia Apnea Hypomagnesemia Hypocalcemia Hyperbilirubinemia	Transposition of great arteries Infant of diabetic mother
Normal: 37–42 wk gestation	SGA	Congenital anomalies Viral infection Thrombocytopenia Maternal drug addiction Neonatal asphyxia Hypoglycemia	
	AGA	—	
	LGA	Birth trauma Hyperbilirubinemia Hypoglycemia—infant of diabetic mother Transposition of great arteries	
Postmature: greater than 42 wk gestation	SGA	Congenital anomalies Viral infection Thrombocytopenia Maternal drug addiction Neonatal asphyxia Aspiration pneumonia Hypoglycemia	
	AGA	—	
	LGA	Birth Trauma Hyperbilirubinemia Hypoglycemia—infant of diabetic mother Transposition great arteries	

This table presents the neonatal problems commonly associated with babies of various size and gestational age. SGA = small for gestational age; AGA = appropriate for gestational age; LGA = large for gestational age.

Table 2-3

Neurologic and External Physical Criteria Used to Assess Gestational Age

Physical	Preterm (<37 wk)	Term (>37 wk)
Ear	Shapeless, pliable	Firm, well formed
Skin	Edematous, thin skin	Thick skin
Sole of foot	Creases only anterior $\frac{1}{3}$	All of foot creased
Breast tissue	Less than 1 mm diameter	More than 5 mm diameter
Genitalia		
Male	Scrotum poorly developed	Scrotum rugated
	Testes undescended	Testes descended
Female	Large clitoris, gaping labia majora	Labia majora developed
Limbs	Hypotonic	Tonic (flexed)
Grasp reflex	Weak grasp	Can be lifted by reflex grasp
Moro relfex	Complete but exhaustible (>32 wk)	Complete
Sucking Reflex	Weak	Strong, synchronous with swallowing

This table presents in very general terms the commonly examined physical and neurological signs. For more detailed examination refer to standard texts.

This is arrived at through a record of the maternal history, but this may be vague or lead to errors in estimating gestational age. Neuromuscular behavior is the best indicator of gestational age, which may also be estimated by examination of special physical characteristics—skin, hair, ears, breasts and external genitalia.[5,6] The Dubowitz scoring system is a well accepted method which combines neurologic and external physical criteria to provide an accurate assessment of gestational age.[7,8] A summary of some of the more significant neurologic and physical signs of maturity is presented in Table 2-3.

Assessment of growth is measured by changes in weight, height, and head circumference. Percentile charts are valuable for following the infant's and child's growth and development. Deviation from growth within the same percentile for a child of any age is of greater significance than any single measurement (Figures 2-1 and 2-2).

Weight, a more sensitive index than length or head circumference, is the most commonly used measurement of growth and is an important indication of well being and illness or poor nutrition in the child. Changes in weight reflect changes in muscle mass, adipose tissue, skeleton, and body water, and thus are non-specific measures of growth.

Infants lose 5–10 percent of their body weight in the first 24-48 hours from loss of body water. In full-term infants, birth weight is regained in 10–14 days. For the full-term newborn a daily increase of 30 grams (210gm/wk) is satisfactory for the first three months. Thereafter, weight gain slows so that at 10–12 months of age it is 70 grams each week. For the full-term infant birth weight is approximately doubled at six months, and tripled at one year. Knowledge of the average weight at various ages is helpful in judging whether there is a possible growth-limiting illness (Table 2-4).

The anesthesiologist should recognize the infant or child whose weight deviates from the normal. Failure to thrive (FTT) indicates that a serious underlying disorder may be present, which could significantly affect the anesthetic procedure. Table 2-5 presents major causes of FTT.

Measurement of length provides the best indicator of skeletal growth, as it is not affected by changes in adipose tissue and water content.

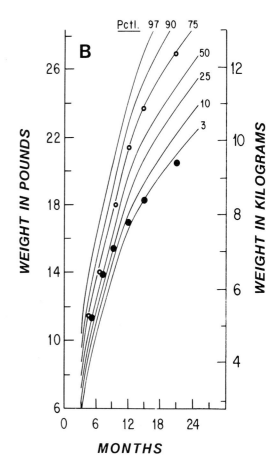

INFANT BOYS

Figure 2-1. Postnatal growth curve (weight) for term male infants. This figure represents normal growth curves. Open circles indicate a normal child. Closed circles demonstrate failure to thrive in a child with severe renal failure.

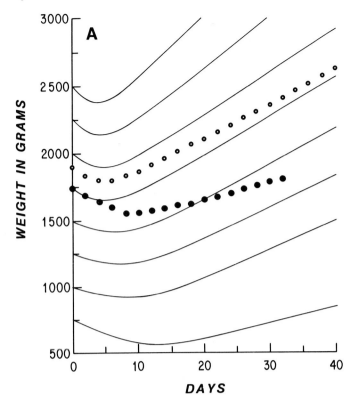

Figure 2-2. Postnatal growth Curve (Weight) for Preterm Infants. This figure represents normal growth curves for preterm infants. Open circles indicate a normal preterm infant. Closed circles demonstrate failure to thrive, in an infant with bronchopulmonary dysplasia.

Table 2-4

The Relationship of Age to Weight

Age (yr)	Weight (kg)
1	10
3	15
5	19
7	23

HEAD CIRCUMFERENCE

Head size reflects growth of the brain, and correlates with intracranial volume and brain weight. Head circumference is a measurement of head growth and it should be appreciated that this reflects only a part of the total body growth process; it may or may not reflect underlying involvement of the brain. The mean expected head circumference for the preterm and full-term newborn is presented in Table 2-6. An abnormally large or small head may indicate abnormal brain development, and this must alert the anesthesiologist to possible neurologic problems. A large head may indicate hydrocephalus or increased intracranial pressure, while a small head may indicate failure of brain development.

During the first year of life, head circumference normally increases 10 cm, and 2.5 cm in the second year. By 6 months of age, head circumference reaches 50 percent of adult size, and by 2 years it is 75 percent. For the first six months of life

Table 2-5

Common Causes of Failure to Thrive (FTT)

Genetic—parental size, chromosomal disorders
Nutritional—inadequate or inappropriate intake, malabsorption, diarrhea, vomiting, cystic fibrosis, celiac disease, carbohydrate intolerance, milk protein allergy
Malformations—especially cardiac or urinary tract
Infections—pulmonary, renal, hepatic, enteral, congenital infections
Metabolic/Endocrine disorders—hypothyroidism, renal tubular acidosis
Preterm and SGA infants
Malignancy

Table 2-6

The Relationship of Gestational Age to Head Circumference

Gestation (wk)	Head Circumference (cm)
28	25
32	29
36	32
40 (full-term)	35

the circumference of the head is greater than the thorax. After two years of age the head circumference increases much less rapidly, i.e., 2–3 cm over the next 10 years. Head circumference is closely followed on standard percentile growth curves. As with weight, deviations of growth of the head within the same percentile is more significant than a single measurement.

The anterior fontanel should be palpated to assess if it is sunken (dehydration) or bulging abnormally, suggesting increased intracranial pressure (hydrocephalus, infection, hemorrhage, increased $PaCO_2$). If bulging, then the sutures should be palpated for abnormal separation due to increased intracranial pressure. The anterior fontanel closes between 9–18 months of age; the posterior fontanel closes by about four months of age. Premature synostosis of sutures may result in an abnormal shape and retard brain growth and development. The head may be abnormal in shape due to genetic, and not necessarily pathological, causes. Cranial molding is seen particularly in LBW infants and is usually of no clinical significance.

THE FACE

While the cranial vault increases rapidly in size, the face and base of the skull develop at a slower rate. At birth the mandible is small, but as the child develops forward growth occurs, reducing the obliquity of the mandibular angle. Failure of prenatal development of the mandible may be associated with severe congenital defects, e.g., Pierre Robin, Treacher-Collins, or Goldenhar's syndromes. These syndromes often have other associated anomalies. After two years of age, while the cranial vault increases relatively little in size, there is a significant change in facial configuration. The upper jaw grows rapidly to accommodate the developing teeth. In addition, the frontal sinuses develop by two to six years, while maxillary, ethmoid and sphenoid sinuses appear after six years of age.

TEETH

The first tooth, usually lower incisor, appears at approximately six months of age (deciduous dentition). Permanent teeth appear at 6 years, with the shedding of the deciduous teeth; this process takes place over the next six to eight years. Poor nutrition and chronic illness may interfere with calcification of deciduous and permanent teeth. Loose teeth should be sought in any child between the ages of five and ten years, or where severe dental caries occur as a result of poor dental hygiene and infection. Appropriate care must be taken when placing an oral airway and performing laryngoscopy in children with loose teeth.

Abnormally developed teeth occur with hereditary disturbances, Down's syndrome, cerebral palsy, and nutritional defects. Normal premature infants may show severe enamel hypoplasia in their primary dentition.[9] Tetracycline administration during the period of calcification in children leads to permanent discoloration.

BODY COMPOSITION

The more immature the infant the greater the relative water content (Table 2-7). Total body water decreases at the expense of the extracellular compartment, with adult levels attained at one year of age.[10] This will have implications regarding drug dosage and distribution in the infant (see Chapters 6 and 7). The male has a higher percentage of water, whereas the female has a slightly higher percentage of fat. The percentage of decrease in extracellular volume is greater than the decrease in total body water because of the simultaneous increase in intracellular water.

DEVELOPMENT OF ORGAN SYSTEMS

RESPIRATORY SYSTEM

In utero the placenta performs the necessary function of gas exchange for the developing fetus, i.e., the delivery of oxygen and removal of carbon dioxide. The fetal lung, while undergoing rhythmic "breathing movements," does not participate in gas exchange but undergoes developmental changes that will allow it to perform this vital function at birth. The airways and terminal air spaces of the fetal lung are filled with fluid (approximately 100–200 ml) which is secreted by the lung. This fluid contains mucopolysaccharides, proteins, and surface-active lipoproteins (surfactant).

Table 2-7

Relationship of Age to Total Body Water

Age	Body Water (%)
Fetus	90
Preterm	80
Full-term	70
6–12 months	60

At birth, physiological adjustments occur with the first breath that ensure the inflation of the lung with air, and maintenance of inflation at the end of expiration. This requires removal of the fluid from the airways and terminal airspaces in the first 4–6 hours of life, and the adequate production of surfactant to maintain alveolar stability. The first breath of air by the newborn infant will generate a negative pressure of 50–70 cm H_2O to move the fluid down the tracheobronchial tree.[11,12] This necessitates overcoming the surface tension forces and viscosity of the fluid in the airways. With repetitive breaths eventually all the fluid is replaced by air. The major portion of the fluid is removed by the pulmonary circulation and lymphatic system. Some of the fluid is expressed orally as the infant's trunk is compressed in the birth canal during delivery, an advantage lost to the infant born by cesarean section who may, as a result, exhibit transient tachypnea from inadequate fluid removal.[13]

The first breath is initiated by many stimuli, which include changes in PaO_2, $PaCO_2$ and pH. However, marked decreases in PaO_2 and increases in $PaCO_2$ from birth asphyxia may cause depression of ventilation. In addition, changes in temperature and tactile stimuli also appear important in initiating respiratory drive.[11]

The preterm infant, however, has much greater difficulty in establishing regular sustained and adequate respirations at birth. This is the result of a less mature central nervous system drive together with inadequate expansion of terminal airspaces. Low levels of surfactant result in an inability to maintain adequate expansion at the end of expiration, leading to a reduced functional residual capacity. The highly compliant chest of the infant also makes inspiratory efforts less effective, and with each breath significant airway closure takes place. Some degree of airway closure occurs in all infants until approximately one year of age.[14]

As the airways and terminal airspaces develop, the pulmonary vascular system is also undergoing development, so that at 24–26 weeks gestation, gaseous exchange across the "alveolar/capillary membrane" may occur, making independent extra-uterine life possible.

Lung growth follows the metabolic needs of the growing child. As the lungs grow there is a rapid multiplication in alveoli until about eight years of age; alveoli increase in number from 24 million at birth to 300 million at eight years.[15] Thereafter growth takes the form of an increase in size of alveoli and airways.[16]

With growth of the lung and airways, compliance increases, but specific compliance (compliance/resting lung volume) remains relatively unchanged throughout life. Resistance to gaseous flow is inversely proportional to the fourth power of the radius (Poiseuille's Law). Therefore, resistance to air flow falls as airway diameter increases.

Oxygen consumption is approximately 7 ml/kg/min.[17] This is about twice that of the adult on a weight basis. This applies, however, only when the infant is in a thermoneutral environment. Hypothermia will markedly increase oxygen consumption and has the potential to compromise the infant. In fact, a fall of only 2°C in the environmental temperature may lead to a two-fold increase in the oxygen consumption of a newborn infant.[18]

Oxygen and carbon dioxide transfer is dependent upon the ventilation/perfusion balance ($\dot{V}/\dot{Q}$) in the lung. Right-to-left shunting of blood in the newborn is higher than it is in the adult due to increased $\dot{V}/\dot{Q}$ inequality within the lung, as well as blood flow through persistent fetal channels (foramen ovale and ductus arteriosus). Right-to-left shunt is approximately 24 percent in the first hour of life, and decreases to 10 percent for the rest of the first week.[19]

Dead space or wasted ventilation of the newborn infant is 2.2 ml/kg, which is similar to the adult. The newborn has a resting tidal volume of 20 ml and dead space ventilation of 7 ml.[20] These dimensions must be considered when using face masks and connections with large amounts of dead space. This is one of the reasons, together with the problems of airway closure and resistance to gas flow through small airways, that newborns under anesthesia should be managed with assisted or controlled ventilation.

Blood gas values evolve rapidly in the newborn infant. The relative hypoxemia of the fetus is corrected in five minutes, the hypercapnia in 20 minutes, and the acidosis (mixed metabolic and respiratory) by 24 hours.[21] The PaO_2 continues to rise to about 75 torr (FIO_2 0.21) in five hours, then stabilizes over the next few days. The $PaCO_2$ decreases over the first day to an average of 33 torr, then rises to approximately 36 torr at one week. The pH rises rapidly in the first 24 hours to 7.32, then continues to increase slowly to 7.35 by the end of the first week. In the newborn, with predominantly fetal hemoglobin, the oxygen dissociation curve is shifted to the left, so that with higher hemoglobin values in the newborn, oxygen transport is proportionately greater than in the adult. This advantage would appear to be somewhat negated, however, by a decrease in oxygen release as a result of oxygen being more tightly bound to fetal hemoglobin. At birth the infant has 60–70 percent fetal hemoglobin, which is replaced with adult hemoglobin over the following 3 months. This would be altered in the infant receiving blood transfusions.

In the neonate as in the adult, PaO_2, $PaCO_2$, and pH control respiration, with PaO_2 acting mainly through peripheral chemoreceptors in the carotid and aortic bodies, and $PaCO_2$ and pH acting on central chemoreceptors in the medulla. The full-term newborn responds to an increase in $PaCO_2$ by an increase in ventilation, in a similar manner to the adult. Preterm infants, however, are significantly less sensitive and have a depressed CO_2 response curve.[22,23] In the newborn, most of the increased ventilation in response to an increased $PaCO_2$ is due to a larger tidal volume, while in adults both tidal volume and frequency increase.

In the newborn, a high concentration of inspired oxygen depresses respiration, while low concentrations stimulate respiration. However, the stimulation effect of hypoxia is transient, following which marked hypoventilation occurs. The preterm infant may respond to hyperoxia and hypoxia with apnea or periodic breathing.[24–27] It usually takes about 10 days for the preterm infant to demonstrate a more mature respiratory response, and this may be delayed in the compromised premature neonate.

The Hering-Breuer reflex, where inflation of the lung results in apnea, is more evident in preterm compared to full-term infants. Inflation may cause an inspiratory gasp before the onset of apnea, and is seen particularly in unstable collapsing lungs. Periodic breathing occurs in 25–50 percent of preterm infants. The breathing pattern is composed of an apneic period (up to 10 seconds) followed by ventilation; this pattern is consistently repeated (Figure 2-3). Periodic breathing is much less frequent after 36 weeks gestational age.[28] By term, a minority of infants will continue to have an abnormal amount of periodic breathing or apnea.

The mechanical aspects of breathing are coordinated between the diaphragmatic and intercostal muscles. The diaphragm is the most important muscle of inspiration. In the neonate any compromise of its function significantly affects the infants breathing. For example, hyperinflation of the lungs flattens and shortens the diaphragm and diminishes its mechanical force (LaPlace's Law). Also, upward displacement of the diaphragm from abdominal distension will affect breathing and gas exchange. This may occur even with simple feedings and is very significant with pathological abdominal distension. As the diaphragm contracts, lung volume increases. This increase in lung volume is compromised in the newborn, and particularly the preterm infant whose chest wall is very compliant and unstable.

The sleep state of the infant may have a profound effect on ventilation. Paradoxical movements of the rib cage develop during rapid eye movement (REM) sleep, due to inhibition of the intercostal muscles while diaphragmatic activity continues.[29] The premature infant spends approximately 65 percent of time in REM sleep, with this proportion diminishing as the infant matures so that at six months adult values of 80 percent quiet and 20 percent REM sleep are reached. In premature infants frequent periods of irregular breathing and apneic spells seen in REM sleep may be significantly reduced by stabilizing the chest wall with continuous positive airway pressure, and by cutaneous or pharmacologic (theophylline) stimulation.[30]

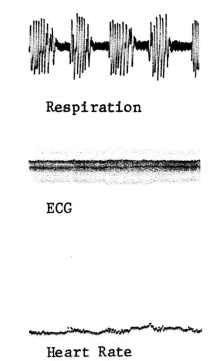

Respiration

ECG

Heart Rate

Figure 2-3. Pneumogram of normal preterm infant. Pneumogram demonstrating the periodic type of respiratory pattern commonly seen in premature infants. Note that there are no changes in the heart rate. (Reproduced with permission of Dorothy Kelly, M.D.)

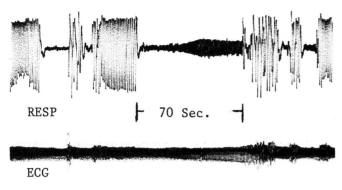

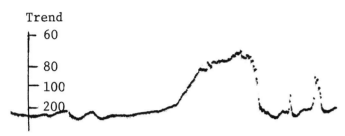

RESP   ├ 70 Sec. ┤

ECG

Trend

├ 60
├ 80
├ 100
├ 200

Figure 2-4. Pneumogram of a former preterm infant demonstrating apnea/bradycardia spells following general anesthesia. Note that severe bradycardia accompanies the apnea. (Reproduced with permission of Dorothy Kelly, M.D.)

The immaturity of the premature infant's mechanisms for control of breathing appear to resurface when the infant (usually within the first six months of life) undergoes anesthesia for a minor surgical procedure. Significant apnea may develop postoperatively, which may be life-threatening (Figure 2-4).[31,32]

CARDIOVASCULAR SYSTEM

Cardiovascular system development, as it relates to changes at the time of birth and myocardial maturation, is discussed in detail in Chapter 15 because of its significance in understanding anesthesia for cardiac surgery. This section considers briefly developmental changes in heart rate, blood pressure, cardiac output, and the electrocardiogram.

Heart Rate

Autonomic control of the heart in utero is mediated predominantly through the parasympathetic nervous system. It is only shortly after birth that sympathetic control appears. In the newborn infant the heart rate may have a wide variation that is within normal limits. In 50 percent of apparently healthy newborns 24 hour electrocardiographic recordings have shown rhythm changes resembling complete, two to one, or Wenckebach sinoatrial block.[33]

In older children a significant number of arrhythmias and conduction abnormalities are also seen, with marked fluctuations in heart rate due to variations in autonomic tone.[34]

Mean heart rate in the newborn in the first 24 hours of life is 120 beats/min. It increases to a mean of 160 beats/min at one month, after which it gradually falls to 75 beats/min at adolescence (Table 2-8).[33]

Table 2-8

The Relationship of Age to Heart Rate

Age	Mean Heart Rate (beats/min)
0–24 hr	120
1–7 d	135
8–30 d	160
3–12 mo	140
1–3 yr	125
3–5 yr	100
8–12 yr	80
2–16 yr	75

Blood Pressure

The mean systolic blood pressure in neonates and infants rises from 65 mm in the first 12 hours of life to 75 mm at four days and 95 mm at six weeks, after which it levels off.[35] There is little change between six weeks and six years, then there is a gradual rise. These measurements apply to infants and children who are awake and quiet. The blood pressure of the preterm infant in the first 12 hours is lower than the full-term infant (Table 2-9).

Cardiac Output in the Newborn

Newborn infants have a resting cardiac output of 180–240 ml/kg/min, which is two to three times adult values. The relatively large cardiac output may reflect the higher metabolic rate and oxygen consumption (7 ml/kg/min) compared to the adult (3.9 ml/kg/min). This may be related to the loss of body heat, which is relatively greater in the newborn because of the larger surface area in relation to body mass.

The Normal Electrocardiogram From Infancy To Adolescence

The electrocardiogram undergoes changes with age. Normal patterns in infants would be distinctly abnormal if seen at a later stage of growth. The P wave reflects atrial depolarization and varies little with age. The P-R interval increases with age (mean value for first year is 0.10 seconds, increasing to 0.14 seconds at 12–16 years). The duration of the QRS complex increases with age, but prolongation above 0.10 seconds is abnormal at any age.

At birth, the QRS axis is right-sided, reflecting the pre-

Table 2-9

The Relationship of Age to Blood Pressure

Age	Normal Blood Pressure (mm Hg)	
	Mean Systolic	Mean Diastolic
0–12 hr (Preterm)	50	35
0–12 hr (Full-term)	65	45
4 d	75	50
6 wk	95	55
1 yr	95	60
2 yr	100	65
9 yr	105	70
12 yr	115	75

dominant right ventricular intrauterine development. It moves leftward significantly in the first month as left ventricular muscle hypertrophies. Thereafter there is a gradual change away from the initial marked right-sided axis.

At birth, T waves are upright in all chest leads. Within hours they become isoelectric or inverted over the left chest. By the seventh day the T waves are inverted in V_4R, V_1, and across to V_4. From then on the T waves stay inverted over the right chest until adolescence, when they become upright over the right chest again. Failure of T waves to become inverted in V_4R and V_1 by seven days may be the earliest ECG evidence of right ventricular hypertrophy.[36,37]

RENAL SYSTEM

In utero, the kidney is an active organ, producing a large volume of urine and helping to maintain amniotic fluid volume. Potter's syndrome, consisting of a disfigured face, pulmonary hypoplasia, and skeletal deformities, is the result of lack of amniotic fluid secondary to renal agenesis. In utero, the fetus maintains its metabolic homeostasis through the placenta, and it is only after birth that the kidney assumes responsibility for metabolic function.

More than 90 percent of newborns will have voided urine within the first 24 hours after birth. All normal infants should have voided within 48 hours.[38]

At birth, glomerular filtration rate (GFR) is 15–30 percent of normal adult values, but reaches 50 percent of the adult value on the fifth to tenth day, and gradually attains adult values at the end of the first year of life.[39]

The low GFR significantly affects the neonate's ability to excrete saline and water loads, as well as drugs. Tubular function develops significantly after 34 weeks gestation.[40] Glomerulotubular balance for glucose appears to be less compromised than previously thought.

The infant's immature kidney responds to stress with changes in its capacity to function; however, the neonatal kidney does not have the reserve to deal with the stress of serious illness.

The "physiological acidemia" of infancy is largely due to a diminished renal tubular threshold for bicarbonate.[41] The infant's kidney concentrates urine to a maximum of 200–800 mOsm/l. This reflects some renal immaturity (fewer and shorter loops of Henle), but is in large part due to the low level of production and excretion of urea by the growing infant. The infant can dilute its urine (to a minimum of 50 mOsm/l) as in the older child; however, the rate of excretion of a water load is less.

The infant's urea production is reduced as a result of growth, and thus the "immature kidney" is able to maintain a normal blood urea nitrogen (BUN) level. When the BUN is elevated, however, this signifies renal failure, excessive dietary intake of protein, or interference with growth due to disease while intake of food has been maintained.

Growth of renal length and cross-sectional area can be related to height or age. Capacity for growth extends into adulthood. For example, if one kidney is removed or destroyed, the remaining normal kidney will hypertrophy; the majority of compensatory growth occurs within six weeks, and is usually complete within six months.

Growth retardation is usually associated with a seriously malfunctioning kidney. When this occurs, a child's rate of growth maybe below the third percentile for their chronological age (Figure 2-1). The reasons for this are not clear.

HEPATIC SYSTEM

Development of the liver and bile ducts begins as an outgrowth of the foregut. By 10 weeks of gestation the biliary tract has completed its development. The vitelline veins give rise to the portal and hepatic veins. Hepatic sinusoids form the ductus venosus—the bridge between the hepatic vein and the inferior vena cava. Most umbilical venous blood from the placenta passes via the ductus venosus to the inferior vena cava. The remainder passes via the portal vein through the liver to the hepatic veins. The portal venous drainage to the left lobe is less than that for the right lobe; this leads to a relative underdevelopment of the left lobe. The ductus venosus closes soon after birth.

Although by late gestation liver cell morphology is similar to that of the adult, the functional development of the liver is somewhat immature in the newborn, and more so in the preterm infant. The liver plays a major role in metabolism, controlling carbohydrate, protein, and lipid delivery to the tissues. At 12 weeks gestation there is evidence of gluconeogenesis and protein synthesis. At 14 weeks glycogen is seen in liver cells.

Toward the end of pregnancy large amounts of glycogen appear in the liver, and as a result the preterm and the SGA infant with smaller stores of glycogen are liable to develop hypoglycemia. Bile acid secretion in the newborn is depressed and malabsorption of fat occurs.

The liver is the site for the synthesis of proteins; this process is active in fetal and neonatal life. In fetal life the main serum protein is alpha-fetoprotein. This protein first appears at six weeks gestation and reaches a peak at 13 weeks. Albumin synthesis starts at three or four months gestation, and approaches adult values at birth; in the preterm infant the level is lower. Proteins involved in clotting are formed in the liver and are at a lower level than normal in the preterm and full term neonate for the first few days of life. The capacity to enzymatically break down proteins is depressed at birth. This is particularly important in the preterm infant, when high protein intake can lead to dangerous levels of serum amino acid concentrations. In the first weeks of life drug metabolism is less efficient than in later life. In addition to less effective hepatic metabolism, altered drug binding by serum proteins and immature renal function contribute to the problem (see Chapters 6 and 7).

Hematopoiesis occurs in the fetal liver, with peak activity at seven months gestation. After six week of age hematopoiesis is confined to the bone marrow, except under pathological conditions (e.g., hemolytic anemia).

Physiologic Jaundice

Hyperbilirubinemia is an especially important consideration in the neonate. The mechanisms for producing jaundice are outlined in Table 2-10.[42]

Increased concentrations of bilirubin occur in the first few days of life. In the term infant, bilirubin levels of 6–7 mg/100 ml are found on the third day of life. In the preterm infant the peak level of 10–12 mg/100 ml occurs on the fifth to seventh day of life. After this period levels gradually decrease to adult levels of less than 1.0 mg/100 ml. In preterm infants the fall is more gradual, taking a month or more. The cause for this hyperbilirubinemia is excessive bilirubin production from breakdown of red blood cells and increased enterohepatic circulation of bilirubin with deficient hepatic conjugation due

Table 2-10

Causes of Jaundice in the Neonate

Excess bilirubin production
Impaired uptake of bilirubin
Impaired conjugation of bilirubin
Defective bilirubin excretion
Increased enterohepatic circulation of bilirubin

Table 2-11

Pathological Causes of Jaundice in the Newborn

- Antibody induced hemolysis (Rh and ABO)
- Hereditary red cell disorders, e.g., glucose-6-phosphate dehydrogenase deficiency (G-6-PD) which gives rise to hemolysis from drugs or infection
- Infections, e.g., neonatal hepatitis, generalized sepsis, severe urinary tract infections
- Hemorrhage into the body, e.g., intracerebral
- Biliary atresia
- Metabolic causes, e.g., hypothyroidism, galactosemia

to depressed glucuronyl transferase activity. The relationship between breast feeding and hyperbilirubinemia has been well documented. It is delayed in onset—after the third day of life—and its cause remains unclear. An earlier hypothesis ascribing it to inhibition of glucuronyl transferase activity has not been substantiated.

Important pathological causes of jaundice in the newborn are presented in Table 2-11. Physiologic jaundice must first be excluded, and the underlying cause is then treated and efforts are directed at preventing bilirubin encephalopathy (kernicterus) by the use of phototherapy and, in selected cases, exchange transfusions. The sick preterm infant is especially at risk for kernicterus, and is more aggressively treated at lower bilirubin levels than the full-term infant.[43] Becoming increasingly common is a form of cholestatic jaundice seen in LBW infants receiving prolonged hyperalimentation. Its mechanism is unclear, but may be due to inhibition of bile flow by amino acids.[44]

THE GASTROINTESTINAL TRACT

In the fetus the digestive tract consists of the developing foregut and hindgut. These rapidly elongate so that a loop of gut is forced into the yolk sac. At five to seven weeks this loop twists around the axis of the superior mesenteric artery, and returns to the abdominal cavity. Maturation occurs gradually from the proximal to the distal end. Blood vessels and nerves (Auerbach's and Meissner's plexus) are developed by 13 weeks gestation, and peristalsis begins. Parotid, sublingual, and submandibular salivary glands arise from the oral mucosa. The pancreas arises from two outgrowths of the foregut. A diverticulum of the foregut gives rise to the liver.

Enzyme levels of enterokinase and lipase increase with gestation, but are lower at birth than in the older child. Nevertheless, the newborn and the preterm infant are able to handle proteins reasonably well. The preterm, however, is unable to tolerate large loads of protein. Fat digestion is limited, particularly in the premature, who absorbs only 65 percent of adult levels.

Anomalies arising from maldevelopment of the gut are listed below, and may be appreciated from an understanding of normal development.

- Esophageal atresia and tracheoesophageal fistula. This occurs when the respiratory tract fails to separate completely from the foregut at four weeks gestation. Failure of separation may be seen as a laryngeal cleft. In its extreme form the cleft may extend from the glottis to the carina.
- Intestinal atresia and stenosis. These are common causes of obstruction in the newborn, particularly in the duodenal region; and this lesion is frequently associated with Down's syndrome. The etiology may be a failure of recanalization

in utero as a result of a vascular accident (intussusception, volvulus, or thrombosis).

- Duplication and diverticulum. These may be blind pouches, or may communicate with the intestinal lumen. Frequently the mucosa is gastric and liable to hemorrhage. Other complications include pressure and obstruction, perforation, and infection. Meckel's diverticulum is relatively common and is due to the persistence of the vitello-intestinal duct.
- Hirschsprung's disease is due to failure of development of Meissner's and Auerbach's plexus.
- Peritoneal bands causing obstruction result from faulty rotation and fixation of the gut, most commonly seen at the duodenojejunal junction.
- Omphalocele and gastroschisis. In these conditions intestine protrudes from the abdominal wall due to failure of closure of the rectus muscles. Gastroschisis is thought to arise possibly as a result of occlusion of the omphalomesenteric artery in utero.

Swallowing

This complex procedure is under central and peripheral control. The reflex is initiated in the medulla, through cranial nerves to the muscles which control the passage of food through the pharyngoesophageal sphincter. In the process, the tongue, soft palate, pharynx, and larynx are all smoothly coordinated. Any pathology of these structures could interfere with normal swallowing. Neuromuscular incoordination, however, is more likely to be responsible for any dysfunction. This is particularly evident when the central nervous system has sustained damage either before or during delivery. With swallowing, pressure in the pharynx rises, the pharyngoesophageal sphincter opens and peristaltic waves in the upper esophagus carry the bolus of food down. Peristaltic waves are absent in the lower esophagus in the infant, although present in the adult. With the immaturity of the pharyngoesophageal sphincter, frequent regurgitation or "spitting" of gastric contents is seen in healthy infants.

Gastroesophageal Reflux

Approximately 40 percent of newborn infants in the first few days of life will regurgitate their food.[45] Lower esophageal pressures are low and take approximately three to six weeks to achieve adult levels. Symptoms of reflux include persistent vomiting, failure to thrive, and in severe cases hematemesis and anemia. Stricture formation may follow. These symptoms are also found with hiatus hernia. Gastroesophageal reflux is one of a number of conditions associated with apnea and bradycardia in the premature infant.[30]

Meconium

Meconium is the material contained in the intestinal tract prior to birth. It consists of desquamated epithelial cells from the intestinal tract and bile, pancreatic and intestinal secretions, and water (70%). Meconium is usually passed in the first few hours after birth, but its passage may be delayed for 48 hours. Meconium in the amniotic fluid usually indicates intrauterine asphyxia. Aspiration of meconium may have serious effects on pulmonary function, leading to pneumonia, pneumothorax, and persistent fetal circulation (PFC).[46,47]

Meconium ileus is associated with cystic fibrosis and occurs in 10 percent of children with the disease. The meconium is inspissated and causes intestinal obstruction. The newborn who fails to pass meconium may also be suffering from Hirschsprung's disease; reduced colonic activity may result in increased water absorption and inspissation of the meconium.

ENDOCRINE (THE PANCREAS)

The placenta is impermeable to both insulin and glucagon. The islets of Langerhans in the fetal pancreas, however, secrete insulin from the eleventh week of fetal life; the amount of insulin secretion increases with age. After birth, insulin response is related to gestational and postnatal age and is more mature in the term infant.

Maternal hyperglycemia, particularly when uncontrolled, results in hypertrophy and hyperplasia of the fetal islets of Langerhans. This leads to increased levels of insulin in the fetus, affecting lipid metabolism and leading to the large, overweight infant characteristic of the poorly controlled diabetic mother. Hyperglycemia alone is not instrumental in this effect; it may also be the result of an increase in serum amino acids found in diabetic mothers.

Meticulous control of the mother's diabetes during pregnancy and delivery has led to a reduction in morbidity and mortality of the infant of the diabetic mother (IDM). Hyperinsulinemia of the fetus will persist after birth and may lead to rapid development of serious hypoglycemia. In addition to severe hypoglycemia, the infant has an increased incidence of congenital anomalies.

SGA infants are frequently hypoglycemic, which may be the result of malnutrition in utero. Some of these infants secrete inappropriately large amounts of insulin in response to glucose, and for this reason may suffer from serious hypoglycemia. In addition, hepatic glycogen stores are inadequate, and deficient gluconeogenesis exists. The premature infant may be hypoglycemic without demonstrable symptoms, therefore necessitating close monitoring of blood glucose levels.

A fasting blood sugar below 35 mg/100 ml for the normal newborn or 25 mg/100 ml for the preterm infant is pathological during the first three days of life. It is important to appreciate that the infant, while showing no symptoms, may develop serious hypoglycemia leading to irreversible central nervous system damage. After the third day of life a fasting blood sugar of less than 45 mg/100 ml is regarded as pathological, and such an infant frequently presents with convulsions—but signs may be subtle, such as lethargy and sommnolence.

HEMOPOIETIC SYSTEM

The blood volume of the full-term newborn infant is dependent upon the time of cord clamping, which modifies the volume of placental transfusion. Blood volume is 93 ml/kg when cord clamping is delayed following delivery, compared with 82 ml/kg with immediate cord clamping.[48,49] Within the first four hours following delivery, however, fluid is lost from the blood and the plasma volume contracts by as much as 25 percent. The larger the placental transfusion, the larger this loss of fluid in the first few hours following birth, with resultant hemoconcentration. The blood volume of the preterm infant is higher (90–105 ml/kg) than the full-term infant because of an increased plasma volume.[48]

The normal hemoglobin range is between 14 gm/100 ml and 20 gm/100 ml. The site of sampling must be considered, however, when interpreting these values for the diagnosis of neonatal anemia or hyperviscosity syndrome. Capillary sampling (e.g., heel stick) will give higher values, as much as 6 gm/100 ml, because of stasis in peripheral vessels leading to loss of plasma and hemoconcentration; thus a venipuncture is required. In 1 percent of infants, fetal–maternal transfusion occurs, and may be responsible for some of the "low normal hemoglobin" values seen.

Erythropoietic activity from the bone marrow decreases immediately after birth in both full-term and preterm infants. The cord blood reticulocyte count of 5 percent persists for a few days and falls below 1 percent by one week. This is followed by a slight increase to one to two percent by the 12th week where it remains throughout childhood. Premature infants have higher reticulocyte counts (up to 10 percent) at birth. Abnormal reticulocyte values reflect hemorrhage or hemolysis. Vitamin E, an anti-peroxidant, is necessary for integrity of the erythrocyte membrane. Preterm infants, especially those less than 1500 gm, are vitamin E deficient and may exhibit a hemolytic anemia at 6–10 weeks of age, further aggravating the existing physiologic anemia.[50]

The hemoglobin concentration falls during the ninth to twelfth week to reach a nadir of 11.0 gm/100 ml (hematocrit 30-33), and then rises. This is due to a decrease in erythropoiesis and to some extent due to a shortened life span of the red blood cell. In premature infants the fall in the hemoglobin level is greater, and is directly related to the degree of prematurity. Also, the nadir is reached earlier (4–8 wk).[51] In infants 800–1000 gm in weight the fall may reach a low of 8 gm/100 ml. This "anemia" is a normal physiological adjustment to extrauterine life. In the preterm infant the "anemia" is greater. Despite the fall in hemoglobin, the oxygen delivery to the tissues is not compromised due to a shift of the oxygen–hemoglobin dissociation curve (to the right), secondary to an increase of 2,3-diphosphoglycerate (2,3-DPG).[52] In addition, fetal hemoglobin is replaced by adult-type hemoglobin, which also results in a shift in the same direction.

After the third month, the hemoglobin level stabilizes at 11.5–12.0 gm/100 ml, until about two years of life. The hemoglobin values of full-term and preterm infants are comparable after the first year. Thereafter there is a gradual increase to mean levels at puberty of 14.0 gm/100 ml for girls and 15.5 gm/100 ml for boys.

The white cell count may normally reach 21,000/mm^3 in the first 24 hours of life and 12,000/mm^3 at the end of the first week, with the number of neutrophils equaling lymphocytes. It then falls gradually, reaching adult levels at puberty.

Table 2-12

Relationship of Motor Milestones to Age

Motor Milestone	Age
Supports head	3 mo
Sits alone	6 mo
Stands alone	12 mo
Balances on one foot	3 yr

Table 2-14

Relationship of Language Milestones to Age

Language Milestones	Age
Squeals	1.5–3.0 mo
Turns to voice	6 mo
Combines 2 words	1.5 yr
Composes short sentences	2 yr
Gives entire name	3 yr

At birth, neutrophil granulocytes predominate but rapidly decrease in number so that during the first week of life, and through four years, the lymphocyte emerges to become the predominant cell. After the fourth year the values approximate the adult.

The neonate has an increased susceptibility to bacterial infection, which is related in part to immaturity of leukocyte function. Sepsis may be associated with a minimal leukocyte response or even with leukopenia. Spurious increases in the white blood cell content may be due to drugs (e.g., epinephrine).

Coagulation in the Infant

At birth, vitamin K-dependent factors, i.e., II, VII, IX and X, are at levels of 20–60 percent of the adult value; in premature infants the value is even less. This results in prolonged prothrombin times seen normally in full-term and preterm infants.

Synthesis of vitamin K-dependent factors occurs in the liver which, being immature, leads to relatively lower levels of the coagulation factors, even with the administration of vitamin K. It takes several weeks for the levels of coagulation factors to reach adult values; the deficit is even more pronounced in the premature infant.

Administration of vitamin K_1 is essential immediately after birth to prevent hemorrhagic disease of the newborn. Its omission could lead to serious and life-threatening consequences, especially if surgery is undertaken.

Infants of mothers who have received anticonvulsant drugs during pregnancy may develop a serious coagulopathy similar to that seen with vitamin K deficiency.[53] Vitamin K_1 administered to the newborn will usually reverse this bleeding tendency, but death has occurred despite therapy.

NEUROLOGIC DEVELOPMENT

The infant's normal mental development depends on maturation of the central nervous system. This development may be affected by physical illness or by inadequate psychosocial support. Delay in development in the preterm

infant, however, may be normal depending on the degree of prematurity.

The rate of brain growth is different from the growth rate of other body systems. There are two spurts of growth—neuronal cell multiplication between 15 and 20 weeks gestation, and glial cell multiplication—commencing at 25 weeks and extending into the second year of life. Myelination continues into the third year. Malnutrition during this phase of neural development may have profound handicapping effects.

The normal newborn shows a variety of primitive reflexes, which include the Moro response and grasp reflex. Milestones of development are useful indicators of mental development and possible deviations from normal. It should be appreciated, however, that these milestones represent the *average*, and infants will vary in their rates of maturation of different body functions and still be within the normal range.[54] The Denver developmental screening test is a useful scheme for assessing these milestones. The test focuses on four areas; (1) gross motor function, (2) fine motor and adaptive skills, (3) language, and (4) personal and social skills.

Gross motor development involves skills of head, trunk, and limb stabilization and postural control (Table 2-12).

Adaptive skills are performed through well coordinated fine motor movements (Table 2-13). Abnormal development may be reflected in a delay in appearance of a particular milestone, or in its pathological persistence with maturation in the child. For example, at 20 weeks a child reaches and retrieves objects, taking virtually everything retrieved into the mouth. As the infant matures, however, this practice usually ceases at 12–13 months of age; in infants with mental abnormality this mouthing continues for a much longer period.

Language development correlates closely with cognitive skills (Table 2-14).

Personal and social skills are modified by environmental factors and cultural patterns (Table 2-15).

Development of walking, speech, and sphincter control are most important. For appropriate evaluation consider familial patterns, level of intelligence, and physical illness. Deafness may cause delayed speech. Incontinence may be due to bladder neck pathology in boys, and an ectopic ureter entering

Table 2-13

Relationship of Fine Motor/Adaptive Milestones to Age

Fine Motor/Adaptive Milestones	Age
Grasps rattle	3 mo
Passes cube hand to hand	6 mo
Pincer grip	1 yr
Imitates vertical line	2 yr
Copies circle	3 yr

Table 2-15

Relationship of Personal-Social Milestones to Age

Personal-Social Milestones	Age
Smiles spontaneously	3 mo
Feeds self crackers	6 mo
Drinks from cup	1 yr
Plays interactive games	2 yr

Table 2-16

Causes of Mental Handicaps

- Infections, e.g., meningitis, encephalitis
- Head injury
- Hypoxemia, e.g., near drowning, carbon monoxide poisoning
- Metabolic, e.g., severe hypoglycemia, hypernatremia, hypothyroidism, phenylketonuria, chronic malnutrition
- Lead poisoning, addicting drugs
- Degenerative disease of the nervous system
- Cerebral tumor, vascular accident
- Congenital malformation

the vagina in girls. For a more detailed analysis and interpretation the anesthesiologist is referred to pediatric texts.

Mental Handicap

The child with mental handicap is late in *all* aspects of development. Smiling in response to the mother, vocalization, sitting, and walking are delayed, as are speech and sphincter control. When there is a delay in the eye following an object, and the head turning in response to sound, blindness and deafness may erroneously be diagnosed. Drooling, common in young infants, is frequently prolonged for years in the mentally abnormal child. Tooth grinding is also common. At first the mentally handicapped infant often appears to be inactive and may be seen as a "good child." Later the child demonstrates constant and sometimes uncontrollable overactivity. In diagnosing mental abnormality, the anesthesiologist must be aware of possible pitfalls:

- The infant born prematurely will be delayed and should be assessed on its conceptual age.
- The infant with cerebral palsy or sensory deficits (auditory and visual) may have normal mental development, but the handicap may interfere with assessment of the mental status.
- Consider the effects of drugs (e.g., barbiturates for epilepsy).

Mental handicaps may be due to a wide range of causes, amongst which those in Table 2-16 should be considered.

REFERENCES

1. Lugo G, Cassady G: Intrauterine Growth Retardation: Clinico-pathologic findings in 233 consecutive infants. *Am J Obstet Gynecol* 109:615–622, 1971
2. Gellis SS, Hsia DYY: The infant of the diabetic mother. *Am J Dis Child* 97:1–41, 1959
3. Kitzmiller JL, Cloherty JP, Younger MD, et al: Diabetic pregnancy and perinatal morbidity. *Am J Obstet Gynecol* 131:560–580, 1978
4. Farquher JW: The infant of the diabetic mother. *Clin Endocrinol Metab* 5:237–264, 1976
5. Farr V, Kerridge DF, Mitchell RG: The value of some external characteristics in the assessment of gestational age at birth. *Dev Med Child Neurol* 8:657–660, 1966
6. Farr V, Mitchell RG, Neligan GA, et al: The definition of some external characteristics used in the assessment of gestational age of the newborn infant. *Dev Med Child Neurol* 8:507–511, 1966
7. Dubowitz LMS, Dubowitz V, Goldberg C: Clinical assessment of gestational age in the newborn infant. *J Pediatr* 77:1–10, 1970
8. Narayanan I, Dua K, Gujral VV, et al: A simple method of assessment of gestational age in newborn infants. *Pediatrics* 69:27–32, 1982
9. Moylan FMB, Seldin EB, Shannon DC, Todres ID: Defective primary dentition in survivors of neonatal mechanical ventilation. *J Pediatr* 96:106–108, 1980
10. Friis-Hansen B: Body composition during growth: In vivo measurements and biochemical data correlated to differential anatomical growth. *Pediatrics* 47:264–274, 1971
11. Karlberg P: The adaptive changes in the immediate postnatal period, with particular reference to respiration. *J Pediatr* 56:585–604, 1960
12. Vyas H, Milner AD, Hopkin IE: Intrathoracic pressure and volume changes during the spontaneous onset of respiration in babies born by cesarean section and by vaginal delivery. *J Pediatr* 99:787–791, 1981
13. Halliday HL, McClure G, McCreid M: Transient tachypnea of the newborn: Two distinct clinical entities? *Arch Dis Child* 56:322–325, 1981
14. Motoyama EK, Brinkmeyer SD, Mutich RL, et al: Reduced FRC in anesthetized infants: Effect of low PEEP. *Anesthesiology* 57:A418, 1982
15. Davies G, Reid L: Growth of the alveoli and pulmonary arteries in childhood. *Thorax* 25:669–681, 1970
16. Charnock EL, Doershuk CF: Development aspects of the human lung. *Pediatr Clin North Am* 20:275–292, 1973
17. Cross KW, Flynn DM, Hill JR: Oxygen consumption in normal newborn infants during moderate hypoxia in warm and cool environments. *Pediatrics* 37:565–576, 1966
18. Hill JR, Rahimtulla KA: Heat balance and the metabolic rate of new-born babies in relation to environmental temperature, and the effect of age and of weight on basal metabolic rate. *J Physiol* 180:239–265, 1965
19. Rudolph AM: The changes in the circulation after birth. Their importance in congenital heart disease. *Circulation* 41:343–359, 1970
20. Nelson NM: Neonatal pulmonary function. *Pediatr Clin North Am* 13:769–799, 1966
21. Koch G, Wendel H: Adjustment of arterial blood gases and acid base balance in the normal newborn infant during the first week of life. *Biol Neonate* 12:136–161, 1968
22. Albersheim S, Boychuk R, Seshia MMK, et al: Effects of CO_2 on immediate ventilatory response to O_2 in preterm infants. *J Appl Physiol* 41:609–611, 1976
23. Frantz ID, Adler SM, Thach BT, et al: Maturational effects on respiratory responses to carbon dioxide in premature infants. *J Appl Physiol* 41:41–45, 1976
24. Rigatto H, Brady JP, Torre Verduzio R: Chemoreceptor reflexes in preterm infants. I. The effect of gestational and postnatal age on the ventilatory response to inhalation of 100% and 15% oxygen. *Pediatrics* 55:604–613, 1975
25. Rigatto H, Torre Verduzco R, Cates DB: Effects of O_2 on the ventilatory response to CO_2 in preterm infants. *J Appl Physiol* 39:896–899, 1975
26. Gerhardt T, Bancalari E: Apnea of prematurity. I. Lung function and regulation of breathing. *Pediatrics* 74:58–62, 1984
27. Gerhardt T, Bancalari E: Apnea of Prematurity. II. Respiratory reflexes. *Pediatrics* 74:63–66, 1984
28. Kelly DH, Shannon DC: Treatment of apnea and excessive periodic breathing in the full-term infant. *Pediatrics* 68:183–186, 1981
29. Henderson-Smart DJ, Read DJC: Depression of respiratory muscles and defective responses to nasal obstruction during active sleep in the newborn. *Aust Paediatr J* 12:261–266, 1976
30. Shannon DC, Gotay F, Stein IM, et al: Prevention of apnea and

bradycardia in low-birthweight infants. *Pediatrics* 55:589–594, 1975

31. Steward DJ: Preterm infants are more prone to complications following minor surgery than are term infants. *Anesthesiology* 56:304–306, 1982

32. Liu LMP, Coté CJ, Goudsouzian NG, et al: Life threatening apnea in infants recovering from anesthesia. *Anesthesiology* 59:506–510, 1983

33. Southall DP, Richards JM, Johnston PGB, Shinebourne EA: Study of cardiac rhythm in healthy newborn infant. *Br Heart J* 41:382, 1979

34. Southall DP, Johnston F, Shinebourne EA, et al: 24-hour electrocardiographic study of heart rate and rhythm patterns in population of healthy children. *Br Heart J* 45:281–291, 1981

35. DeSwiet M, Fayers P, Shinebourne EA: Systolic blood pressure in a population of infants in the first year of life: The Brompton study. *Pediatrics* 65:1028–1035, 1979

36. Southall DP, Vulliamy DG, Davies MJ, et al: A new look at the neonatal electrocardiogram. *Br Med J* 2:615–618, 1976

37. Rautaharju PM, Davignon A, Soumis F, et al: Evolution of QRS-T Relationship from birth to adolescence in Frank-lead orthogonal electrocardiograms of 1492 normal children. *Circulation* 60:196–204, 1979

38. Clark DA: Times of first void and first stool in 500 newborns. *Pediatrics* 60:457–459, 1977

39. Leake RD, Trygstad CW, Oh W: Inulin clearance in the newborn infant: Relationship to gestational age and postnatal age. *Pediatr Res* 10:759–762, 1976

40. Arant BS: Developmental patterns of renal functional maturation compared in the human neonate. *J Pediatr* 92:705–712, 1978

41. Edelman CM, Spitzer A: The maturing kidney. *J Pediatr* 75:509–519, 1969

42. Oski FA: Jaundice, in Avery, ME Taeusch HW, Jr. (Eds): Diseases of the newborn, 5th ed. Philadelphia, W.B. Saunders, 1984, pp 622–650

43. Seligmin JW: Recent and changing concepts of hyperbilirubinemia and its management in the newborn. *Pediatr Clin N Am* 24:509–527, 1977

44. Touloukian RJ, Downing SE: Cholestasis associated with long-term parenteral hyperalimentation. *Arch Surg* 106:58–62, 1973

45. Winter HS, Grand RJ: Gastroesophageal reflux. *Pediatrics* 68:134–136, 1981

46. Levin DL, Gregory GA: The effect of tolazoline on right-to-left shunting via a patent ductus arteriosus in meconium aspiration syndrome. *Crit Care Med* 4:304–307, 1976

47. Marshall R, Tyrala E, McAlister W, et al: Meconium aspiration syndrome. Neonatal and follow-up study. *Am J Obstet Gynecol* 131:672–676, 1978

48. Usher R, Lind J: Blood volume of the newborn premature infant. *Acta Paediatr Scand* 54:419–431, 1965

49. Usher R, Shephard M, Lind J: The blood volume of the newborn infant and placental transfusion. *Acta Paediatr Scand* 52:497–512, 1963

50. Oski FA, Barness LA: Vitamin E deficiency: A previously unrecognized cause of hemolytic anemia in the premature infant. *J Pediatr* 70:211–220, 1967

51. O'Brien RT, Pearson HA: Physiologic anemia of the newborn infant. *J Pediatr* 79:132–138, 1971

52. Delivoria-Papadopoulos M, Roncevic N, Oski FA: Postnatal changes in oxygen transport of term, premature and sick infants: The role of red cell 2-3 diphosphoglycerate and adult hemoglobin. *Pediatr Res* 5:235–245, 1971

53. Mountain KR, Hirsh J, Gallus AS: Neonatal coagulation defect due to anticonvulsant drug treatment in pregnancy. *Lancet* 1:265–268, 1970

54. Illingworth RS: *Development of the Infant and Young Child*, 7th ed. Baltimore, Williams and Wilkins, 1980

3

Temperature Regulation

Francis X. Vacanti
John F. Ryan

BASIC PHYSIOLOGY

HOMEOSTASIS

Body temperature is the result of the balance between the factors leading to heat loss and gain, and the distribution of heat within the body.[1] Body temperature remains constant when the net heat loss is equal to the net heat gain if there are no changes in the distribution of heat within the body. An increase in heat loss or a decrease in heat gain, if unopposed or inadequately opposed, leads to hypothermia, with decreasing temperature until a new equilibrium is reached. The potential exists for the unstable conditions to progress to a positive feedback cycle, where the decrease in body temperature will lead to a decrease in the metabolic rate, leading to further heat loss and diminution in metabolic rate. The body safeguards against this unstable state by initiating an increase in metabolic rate (e.g. shivering) during the initial exposure to a cold environment, or by reducing heat loss by vasoconstriction.[2]

The central nervous system (CNS) receives multiple sensory inputs concerning the state of thermal balance throughout the body.[2,3] The CNS interprets the data and activates effector mechanisms to adjust the balance of heat loss and heat gain.[4] Under extreme conditions, the central integrating system may receive conflicting data on the thermal state of the body and may make incorrect adjustments of the temperature regulating mechanism (e.g., a cold patient who is covered with a warm blanket stops shivering).[2,5] The temperature which the body strives to maintain can also be altered pharmacologically.[6]

Temperature receptors are more sensitive to rapid than to gradual temperature change. They are found in varied locations throughout the body, including the hypothalamus, skin, spinal cord, gastrointestinal tract, and the respiratory tract. The anterior hypothalamus responds to heat, while the posterior hypothalamus responds to cold. The hypothalamus controls temperature by adjustments of the body's activity, cutaneous circulation, sweating, and pulmonary ventilation.[2]

FACTORS IN NEWBORN INFANTS

The newborn infant has an intact central temperature control mechanism, but is limited, however, by certain anatomic and physiologic factors. The infant attempts to maintain a constant body temperature, but can only succeed within a narrow range of environmental conditions. A full-term infant starts developing hypothermia at an ambient temperature of 23°C. An infant readily loses heat to the environment from his relatively large surface area, whereas the potential for producing heat is limited. In this respect, premature infants are more vulnerable, thus they require a higher environmental temperature to maintain normothermia.[7]

The important mechanisms of increasing heat production are activity, shivering, and non-shivering thermogenesis. Obviously, the anesthetized infant cannot increase his heat production by increased activity. Shivering is practically absent in infants under the age of three months. Consequently, the only available mechanism in the anesthetized infant is non-shivering thermogenesis, which is achieved principally through brown fat metabolism.

Brown fat comprises two to three percent of the body weight of the infant. It is present mainly between the scapulae, in the neck, in the mediastinum around the internal mammary arteries, as well as around the kidneys and adrenals. Brown fat is a highly specialized tissue with abundant blood supply and a large number of mitochondrial cytochromes, which provide this tissue its brown color. These cells have several small vacuoles of fat and are richly supplied with sympathetic nerve endings.

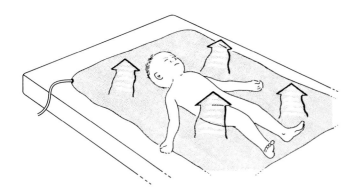

Figure 3-1. In the operating room the heating blanket is of value in maintaining temperature in children of 0.5m² BSA or less (approximately 10 kg and 15 months of age). In chronic disease states which result in retarded growth, weight rather than age is more important in determining the efficacy of a heating blanket. (Reproduced from Goudsouzian NG et al: The effects of a warming blanket on the maintenance of body temperature in anesthetized infants and children. Anesthesiology, 39:351–353, 1973. With permission.)

When an infant is exposed to a cold environment, there is an increase in norepinephrine production which in turn increases the metabolism of the brown fat.[8] Once norepinephrine is released, it acts on the alpha and beta adrenergic receptors of the brown adipocytes. This stimulates the release of lipase which in turn splits the triglycerides into glycerol and fatty acids, thus increasing heat production.[9] The increase in brown fat metabolism is accompanied by an increase in the proportion of cardiac output diverted through the brown fat. This may reach as much as 25 percent of cardiac output, which in turn facilitates the direct warming of blood.

The increased norepinephrine levels produce pulmonary and peripheral vasoconstriction. The rise in pulmonary arterial pressure will predispose to increased right to left shunting through the foramen ovale and ductus arteriosus, potentially leading to hypoxemia. The peripheral vasoconstriction produces a mottled appearance to the skin.

HEAT EXCHANGE

Heat is exchanged between the body and its environment in both directions by conduction, convection, evaporation and condensation, and radiation. The net effect of each of the methods is dependent on the balance of the rate of heat transfer into and out of the body.

Conduction

The kinetic energy of the vibratory motion of the molecules at the surface of the skin or other exposed surfaces is transmitted to the molecules of the medium immediately adjacent to the skin. The rate of heat transfer to the body's environment is related to the temperature difference between the skin and its environment. As the temperature of the environment is increased by its interaction with the body's surface, the rate of heat loss from the body is decreased.

Increasing the temperature of the conducting medium at its interface with the exposed surfaces minimizes the rate of heat loss by conduction. This can be achieved by two mechanisms.

The first method involves warming the entire conducting medium. This is done clinically by the use of warm blankets, a warm water mattress, and warm irrigating solutions intraoperatively.[10,11]

Warming the conduction medium seems to be more effective in maintaining body temperature in infants than in older children. The relatively large surface area of the infant allows for the relatively rapid rate of heat loss to a cold environment and for a relatively rapid rate of heat gain from a warm environment. Consequently, the warming blanket is more effective in maintaining body temperature in children with less than 0.5 m² body surface area (i.e, approximately 10 kg) than in larger children (see Fig. 1).

The second method of decreasing conductive heat loss is by use of thermal insulation. A good thermal insulator will conduct heat poorly from its surface that is in contact with the body. As a result of this resistance to heat flow, a temperature gradient is maintained throughout the thickness of the insulation. The temperature will be highest at its interface with the body's surface and lowest at its interface with the environment. Because of the warmer temperature of the surface of the insulation that is in contact with the body, the rate of heat loss by conduction is decreased. Reduction of heat loss by this mechanism can be accomplished with the use of blankets, O.R. drapes, and covering the head. The latter is particularly important, since the heat loss from the uncovered head of an infant may represent as much as 60 percent of total heat loss in an operating room.

Convection

Air is an effective thermal insulator as long as it is not moving. The efficiency of static air as an insulator is illustrated by the use of air in both natural and man-made insulation such as down and fiberglass. The bulk of the volume of these insulators is trapped air, which is prevented from moving by the surrounding matrix of insulation.

Under usual operating room conditions, air is able to move freely. Air that is warmed by exposure to the surface of the body rises and is replaced by the cooler air from the environment. This movement of air by convection results in an effective loss of heat because it results in the maintenance of a temperature gradient between the body surface and its immediately adjacent environment. The rapid turnover rate of air in modern O.R.'s adds to convectional heat loss. The O.R. temperature should therefore be kept elevated with higher levels for the smaller infants (Table 1).

Table 3-1

Operating Room Temperature

Newborns and small neonates	80°F (26.6°C)
Infants to 6 months	78°F (25.5°C)
6 months to 2 years	76°F (24.4°C)

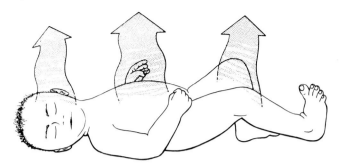

Figure 3-2. (Reproduced from Dick W, et al: Prevention of heat loss during anesthesia and operation in the newborn baby and small infants. *Acta Anaesth Scand,* Suppl 37:134–139, 1970. With permission.)

Heat loss by convection can be reduced by keeping the infant in the incubator until it is necessary to remove him to prepare for the operation. Convective heat loss can also be reduced by keeping the infant covered with a blanket when possible, keeping the doors closed to reduce drafts, covering the head, and by surgical drapes.

Consequently, neutral thermal conditions in a baby can be provided at even 25°C when he is well wrapped, whereas at least 32.5°C is required when naked.[12]

Radiation

All objects that are above absolute zero in temperature give off electromagnetic radiation. The radiation emitted from the human body is in the infrared region of the electromagnetic spectrum. The walls and other objects around the body also emit infrared radiation, the quantity of which is related to the temperature of these objects. If the temperature of these objects is less than the temperature of the body, as is usually the case, then the rate of heat radiated from the body to the surrounding objects is more than the rate of radiation from the objects to the body, and there is a net loss of heat from the body to the environment by radiation. Radiation is the major mechanism of heat loss under normal conditions (Fig. 2), but under conditions of elevated body temperature there is little capacity for increasing heat loss by increasing the rate of radiant heat loss.

If an incubator is in a cold room, an infant may become hypothermic even if a warm temperature is maintained inside the incubator. This is because the walls of the incubator will be at a lower temperature than the air inside the incubator, and the naked infant will radiate heat through the air to the walls of the incubator. This effect can be minimized by placing a shell of transparent plexiglas inside the incubator around the infant. The temperature of the inner shell is maintained at a temperature higher than that of the outer shell, thereby reducing radiant heat loss (Fig. 3). Radiant heat loss can be reduced by increasing the temperature of the room, thereby increasing the temperature of the surrounding walls. Net loss can also be reduced by use of a radiant heat lamp (Fig. 4), but care must be taken to keep the lamp at an adequate distance from the skin, and the skin temperature should be monitored to prevent burns.[13]

Covering the infant with a thermal insulator such as a blanket will reduce radiant heat loss because the inner surface of the blanket will rapidly approach a temperature close to that of the skin and thereby reduce the rate of radiant loss from the

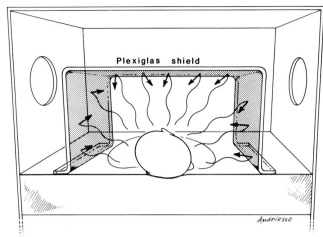

Figure 3-3. Use of a transparent shell inside the incubator can be of great importance to minimize radiant heat loss during transport of the infant. This is true whether the transport is from hospital to hospital or from the intensive care unit to the operating room. The warmth of the incubator should be maintained during the operation to provide a safe environment for the return trip to the intensive care unit.

skin to the surrounding blanket. Because of the resistance to heat flow through the blanket, the outer surface of the blanket will maintain a temperature near that of the environment and will therefore radiate slowly to the surrounding walls. Because visual observation is important, the blanket can be replaced by a single layer of clear plastic or by a cover of clear plastic packing material with dead air spaces trapped between two layers of plastic to serve as insulation.[14]

Reflecting the emitted radiation back to the skin will also decrease the rate of heat loss by radiation. This can be accomplished by covering or wrapping the infant in a blanket made of a thin sheet of aluminized plastic such as polyethylene. Care must be taken to prevent pooling of prep solutions inside the wrap.[11]

Evaporation

Each gram of water that evaporates from the surface of the body carries with it 0.58 kcal of heat that it obtains from its environment as the heat of vaporization. Under normal conditions, approximately 20 percent of the total body heat loss is

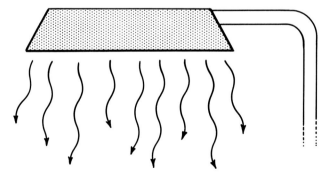

Figure 3-4. Radiant heat lamps and radiant warmers are useful in maintaining body temperature. Care must be taken to maintain an adequate distance from the skin and to monitor skin temperature in order to prevent injury.

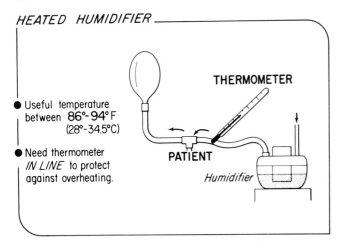

Figure 3-5. Temperature of the gases leaving the heated humidifier should be monitored close to the patient's airway. This provides adequate saturation and protects against overheating of the airway. In our operating rooms, the heated humidifier is the second most important adjunct of maintaining the infant's body temperature. The most important factor is room temperature.

due to evaporation, but when stressed by a warm environment, the rate of heat loss can be increased by sweating. The driving force for evaporation is the difference between the vapor pressure at the body surface and the environment.

Heat exchange with the environment is significant at the surfaces of both the skin and the lungs. Since the infant's skin is thinner and more permeable than the older child's or adult's, evaporative heat loss from the skin is greater.

In the spontaneously breathing individual, the temperature of the inspired gases reaches 32°C at the pharynx, with a relative humidity of 86 percent. Full saturation is achieved in the distal bronchi. In the anesthetized patient, an open breathing system delivers gases that are practically devoid of humidity. The minute ventilation (relative to body weight) is high in an infant, thus increasing evaporative heat loss through the respiratory system. The rate of respiratory evaporative heat loss is increased by breathing cool dry gases, since these gases have a low vapor pressure. It can be calculated that a 3 kg infant with a minute ventilation of 500 ml/min will expend 0.0035 kcal/min to raise the temperature of the inspired gases to body temperature. To saturate the gases with water vapor, about 0.012 kcal/min is needed. The total heat to warm and humidify the inspired gases is 0.015 kcal/min, or approximately 1 kcal/hr. This represents 8–10 percent of the total caloric expenditure of the infant.[15] With a closed system, relative humidity can be raised to 80 percent at 20°C (water content 14 mg/l).[16] The introduction of a heated humidifier into this system can provide a water content of 30 mg/l at 30°C.[17] Such humidification is similar to that occurring normally at the pharynx, and minimizes the calories lost through the respiratory system (Fig. 5).[18]

TEMPERATURE MONITORING

A variety of methods for monitoring temperature are available, each with its own advantages and disadvantages. There is no one best procedure, so a method must be chosen, based on a consideration of the needs of each patient weighed against the advantages and disadvantages of that system. The available techniques monitor either central temperature or non-central temperature.

CENTRAL TEMPERATURE MONITORING

The temperature sensed by the temperature regulating center of the hypothalamus is the central or core temperature. It is the temperature of the blood flowing through the branches of the internal carotid artery to the hypothalamus. Central temperature probes monitor the temperature of blood that is close to the internal carotid artery temperature.

Nasopharyngeal temperature probes are warmed by branches of the internal carotid artery. When properly placed they may reflect the central temperature accurately. This probe can easily be displaced into the esophagus, however, to be cooled by the inspired gases; therefore care must be exercised to maintain the proper placement of the probe. Even when properly placed, the probe may be influenced by air flow over it.

Tympanic temperature probes monitor the temperature of blood flowing adjacent to the tympanic membrane.[19] This blood is similar in temperature to the blood flowing to the hypothalamic centers. It is not frequently used during anesthesia because of the risk of damaging the tympanic membrane, as evidenced sometimes by the appearance of blood after removal of the probe.

Esophageal temperature probes should be placed in the lower third of the esophagus. In this location they sense the temperature of the aortic blood, and are not influenced by the cooling effect of gases flowing through the endotracheal tube. Movement of the temperature probe to its proper position may result in an increase in measured temperature by a full degree celsius. This method is more readily maintained than a nasopharyngeal temperature probe, and is appropriate during endotracheal anesthesia.

PERIPHERAL TEMPERATURE MONITORING

Noncentral probes do not measure core temperature but rather regional temperature, and they are influenced by a variety of factors, including regional blood flow. They are convenient and useful for monitoring changes and trends in temperature.

Axillary temperature monitoring is a useful guide to measure trends, and is optimally used if the arm of the patient is fully adducted to prevent cooling of the probe by the surrounding air. In an infant, a rapidly flowing IV in the arm can falsely lower the measured value.

Rectal temperature reflects the temperature of tissue perfused by the inferior hemorrhoidal artery. It sometimes deviates from central temperature when the patient is subjected to thermal stress, and during cystoscopy.[20]

Liquid crystal temperature sensors placed on the forehead are available that sense changes of 0.5°C. During mild hypothermia or severe vasoconstriction in the skin of the forehead, the liquid crystals read temperatures that are about 2–3°C below tympanic temperature and may be unreliable.[21]

As a general rule when any probe is introduced into a body cavity, due care must be exercised to prevent damage or perforation of that cavity.

SUMMARY

It is important to monitor temperature, especially in the newborn or neonate, to prevent hypothermia (Table 2). Decreased body temperature is initially compensated for by increased metabolism. If this compensation fails and temperature continues to decrease, regional blood flow shifts, causing a metabolic acidosis, and eventually apnea. To prevent hypothermia, it is mandatory to monitor temperature in infants, whether in the intensive care unit or the operating room. A thorough understanding of the physiology of temperature homeostasis will lead to a rational approach to effective maintenance of body temperature.

Table 3-2

Prevention of Hypothermia

1	Monitoring
2	Heating blanket
3	Steri-drape
4	Radiant heat
5	Heating of fluids
6	Anesthesia system
7	Room temperature

REFERENCES

1. Rackow H, Salanitre E: Modern concepts in pediatric anesthesiology. *Anesthesiology*, 30:208–234, 1969
2. Benzinger TH: Heat regulation: Homeostasis of central temperature in man. *Physiological Reviews*, 49:671–759, 1969
3. Poulos DA: Central processing of cutaneous temperature information. *Federation Proceedings*, 40:2825–2829, 1981
4. Hense H: Neural processes in long-term thermal adaptation. *Federation Proceedings*, 40:2830–2834, 1981
5. Heiser MS, Downes JJ: Temperature regulation in the pediatric patient. *Seminars in Anesthesia*, 2 (1):37–42, 1984
6. Carpenter DO: Ionic and metabolic basis of neuronal thermosensitivity. *Federation Proceedings*, 40:2808–2813, 1981
7. Brueck K: Temperature regulation in the newborn infant. *Biologica Neonatorum*, 3:65–119, 1961
8. Schiff D, Stern L, Leduc J: Chemical thermogensis in newborn infants. Catecholamine excretion and the plasma nonesterified fatty acid response to cold exposure. *Pediatrics*, 37:577–582, 1966
9. Himms-Hoge L: Cellular thermogenesis. *Ann Rev Physiol*, 38:315–335, 1976
10. Goudsouzian NG, Morris RH, Ryan JF: The effects of a warming blanket on the maintenance of body temperature in anesthetized infants and children. *Anesthesiology*, 39:351–353, 1973
11. Dick W, Kreuscher H, Luhken D: Prevention of heat loss during anesthesia and operation in the newborn baby and small infants. *Acta Anaesth Scand*, suppl 37:134–139, 1970
12. Hey EN, O'Connell B: Oxygen consumption and heat balance in the cot-nursed baby. *Arch Dis Child*, 45:335–343, 1970
13. Day RL, Caliguiri L, Kamenski C, Ehrlich F: Body temperature and survival of premature infants. *Pediatrics*, 34:171–181, 1964
14. Baumgart S: Reduction of oxygen consumption insensible water loss and radiant heat demand with use of a plastic blanket for low birth weight infants under radiant warmers. *Anesthesiology*, 74:1022–1028, 1984
15. Goudsouzian N: Anatomical differences between the child and the adult and their clinical sequelae, in R. Salem, (ed): *Pediatric Anesthesia Current Practice*. New York, Academic Press, 1981, pp 1–3
16. Weeks DB, Bromark E: A method of quantitiating humidity in the anesthesia circuit by temperature control semiclosed circle. *Anesth Analg*, 49:292–296, 1970
17. Epstein RA: Humidification during positive pressure ventilation in infants. *Anesthesiology*, 35:532–536, 1971
18. Fonkalsrud EW, Calmes S, Barcliff LT, et al: Reduction of operative heat loss and pulmonary secretions in neonates by use of heated and humidified anesthetic gases. *J Thorac Cardiovasc Surg*, 80:718–723, 1980
19. Benzinger M: Tympanic thermometry in surgery and anesthesia. *JAMA*, 209:1207–1211, 1969
20. Roe CF: Effect of bowel exposure on body temperature during surgical operations. *Am J of Surg*, 122:13–15, 1971
21. Gravenstein JS, Newbower RS, Ream AK, et al (eds): Essential Noninvasive Monitoring. New York, Grune and Stratton, 1980, p 177

4

The Preoperative Evaluation of Pediatric Patients

Charles J. Coté
I. David Todres
John F. Ryan

The preoperative evaluation and preparation of the pediatric patient is basically similar to that of the adult from the physiological standpoint. In the psychological preparation of the infant and child, however, there is a great difference from the adult. The child does not have the experience to place the hospital, with its overwhelming size, smells, and noise levels, in perspective. The child will fear separation from the parents, and may also have difficulty in comprehending the need for hospitalization. Therefore, a special approach by the anesthesiologist, surgeon, nurses, and parents is required. The preoperative evaluation is usually simplified once some of the basic concepts of how to evaluate a child are established.

PSYCHOLOGICAL PREPARATION OF THE CHILD FOR SURGERY

Many hospitals have either an open house or a brochure that is given to describe the preoperative preparative programs to the parents prior to their child's admission. The anesthesiologist should participate in the design of such programs so that they accurately reflect the anesthetic practice of that institution. The preoperative anesthetic experience begins at the time that the parents are first told by the surgeon that their child is to have surgery. This is the most appropriate time to introduce the parents to these preparative programs, rather than waiting for a hasty, and often inadequate, last minute talk to a nervous and preoccupied couple. Being prepared enables the parents to answer the child's questions and thus paves the way for a smooth preoperative course. The greater understanding and amount of information that the parents have, the

less will be their anxiety; this in turn will be reflected in the child. Inadequate preparation of the child and family will often make the anesthetic induction traumatic and difficult for both the child and the anesthesiologist, with significant likelihood of postoperative psychological disturbances.

Special aspects of the child's perception of anesthesia should be anticipated. It is important to reassure the child that anesthesia will be a type of deep sleep, not the same as the usual nightly sleep, but rather a special type during which there will be no pain from surgery, and from which the child will very definitely be awakened. Another fear that many children have is the possibility that they will wake up in the middle of the anesthetic and surgical process. They should be reassured that they will awaken *only* when the surgery and anesthesia are completed. The reason and need for a surgical procedure should also be carefully explained to the child.

The words the anesthesiologist uses to describe what can be anticipated must be carefully chosen, since children think concretely and tend to interpret literally. Examples of this are presented by the following anecdotes:

A four year old child was informed that in the morning he would receive a "shot" which would "put him to sleep." That night a frantic call was received from the mother describing a very upset child; the child thought he was going to be "put to sleep" like the veterinarian had "put to sleep" his sick pet.

A five year old child was admitted to the hospital for elective inguinal herniorrhaphy. He received a heavy premedication and was sleeping upon arrival in the operating room. After discharge, the parents frequently discovered him wandering about the house at night. Upon questioning, the child stated that he was protecting his family. "I don't want anyone sneaking up on you and operating while you are sleeping."

In the first example, the anesthesiologist's choice of words was misunderstood by the child's concrete thought processes, while the second case represents a problem of communication; the child was never told he would have an operation.

The importance of proper psychological preparation for surgery should not be underestimated.[1,2] Often little has been explained to either patient or parent. The anesthesiologist can play a key role in alleviating fear of the unknown through an understanding of the child's perception of anesthesia and surgery. This can be accomplished by a calm, friendly face, a warm introduction, touching the patient in a reassuring manner (holding the child's or parent's hand), and being completely honest with both. Children respond positively to an honest description of exactly what they can anticipate. This includes informing the child of the slight discomfort of starting an intravenous line, an intramuscular premedication, or a mask induction for anesthesia. This is important, as the anesthesiologist who condescendingly tells the child that there will be no pain finds that when there is pain, credibility is lost.

The postsurgical process, from the operating room to the recovery room and the onset of postoperative pain, should be described. Encourage the patient to ask any questions he or she may have. The patient must be told that everything possible will be done to maintain comfort. Allowing a favorite "security" blanket or "teddy bear" to accompany the child to the operating room may also be a great help.

One of the very important features of the preoperative evaluation and preparation of the child is not only preparation for this unique experience in the child's life, but also for any repeat anesthetic and surgical procedures. Close cooperation between the anesthesiologist and the parents in preparing the child is vital to a favorable outcome.

While focusing on the preparation of the child, it is crucial to appreciate that the most favorable outcome will depend upon preparation of the whole family unit, that is, child, siblings, and parents. In certain circumstances, parents will want to accompany their child from the wards to the operating room environment. If they can be accommodated and if this is judged to be in the child's best interest, the anesthesiologist should support the parents' decision. What eases the parents calms the child, and this can only enhance patient care.

Prior to surgery it is essential to discuss in clear terms the anesthetic risks. This should be carried out in a reassuring manner by describing to the parents exactly what measures are being taken to closely monitor the safety of their child. Mentioning details such as a blood pressure cuff, EKG monitors to "watch the heart beat," stethoscopes "to listen to the heart tones," IV's to be able to give fluid and medications, is important to reassure the parents that their child will be anesthetized with the utmost safety and care. Parents should be given ample opportunity to ask questions.

The anesthetic–surgical experience has often been associated with children who return home and then relive unpleasant memories in the form of nightmares. In addition, some children will exhibit psychosomatic manifestations of this experience, such as the development of tics, agitation, lack of concentration, or bedwetting. Therefore, attention toward reducing anxiety and unpleasant experiences is most impor-

tant. Fortunately, many of these problems resolve themselves after a short time.

HISTORY OF PRESENT ILLNESS

In most situations the history of the present illness will be related to physicians by the parents. If the child is old enough, it is helpful to obtain the child's corroboration. The history should focus on:

- The relevant organ systems involved
- Medications related to and taken prior to the present illness
- Previous surgical and hospital experiences related to the current problem
- The time of last oral intake and its relation to the illness or injury (It is essential to appreciate that decreased gastrointestinal motility often begins with the illness or injury. A child who has had an accident within several hours of eating should be considered to have a full stomach, even though the surgical procedure may be planned for many hours after the accident. This will be considered in greater detail later in this chapter)
- Review of all other body systems should also be made (Table 4-1), with special emphasis on history of a recent upper respiratory infection, allergic reactions, bleeding tendencies (bruising), fever, anemia, seizures, diarrhea, and vomiting (The latter being particularly important in the young infant because of the rapid fluid turnover and increased risk of hypovolemia)

THE NEONATE

The medical history of a pediatric patient begins in utero; problems that may have been present during gestation and birth may still be relevant in the neonatal period (Table 4-2). This history is especially important to the neonate who requires an urgent surgical procedure. The problems one expects in a full-term baby of normal birth weight are different from those anticipated in a full-term baby who is small for gestational age (SGA). These considerations are magnified for a premature baby of appropriate weight, and are markedly intensified for a baby who is both premature and SGA (Chapter 2). A careful neonatal and gestational history often enables the anesthesiologist to anticipate problems which could prove potentially dangerous during anesthesia. Several complex scoring systems for both physical characteristics and neurological examination provide good estimates of gestational age.[3–6] Chapter 2 presents the most common physical characteristics of babies of varying gestational ages. By plotting gestational age against birth weight one is able to define categories, each with its own risk for associated neonatal problems. For example, a 2000 gm baby with characteristics of 29 weeks gestation would be large for gestational age (LGA), whereas at 35 weeks gestation the child would be appropriate for gestational age (AGA). The same weight in a child of 40 weeks gestation would be considered small for gestational age (SGA). Thus weight alone is not the sole criteria for determining prematurity. The maternal medical and pharmacologic history may also provide invaluable data for the management of the neonate requiring surgery (Table 4-2).

Table 4-1

Review of Systems—Anesthetic Implications

System	Questions to Ask	Possible Anesthetic Implications
Respiratory	Bronchitis, cough, asthma	Irritable airway, bronchospasm, medication history
	Recent cold	Atelectasis, infiltrate
	Croup	Possible subglottic narrowing
	Apnea/bradycardia	Postoperative apnea/bradycardia
Cardiovascular	Murmur	Possible septal defect, avoid air bubbles in IV
	Cyanosis	Right to left shunt
	History of squatting	Possible Fallot's tetrology
	Hypertension	Possible coarctation, renal disease
	Rheumatic fever	Valvular heart disease
	Excercise intolerance	Congestive heart failure, cyanosis
Neurological	Seizures	Medications, metabolic derangement
	Head trauma	Intracranial hypertension
	Swallowing ability (chokes during feeding)	Possible aspiration, esophageal reflux, hiatus hernia
	Neuromuscular disease	Neuromuscular relaxant drug sensitivity, malignant hyperpyrexia
Gastrointestinal/ hepatic	Vomiting, diarrhea	Electrolyte imbalance, dehydration, full stomach
	Malabsorption	Anemia
	Black stools	Anemia, hypovolemia
	Reflux	Treat like full stomach
	Jaundice	Drug metabolism/hypoglycemia
Genitourinary	Frequency	Urinary tract infection, diabetes, hypercalcemia
	Time of last urination	State of hydration
	Frequent urinary tract infections	Evaluate renal function
Endocrine/ metabolic	Abnormal development	Possible endocrinopathy, hypothyroid, diabetes, etc.
	Hypoglycemia, steroid therapy	Hypoglycemia, adrenal insufficiency
Hematologic	Anemia	Possible need for transfusion
	Bruising, excess bleeding	Coagulopathy, thrombocytopenia, thrombocytopathy
	Sickle cell disease	Hydration, possible exchange transfusion
Allergies	Medication	Possible drug interaction
Dental	Loose teeth	Aspirate loose teeth
	Carious teeth	Possible subacute bacterial endocarditis prophylaxis

PAST MEDICAL HISTORY

This should include a history of all previous hospitalizations or surgery, prior immunizations, childhood illnesses, and possible contacts with infectious diseases. A history of prematurity and apnea and/or bradycardic spells is highly significant.

FAMILY HISTORY

It is important to inquire if there is a familial history of (1) prolonged paralysis associated with anesthesia (possible pseudocholinesterase deficiency), (2) unexpected deaths (possible sudden infant death syndrome, malignant hyperthermia), (3) genetic defects, (4) familial medical conditions, e.g., muscular dystrophy, cystic fibrosis, sickle cell disease, bleeding tendencies (hemophilia), and (5) allergic reactions.

OTHER DATA

Examination of previous medical, surgical, and anesthetic records will assist in planning the anesthetic procedure. Special note should be taken of any difficulties previously encountered before, during and after surgery. Specific attention should be paid to airway problems, tracheal intubation, venous access, hypotension, bradycardia, cyanosis, or agitation.

PHYSICAL EXAMINATION

A great deal of knowledge can be gained during the physical examination by observing how the child interacts with parents and physicians. While observing the child and talking to the family, we are gaining the child's acceptance. A child is not examined in the same way as an adult. Examination starts with careful, nonthreatening observations and proceeds to the

Table 4-2

Maternal History with Commonly Associated Neonatal Problems

Maternal History	Commonly Expected Problems With Neonate
Rh–ABO Incompatibility	Hemolytic anemia, hyperbilirubinemia, kernicterus
Toxemia	SGA and its associated problems (Table 2-2), muscle relaxant interaction with magnesium therapy
Hypertension	SGA and its associated problems (Table 2-2)
Drug Addiction	Withdrawal, SGA
Infection	Sepsis, thrombocytopenia, viral infection
Hemorrhage	Anemia, shock
Diabetes	Hypoglycemia, birth trauma, LGA, SGA, and associated problems (Table 2-2)
Polyhydramnios	Tracheoesophageal fistula, anencephaly, multiple anomalies
Oligohydramnios	Renal hypoplasia, pulmonary hypoplasia
Cephalopelvic Disproportion	Birth trauma, hyperbilirubinemia, fractures
Alcoholism	Hypoglycemia, congenital malformation, fetal alcohol syndrome, SGA and associated problems (Table 2-2)

SGA = small for gestational age; LGA = large for gestational age.

physical examination according to the child's interaction with the anesthesiologist.

While looking at the patient observe the skin and facies for obvious signs of pallor, cyanosis, sweating, jaundice, apprehension, pain, or signs of previous surgery. Does the child have an obvious upper respiratory tract infection? Is the child having respiratory difficulty—nasal flaring, grunting respirations, stridor, retractions, or wheezing? Is there any abdominal distension? Are there any congenital abnormalities? It is important to be alert to any unusual features, since these may represent a specific syndrome. *When there is one congenital malformation there is a greater likelihood of another.*

We must also consider the child's environment. The devices that are attached to the child may provide important clues to underlying conditions and ongoing therapy, e.g., endotracheal tubes, respirators, intravenous lines, urinary catheters, nasogastric tubes, or respiratory and cardiac monitors.

Having talked with the parents and observed the child, the examination proceeds in a manner similar to that performed in the adult, but there are special differences. It is important to warm the stethoscope and the examining hands.

Begin with the less painful areas; listen to the heart and lungs, and defer the throat examination and potentially painful examinations to the end. Special points of interest include (1) fever, (2) missing or loose teeth (possible dislodgement during laryngoscopy), (3) micrognathia (difficult intubation), (4) nasal speech or mouth breathing (hypertrophied adenoids, tonsils, difficult induction, potential bleeding with nasogastric tube or nasotracheal intubation), (5) heart murmurs (take care to avoid air bubbles in IV lines), (6) abdominal distension (full stomach, impeded respiration), (7) the child's neurologic status (increased intracranial pressure, loss of gag reflex, control of the airway and breathing), and (8) edema (congestive heart failure, nephrotic syndrome, hypoproteinemia, renal failure). Because fluid turnover is much more rapid in the infant than in the adult, special emphasis must be paid to hydration (dry mouth, loss of tears, tenting of the skin, sunken fontanelle and eyeballs, mottled skin—see Chapter 10).

In the very young infant one must take special care during the examination to avoid dangerous hypothermia with prolonged periods of undress. The anesthesiologist may readily evaluate such an infant in the incubator or isolette. A rapid assessment of gestational age may be made by examining specific physical and neurological characteristics (Table 2-3).[7]

LABORATORY DATA

The amount of laboratory data gathered should be appropriate to the history, illness, and surgical procedure. Minimum routine tests in most hospitals include a hematocrit and urinalysis. In general a routine chest X-ray is not necessary; recent studies have confirmed the cost ineffectiveness of routine chest X-rays in children.[8,9] If, however, there is a history of a recent respiratory tract infection (within one month), it may be advantageous to obtain a chest X-ray to rule out an asymptomatic infiltrate or an area of atelectasis.[10] If major reconstructive surgery is contemplated, a bleeding profile (platelet count, prothrombin time, and partial thromboplastin time) should be obtained; a bleeding time should also be performed on children taking medications containing aspirin. Special laboratory data, such as electrolytes, blood sugar, renal function tests, blood gas analysis, an EKG, ECHO, liver function tests, CAT scan, or pulmonary function tests, should be obtained when appropriate.

Finally, the patient's history, physical examination, medications, and laboratory data must be synthesized into an anesthetic plan that combines the psychological needs of the patient, and the anesthesiologist's concerns for patient safety, with optimum operating conditions for the surgeon.

SPECIAL PROBLEMS

THE FULL STOMACH

This is probably the most common problem in pediatric anesthesia. There is never a time when a child can be trusted to fast. Therefore, the anesthesiologist must always be suspicious and must ask the child just prior to induction if anything has been eaten. It is not unusual to find bubble gum, candy, or other food in a child's mouth. When the anesthesiologist suspects a full stomach, induction of anesthesia must be managed appropriately. The preferred method under these circumstances is a rapid intravenous induction. Before this is undertaken the anesthesiologist must ensure that the proper equipment is at hand, i.e., two functioning laryngoscope blades and handles (should a bulb or contact fail, a spare is available), two suctions (should the suction be blocked by vomitus or blood, a second is available), appropriate drugs, a leak-free anesthesia circuit, appropriately sized endotracheal tubes, and stylette. After an IV is started the child is given atropine 0.02 mg/kg IV, and is denitrogenated with 100 percent oxygen ("preoxygenated") for three minutes. Even with a crying child it is possible to increase the PaO_2 by enriching the immediate environment with high flows of oxygen. It is important to adequately preoxygenate the patient in order to avoid positive-pressure ventilation prior to intubation; this may result in distension of an already full stomach, with possible regurgitation and aspiration. The child is then given 5–6 mg/kg thiopental IV, followed immediately with 1–2 mg/kg succinylcholine.[11] If the fluid volume status of the child is marginal, then a much smaller dose of thiopental is advised, or alternately ketamine in a dose of 1 mg/kg IV. The child should have cricoid pressure (Sellick maneuver) applied as he falls asleep, and pressure should be maintained until an endotracheal tube is safely inserted and the lungs are inflated.[12,13] Finally, a neonate may be intubated awake; this may provide a greater margin of safety because it preserves spontaneous ventilation as well as the gag reflex.

FASTING

Patients are ordered to fast in order to minimize the dangers of aspiration. Fasting merely protects against aspiration of particulate matter. The period of time that a child can safely fast is variable, and usually is dependent on the child's age, weight, and nutritional status.[14] As a general rule, most pediatric anesthesiologists would request an eight-hour period free of milk and solids. Term newborns, and children up to six months of age, have small glycogen stores and therefore should be offered clear liquids (sugar water, ginger ale, plain gelatin) up to four hours prior to surgery. This should be reduced to two hours for premature babies. Children six months to three years of age may be kept fasting six hours, and children three to six years, eight hours. It is important to explain to the child why he or she must not eat or drink; however, even though instructed to fast, partially digested food is frequently discovered in the stomach.

A study of children anesthetized for elective surgery found that even with strict abstinence of fluids and solids 75 percent had a gastric residual volume greater than 0.4 ml/kg and a pH less than 2.5, factors which put these children at risk of acid aspiration (Mendelson's syndrome).[15] Oral cimetidine 7.5 mg/kg one hour prior to surgery has proven to be a safe and effective agent in reducing both gastric residual volume and acid content in children. This should be considered for children with gastroesophageal reflux, hiatus hernia, anticipated airway difficulty, and children scheduled for bronchoscopy.[16]

Not infrequently the scheduled surgery may be delayed, thus extending the period of fasting to a point which may be potentially dangerous (inducing, for example, hypoglycemia or hypovolemia). Therefore, we recommend that an IV be started and appropriate fluids administered prior to induction of anesthesia. This is particularly important in the premature infant and neonate.

ANEMIA

There is little data regarding the minimum hematocrit necessary to ensure adequate oxygen transport and delivery in the pediatric patient. It is recognized that patients with chronic anemia, such as renal failure, do not need to be transfused for minor procedures because of compensatory mechanisms such as increased 2,3-diphosphoglycerate, oxygen extraction, and cardiac output. Elective surgery on the anemic pediatric patient is a controversial area. Consideration must be given to what type of surgery is planned and how urgent it is. Most pediatric anesthesiologists would recommend a hematocrit above 30, but under special circumstances (e.g., physiologic anemia between 2–4 months of age, or renal failure) a lower value may be acceptable. If significant blood loss is anticipated, and the surgery is elective, then the cause of anemia should be investigated, treated, and the surgery postponed until the hematocrit is restored to the normal range. *Children should not receive blood transfusions for elective surgery in order to bring their hematocrit up to 30 because of the potential risk of contracting hepatitis and acquired immune deficiency syndrome (AIDS).*

UPPER RESPIRATORY INFECTION (URI)

Another common problem faced by the pediatric anesthesiologist is the safety of anesthetizing a child who has, or is recovering from, an upper respiratory tract infection (URI). There is little data regarding this problem. One study has demonstrated no correlation of post-intubation croup in children who had an active URI as opposed to noninfected patients.[17] A retrospective study has revealed a significant correlation of intraoperative complications, such as atelectasis and cyanosis, with a history of a recent URI.[10] Therefore, if the patient has fever, a recent onset of purulent nasal discharge, or cough, one should consider postponing elective surgery; these symptoms may represent the prodromal stage of an infectious disease. If the child is recovering from an URI, there should be a normal physical examination and a normal white blood cell count prior to anesthesia. It is our clinical impression that infected airways tend to be more prone to laryngospasm and bronchospasm, and for these reasons we tend to postpone elective operations on patients with an active infection.

Allergic rhinitis tends to be seasonal in nature, has a clear nasal discharge, no fever, and probably has no higher incidence of intraoperative anesthetic complications and is not a contraindication to general anesthesia.

FEVER

It is not uncommon for a child to have a low-grade fever prior to surgery, and it is nearly always a dilemma as to what to do about it. In general, if the child only has 0.5–1.0°C fever and no other symptoms, such a fever is not a contraindication to general anesthesia. If, on the other hand, the fever is associated with a recent onset of rhinitis, pharyngitis, otitis media, dehydration, or any other sign of impending illness, one must consider postponing the procedure. On occasion it is necessary to anesthetize a child with fever, and in this situation some effort should be made to reduce the fever prior to induction of anesthesia, primarily to reduce oxygen demands.[18] Reduction of the fever should not include aspirin since this may interfere with platelet function. There is no

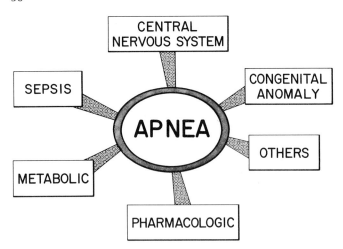

Figure 4-1. Apnea, defined as the absence of movement of air at the mouth or nose, may have many etiologies. Those which anesthesiologists are most often involved with concern metabolic, pharmacologic, or respiratory causes.

evidence that an existing fever predisposes the patient toward malignant hyperpyrexia.[19] One useful tool in lowering temperature and providing fluid and electrolytes is to infuse cold lactated Ringer's or normal saline through a peripheral venous line. Thermoregulation is considered in greater detail in Chapter 3.

SICKLE CELL DISEASE

Whenever sickle cell disease or trait is a possibility the anesthetic and postanesthetic management is modified.[20] It is important to obtain a good family history, and a sickle cell preparation. It must be emphasized that the status of hydration and oxygenation is critical in all sickle cell patients. Thus a secure intravenous route with hydration of at least one and a half times maintenance should be continued well into the postoperative period, especially following procedures where ileus may result (third space losses). Meticulous attention to detail to ensure a stable cardiovascular status and adequate ventilation will result in adequate oxygenation to prevent sickling. Children with hemoglobin SC are especially at risk because they have a relatively normal hemoglobin level, yet are extremely vulnerable to the complications of sickle cell crisis.[21] Children with sickle cell disease (SS) should have hematologic consultation regarding prophylactic preoperative exchange transfusion.

THE MENTALLY HANDICAPPED CHILD

Mentally handicapped children may be the most challenging patients to anesthetize because one of our most important tools, our ability to explain procedures and reassure the patient, may be useless. If a child has a bad hospital experience this will greatly magnify the difficulties of future admissions. Therefore the care of these children requires the utmost in patience, understanding, preparation, and cooperation among the family, pediatrician, surgeon, anesthesiologist, and nursing staff. Sedating such a child prior to surgery is often indicated, and may be accomplished with oral diazepam 0.2–0.3 mg/kg, or rectal methohexital.[22] We prefer the latter technique since it has the advantages of minimal trauma to the child, and parental participation in the process.

The mentally handicapped child is often limited in the ability to relate to people outside the family. In these situations we try to have the family near when the child awakens in the recovery room. Traditional exclusion of the parents of such a child from this area of the hospital may not be in the child's best interests.

PREMATURITY AND RETROLENTAL FIBROPLASIA (RLF)

At present it appears that there is a relationship between oxygen administration and RLF. This condition, however, has also appeared in stillborns and infants with cyanotic congenital heart disease.[23] Multicenter studies have shown that the disease occurs especially in the sick low-birth-weight infant (less than 1000 gm) who was exposed to oxygen therapy for a prolonged period. No significant correlation could be shown with levels of arterial PaO_2.[24–26] The dilemma presented to the anesthesiologist is to balance the administration of oxygen during anesthesia, to provide an adequate concentration to the vital organs (e.g., the brain and heart), while avoiding potentially damaging effects on the retina. Knowledge of retinal maturation may provide us with a rational approach to some of these problems. The infant's retina does not mature until 42–44 weeks of gestation.[27] A prospective study of term infants coming to elective surgery revealed that only those infants greater than 44 weeks gestation had fully matured retinas.[28] This would suggest that it may be advisable to delay *elective* surgery until after retinal maturation, i.e., after 44 weeks of gestation. This will be considered in greater detail in Chapter 7.

APNEA

In the evaluation of the infant with a history of prematurity, the anesthesiologist must be aware that there is a group of infants who may develop perioperative respiratory complications.[29] Prematurely born infants who have a history of idiopathic apnea are more prone than term infants to experiencing life-threatening apnea postoperatively.[30] At the time surgery is scheduled these children may or may not continue to have intermittent apnea spells, and will often appear normal for their age. The infants at greatest risk are those with a history of prematurity and a history of apnea/bradycardia spells who are less than 44 weeks conceptual age.[30] If the child is taking theophylline preoperatively this therapy should be continued into the postoperative period. A serum concentration between 5–15 µg/ml is considered to be a therapeutic level.[31] Therefore, these children must not be anesthetized as outpatients.

Apnea may be related to many causes (Fig. 4-1). The most common following an operative procedure, however, relate to metabolic derangements, pharmacologic effects, or central nervous system immaturity. Metabolic causes of apnea such as hypothermia, hypoglycemia, hypocalcemia, acidosis, and hypoxemia, can be avoided by meticulous attention to the details of the anesthetic management of neonates (see Chapter 13). Pharmacologic effects cannot be avoided, since administering anesthesia requires the use of drugs, and most drugs used in anesthesia affect the respiratory system directly or indirectly. Most inhalational agents, narcotics, and sedatives have been demonstrated in a dose-related fashion to depress the central response to CO_2 in adults.[32] Few studies have examined this problem in neonates. Such respiratory depression, however, is probably more likely to occur in neonates who have an immature respiratory center. Studies in adults have demonstrated ablation of both the response to hypoxia, and the potentiation of that response by hypercarbia in the presence of halothane in concentrations as low as 0.1 percent; thus residual anesthetic action may contribute to the development of apnea in babies.[33] In addition, most pharmacologic agents used in anesthesia will decrease muscle tone of the upper airway, thus contributing to the development of upper airway obstruction, more labored breathing, fatigue, and apnea. Potent inhalational anesthetic agents decrease intercostal muscle tone, thus reducing functional residual capacity, and therefore increasing the propensity to develop hypoxemia.[34,35] Figure 4-2 presents several possible sequences of events leading to the development of apnea. Thus, there does not appear to be an "ideal" anesthetic technique for the neonate, and these infants should, therefore, be cared for only in a facility that has the proper operating room equipment and a neonatal intensive care unit to which the child can be admitted postoperatively for 24-hour monitoring for postoperative cardiorespiratory problems.[29,30] This monitoring should be continued until the child is free of apnea for 24 hours.

BRONCHOPULMONARY DYSPLASIA (BPD)

Bronchopulmonary dysplasia is a common result of prolonged ventilation of the premature neonate with hyaline membrane disease. Infants with BPD suffer from chronic hypoxemia, hypercarbia, and increased pulmonary vascular resistance.[36–40] The latter may lead to cor pulmonale and congestive heart failure. In addition, variations in pulmonary interstitial edema increases the possibility of respiratory failure. Frequently these infants are on diuretic therapy.[41] In evaluating these infants for anesthesia and surgery, adequate preoperative preparation must be carried out (in some cases over several days) to optimize oxygenation and myocardial function. These children, therefore, require special attention to fluid and electrolyte balance and careful titration of intraoperative fluids. In addition, chronic air trapping should alert the anesthesiologist to the potential dangers of N_2O.[42] It is also important *to allow adequate expiratory time and to avoid excessive positive pressure ventilation.* These changes in lung function and structure may persist long beyond the first year of life, and may be slightly improved with the use of bronchodilators.[43] There is a seven-fold greater incidence of sudden infant death syndrome in these patients, which would suggest the need for postoperative apnea monitoring.[44]

THE DIABETIC CHILD

Diabetes is a relatively common childhood disease and when such patients come to surgery careful management of their insulin therapy must be continued. Knowledge of insulin schedule, normal serum glucose curves, and time of glucosuria is important. The patient's normal diet and insulin regimen should be maintained up to and including the day prior to surgery. In general, an attempt should be made to schedule a diabetic patient as the first case of the day. An IV with 5 percent glucose at maintenance should be started on the ward to avoid dangerous hypoglycemia. We usually administer one half the normal insulin dosage the morning of surgery *after* the

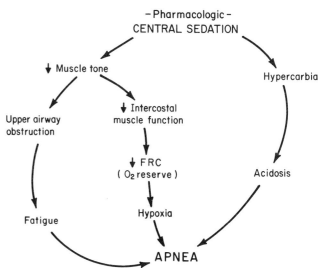

Figure 4-2. Pharmacologic interventions may result in several sequences of events.

IV is started. 5 percent glucose is continued throughout the surgical procedure. Serum glucose should be monitored both intraoperatively and postoperatively (Dextrostix* and blood sugar) until the child is back on a routine schedule.

An alternative to the above regimen is to use a continuous infusion of glucose and insulin. To date there is little published data for the use of continuous insulin infusions for patients undergoing elective surgery, especially children. One study in adults found better control of glucose levels, but it was necessary to alter the infusions in order to prevent hypoglycemia.[45]

Emergency surgery, and the resultant stress on diabetic patients (e.g., appendectomy), may result in marked alteration in glucose–insulin response and acid–base status. Hydration and efforts to correct hyperglycemia and ketoacidosis should be made prior to induction of general anesthesia. Serum glucose and potassium levels must be closely monitored (at least hourly), and appropriate doses of insulin administered until they are stable.

There are two generally accepted methods for correction of keto-acidosis. The first is the standard loading dose of insulin, half intravenously and half subcutaneously, with increments given every 1–2 hours as indicated. The second method utilizes a loading dose of insulin followed by a constant infusion. The latter method purportedly provides a smoother correction; however, no studies have proven one method superior to the other. Both methods require meticulous attention to glucose and potassium levels; the latter method may have a lower incidence of these problems.[46–49]

SEIZURE DISORDERS

The management of the child with a seizure disorder requires knowledge of the medication the child is taking, the medication schedule, and possible interaction between the patient's medications and anesthetic drugs. The stress of surgery and anesthesia may alter the seizure threshold and

---

* Ames & Co., a division of Miles Laboratories, Inc., Elkhart, Indiana.

result in increased seizure activity. We continue seizure medications, therefore, up to the immediate time of elective surgery, allowing the child to take his medications with a sip of water the morning of surgery. For emergency procedures, missing one or two doses usually will not result in serious alteration of pharmacologic drug levels; however, if the medications will be interrupted for a longer period of time, intravenous or intramuscular therapy must be instituted. Blood levels of anticonvulsant drugs should be monitored for proper therapeutic effect.

HYPERALIMENTATION

Intravenous alimentation is frequently used as a means of life support and to prepare patients for surgery.[50] It is important for the anesthesiologist to know the composition and rate of administration of these fluids so that potential intraoperative complications may be avoided. Most of these solutions are hypertonic with a high glucose content and must be administered through a centrally placed intravenous route. Basic principles of care are:

- Avoid contamination of the line by puncturing it for medications or changing fluids without first communicating with the managing physicians. If a line change at the end of surgery is appropriate, then the present line may be used intraoperatively.
- Do not suddenly stop the hyperalimentation fluid, since this will leave the child in a relative hyperinsulinemic state, which may result in profound hypoglycemia, the signs of which may be masked by general anesthesia.
- Use an infusion device at all times so that the rate of infusion is constant. Accidental rapid infusion of large amounts of hyperalimentation fluid may cause hypertonic nonketotic coma.[50]
- Careful monitoring of serum glucose, potassium, sodium, calcium, and acid–base status is important preoperatively, intraoperatively, and postoperatively.
- A preoperative check of line placement is also important to avoid intraoperative complications such as hydrothorax or hemothorax.

THE ASTHMATIC PATIENT

Asthmatic patients coming to elective surgery should be free of significant wheezing. A history of prior emergency room visits and hospitalizations should be obtained. Specific information regarding possible pneumothorax, respiratory arrests, steroid therapy, and drug overdose should be sought. All asthmatic medications should be maintained up to and including the morning of surgery. Theophylline levels should be in the 10–20 μg/ml range in order to have optimal therapeutic effect.[51] Baseline EKG and chest X-rays should be obtained.

Emergency surgery may necessitate anesthesia in spite of bronchospasm. In this situation the urgency of the surgery must be balanced against the severity of the bronchospasm. Some control of bronchospasm should ideally be instituted prior to anesthesia (oxygen administration, hydration, subcutaneous epinephrine, aminophylline infusion, beta$_2$ agonist therapy, steroids, and antibiotics). Baseline blood gas analysis may be critical to differentiate moderate from severe airway obstruction. Any asthmatic with a $PaCO_2$ above 45 torr must be considered to have incipient respiratory failure.[52]

OUTPATIENT SURGERY

No other area of pediatric anesthesia has expanded so greatly in recent years as outpatient surgery.[53] Cost effectiveness and minimal psychologic trauma are the major benefits of such programs. In fact, more than half of our anesthetics are delivered to outpatients.

It is therefore important to have a smoothly functioning outpatient facility with adequate space for a play area and patient examination rooms, easy access to basic laboratory studies (hematocrit, urinalysis), and recovery areas for both immediate postanesthesia and long-term postsurgical observation. A clear agreement with the surgeons that only healthy American Society of Anesthesiologists (ASA) Class 1 and 2 patients are appropriate candidates for outpatient surgery is important. Under special prearranged and well-planned circumstances, an ASA Class 3 patient may be anesthetized as an outpatient.

The goal of outpatient anesthetic management is an alert, comfortable patient, capable of going home within several hours of surgery. In our experience rectal methohexital (20–30 mg/kg) has proven most effective as a premedication for smaller outpatients without significant prolongation of hospital stay.[22] Oral premedication using atropine 0.02 mg/kg, meperidine 1.5 mg/kg, and diazepam 0.1 mg/kg, has been reported, also without significant delay of discharge.[54]

All patients, except those having the briefest surgical procedures (e.g., myringotomy), have an IV started during anesthesia to compensate for the period of fasting. In addition, we make maximal use of intraoperative nerve blocks to diminish postoperative pain. Penile and ileoinguinal nerve blocks are particularly useful for circumcisions, hypospadias repair, and herniorrhaphy.

After leaving the postanesthetic recovery room, children are observed for several hours to ensure that they are afebrile, able to tolerate fluids, and do not have problems with the surgical site. Parents are instructed to notify us immediately if there are any problems after discharge.

REFERENCES

1. Azarnoff P, Woody PD: Preparation of children for hospitalization in acute care hospitals in the United States. *Pediatrics* 68:361–368, 1981
2. Egbert LD, Battit GE, Turndorf H, et al: The value of the preoperative visit by an anesthetist. *JAMA* 185:553–555, 1963
3. Battaglia FC, Lubchenco LO: A practical classification of newborn infants by weight and gestational age. *J Pediatr* 71:159–163, 1967
4. Farr V, Kerridge DF, Mitchell RG: The value of some external characteristics in the assessment of gestational age at birth. *Dev Med Child Neurol* 8:657–660, 1966
5. Farr V, Mitchell RG, Neligan GA, et al: The definition of some external characteristics used in the assessment of gestational age of the newborn infant. *Dev Med Child Neurol* 8:507–511, 1966
6. Dubowitz LMS, Dubowitz V, Goldberg C: Clinical assessment of gestational age in the newborn infant. *J Pediatr* 77:1–10, 1970
7. Narayanan I, Dua K, Gujral VV, et al: A simple method of assessment of gestational age in newborn infants. *Pediatrics* 69:27–32, 1982
8. Sane SM, Worsing RA, Wiens CW, et al: Value of preoperative chest x-ray examinations in children. *Pediatrics* 60:669–672, 1977
9. Wood RA, Hoekelman RA: Value of the chest x-ray as a

screening test for elective surgery in children. *Pediatrics* 67: 447–452, 1981

10. McGill WA, Coveler LA, Epstein BS: Subacute upper respiratory infection in small children. *Anesth Analg* 58:331–333, 1979

11. Coté CJ, Goudsouzian NG, Liu LMP, et al: The dose response of intravenous thiopental for the induction of general anesthesia in unpremedicated children. *Anesthesiology* 55:703–705, 1981

12. Sellick BA: Cricoid pressure to control regurgitation of stomach contents during induction of anesthesia. *Lancet* 2:404–406, 1961

13. Salem MR, Wong AY, Fizzotti GF: Efficacy of cricoid pressure in preventing aspiration of gastric contents in paediatric patients. *Br J Anaesth* 44:401–404, 1972

14. Watson BG: Blood glucose levels in children during surgery. *Br J Anaesth* 44:712–715, 1972

15. Coté CJ, Goudsouzian NG, Liu LMP, et al: Assessment of risk factors related to the acid aspiration syndrome in pediatric patients—gastric pH and residual volume. *Anesthesiology* 56:70–72, 1982

16. Goudsouzian NG, Coté CJ, Liu LMP, et al: The dose response effects of oral cimetidine on gastric pH and volume in children. *Anesthesiology* 55:533–536, 1981

17. Koka BV, Jeon IS, Andre JM, et al: Postintubation croup in children. *Anesth Analg* 56:501–505, 1977

18. Stern RC: Pathophysiologic basis for the symptomatic treatment of fever. *Pediatrics* 59:92–98, 1977

19. Steward DJ: Malignant hyperthermia—the acute crisis, in Britt BA (ed): *International Anesthesiology Clinics*, vol 17, no 4. Boston, Little, Brown, 1979, pp 1–9

20. Howells TH, Huntsman RG, Boys JE, et al: Anaesthesia and sickle cell haemoglobin. *Br J Anaesth* 44:975–987, 1972

21. Rockoff AS, Christy D, Zeldis N, et al: Myocardial necrosis following general anesthesia in hemoglobin SC disease. *Pediatrics* 61:73–76, 1978

22. Liu LMP, Goudsouzian NG, Liu PL: Rectal methohexital premedication in children, a dose comparison study. *Anesthesiology* 53:343–345, 1980

23. Kalina RE, Hodson WA, Morgan BC: Retrolental fibroplasia in a cyanotic infant. *Pediatrics* 50:765–768, 1972

24. James LS, Lanman JT: History of oxygen therapy and retrolental fibroplasia. *Pediatrics* 57(suppl):591–642, 1976

25. Phelps DL: Retinopathy of prematurity: An estimate of vision loss in the United States—1979. *Pediatrics* 67:924–926, 1981

26. Gunn TR, Easdown J, Outerbridge EW: Risk factors in retrolental fibroplasia. *Pediatrics* 65:1096–1100, 1980

27. Patz A: Retrolental fibroplasia. *Surv Ophthalmo* 14:1–29, 1969

28. Quinn GE, Betts EK, Diamond GR, et al: Neonatal age (human) at retinal maturation. *Anesthesiology* 55:A326, 1981

29. Steward DJ: Preterm infants are more prone to complications following minor surgery than are term infants. *Anesthesiology* 56:304–306, 1982

30. Liu LMP, Coté CJ, Goudsouzian NG, et al: Life threatening apnea in infants recovering from anesthesia. *Anesthesiology* 59:506–510, 1983

31. Kelly DH, Shannon DC: Treatment of apnea and excessive periodic breathing in the full-term infant. *Pediatrics* 68:183–186, 1981

32. Kafer ER, Marsh HM: The effect of anesthetic drugs and disease on the chemical regulation of ventilation. *Int Anesthesiol Clin*, 15:1–38, 1977

33. Knill RL, Gelb AW: Ventilatory responses to hypoxia and hypercapnia during halothane sedation and anesthesia in man. *Anesthesiology* 49:244–251, 1978

34. Tusiewicz K, Bryan AC, Froese AB: Contributions of changing rib cage–diaphragm interactions to the ventilatory depression of halothane anesthesia. *Anesthesiology* 47:327–337, 1977

35. Motoyama EK, Brinkmeyer SD, Mutich RL et al: Reduced FRC in anesthetized infants: effect of low PEEP. *Anesthesiology* 57:A418, 1982

36. Moylan FMB, Shannon DC: Preferential distribution of lobar empyema and atelectasis in bronchopulmonary dysplasia. *Pediatrics* 63:130–134, 1979

37. Bryan HM, Hardie MJ, Reilly BJ, et al: Pulmonary function studies during the first year of life in infants recovering from respiratory distress syndrome. *Pediatrics* 52:169–178, 1973

38. Fitzhardinge PM, Pape K, Arstikaitis M, et al: Mechanical ventilation of infants of less than 1,501 gm birth weight: Health, growth, and neurologic sequelae. *J Pediatr* 88:531–541, 1976

39. Johnson JD, Malachowski NC, Grobstein R, et al: Prognosis of children surviving with the aid of mechanical ventilation in the newborn period. *J Pediatr* 84:272–276, 1974

40. Berman W, Yabek SM, Dillon T, et al: Evaluation of infants with bronchopulmonary dysplasia using cardiac catheterization. *Pediatrics* 70:708–712, 1982

41. Moylan FMB, O'Connell KC, Todres ID, et al: Edema of the pulmonary interstitium in infants and children. *Pediatrics* 55:783–787, 1975

42. Gold MI, Joseph SI: Bilateral tension pneumothorax following induction of anesthesia in two patients with chronic obstructive airway disease. *Anesthesiology* 38:93–97, 1973

43. Smyth JA, Tabachnik E, Duncan WJ, et al: Pulmonary function and bronchial hyperreactivity in long-term survivors of bronchopulmonary dysplasia. *Pediatrics* 68:336–340, 1981

44. Werthammer J, Brown ER, Neff RK, et al: Sudden infant death syndrome in infants with bronchopulmonary dysplasia. *Pediatrics* 69:301–304, 1982

45. Taitelman U, Reece EA, Bessman AN: Insulin in the management of the diabetic surgical patient—continuous infusion vs subcutaneous administration. *JAMA* 237:658–660, 1977

46. Martin MM, Martin ALA: Continuous infusion of insulin in the treatment of diabetic ketoacidosis in children. *J Pediatr* 89: 560–564, 1976

47. Edwards GA, Kohaut EC, Wehring B, et al: Effectiveness of low-dose continuous intravenous insulin infusion in diabetic ketoacidosis. *J Pediatr* 91:701–705, 1977

48. Perkin RM, Marks JF: Low-dose continuous insulin infusion in childhood ketoacidosis. *Clin Pediatr* 18:540–548, 1979

49. Weber ME, Abbassi V: Continuous intravenous insulin therapy in severe diabetic ketoacidosis: Variations in dosage requirements. *J Pediatr* 91:755–756, 1977

50. Blackburn GL, Maini BS, Pierce EC: Nutrition in the critically ill patient. *Anesthesiology* 47:181–194, 1977

51. Weinberger M: Theophylline for treatment of asthma. *J Pediatr* 92:1–7, 1978

52. Downes JJ, Wood DW, Striker TW, et al: Arterial blood gas and acid–base disorders in infants and children with status asthmaticus. *Pediatrics* 42:238–249, 1968

53. Steward DJ: Outpatient pediatric anesthesia. *Anesthesiology* 43: 268–276, 1975

54. Brzustowicz RM, Nelson DA, Betts EK, et al: Efficacy of oral premedication in children for out-patient surgery. *Anesthesiology* 55:A328, 1981

5

The Pediatric Airway

Charles J. Coté
I. David Todres

An understanding of the pathologic airway conditions of infants and children rests upon a knowledge of normal developmental anatomy, physiological function, and the special differences between the adult and pediatric airway.

FUNCTIONAL ANATOMY

The classic work of Negus, Bergman, Bayeux, and Galatti as quoted by Eckenhoff, Fink, and Demarest, forms the foundation of what we know about structure and function of the airway.[1-3] The larynx is composed of a series of cartilages (the hyoid, thyroid, cricoid, and arytenoid) which are suspended from the base of the skull by ligaments. The body of the cricoid cartilage articulates posteriorly with the inferior cornu of the thyroid cartilage by means of a synovial joint. The paired triangular arytenoid cartilages rest on top of and articulate with the superior posterior aspect of the cricoid cartilage, also by means of a synovia-filled joint. The arytenoid cartilages are protected by the thyroid cartilage (Figure 5-1).

These cartilages are covered by tissue folds and muscles. Contraction of the intrinsic laryngeal muscles alters the position and configuration of these tissue folds, thus influencing laryngeal function during respiration, forced voluntary glottic closure, and reflex laryngospasm, swallowing, and phonation (Figure 5-2A & B).

The laryngeal tissue folds are:

1. Paired aryepiglottic folds extending from the anterior epiglottis posteriorly to the superior surface of the arytenoids
2. Paired vestibular folds (false vocal cords) extending from the thyroid cartilage posteriorly to the superior surface of the arytenoids
3. Paired vocal folds (true vocal cords) extending from the posterior surface of the thyroid plate to the anterior projection or vocal process of the arytenoids
4. A single interarytenoid fold (composed of the interarytenoid muscle covered by tissue) bridging the arytenoid cartilages
5. A single thyrohyoid fold extending from hyoid bone to thyroid cartilage

INSPIRATION

With inspiration the larynx is pulled downward due to the negative intrathoracic pressure generated by the descent of the diaphragm and contraction of the intercostal muscles. With deep inspiration the larynx moves a distance of 1–2 vertebral bodies from its normal resting position. This leads to longitudinal stretching of the larynx (analogous to the opening of a jack-in-the-box), thus increasing the distance between aryepiglottic and vestibular folds as well as the distance between the vestibular and vocal folds. Contraction of the intrinsic muscles within the larynx results in lateral movement and posterior displacement of the arytenoids, causing an increase in the interarytenoid distance, and separation as well as stretching of the paired aryepiglottic, vestibular, and vocal folds. This results in an overall enlargement of the laryngeal opening, allowing free passage of air.

EXPIRATION

At the end of expiration, the larynx reverts to its resting position (analogous to the closing of a jack-in-the-box) with longitudinal shortening of the distance between the aryepiglottic, vestibular, and vocal folds. The arytenoids return simultaneously to their resting position by rotating medially and rocking forward, thus decreasing the interarytenoid dis-

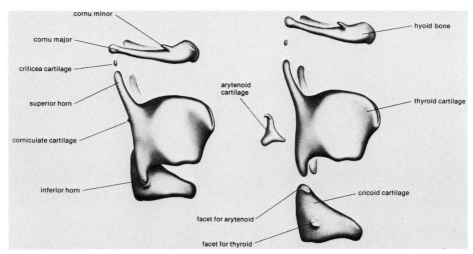

Figure 5-1. Laryngeal cartilages. The natural positions of the laryngeal cartilages are presented on the left, with the individual cartilages separated on the right. (From Fink BR, Demarest RJ: Laryngeal Biomechanics. Cambridge, MA, Harvard University Press, Copyright (C) 1978 by the President and Fellows of Harvard College.)

tance and reducing the tension on and causing thickening of the paired aryepiglottic, vestibular, and vocal folds.

FORCED GLOTTIC CLOSURE AND LARYNGOSPASM

Glottic closure during forced expiration (Valsalva maneuver) is voluntary laryngeal closure, and is similar in its effects to involuntary laryngeal closure (laryngospasm). Forced glottic closure occurs at several levels. Contraction of intrinsic laryngeal muscles results in (1) a marked reduction in the interarytenoid distance, (2) anterior rocking and medial movement of the arytenoids causing apposition of the paired vocal, vestibular, and aryepiglottic folds, (3) longitudinal shortening

of the larynx (further closing of the jack-in-the-box), obliterating the space between the aryepiglottic, vestibular, and vocal folds, (4) contraction of the thyrohyoid muscle pulling the hyoid bone downward and thyroid cartilage upward, leading to further closure.[1,3–8]

Closure of the larynx during laryngospasm is similar to that described above for voluntary forced glottic closure except for an inspiratory effort which separates longitudinally the vocal from the vestibular folds. In addition, minimal apposition of the aryepiglottic folds and median thyrohyoid fold occurs because contraction of the thyroarytenoid and thyrohyoid muscles does not occur. This may leave the upper part of the larynx partially open, thus accounting for the inspiratory stridor of partial laryngospasm.[1,4] Anterior and

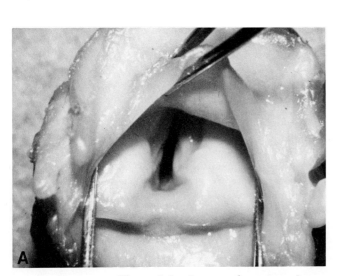

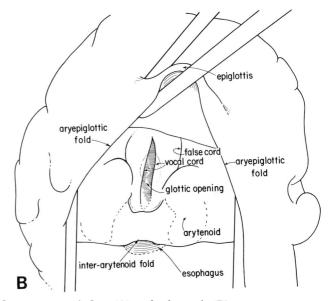

Figure 5-2. Laryngeal anatomy. Larynx of a premature infant (A) and schematic (B).

upward displacement of the mandible will also separate longitudinally the base of the tongue, the epiglottis, and the aryepiglottic folds from the vocal folds, thus helping to relieve laryngospasm.[5]

SWALLOWING

Glottic closure during swallowing is similar to that which occurs with forced glottic closure. Protection of the glottic opening results primarily from apposition of the laryngeal folds. In addition, an upward movement of the larynx occurs, causing close thyroid–hyoid approximation and secondary folding of the epiglottis over the glottis.[1,6,7] With loss of consciousness, local anesthesia, or sedation, the normal protective mechanism of the larynx may be lost or obtunded, thus predisposing to pulmonary aspiration of pharyngeal contents.

PHONATION

Phonation comprises a complex series of maneuvers resulting in fine alterations in vocal fold tension during movement of air, causing vibration of the vocal folds. This is accomplished by alteration of the angle between the thyroid and cricoid cartilages and medial movement of the arytenoids during expiration.[1,9,10] Phonation is the only maneuver which alters the cricothyroid angle.[1] Lesions or malfunction of the vocal folds (e.g., inflammation, papilloma, or paresis) thereby affect phonation. Despite significant airway obstruction during inspiration, however, it may be possible to phonate.

HISTOLOGY

The highly vascular mucosa of the mouth is continuous with that of the larynx and trachea. This mucosa is covered with squamous and pseudostratified ciliated epithelium, loosely adherent to the underlying structures in most areas, but tightly adherent to the vocal cords and laryngeal surface of the epiglottis. The vocal cords are covered with stratified epithelium.[11,12] This mucosa is also rich in lymphatic vessels and seromucous secreting glands which lubricate the laryngeal folds. The submucosa consists of loose, fibrous stroma, except on the tracheal surface of the epiglottis and the vocal cords. For this reason most inflammatory processes of the airway above the level of the vocal cords are limited by the barrier formed by the firm adherence of the mucosa to the vocal cords.[12] Thus, epiglottitis is usually limited to the supraglottic structures, and the loosely adherent mucosa explains the ease with which localized swelling occurs. In a similar manner, an inflammatory process of the subglottic region (laryngotracheobronchitis) results in significant subglottic edema in the loosely adherent mucosa of the airway below the vocal cords, but does not usually spread above the level of the vocal cords.[11]

SENSORY AND MOTOR INNERVATION OF INFANT LARYNX

The sensory innervation of the larynx is derived from the internal branch of the superior laryngeal nerve and the recurrent laryngeal nerve. The superior laryngeal nerve innervates the supraglottic region while the inferior laryngeal nerve innervates the infraglottic region. The motor innervation of the larynx is accomplished through the recurrent laryngeal nerves, which supply all the intrinsic muscles of the larynx except the cricothyroidei. The external branch of the superior layngeal nerve supplies the cricothyroidei. Thus, anesthetic agents injected to block the superior laryngeal nerve will result in anesthesia of the supraglottic region down to the inferior margin of the epiglottis, whereas motor blockade of the cricothyroidei will result in a relaxation of the vocal cords. Transtracheal injection of local anesthetic, or a specific recurrent laryngeal nerve block, is required for tracheal anesthesia.[10,11]

BLOOD SUPPLY

The blood supply to the larynx is provided by laryngeal branches of the superior and inferior thyroid arteries. The inferior laryngeal nerve and artery lie in close proximity to each other, thus accounting for vocal cord paresis during attempts to control bleeding during thyroidectomy.[13]

DEVELOPMENTAL ANATOMY

Five major differences pertain between the neonatal and adult airway.[2,3,8]

TONGUE

The infant tongue is relatively large in proportion to the rest of the oral cavity, thus more easily obstructing the airway, especially in the neonate. The tongue is more difficult to manipulate and stabilize with a laryngoscope blade.

POSITION OF LARYNX

The infant larynx is higher in the neck (C_{3-4}) compared to the adult (C_{4-5}) (Figure 5-3). Thus, the tongue is closer to the roof of the mouth and easily obstructs the airway. The more rostral location also creates difficulty in visualization of laryngeal structures; a straight laryngoscope blade better facilitates visualization of the larynx.

EPIGLOTTIS

The adult epiglottis is broad, and its axis is parallel to that of the trachea (Figure 5-4). The infant epiglottis is narrower, shorter, and angled away from the axis of the trachea (Figure 5-5) and therefore it is more difficult to lift the epiglottis with the tip of a laryngoscope blade.

VOCAL FOLDS

The infant vocal folds have a lower attachment anteriorly than posteriorly (angled), whereas in the adult, the axis of the vocal folds is perpendicular to that of the trachea. This anatomical feature occasionally leads to difficulty in intubation, i.e., the tip of the endotracheal tube is caught at the anterior commissure of the vocal folds.

SUBGLOTTIC AREA

The narrowest portion of the infant larynx is the nondistensible cricoid cartilage; in the adult, it is the rima glottidis. In the adult, therefore, an endotracheal tube which

GLOTTIC OPENING RELATIVE TO CERVICAL VERTEBRA (C)

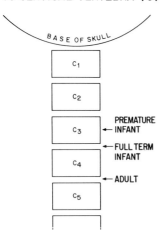

Figure 5-3. The premature infant larynx is located at the middle of the third cervical vertebra (C_3), the full-term infant larynx is at the C_{3-4} interspace, while the adult larynx is at the C_{4-5} interspace. (Adapted from Negus VE: The Comparative Anatomy and Physiology of the Larynx. New York, Grune & Stratton, 1949.)

traverses the glottis will pass freely into the trachea because the airway beyond is of larger diameter. In the child, however, an endotracheal tube might easily pass through the vocal folds but not through the subglottis (Figure 5-6). A tightly fitting endotracheal tube that compresses tracheal mucosa may cause edema in subglottic structures (cricoid cartilage), leading to a significant increase in airway resistance upon extubation. For example, if the diameter of the trachea at this point is 4.0 mm, and 1.0 mm of circumferential edema forms, 75 percent of the cross-sectional area would be lost (Figure 5-7).[2] This increases the resistance component of the work of breathing by a factor inversely proportional to the radius of the lumen to the fourth power. With turbulent flow, this resistance will be further increased.[14] As the child matures (by approximately 10–12 years of age) the cricoid and thyroid cartilages grow, thus eliminating both the angulation of the vocal cords and the narrow subglottic area.

PHYSIOLOGY

OBLIGATE NASAL BREATHING

The infant is an obligate nasal breather.[15,16] Thus, obstruction of the anterior or posterior nares (choanal atresia,

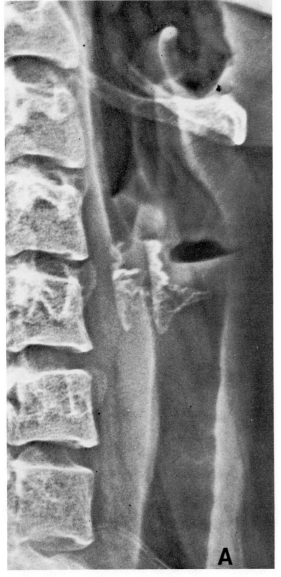

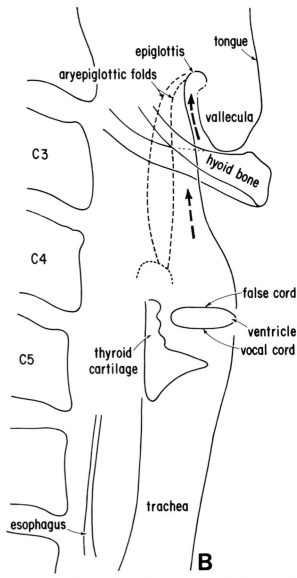

Figure 5-4. Lateral neck xerogram (A) and schematic (B) of the adult larynx. Note the relatively thin, broad epiglottis, the axis of which is parallel to the trachea. The hyoid bone "hugs" the epiglottis; there is no subglottic narrowing.

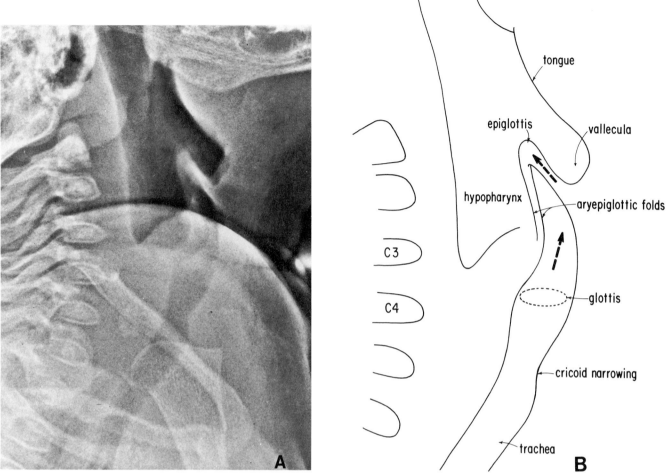

Figure 5-5. Lateral neck xerogram (A) and schematic (B) of the infant larynx. Note the short, angled epiglottis and the narrow cricoid cartilage.

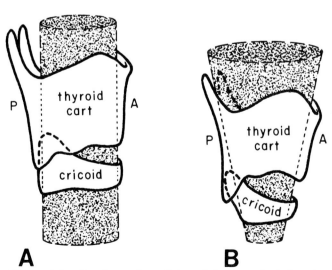

Figure 5-6. Configuration of the adult (A) v the infant larynx (B). Note cylinder shape of adult larynx; infant larynx is funnel shaped due to narrow undeveloped cricoid cartilage.

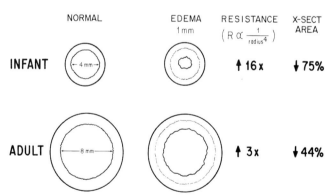

Figure 5-7. Relative effects of airway edema in the infant and adult. The normal infant and adult airways are presented on the left, edematous airways (1 mm circumferential) on the right. Note that resistance to flow is inversely proportional to radius of the lumen to the fourth power for laminar flow, and the radius of the lumen to the fifth power for turbulent flow. The net result in the infant is a 75 percent reduction in cross-sectional area, and 16-fold increase in resistance, as compared to a 44 percent reduction in cross-sectional area and a 3-fold increase in resistance in the adult.

39

stenosis, nasal congestion) may lead to asphyxia.[17–19] Immaturity of coordination between respiratory efforts and oropharyngeal motor/sensory input accounts in part for obligate nasal breathing.[20] Furthermore, with the larynx more rostral in the neck of the infant, the distances between the tongue, hyoid bone, epiglottis, and the roof of the mouth are shorter than in the older child or adult. During quiet respiration the tongue rests against the roof of the mouth, resulting in oral airway obstruction.[16,20] As the infant matures the ability to coordinate respiratory and oral function develops; the larynx enlarges, its position moves lower in the neck as the cervical spine lengthens, and the infant becomes able to breathe adequately through the mouth. This maturation takes 3–5 months to develop.[20]

TRACHEAL AND BRONCHIAL FUNCTION

Tracheal and bronchial diameters are a function of elasticity, and distending or compressive forces. The infant larynx, trachea, and bronchi are much more compliant than the adult, and therefore more subject to the effects of distending and compressive forces.[15,21,22] The intrathoracic trachea is subject to different stresses compared to the extrathoracic portion.[21] On expiration intrathoracic pressure remains slightly negative, thus maintaining patency of the intrathoracic trachea and bronchi (Figure 5-8A). On inspiration a greater negative intrathoracic pressure dilates and stretches the *intrathoracic* trachea.[23] The *extrathoracic* trachea is slightly narrowed (by dynamic compression) as a result of a differential in pressure between intratracheal pressures and atmospheric pressures; patency is ensured by the muscles and soft tissues of the neck (Figure 5-8B). Obstruction of the extrathoracic upper airway (e.g., epiglottitis, laryngotracheobronchitis, or a foreign body) alters normal airway dynamics. Inspiration against an obstruction results in the development of greater negative intrathoracic pressure, thus dilating the intrathoracic airways to a greater degree. More important clinically is the increased tendency toward dynamic collapse of the extrathoracic trachea below the level of the obstruction. This collapse is greatest at the thoracic inlet where the highest pressure gradient exists between negative intratracheal and normal atmospheric pressures, thus aggravating the inspiratory stridor (Figure 5-8C).[21,24–29] With intrathoracic tracheal obstruction (e.g., a foreign body or vascular ring), stridor may occur on both inspiration and expiration.[29–32] In lower airway obstruction (e.g., asthma or bronchiolitis) significant intrathoracic tracheal and bronchial collapse may occur owing to the prolonged expiratory phase and greatly increased positive extraluminal pressure (Figure 5-8D).[33] In addition, because the child's airways are highly compliant, they may be more susceptible to closure during smooth muscle contraction.

Dynamic airway collapse is particularly important when considering the highly compliant trachea and bronchi of an infant or child, and the extremes of transluminal pressures that occur when the child is crying. Thus, due to dynamic airway collapse, the degree of airway obstruction is aggravated during crying. For this reason it is very important to keep a child with airway obstruction content and quiet with the help of assurance, distraction, comfort, and his or her parents. *The use of sedatives and narcotics, prior to control of the airway, (endotracheal tube inserted) can result in significant morbidity or mortality, as the critical voluntary efforts to breathe are depressed.*

THE WORK OF BREATHING

The nasal passages account for 25 percent of the total resistance to air flow in the neonate, compared to 60 percent in the adult.[16,34] In the infant, the majority of resistance occurs in the bronchial and small airways, primarily as a function of small airway diameter and lack of supporting structures.[14,15,35,36] The chest wall of the neonate is highly compliant. Thus, the ribs provide little support for the lung by way of maintaining negative intrathoracic pressure. This leads to functional airway closure with every breath.[37–39] In the infant and child, therefore, small airway resistance accounts for the majority of the work of breathing, whereas in the adult the nasal passages provide the majority of flow resistance.[16,34,37,38,40–50] The work of breathing for each kilogram of body weight is the same in the infant or adult. However, the greater oxygen consumption for each kilogram of body weight in the infant accounts for the increased respiratory frequency. The oxygen consumption of the neonate (4–6 ml/kg/min) is twice that of the adult (2–3 ml/kg/min).[51] In premature infants the metabolic cost of breathing is three times that of the adult (6 percent v 2 percent of total oxygen consumption).[52] Any pathologic alteration of the airway which increases the work of breathing may result in respiratory failure. As discussed earlier, the resistance component of respiratory work is increased by the power of four, and is inversely proportional to the radius of the lumen involved. Because infants have smaller airways than adults, any pathologic airway narrowing will have greater adverse effects on their work of breathing, compared to similar pathology in adults. An increase in the work of breathing may also result from employment of a long endotracheal tube of small diameter, a partially obstructed endotracheal tube, or a narrowed airway. These situations all result in increased oxygen consumption, which in turn increase oxygen demand.[53] The increased oxygen demand is initially met by an increase in respiratory rate, but the increased work of breathing may result in exhaustion and lead to respiratory failure (CO_2 retention and hypoxemia).

Another important consideration is the difference in muscle histology of the diaphragm and intercostal muscles of premature and term infants compared to older children. Type I muscle fibers permit prolonged repetitive movement (e.g. the long distance runner through repeated exercise increases type I muscle fibers in the legs). Fewer type I muscle fibers are present in the diaphragm and intercostal muscles of the premature than the term baby, and the term infant has fewer than the two year old child (Figure 5-9). Thus, any condition which increases the work of breathing may easily fatigue the respiratory muscles and result in respiratory failure.[54]

CLINICAL, RADIOLOGIC, AND LABORATORY EVALUATION OF THE AIRWAY

A history and physical examination with specific reference to the airway should be performed in all pediatric patients scheduled for surgery. In special situations, radiologic and biochemical studies are also required to evaluate a disorder revealed by the history and physical examination.

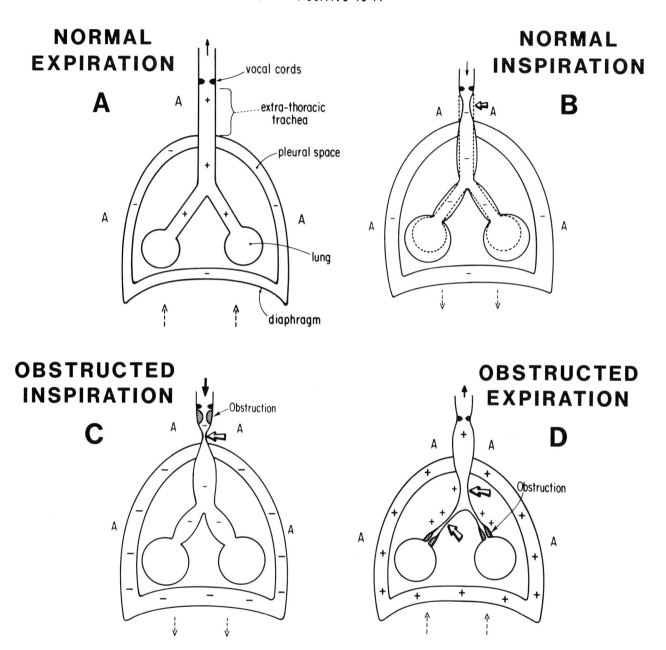

A = Atmospheric pressure

— = Negative to A

+ = Positive to A

NORMAL EXPIRATION

A

vocal cords
extra-thoracic trachea
pleural space
lung
diaphragm

NORMAL INSPIRATION

B

OBSTRUCTED INSPIRATION

C

Obstruction

OBSTRUCTED EXPIRATION

D

Obstruction

Figure 5-8. (A, normal expiration) The normal sequence of events at end-expiration is a slight negative intrapleural pressure stenting the airways open. In infants the highly compliant chest does not provide the support required; thus, airway closure occurs with each breath. Intraluminal pressures are slightly positive in relation to atmospheric pressure, resulting in air being forced out of the lungs. With descent of the diaphragm and contraction of the intercostal muscles a greater negative intrathoracic pressure relative to intraluminal and atmospheric pressure is developed (B, normal inspiration). The net result is a stretching longitudinally of the larynx and trachea, dilatation of the intrathoracic trachea and bronchi, movement of air into the lungs, and some dynamic collapse of the extrathoracic trachea (open arrow). The dynamic collapse is due to the highly compliant trachea and the negative intraluminal pressure in relation to atmospheric pressure (C, obstructed inspiration). Note the severe dynamic collapse of the extrathoracic trachea below the level of obstruction. This collapse is greatest at the thoracic inlet where the largest pressure gradient exists between negative intratracheal pressure and atmospheric pressure (open arrow).[21] (D, obstructed expiration.) Breathing against an obstructed lower airway (bronchiolitis, asthma) results in greater positive intrathoracic pressures, with dynamic collapse of the intrathoracic airways [prolonged expiration or wheezing (open arrows)].

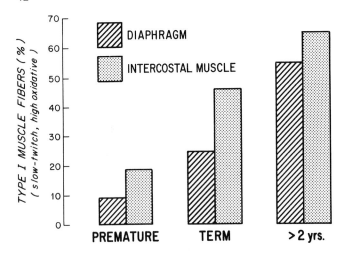

Figure 5-9. Muscle fiber composition of diaphragm and intercostal muscles related to age. Note that the premature infant's diaphragm and intercostal muscles have fewer type I fibers compared to term newborns and older children. The data suggest a possible mechanism for early fatigue in premature and term babies when the work of breathing is increased. (Data abstracted from Keens TG, et al: Developmental pattern of muscle fibers in human ventilatory muscles J Appl Physiol 44:909–913, 1978.)

CLINICAL EVALUATION

The medical history should investigate the following:

- Presence of an upper respiratory infection (indicates a predisposition to coughing and bronchospasm during anesthesia, or potential post-intubation subglottic edema)
- Snoring or noisy breathing (possible adenoidal hypertrophy)
- Nature of cough (croupy cough, brassy, productive), and whether it is acute or chronic (possible foreign body aspiration)
- Past episodes of croup (potential post-intubation croup)
- Inspiratory stridor, usually of high pitch, with or without effort (possible subglottic narrowing)
- Hoarse voice (possible vocal cord palsy, papilloma, granuloma, laryngitis)
- Asthma or bronchodilator therapy (potential bronchospasm)
- Repeated pneumonias (possible incompetent larynx, bronchiectasis, cystic fibrosis)
- History of foreign body aspiration
- Previous anesthetic problems, particularly related to the airway (potential difficult intubation)
- Atopy, allergy

The physical examination should include the following observations:

- Facial expression
- Mouth breathing
- Color of mucous membranes
- Nasal flaring
- Retractions (suprasternal, intercostal, subcostal)
- Respiratory rate

- Voice change
- How far the child can open the mouth (Figure 5-10A)
- Size of the mouth
- Size of the tongue
- Loose or missing teeth (Figure 5-10B)
- Size and configuration of palate
- Size and configuration of mandible
- Location of larynx (Figure 5-10C)
- Is stridor predominantly inspiratory suggesting an upper airway (extrathoracic) lesion?
- Is stridor both inspiratory and expiratory suggesting an intrathoracic lesion (vascular ring, foreign body)?
- Is the expiratory phase prolonged, or stridor predominantly expiratory, suggesting lower airway disease?
- Are there obvious congenital anomalies which may fit a recognizable syndrome? *The finding of one anomaly mandates a search for other anomalies.* If a congenital syndrome is diagnosed, all anesthetic implications must be considered (see Appendix 5-1).

RADIOLOGIC AND LABORATORY EVALUATION

Routine evaluation of the airway requires only a careful history and physical examination. With airway pathology, however, laboratory and radiologic evaluation may be invaluable. X-rays of the upper airway (anterior, posterior, and lateral films and fluoroscopy) may provide evidence as to the site and cause of airway obstruction. Tomograms and xerograms may provide more detailed information.[55–62] *Radiologic airway examination in a child with a compromised airway must be undertaken only when there is no immediate threat to the child's safety, and only in the presence of skilled and appropriately equipped personnel able to manage the airway.* Securing the airway through endotracheal intubation must not be postponed in order to obtain a radiologic diagnosis when it is obvious that the patient has severely compromised air exchange. Occasionally blood gas analysis is of special value in assessing the degree of physiologic compromise, especially with chronic airway obstruction and compensated respiratory acidosis. Obtaining an arterial puncture for blood gas analysis, however, while providing useful information, is often upsetting to the child and may possibly aggravate the underlying airway obstruction through dynamic airway collapse. Candidates for blood gas analysis, therefore, must be carefully selected, and the procedure skillfully and gently performed. Starting an IV must likewise be performed carefully and skillfully, preferably with local anesthetic supplementation so as to avoid patient anxiety. In most circumstances it is preferable to start the IV in the operating room after the patient is anesthetized.

TRACHEAL INTUBATION

NORMAL AIRWAY

Major differences exist in the techniques for intubating the trachea of the infant and child as compared to the adult.[2,3,63,64] The adult's and older child's trachea is most easily intubated when a folded blanket or pillow is placed beneath

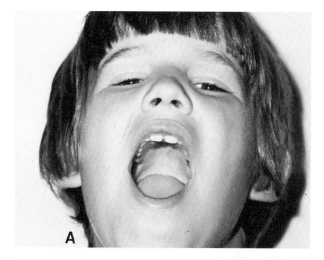

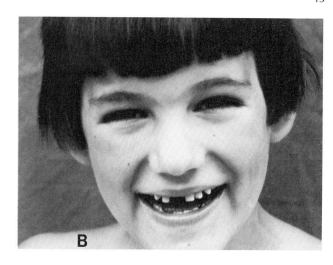

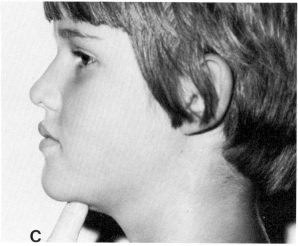

Figure 5-10. (A) How far can the child open his mouth? Are there any abnormalities of the mouth, tongue, palate, mandible? (B) Are there any loose or missing teeth? (C) Is the mandible of normal configuration? How much space is there between the genu of the mandible and the thyroid cartilage? This space is an indication of the extent of anterior displacement of the larynx; normally there should be at least one finger's breadth in the newborn, and three in the adolescent.

the occiput of the head, resulting in the "sniffing" position, i.e., anterior displacement of the cervical spine with extension of the head at the atlanto-occipital joint.[13,65] This results in alignment of the axes of the structures of the mouth, oropharynx, and trachea, and permits more direct visualization of laryngeal structures. Figures 5-11A–F demonstrate maneuvers for positioning of the head during airway management. In infants and children younger than three years of age the head is large in proportion to the trunk, and as a result it is usually unnecessary to elevate the occiput; head extension at the atlanto-occipital joint alone will align the airway axes. When head elevation is unnecessarily performed it may actually hinder exposure of the glottis. In newborns it is sometimes helpful to have an assistant hold the shoulders flat on the operating room table with the head slightly extended. Excessive extension of the neonatal head may stretch the immature trachea, resulting in tracheal compression and airway obstruction.

AIRWAY SELECTION

The infant tongue is relatively large in proportion to the oropharynx and often obstructs the airway during induction

of anesthesia or loss of consciousness from any cause. It is important therefore to select an oropharyngeal airway of proper size to achieve unobstructed air exchange. An oral airway is often used to protect an oral endotracheal tube from compression between the teeth, and will also facilitate oropharyngeal suctioning. By holding the airway as shown in Figures 5-12A & B, one can choose the appropriate size; an airway one size larger and smaller should also be readily available. Airway insertion is facilitated with a tongue depressor, which prevents folding of the tongue upon itself or thrusting the tongue into the pharynx and thus causing complications of impaired venous and lymphatic drainage, macroglossia, and airway obstruction. If the airway extends too deeply the tip may push the epiglottis down, causing traumatic epiglottitis, or the tip may impinge upon the uvula, causing uvular swelling and airway obstruction (Figures 5-12C & D).[66–69] If the airway is too short it will come to rest against the base of the tongue, forcing it posteriorly, and thus further contributing to airway obstruction (Figures 5-12E & F). Care must also be taken to avoid catching the lips and tongue between the teeth and airways.

Nasopharyngeal airways are occasionally of value in pediatric patients; the proper size may be measured against the side of the face and neck. Usually a shortened endotracheal tube will serve this purpose, since rubber airways are not made

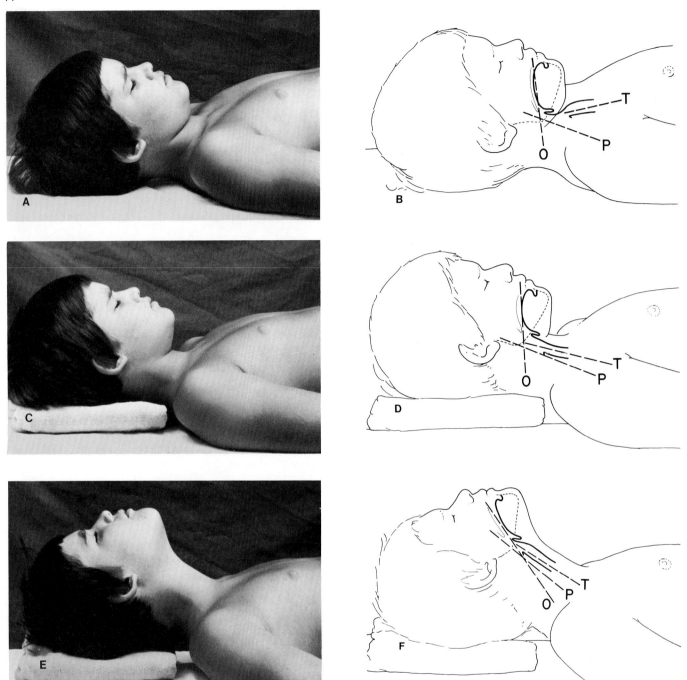

Figure 5-11.   Positioning for ventilation and tracheal intubation. With the patient flat on the bed or operating table (A) the oral (O), pharyngeal (P) and tracheal (T) axes pass through three divergent planes (B). A folded sheet or towel placed under the occiput of the head (C) will align the pharyngeal (P) and tracheal (T) axes (D). A folded sheet or towel under the occiput of the head plus extension of the atlanto-occipital joint (E) results in alignment of the oral (O), pharyngeal (P), and tracheal (T) axes (F).

for pediatric use. Under most circumstances, however, nasopharyngeal airways are avoided to prevent traumatic bleeding of hypertrophied adenoids.

ENDOTRACHEAL TUBE SELECTION

The selection of a proper size endotracheal tube depends on the individual patient for whom it is intended.[70] The only

requirement for manufacturers is that they standardize the internal diameter (ID) of an endotracheal tube. The external diameter may vary according to the material from which the tube is constructed, and its manufacturer. This mandates familiarity with various types and makes of tubes. An appropriate size uncuffed endotracheal tube may be approximated according to age (Table 5-1).[71] In general, it is desirable to select an uncuffed tube which would result in an air leak around the

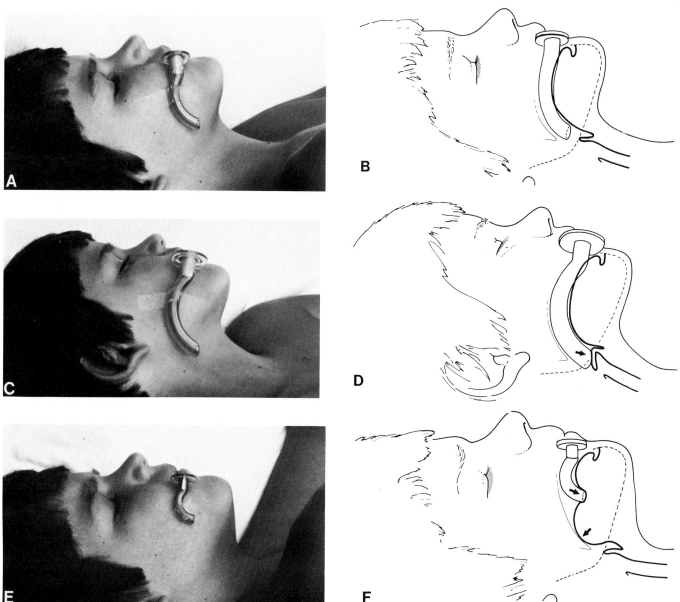

Figure 5-12. Proper airway selection. The proper size of the airway should relieve airway obstruction secondary to the tongue without damaging laryngeal structures. The appropriate size can be estimated by holding the airway next to the child's face; the tip of the airway should end just cephalad to the angle of the mandible (A). This should result in proper alignment with the glottic opening (B). If too large an oral airway is inserted, the tip will line up posterior to the angle of the mandible (C) and obstruct the glottic opening by pushing the epiglottis down (D, arrow). If too small an oral airway is inserted, the tip will line up well above the angle of the mandible (E); this will exacerbate airway obstruction by kinking the tongue (F, arrows).

tube at 20–30 cm H_2O peak inflation pressure (PIP) in children under 10 years of age. An uncuffed tube is also of value because an endotracheal tube of larger ID can be passed beyond the nondistensible cricoid cartilage resulting in less airway resistance.[14,72,73] In addition, with an uncuffed tube and an air leak, minimal pressure is apposed to the internal surface of the cricoid cartilage, with less risk for post-intubation edema formation. If a cuffed endotracheal tube is passed, a smaller internal diameter tube must be selected to compensate for the room taken up at the cricoid barrier by the endotracheal tube cuff. In addition, inflation of the cuff will apply pressure and possibly cause pathologic edema at this narrow portion of the trachea.

In general, we select the size of endotracheal tube according to Table 5-1, and have available tubes of a half ID size above and below the chosen size. After intubation and stabilization of the child, if there is no leak below 30 cm H_2O PIP, we change the tube to the next half size smaller.

SELECTION OF LARYNGOSCOPE BLADE

A straight blade is generally more suitable in infants and young children than the curved blade because the larynx is located higher in the neck, thus making it easier to lift the base of the tongue or fix the epiglottis. The blade is usually advanced beyond the epiglottis into the esophagus, with laryn-

Table 5-1

Internal Diameter of Endotracheal
Tubes (mm I.D.) Used in Infants and
Children

Age	Size (I.D.)
Premature	
1000 gm	2.5
1000–2500 gm	3.0
Neonate to 6 mo	3.0–3.5
6 months to 1 yr	3.5–4.0
1–2 yr	4.0–5.0
Beyond 2 yr	$\dfrac{\text{age (yrs)} + 16}{4}$

Table 5-2

The Size of Laryngoscope Blades Used in Infants and
Children

Age	Blade Size		
	Miller	Wis-Hippel	Macintosh
Premature	0	—	—
Neonate	0	—	—
Neonate–2 yr	1	—	—
2–6 yr	—	1.5	—
6–12 yr	2	—	2
Over 12 yr	3	—	3

geal visualization achieved during withdrawal of the blade. This can result in laryngeal trauma when the tip of the blade scrapes the arytenoids and aryepiglottic folds. A less traumatic technique is to place the tip of the blade directly in the vallecula in a motion similar to that for the curved blade in adults. One can thus lift the base of the tongue, which in turn lifts the epiglottis, exposing the glottic opening. This maneuver avoids unnecessary laryngeal trauma caused by the withdrawal of the blade from the esophagus. If this technique is unsuccessful then one may lift the epiglottis with the tip of the blade. Care must always be taken to avoid using the laryngoscope as a fulcrum with pressure on the teeth or

alveolar ridge. Curved blades prove satisfactory for use in older children and adolescents. The size blade chosen depends on the body mass of the patient and preference of the anesthesiologist. Table 5-2 presents the ranges commonly used.

INSERTION DISTANCE

The length of the trachea (vocal cords to carina) in neonates and children up to one year of age varies from 5–9 cm.[23] In most infants three months to one year of age, if the 10-cm mark of the endotracheal tube is placed at the alveolar ridge, the tip of the tube will rest above the carina. In the premature or term infant the distance is less. In children two

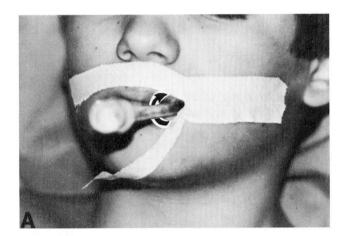

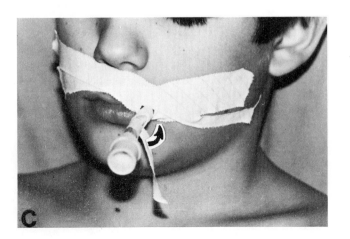

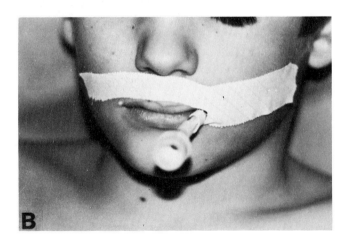

Figure 5-13. Securing the endotracheal tube. After insertion of the oral endotracheal tube and examination for proper position, the area between the nose and upper lip and both cheeks is coated with tincture of benzoin. After the benzoin is dry, tape that has been slit up the middle is applied to the cheek, and the endotracheal tube is placed at the division of the torn tape (A). One half is wrapped circumferentially around the tube and the other half applied to the space above the upper lip (B). A second piece of tape is applied in similar fashion from the opposite direction (C). A nasal endotracheal tube may also be secured with this technique.

years old, 12 cm is usually appropriate. After this the correct length of insertion (cm) for oral intubation can be approximated by the formula:[74–76]

$$\frac{age\ (yrs)}{2} + 12$$

An alternate formula is

$$\frac{weight\ (kg)}{5} + 12$$

After the endotracheal tube is inserted and the first strip of adhesive tape applied to secure it, one must observe for symmetry of chest expansion and listen for equality of breath sounds high in the midaxillae and apices. It is also important to listen over the stomach and to observe for cyanosis. Once satisfactory position is achieved a second strip of tape will assure secure fixation (Figure 5-13).

TECHNIQUE

Laryngoscopy may be performed with the patient awake, anesthetized and breathing, or with neuromuscular blockade (by means of thiopental and succinylcholine). Most intubations in children who are awake are performed in neonates, an approach not feasible or humane in older awake and uncooperative children. On occasion a blind nasal intubation may be accomplished in the older child, but this requires good topical anesthesia as well as adequate sedation. The use of a neuromuscular blockade and intravenous barbiturate anesthesia is most commonly utilized, usually providing optimal conditions. However, *if airway obstruction or the potential for airway obstruction exists, neuromuscular blockade should not be used.* Complete relaxation often accentuates obstruction by causing relaxation of cervical tissues. Spontaneously assisted ventilation during general anesthesia is the preferred technique when abnormal airway anatomy is present; this allows adequate exchange of oxygen while the airway is examined for appropriate approach to intubation.

THE ABNORMAL AIRWAY

For any laryngoscopy, but especially for a difficult airway, the proper array of equipment must always be available (Table 5-3). The approach to the difficult airway, as described earlier, must include careful physical examination and when feasible radiologic evaluation.[55–62] Lateral neck xerograms are particularly helpful in delineating anatomical aberrations.[59–62] Past medical, surgical, and anesthetic histories, chest x-ray, and blood gas analysis must also be sought when necessary. In addition to the airway pathology, knowledge of the pathophysiology of the congenital syndrome or disease process must be fully understood (see Appendix 5-1, Tables 5-4 and 5-5).

It is important to recognize those circumstances that may cause the obstruction of the airway of an infant or child. Conditions which predispose to airway problems may be grouped according to anatomic location, and may result from congenital malformation, or inflammatory, traumatic, metabolic, or neoplastic disorders. Tables 5-4 and 5-5 list the more common pediatric airway problems according to anatomic location. Appendix 5-1 lists the more common pediatric syndromes and associated anesthetic considerations; more complete information may be obtained from standard pediatric textbooks.[77–80]

The safest approach to managing the difficult airway is to formulate a plan and have skilled help available, especially a surgeon experienced in performance of pediatric bronchoscopy and tracheostomy. Spontaneous ventilation should always be maintained.[185–188] There are two reasons for maintaining spontaneous gas exchange. First, should neuromuscular blockade be administered to facilitate intubation, total airway obstruction can result because the muscle tone of tongue, cervical and laryngeal muscles, and suspensory ligaments is lost; this obstruction may not be alleviated via manual ventilation of the lungs. Second, if the patient is paralyzed, a valuable guide to locating the glottis (spontaneous breath sounds) is lost. It is not unusual with syndromes such as Goldenhar's, Pierre Robin, Treacher-Collins, or cervical burn contracture, to be able to visualize only the tip of the epiglottis. By shaping the endotracheal tube with a stylette, placing the tip behind the epiglottis, and then listening for breath sounds with the ear at the proximal end of the tracheal tube, one is often able to "blindly" locate the glottis and trachea.

SPECIAL TECHNIQUES FOR THE DIFFICULT AIRWAY

Many techniques for managing the difficult airway have been suggested (Table 5-6). Fiberoptic laryngoscopes, bronchoscopes, and modified endotracheal tubes have also been employed.[183–193] Transtracheal passage of an intravenous catheter through the cricothyroid membrane into the larynx, or retrograde passage of a guide wire from a Seldinger vascular cannulation set have also been recommended.[194–199] Adding 5 percent CO_2, or the use of doxapram hydrochloride to induce hyperpnea (augmenting breath sounds), have been utilized, but with modest success.[200–202] Each technique offers

Table 5-3

Minimal Equipment For Difficult Airway Management

Oxygen source
Mask and bag (proper size)
Oral airways (proper size)
Suction catheters (proper size)
At least two functioning suction systems
Endotracheal tubes of various sizes
Proper size stylette
Extra laryngoscope blades and handles, Oxyscope*
Premedication
    cimetidine
    glycopyrrolate
Drugs
    atropine
    thiopental
    ketamine
    succinylcholine
    curare
    pancuronium
    atracurium
    vecuronium

* Foregger, Langhorn PA

Table 5-4

Pediatric Airway Pathology Related to Anatomic Location

Anatomical Site	Etiology	Clinical Condition
Nasopharynx	Congenital	Choanal atresia, stenosis,[17,18] encephalocoele[81]
	Traumatic	Foreign body, trauma
	Inflammatory	Adenoidal hypertrophy,[82] nasal congestion[19]
	Neoplastic	Teratoma
Tongue	Congenital	Hemangioma, Down's syndrome[83–86]
	Traumatic	Burn, laceration, lymphatic/venous obstruction[66–69]
	Metabolic	Beckwith-Wiedemann Syndrome,[87–88] hypothyroidism, mucopolysaccharidosis,[89–90] glycogen storage disease,[91] gangliosidosis[92]
	Neoplastic	Cystic hygroma,[93–94] cystic teratoma
Mandible/Maxilla	Congenital hypoplasia	Pierre Robin syndrome,[95–103] Treacher-Collins syndrome,[104–108] Goldenhar's syndrome,[109] Apert's syndrome,[110] achondroplasia,[111–112] Turner's syndrome,[113–114] Cornelia DeLange syndrome[115–116] Smith-Lemli-Opitz syndrome[117] Hallermann-Streiff syndrome[118]
	Traumatic	Fracture,[119] neck burn with contractures
	Inflammatory	Juvenile rheumatoid arthritis[120–124]
	Neoplastic	Tumors, cherubism[125]
Pharynx/Larynx	Congenital	Laryngeal web, laryngeal stenosis,[126] laryngocoele,[127] laryngomalacia (infantile larynx)[127]
	Traumatic	Dislocated/fractured larynx,[128–132] foreign body,[29,30,133–136] inhalation injury (burn),[137–142] post intubation edema/ granuloma/stenosis,[143–154] swelling of uvula,[66–68] soft palate trauma
	Inflammatory	Epiglottitis,[25–27,155–167] acute tonsillitis,[82] peritonsillar abscess,[168,169] retropharyngeal abscess, diphtheritic membrane, laryngeal polyposis[170–172]
	Metabolic	Hypocalcemic laryngospasm[22]
	Neoplastic	Tumors
	Neurologic	Vocal cord paralysis, Arnold-Chiari malformation[173–175]

Table 5-4 (continued)

Anatomical Site	Etiology	Clinical Condition
Trachea	Congenital	Vascular ring,[31,32] tracheal stenosis,[176] tracheomalacia[127,128,159]
	Inflammatory	Laryngotracheobronchitis[27,28,177–181]
	Neoplastic	Mediastinal tumors–neurofibroma,[182] paratracheal nodes (lymphoma)

Table 5-5

Cervical Spine Anomalies

Etiology	Clinical Condition
Congenital	Klippel-Feil malformation,[183] Goldenhar's syndrome,[109] torticollis
Traumatic	Fracture, subluxation,[128–132,184] neck burn contracture
Inflammatory	Rheumatoid arthritis[120–124]
Metabolic	Mucopolysaccharidosis (Morquio's)[89,90]

Abnormalities of the cervical spine may limit extension and flexion thus contributing to the difficulties of airway management.

Table 5-6

Adjuncts and Equipment for the very Difficult Airway

Fiberoptic bronchoscope/laryngoscope—pediatric size
Surgeon skilled at pediatric tracheostomy
Tracheostomy tubes (proper size and connectors)
Equipment for Seldinger technique
Equipment for percutaneous cricothyroidotomy
5 % carbon dioxide
Doxapram hydrochloride

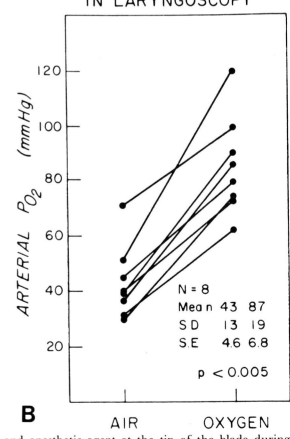

Figure 5-14. Modified laryngoscope. The Oxyscope delivers oxygen and anesthetic agent at the tip of the blade during laryngoscopy (A). Increased PaO_2 levels were achieved during laryngoscopy of infants (B). (Reproduced with permission, Todres ID et al: Crit Care Med 9:544–545, 1981.)

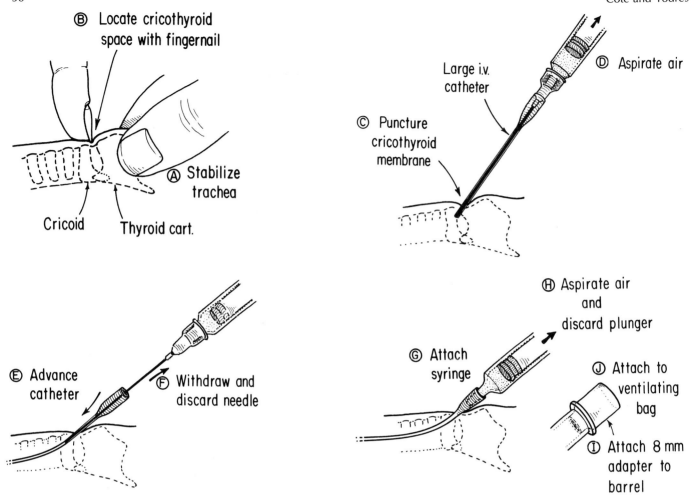

Figure 5-15. Percutaneous cricothyroidotomy. Extend the head in the midline with a rolled towel or folded sheet transversely beneath the shoulders. Stabilize trachea (A). The cricothyroid membrane is located with the fingertip between the thyroid and cricoid cartilages (B). This space is so narrow (1 mm) that only a fingernail can palpate it in an infant. A large intravenous catheter (12–14 gauge) is inserted through the cricothyroid membrane (C) and air aspirated (D). The catheter is advanced into the trachea through the membrane (E) and the needle discarded (F); intraluminal position is reconfirmed by attaching a 3 ml syringe (G) and aspirating for air (H). The 3 ml syringe barrel *without plunger* is attached to the catheter (I). An 8 mm endotracheal tube adaptor is attached to the syringe barrel (J). (Reprinted from Stinson TW III: A simple connector for transtracheal ventilation. *Anesthesiology* 47:232, 1977. With permission.) Connections are made to standard anesthetic equipment (15 mm connections). As an alternative, a 3 mm airway adapter will fit any IV catheter.

merits and drawbacks. Doxapram or CO_2 may induce cardiac arrhythmias, and for this reason are infrequently employed. Fiberoptic laryngoscopes, bronchoscopes, and modified endotracheal tubes are rarely used by most anesthesiologists, and therefore should not be the first choice during a difficult airway situation unless the operator is thoroughly familiar with their use. Previous experience with such equipment on normal airways can render these devices valuable adjuncts in difficult airway management. The size of these bronchoscopes and laryngoscopes may limit usefulness to endotracheal tube sizes 3.5 mm ID or greater. Retrograde transtracheal passage of a catheter has been reported as very useful, but the large needle required may cause damage to the infant larynx. Use of the Seldinger technique may minimize tracheal damage by utilizing a smaller, thin-walled needle. Employment of an Oxyscope* will provide an increased FIO_2 and is particularly useful for intubation in the conscious neonate whose oxygen

consumption is high, and in whom cyanosis can rapidly develop (Figures 5-14A & B).[203]

Finally, if one is unable to intubate the airway it is important to recognize the limits of one's ability. In this circumstance one should not hesitate to seek assistance from a colleague, or ask the surgeon to perform a tracheostomy or bronchoscopy. As an alternative the child could be referred to a major pediatric center. In an urgent situation, percutaneous cricothyroidotomy may be lifesaving.

PERCUTANEOUS CRICOTHYROIDOTOMY

The cricothyroid membrane is of small width in infants and children. Thus, cricothyroidotomy may readily damage cricoid and thyroid cartilages, resulting in subsequent laryngeal stenosis and permanent damage to the speech mechanism. This procedure should be reserved for use only under emergency circumstances.[204–206] A schema of this procedure is presented in Figure 5-15A–J.

_____
* Foregger Co, Inc., Smithtown, NY 11787

This technique will provide only a means for oxygen insufflation, but will not provide adequate ventilation in older children; the lumen *may* be large enough to permit ventilation of an infant's lungs. With inadequate alveolar ventilation, but temporary oxygenation, hypercarbia is generally well-tolerated by healthy children until more effective ventilation is established.[206]

ACKNOWLEDGMENT

The authors wish to express special thanks to Dr. Leroy D. Vandam for his thoughtful help and advice.

REFERENCES

1. Fink RB, Demarest RJ: *Laryngeal Biomechanics.* Cambridge, MA, Harvard University Press, 1978

2. Eckenhoff JE: Some anatomic considerations of the infant larynx influencing endotracheal anesthesia. *Anesthesiology* 12:401–410, 1951

3. Negus VE: *The Comparative Anatomy and Physiology of the Larynx.* New York, Grune & Stratton, 1949

4. Fink BR: The mechanism of closure of the human larynx. *Trans Amer Acad Otolaryng Ophthal* 60:117–129, 1956

5. Fink BR: The etiology and treatment of laryngeal spasm. *Anesthesiology* 17:569–577, 1956

6. Ardran GM, Kemp FH, Manen L: Closure of the larynx. *Br J Radiol* 26:497–509, 1953

7. Ardran GM, Kemp FH: The mechanism of the larynx. II. The epiglottis and closure of the larynx. *Br J Radiol* 40:372–389, 1967

8. Wilson TG: Some observations on the anatomy of the infantile larynx. *Acta Otolaryngol* 43:95–99, 1953

9. Cavagna GA, Margaria R: An analysis of the mechanics of phonation. *J Appl Physiol* 20:301–307, 1965

10. Pressman JJ, Kelemen G: Physiology of the larynx. *Physiol Rev* 35:506–554, 1955

11. Jones HM: Acute epiglottitis: A personal study over twenty years. *Proc R Soc Med* 63:14–22, 1970

12. Ballenger JJ: Anatomy of the Larynx, in Diseases of the Nose, Throat, and Ear. John J. Ballenger, Ed. Lea & Febiger, Philadelphia, 1977. Edition 12, pp. 330–336

13. Vandam LD: Functional anatomy of the larynx. *Week Anesthesiol Update* 1:2–6, 1977

14. Macintosh R, Mushin WW, Epstein HG: *Physics for the Anaesthetist,* 2nd ed. Oxford, Blackwell Scientific Publications, pp. 156–191, 1958

15. Polgar G: Airway resistance in the newborn infant. *J Pediatr* 59:915–921, 1961

16. Polgar G, Kong GP: Nasal resistance of newborn infants. *J Pediatr* 67:557–567, 1965

17. Hobolth N, Buchmann G, Sandberg LE: Congenital choanal atresia. *Acta Paediatr Scand* 56:286–294, 1967

18. Maniglia AJ, Goodwin WJ Jr: Congenital choanal atresia. *Otolaryngol Clin North Am* 14:167–173, 1981

19. Passy V, Newcron S, Snyder S: Rhinorrhea with airway obstruction. *Laryngoscope* 85:888–895, 1975

20. Bosma JF: Introduction to the symposium, in: Bosma JF, Showacre J (eds): *Symposium on Development of Upper Respiratory Anatomy and Function: Implications of Sudden Infant Death Syndrome.* Washington DC, U.S. Government Printing Office, 1974, pp 5–49

21. Wittenborg MH, Gyepes MT, Crocker D: Tracheal dynamics in infants with respiratory distress, stridor, and collapsing trachea. *Radiology* 88:653–662, 1967

22. Wilson TG: Stridor in infancy. *J Laryngol Otol* 66:437–451, 1952

23. Fearon B, Whalen JS: Tracheal dimensions in the living infant. *Ann Otol* 76:965–974, 1967

24. Maze A, Bloch E: Stridor in pediatric patients. *Anesthesiology* 50:132–145, 1979

25. Lazoritz S, Saunders BS, Bason WM: Management of acute epiglottitis. *Crit Care Med* 7:285–290, 1979

26. Schloss MD, Hannallah R, Baxter JD: Acute epiglottitis: 26 years' experience at the Montreal Children's Hospital. *J Otolaryngol* 8:259–265, 1979

27. Davis HW, Gartner JC, Galvis AG, et al: Acute upper airway obstruction: Croup and epiglottitis. *Pediatr Clin North Am* 28:859–880, 1981

28. Baker SR: Laryngotracheobronchitis—a continuing challenge in child health care. *J Otolaryngol* 8:494–500, 1979

29. Cohen SR, Herbert WI, Lewis GB Jr, et al: Foreign bodies in the airway: Five year retrospective study with special reference to management. *Ann Otol Rhino Laryngol* 89:437–442, 1980

30. Stark DC, Biller HF: Aspiration of foreign bodies: Diagnosis and management. *Int Anesthesiol Clin* 15:117–145, 1977

31. Mustard WJ, Bayliss CE, Fearon B, et al: Tracheal compression by the innominate artery in children. *Ann Thorac Surg* 8:312–319, 1969

32. Fearon B, Shortreed R: Tracheobronchial compression by congenital cardiovascular anomalies in children: Syndrome of apnea. *Ann Otol Rhino Laryngol* 72:949–969, 1963

33. Wohl MEB, Stigol LC, Mead J: Resistance of the total respiratory system in healthy infants and infants with bronchiolitis. *Pediatrics* 43:495–509, 1969

34. Butler J: The work of breathing through the nose. *Clin Sci* 19:55–62, 1960

35. Briscoe WA, DuBois AB: The relationship between airway resistance, airway conductance, and lung volume in subjects of different age and body size. *J Clin Invest* 37:1279–1285, 1958

36. Cook CD, Sutherland JM, Segal S, et al: Studies of respiratory physiology in the newborn infant. III. Measurements of mechanics of respiration. *J Clin Invest* 36:440–448, 1957

37. Mansell A, Bryan C, Levison H: Airway closure in children. *J Appl Physiol* 33:711–714, 1972

38. Anthonisen NR, Danson J, Robertson PC, et al: Airway closure as a function of age. *Respir Physiol* 8:58–65, 1969

39. Motoyama EK, Brinkmeyer SD, Mutich RL, et al: Reduced FRC in anesthetized infants: Effect of low PEEP. *Anesthesiology* 57:A418, 1982

40. Sharp JT, Druz WS, Balagot RC, et al: Total respiratory compliance in infants and children. *J Appl Physiol* 29:775–779, 1970

41. Lacourt G, Polgar G: Interaction between nasal and pulmonary resistance in newborn infants. *J Appl Physiol* 30:870–873, 1971

42. Doershuk CF, Matthews LW: Airway resistance and lung volume in the newborn infant. *Pediatr Res* 3:128–134, 1969

43. Nelson NM, Prodhom LS, Cherry RB, et al: Pulmonary function in the newborn infant: The alveolar–arterial oxygen gradient. *J Appl Physiol* 18:534–538, 1963

44. Phelan PD, Williams HE: Ventilatory studies in healthy infants. *Pediatr Res* 3:425–432, 1969

45. Auld PAM, Nelson NM, Cherry RB, et al: Measurement of thoracic gas volume in the newborn infant. *J Clin Invest* 42:476–483, 1963

46. Swyer PR, Reiman RC, Wright JJ: Ventilation and ventilatory mechanics in the newborn. *J Pediatr* 56:612–622, 1960

47. Nelson NM: Respiration and circulation after birth, in Smith CA, Nelson NM (eds): *The Physiology of the Newborn Infant.* Springfield, IL, Charles C. Thomas, 1977

48. Chernick V, Avery ME: The functional basis of respiratory pathology, in Kendig EL Jr, Chernick V (eds): *Disorders of the Respiratory Tract,* 3rd ed. Philadelphia, Saunders, 1977

49. Sutherland JM, Ratcliff JW: Crying vital capacity. *Am J Dis Child* 101:67–74, 1961

50. Krieger I: Studies on mechanics of respiration in infancy. *Am J Dis Child* 105:439–448, 1963

51. Cross KW, Tizard JPM, Trythall DAH: The gaseous metabolism of the newborn infant. *Acta Paediatr* 46:265–285, 1957

52. Thibeault DW, Clutario B, Auld PAM: The oxygen cost of breathing in the premature infant. *Pediatrics* 37:954–959, 1966

53. Epstein RA, Hyman AI: Ventilatory requirements of critically ill neonates. *Anesthesiology* 53:379–384, 1980

54. Keens TG, Bryan AC, Levison H, et al: Developmental pattern of muscle fiber types in human ventilatory muscles. *J Appl Physiol* 44:909–913, 1978

55. Slovis TL, Haller JO, Berdon WE, et al: Noninvasive visualization of the pediatric airway. *Curr Probl Diagn Radiol* 8:1–67, 1979

56. Dunbar JS, Kramer SS: Radiology of trauma to the pediatric larynx. *Ear Nose Throat J* 60:356–365, 1981

57. Grunebaum M, Adler S, Varsano I: The paradoxical movement of the mediastinum: A diagnostic sign of foreign body aspiration during childhood. *Pediatr Radiol* 8:213–218, 1979

58. Kushner DC, Harris GB: Obstructing lesions of the larynx and trachea in infants and children. *Radiol Clin North Am* 16:181–194, 1978

59. Doust BD, Ting YM: Xeroradiography of the larynx. *Radiology* 110:727–730, 1974

60. Rosenfield NS, Peck DR, Lowman RM: Xeroradiography in the evaluation of acquired airway abnormalities in children. *Am J Dis Child* 132:1177–1180, 1978

61. Moorthy SS, LoSasso AM, King H, et al: Evaluation of larynx and trachea by xeroradiography. *Anesth Analg* 55:598–600, 1976

62. Holinger PH, Lutterbeck EF, Bulger R: Xeroradiography of the larynx. *Ann Otol Rhino Laryngol* 81:806–808, 1972

63. Davenport HT, Rosales JK: Endotracheal intubation in infants and children. *Can Anaesth Soc J* 6:65–74, 1959

64. Gillespie NA: Endotracheal anaesthesia in infants. *Br J Anaesth* 17:2–12, 1939

65. Gordon RA: Anesthetic management of patients with airway problems. *Int Anesthesiol Clin* 10:37–59, 1972

66. Haselby KA, McNiece WL: Respiratory obstruction from uvular edema in a pediatric patient. *Anesth Analg* 62:1127–1128, 1983

67. Bennett RL, Lee TS, Wright BD: Airway-obstructing supraglottic edema following anesthesia with the head positioned in forced flexion. *Anesthesiology* 54:78–80, 1981

68. Ravindran R, Priddy S: Uvular edema, a rare complication of endotracheal intubation. *Anesthesiology* 48:374, 1978

69. Moore MW, Rauscher LA: A complication of oropharyngeal airway placement. *Anesthesiology* 47:526, 1977

70. Slater HM, Sheridan CA, Ferguson RH: Endotracheal tube sizes for infants and children. *Anesthesiology* 16:950–952, 1955

71. Corfield HMC: Orotracheal tubes and the metric system. *Br J Anaesth* 35:34, 1963

72. Glauser EM, Cook CD, Bourgas TP: Pressure-flow characteristics and dead spaces of endotracheal tubes used in infants. *Anesthesiology* 22:339–341, 1961

73. Hall JE: The physiology of respiration in infants and young children. *Proc R Soc Med* 48:761–764, 1955

74. Cole F: Pediatric formulas for the anesthesiologist. *Am J Dis Child* 94:672–673, 1957

75. Morgan GAR, Steward DJ: Linear airway dimensions in children: Including those with cleft palate. *Can Anaesth Soc J* 29:1–8, 1982

76. Morgan GAR, Steward DJ: A preformed paediatric orotracheal tube design based on anatomical measurements. *Can Anaesth Soc J* 29:9–11, 1982

77. Smith DW: *Recognizable Patterns of Human Malformation* 2nd ed. Philadelphia, W.B. Saunders, 1976

78. Jones AEP, Pelton DA: An index of syndromes and their anesthetic implications. *Can Anaesth Soc J* 23:207–266, 1976

79. Vaughan VC III, McKay RJ, Nelson WE (eds): *Nelson Textbook of Pediatrics*. Philadelphia, W.B. Saunders, 1975

80. Barnett HL (ed): *Pediatrics*. New York, Appleton Century Crofts, 1972

81. Creighton RE, Relton JE, Miridy HW: Anaesthesia for occipital encephalocoele. *Can Anaesth Soc J* 21:403–406, 1974

82. Meyers EF, Krupin B: Anesthetic management of emergency tonsilectomy and adenoidectomy in infectious mononucleosis. *Anesthesiology* 42:490–491, 1975

83. Coleman M: Down's syndrome. *Pediatr Ann* 7:90–103, 1978

84. Clark RW, Schmidt HS, Schuller DE: Sleep induced ventilatory dysfunction in Down's syndrome. *Arch Intern Med* 140:45–50, 1980

85. Levine OR, Simpser M: Alveolar hypoventilation and cor pulmonale associated with chronic airway obstruction in infants with Down's syndrome. *Clin Pediatr (Phila)* 21:25–29, 1982

86. Kobel M, Creighton RE, Steward DJ: Anaesthesia considerations in Down's syndrome: Experience with 100 patients and a review of the literature. *Can Anaesth Soc J* 29:593–599, 1982

87. Smith DF, Mihm FG, Flynn M: Chronic alveolar hypoventilation secondary to macroglossia in the Beckwith-Wiedemann Syndrome. *Pediatrics* 70:695–697, 1982

88. Combs JT, Grunt JA, Brandt IK: New syndrome of neonatal hypoglycemia associated with visceromegaly, macroglossia, microcephaly and abnormal umbilicus. *N Engl J Med* 275:236–243, 1966

89. Jones AEP, Crowley TF: Morquio syndrome and anesthesia. *Anesthesiology* 51:261–262, 1979

90. Birkinshaw KJ: Anaesthesia in a patient with an unstable neck: Morquio's syndrome. *Anaesthesia* 30:46–49, 1975

91. Cox JM: Anesthesia and glycogen storage disease. *Anesthesiology* 29:1221–1225, 1968

92. Bougas TP, Smith RM: Pathologic airway obstruction in children. *Anesth Analg* 37:137–146, 1958

93. Weller RM: Anaesthesia for cystic hygroma in a neonate. *Anaesthesia* 29:588–594, 1974

94. MacDonald DJF: Cystic hygroma: An anaesthetic and surgical problem. *Anaesthesia* 21:66–71, 1966

95. Fletcher MM, Blum SL, Blanchard CL: Pierre Robin syndrome, pathophysiology of obstructive episodes. *Laryngoscope* 79:547–560, 1969

96. Lapidot A, Rezvani F, Terrefe D et al: A new functional approach to the surgical management of Pierre Robin syndrome: experimental and clinical report. *Laryngoscope* 86:979–983, 1976

97. Hawkins DB, Simpson JV: Micrognathia and glossoptosis in the newborn. Surgical tacking of the tongue in small jaw syndromes. *Clin Pediatr* 13:1066–1073, 1974

98. Khouw YH, Kleine JW: A difficult intubation. *Acta Anaesthesiol Belg* 26:78–80, 1975

99. Cogswell JJ, Easton DM: Cor pulmonale in the Pierre Robin syndrome. *Arch Dis Child* 49:905–908, 1974

100. Heaf DP, Helms PJ, Dinwiddie R, et al: Nasopharyngeal airways in Pierre Robin syndrome. *J Pediatr* 100:698–703, 1982

101. Stern LM, Fonkalsrud EW, Hassakis P, et al: Management of Pierre Robin syndrome in infancy by prolonged nasopharyngeal intubation. *Am J Dis Child* 124:78–80, 1972

102. Lewis MB, Pashayan HM: Management of infants with Robin anomaly. *Clin Pediatr (Phila)* 19:519–521, 525–528, 1981

103. Mallory SB, Paradise JL: Glossoptosis revisited: On the development and resolution of airway obstruction in the Pierre Robin syndrome. *Pediatrics* 64:946–948, 1979

104. MacLennan FM, Robertson GS: Ketamine for induction and intubation in Treacher-Collins syndrome. *Anaesthesia* 36:196–198, 1981

105. Johnson C, Taussig LM, Koopman C, et al: Obstructive sleep apnea in Treacher-Collins syndrome. *Cleft Palate J* 18:39–44, 1981

106. Divekar VM, Sircar BN: Anesthetic management in Treacher-Collins syndrome. *Anesthesiology* 26:692–693, 1965

107. Sklar GS, King BD: Endotracheal intubation and Treacher-Collins syndrome. *Anesthesiology* 44:247–249, 1976

108. Ross EDT: Treacher-Collins syndrome an anaesthetic hazard. *Anaesthesia* 18:350–354, 1963

109. Stelling L: Goldenhar syndrome and airway management. *Am J Dis Child* 132:818, 1978

110. Walts LF, Finerman G, Wyatt GM: Anaesthesia for dwarfs and other patients of pathological small stature. *Can Anaesth Soc J* 22:703–709, 1975

111. Mather JS: Impossible direct laryngoscopy in achondroplasia: A case report. *Anaesthesia* 21:244–248, 1966

112. Allansmith M, Senz E: Chondrodystrophia congenita punctata (Conradi's Disease). *Am J Dis Child* 100:133–140, 1960

113. Noonan JA: Hypertelorism with Turner phenotype. *Am J Dis Child* 116:373–380, 1968

114. Nora JJ, Torres FG, Sinha AK, et al: Characteristic cardiovascular anomalies of XO Turner syndrome, XX and XY phenotype and XO/XX Turner mosaic. *Am J Cardiol* 25:639–641, 1970

115. Ptacek LJ, Opitz JM, Smith DW, et al: The Cornelia de Lange syndrome. *J Pediatr* 63:1000–1020, 1963

116. Jervis GA, Stimson CW: De Lange syndrome. *J Pediatr* 63:634–645, 1963

117. Smith DW, Lemli L, Opitz JM: A newly recognized syndrome of multiple congenital anomalies. *J Pediatr* 64:210–217, 1964

118. Hoefnagel D, Benirschke K: Dyscephalia mandibulo-oculo-facialis (Hallermann-Streiff Syndrome). *Arch Dis Child* 40:57–61, 1965

119. Holinger PH, Schild JA: Pharyngeal, laryngeal, and tracheal injuries in the pediatric age group. *Ann Otol Rhino Laryngol* 81:811–817, 1972

120. Jacobs JC, Hui RM: Cricoarytenoid arthritis and airway obstruction in juvenile rheumatoid arthritis. *Pediatrics* 59:292–293, 1977

121. D'Arcy EJ, Fell RH, Ansell BM, et al: Ketamine and juvenile chronic polyarthritis (Still's disease). Anaesthetic problems in Still's disease and allied disorders. *Anaesthesia* 31:624–632, 1976

122. Jenkins LC, McGraw RW: Anaesthetic management of the patient with rheumatoid arthritis. *Can Anaesth Soc J* 16:407–415, 1969

123. Edeilist G: Principles of anesthetic management in rheumatoid arthritic patients. *Anaesth Analg* 43:227–231, 1964

124. Gardner DL, Holmes F: Anaesthetic and post-operative hazards in rheumatoid arthritis. *Br J Anaesth* 33:258–264, 1961

125. Hamner JE III, Ketcham AS: Cherubism: An analysis of treatment. *Cancer* 23:1133–1143, 1969

126. Holinger PH, Johnston KC: Factors responsible for laryngeal obstruction in infants. *JAMA* 143:1229–1232, 1950

127. Holinger PH, Brown WT: Congenital webs, cysts, laryngocoeles and other anomalies of the larynx. *Ann Otol Rhinol Laryngol* 76:744–752, 1967

128. Seed RF: Traumatic injury to the larynx and trachea. *Anaesthesia* 26:55–65, 1971

129. Saletta JD, Folk FA, Freeark RJ: Trauma to the neck region. *Surg Clin North Am* 53:73–86, 1971

130. Curtin JW, Holinger PH, Greeley PW: Blunt trauma to the larynx and upper trachea: Immediate treatment, complications, and late reconstructive procedures. *J Trauma* 6:493–502, 1966

131. Dalal FY, Schmidt GB, Bennett EJ, et al: Fractures of the larynx in children. *Can Anaesth Soc J* 21:376–378, 1974

132. Ellis FR: The management of the cut-throat. *Anaesthesia* 21:253–260, 1966

133. Kim IG, Brummitt WM, Humphry A, et al: Foreign body in the airway: A review of 202 cases. *Laryngoscope* 83:347–354, 1973

134. Steichen FM, Fellini A, Einhorn AH: Acute foreign body laryngotracheal obstruction: A cause for sudden and unexpected death in children. *Pediatrics* 48:281–285, 1971

135. Chatterji S, Chatterji P: The management of foreign bodies in air passages. *Anaesthesia* 27:390–395, 1972

136. Baraka A: Bronchoscopic removal of inhaled foreign bodies in children. *Br J Anaesth* 46:124–126, 1974

137. Moylan JA, Chan AK: Inhalation injury—an increasing problem. *Ann Surg* 185:34–37, 1978

138. Chu CS: New concepts of pulmonary burn injury. *J Trauma* 21:958–961, 1981

139. Trunkey DD: Inhalation injury. *Surg Clin North Am* 58:1133–1140, 1978

140. Mellins RB, Park S: Respiratory complications of smoke inhalation in victims of fires. *J Pediatr* 87:1–7, 1975

141. Fein A, Leff A, Hopewell PC: Pathophysiology and management of the complications resulting from fire and the inhaled products of combustion: Review of the literature. *Crit Care Med* 8:94–98, 1980

142. Hunt JL, Agee RN, Pruitt BA Jr: Fiberoptic bronchoscopy in acute inhalation injury. *J Trauma* 15:641–649, 1975

143. Allen TH, Steven IM: Prolonged nasotracheal intubation in infants and children. *Br J Anaesth* 44:835–840, 1972

144. Bain JA: Late complications of tracheostomy and prolonged endotracheal intubation. *Int Anesthesiol Clin* 10:225–244, 1972

145. Komorn RM, Smith CP, Erwin JR: Acute laryngeal injury with short term endotracheal anesthesia. *Laryngoscope* 83:683–690, 1973

146. Markham WG, Blackwood MJA, Conn AW: Prolonged nasotracheal intubation in infants and children. *Can Anaesth Soc J* 14:11–21, 1967

147. Lewis RN, Swerdlow M: Hazards of endotracheal anaesthesia. *Br J Anaesth* 36:504–515, 1964

148. Hatch DJ: Prolonged nasotracheal intubation in infants and children. *Lancet* 1:1272–1275, 1968

149. Blanc VF, Tremblay NA: The complications of tracheal intubation: A new classification with a review of the literature. *Anesth Analg* 53:202–213, 1974

150. Joshi VV, Mandavia SG, Stern L, et al: Acute lesions induced by endotracheal intubation occurrence in the upper respiratory tract of newborn infants with respiratory distress syndrome. *Am J Dis Child* 124:646–649, 1972

151. Hawkins DB: Glottic and subglottic stenosis from endotracheal intubation. *Laryngoscope* 87:339–346, 1977

152. Grillo HC: Surgical treatment of postintubation tracheal injuries. *J Thorac Cardiovasc Surg* 78:860–875, 1979

153. Morrison MD, Maber BR: Crico-arytenoid joint obliteration following long term intubation in the premature infant. *J Otolaryngol* 6:277–283, 1977

154. Othersen HB Jr: Intubation injuries of the trachea in children: Management and prevention. *Ann Surg* 189:601–606, 1979

155. Oh TH, Motoyama EK: Comparison of nasotracheal intubation and tracheostomy in management of acute epiglottitis. *Anesthesiology* 46:214–216, 1977

156. Baxter JD, Pashley NR: Acute epiglottitis—25 years experience in management, the Montreal Children's Hospital. *J Otolaryngol* 6:473–476, 1977

157. Schuller DE, Birck HG: The safety of intubation in croup and epiglottitis in an eight-year follow-up. *Laryngoscope* 85:33–46, 1975

158. Travis KW, Todres ID, Shannon DC: Pulmonary edema associated with croup and epiglottitis. *Pediatrics* 59:695–698, 1977

159. Davison FW: Acute laryngeal obstruction in children. A fifty year review. *Ann Otol Rhinol Laryngol* 87:606–613, 1978

160. Phelan PD, Mullins GC, Laundau LI, et al: The period of nasotracheal intubation in acute epiglottitis. *Anaesth Intensive Care* 8:402–403, 1980

161. Enoksen A, Bryne H, Hoel TM, et al: Epiglottitis acuta treated with nasotracheal intubation. *Acta Anaesth Scand* 23:422–426, 1979

162. Bottenfield GW, Arcinue EL, Sarnaik A, et al: Diagnosis and

management of acute epiglottitis—Report of 90 consecutive cases. *Laryngoscope* 90:822–825, 1980

163. Battaglia JD, Lockhart CH: Management of acute epiglottitis by nasotracheal intubation. *Am J Dis Child* 129:334–336, 1975

164. Adair JC, Ring WH: Management of epiglottitis in children. *Anesth Analg* 54:622–625, 1975

165. Milko DA, Marshak G, Striker TW: Nasotracheal intubation in the treatment of acute epiglottitis. *Pediatrics* 53:674–677, 1974

166. Blanc VF, Weber MC, LeDuc C, et al: Acute epiglottitis in children: Management of 27 consecutive cases with nasotracheal intubation, with special emphasis on anaesthetic considerations. *Can Anaesth Soc J* 24:1–11, 1977

167. Weber ML, Desjardins R, Perreault G, et al: Acute epiglottitis in children—treatment with nasotracheal intubation: Report of 14 consecutive cases. *Pediatrics* 57:152–155, 1976

168. Sumner E: Quinsy tonsillectomy: A safe procedure. *Anaesthesia* 28:558–561, 1973

169. Beeden AG, Evans JN: Quinsy tonsillectomy—a further report. *J Laryngol Otol* 84:443–448, 1970

170. Kloss J, Petty C: Obstruction of endotracheal intubation by a mobile pedunculated polyp. *Anesthesiology* 43:380, 1975

171. Stein AA, Volk BM: Papillomatosis of trachea and lung. *Arch Pathol* 68:468–472, 1959

172. Hitz HB, Oesterlin E: A case of multiple papillomata of the larynx with aerial metastases to lungs. *Am J Pathol* 8:333–339, 1932

173. Fitzsimmons JS: Laryngeal stridor and respiratory obstruction associated with mylomeningocele. *Dev Med Child Neurol* 15:533–536, 1973

174. Holinger PC, Holinger LD, Reichert TJ, et al: Respiratory obstruction and apnea in infants with bilateral abductor vocal cord paralysis, meningomyelocele, hydrocephalus, and Arnold-Chiari malformation. *J Pediatr* 92:368–373, 1978

175. Bluestone CD, Delerme AN, Samuelson GH: Airway obstruction due to vocal cord paralysis in infants with hydrocelphalus and meningomyelocoele. *Ann Otol Rhinol Laryngol* 81:778–783, 1972

176. Steward DJ: Congenital abnormalities as a possible factor in the aetiology of post-intubation subglottic stenosis. *Can Anaesth Soc J* 17:388–390, 1970

177. Koka BV, Jean IS, Andre JM, et al: Post intubation croup in children. *Anesth Analg* 56:501–505, 1977

178. Davison FW: Acute laryngeal obstruction in children. *JAMA* 171:1301–1305, 1959

179. Taussig LM, Castro O, Beaudry PH, et al: Treatment of laryngotracheo-bronchitis (croup). Use of intermittent positive-pressure breathing and racemic epinephrine. *Am J Dis Child* 129:790–793, 1975

180. Mitchell DP, Thomas RL: Secondary airway support in the management of croup. *J Otolaryngol* 9:419–422, 1980

181. Duncan PG: Efficacy of helium-oxygen mixtures in the management of severe viral and post-intubation croup. *Can Anaesth Soc J* 26:206–212, 1979

182. Bray RJ, Fernandes FJ: Mediastinal tumor causing airway obstruction in anaesthetized children. *Anaesthesia* 37:571–575, 1982

183. Gunderson CH, Greenspan RH, Glaser GH, et al: The Klippel-Feil Syndrome: Genetic and clinical reevaluation of cervical fusion. *Medicine* 46:491–512, 1967

184. Schneider RC: Concommitant cranio-cerebral and spinal trauma, with special reference to the cervico medullary region. *Clin Neurosurg* 17:266–309, 1970

185. Pelton DA, Whalen JS: Airway obstruction in infants and children, in Spoerel WE (ed). *Problems of the Upper Airway.* Int Anesth Clin 10:123–150, 1972, Little, Brown

186. Salem MR, Mathrubhutham M, Bennet EJ: Current concepts: Difficult intubation. *N Engl J Med* 295:879–881, 1976

187. Gordon RA: Anesthetic management of patients with airway problems, in Spoerel WE (ed). Problems of the Upper Airway. Int Anesth Clin 10:37–59, 1972, Little, Brown

188. Webster AC: Anesthesia for operations on the upper airway, in Spoerel WE (ed). Problems of the Upper Airway. Int Anesth Clin 10:61–122, 1972, Little, Brown

189. Fan LL, Flynn JW: Laryngoscopy in neonates and infants: Experience with the flexible fiberoptic bronchoscope. *Laryngoscope* 91:451–456, 1981

190. Taylor PA, Towey RM: The broncho-fiberscope as an aid to endotracheal intubation. *Br J Anaesth* 44:611–612, 1972

191. Davis NJ: A new fiberoptic laryngoscope for nasal intubation. *Anesth Analg* 52:807–808, 1973

192. Aro L, Takki S, Aromaa U: Technique for difficult intubation. *Br J Anaesth* 43:1081–1083, 1971

193. Katz RL, Berci G: The optical stylet—a new intubation technique for adults and children with specific reference to teaching. *Anesthesiology* 51:251–254, 1979

194. Bourke D, Levesque PR: Modification of retrograde guide for endotracheal intubation. *Anesth Analg* 53:1013–1014, 1974

195. Waters DJ: Guided blind endotracheal intubation for patients with deformities of the upper airway. *Anaesthesia* 18:158–162, 1963

196. Borland LM, Swan DM, Leff S: Difficult pediatric intubation: A new approach to the retrograde technique. *Anesthesiology* 55:577–578, 1981

197. Duncan JAT: Intubation of the trachea in the conscious patient. *Br J Anaesth* 49:619–623, 1977

198. Rosenberg MB, Levesque PR, Bourke DL: Use of the LTA(R) kit as a guide for endotracheal intubation. *Anesth Analg* 56:287–288, 1977

199. Roberts KW: New use for Swan-Ganz introducer wire. *Anesth Analg* 60:67, 1981

200. Magill IW: Endotracheal anesthesia. *Am J Surg* 34:450–455, 1936

201. Gillespie NA: *Endotracheal Anesthesia*, 3rd ed. Madison, University of Wisconsin Press, 1963

202. Davies JAH: Blind nasal intubation using doxapram hydrochloride. *Br J Anaesth* 40:361–364, 1968

203. Todres ID, Crone RK: Experience with a modified laryngoscope in sick infants. *Crit Care Med* 9:544–545, 1981

204. Smith RB, Schaer WB, Pfaeffle H: Percutaneous transtracheal ventilation for anaesthesia and resuscitation: A review and report of complications. *Can Anaesth Soc J* 22:607–612, 1975

205. Stinson TW III: A simple connector for transtracheal ventilation. *Anesthesiology* 47:232, 1977

206. Frumin MJ, Epstein RM, Cohen G: Apneic oxygenation in man. *Anesthesiology* 20:789–798, 1959

Appendix 5-1

Syndromes and Disease Processes with Associated Airway Difficulties

Syndrome	Airway	Cerebral	Cardiac	Renal	GI	Endocrine Metabolic	Musculo-skeletal	Anesthetic Considerations
Achondroplasia	mid-facial hypoplasia, small nasal passages & mouth	Megacephaly ± hydrocephalus 2° to narrow foramen magnum					dwarfism	1. difficult intubation 2. ± hydrocephalus
Apert's Syndrome	maxillary hypoplasia, narrow palate ± cleft palate	craniosynostosis, flat facies, hyperteleorism	± CHD	± hydronephrosis, ± polycystic kidney	± esophageal atresia		syndactyly	1. difficult intubation 2. associated cardiac & renal problems
Arthrogryposis Multiplex Congenita (multiple congenital contractures)	Associated hypoplastic mandible, cleft palate, Klippel-Feil Syndrome, torticollis		± VSD				thoracolumbar scoliosis	1. difficult intubation 2. associated cardiac disease 3. minimal muscle relaxant required 4. ± malignant hyperthermia
Beckwith-Wiedemann Syndrome (visceromegaly)	macroglossia-regresses with age—may require partial glossectomy	± mental retardation 2° to hypoglycemia	large heart	enlarged kidneys	omphalocoele, hepato-splenomegaly	hypoglycemia up to 4 months of age, polycythemia	eventration diaphragm	1. difficult intubation 2. asymptomatic hypoglycemia 3. omphalocoele 4. neonatal polycythemia
Cherubism (fibrous dysplasia of jaw)	bilateral painless mandibular and maxillary swelling may progress to airway obstruction							1. difficult intubation 2° to intraoral masses
Cornelia De Lange Syndrome	high arch palate, micrognathia, spurs at anterior angle of mandible, large tongue, ± cleft palate, short neck	mental deficiency	± CHD					1. difficult intubation 2. associated cardiac disease
Craniofacial Dysostosis of Crouzon	maxillary hypoplasia with inverted v-shaped palate, ± large tongue	ocular proptosis 2° to shallow orbits, cranio-synostosis						1. difficult intubation 2. eye injury
Cretinism (congenital hypothyroid)	large tongue	may be mentally deficient					hypothermia hypometabolic	umbilical hernia	1. difficult intubation 2. hypothermia

55

Appendix (continued)

Syndrome	Airway/Physical features	Cardiovascular	Other systemic	Anesthetic considerations
				3. decreased drug metabolism
Epidermolysis Bullosa	pressure lesions to airway			1. need gentle intubation with small tube 2. postop laryngeal obstruction 2° to bulla formation
Goldenhar's Syndrome (oculoauriculovertebral syndrome)	hypoplastic zygomatic arch, mandibular hypoplasia, macrostomia, ± cleft tongue, palate		occipitalization of atlas, cervical vertebral defects	1. difficult intubation 2. cervical spine defects
Hallerman-Streiff Syndrome (oculomandibulo-dyscephaly)	malar hypoplasia, micrognathia, hypoplasia of rami and anterior displacement of temperomandibular joint, narrow high arch palate			1. difficult intubation
Marfan's Syndrome	narrow facies with narrow palate	dissecting aortic aneurysm, aortic insufficiency	scoliosis, kyphosis	1. difficult intubation 2. associated cardiac, pulmonary disease
Papillomatosis Larynx and Trachea	difficult laryngoscopy			1. difficult intubation 2. care not to seed tissue into trachea
Pierre Robin Syndrome	hypoplastic mandible, pseudomacroglossia, ± high arched, cleft palate			1. difficult intubation
Pompe's Disease (cardiomuscular glycogen storage disease)	large tongue	cardiomyopathy	muscle weakness	1. difficult intubation 2. muscle weakness sensitive to muscle relaxants 3. congestive heart failure, sensitive to myocardial depressants
Rheumatoid Arthritis	temperomandibular joint mobility limited,	myocarditis, valvular disease	cervical spine subluxation, steroid therapy,	1. difficult intubation 2. associated heart

Syndrome	Airway / Physical	CNS	Cardiac	GI/GU	Other	Systemic	Spine	Anesthetic considerations
	hypoplastic mandible, cricoarytenoid arthritis with narrow larynx		esp. aortic insufficiency			anemia	rigid cervical spine	disease 3. problems with positioning 4. steroid therapy
Rubinstein-Taybi Syndrome	maxillary hypoplasia narrow palate	mental deficiency	± CHD				associated cervical vertebral anomalies	1. difficult intubation 2. cervical spine instability 3. associated cardiac disease
Scleroderma	extensive scarring mouth, face, body					steroid therapy		1. difficult intubation 2. decreased pulmonary compliance 3. steroid therapy
Smith-Lemli-Opitz Syndrome	micrognathia, ± cleft palate, recurrent pneumonia	moderate mental deficiency, microcephaly	± CHD					1. difficult intubation 2. associated cardiac disease
Stevens-Johnson Syndrome	laryngeal, tracheal, bronchial bullae, pneumothorax, pleural effusion		myocarditis	esophagitis, fluid shifts	urethritis	temperature elevations		1. difficult intubation 2. fluid balance 3. myocarditis 4. temperature control 5. avoid intubation if possible
Thalassemia Major (Cooley's anemia)	malar hypoplasia causes relative mandibular hypoplasia				hemosiderosis			1. may be difficult intubation 2. anemia 3. associated cardiac disease
Treacher-Collins Syndrome	malar, mandibular hypoplasia, ± cleft lip, ± choanal atresia, ± macro or microstomia		± CHD				± cervical spine deformity	1. difficult intubation 2. associated cardiac disease
Trisomy 21-Down's Syndrome	small mouth, hypoplastic mandible, protruding tongue	mental retardation	A-V communis VSD, ASD	duodenal atresia			hypotonia	1. may be difficult intubation 2. associated cardiac disease 3. ? less muscle relaxant
Turner's Syndrome (Noonan Syndrome)	narrow maxilla, small mandible, short neck	mental deficiency	coarctation aorta-females, pulmonary artery coarctation-males		idiopathic hypertension	hypogonadism		1. difficult intubation 2. associated cardiac disease 3. hypertension

6

Pediatric Clinical Pharmacokinetics—Principles and Concepts

J.A. Jeevendra Martyn

Significant differences exist among neonates, infants, children, and adults in the way the body handles drugs. From infancy on, the body and organs are in a continuous state of development, and multiple, concomitant physiologic changes occur with age. In the neonate, for example, the brain and liver are large relative to body size, the brain contains less myelin, and the enzyme systems of the liver are undeveloped. Neonates also have less adipose tissue than the adult or older child, and the size of the body water compartments changes with age, as does blood pressure, which reflects alterations in blood flow and resistance. All of these physiologic factors can modify the pharmacokinetics and the pharmacodynamic actions of drugs. This chapter reviews the physiology of the child and basic principles of pharmacokinetics, providing a conceptual framework for understanding the disposition and effect of intravenous drugs in the pediatric patient. The pharmacology of the anesthetic agents, narcotics, and sedatives is discussed in chapter 7.

During the last ten years, the development of new, sensitive techniques for assaying drugs and drug metabolites, together with progress in computer technology, have made possible remarkable advances in pharmacokinetic studies. Despite these advances, however, most regimens for drugs used in children are determined merely by fractionating adult doses according to the weight, age, or body surface area of the child. This lack of knowledge of pharmacokinetic action in children exists in large part because of technical, ethical, and complex medicolegal issues that hinder or prevent evaluation in children.[1] Thus, the pediatric patient is something of a "therapeutic orphan." The few pharmacologic studies conducted in children suggest that pediatric patients handle drugs quite differently than adults. In the absence of hard data, therefore, a review of pediatric physiology (with respect to absorption, distribution, metabolism, and excretion) and basic pharma-cokinetic principles (e.g., one-compartment model, first-order kinetics, elimination, half-life, and so forth) should shed light on drug disposition and usage in the newborn and older child.[2–7]

ABSORPTION

ORAL

The oral route is the commonest and simplest way to administer a drug. Absorption occurs by passive diffusion across a concentration gradient. Dissolution from tablet form, although often important, does not play a significant role in pediatrics, because most drugs are administered in the fluid form. Two main factors, pH-dependent diffusion and gastric emptying time, regulate the gastrointestinal absorption of drugs.[2,8] Other factors include the degree of ionization, lipid solubility, and molecular size. Generally speaking, in an acidic medium (e.g., the stomach) acidic drugs are nonionized, and therefore absorption is favored. In an alkaline medium (e.g., the intestine) basic drugs are more rapidly absorbed. In the neonate, the gastric pH undergoes maturational changes and is markedly different from pH values present in older children and adults.[7] At birth, the gastric pH usually ranges between 6 and 8, but it drops quickly within 24 hours to a value between 1 and 3. This decrease in pH is difficult to explain, since the gastric mucosa in the neonate is not mature enough to secrete acid. Over the next seven to ten days, almost no acid is secreted. Adult values for gastric acidity (pH) usually are not reached until two years of age.[7,8]

In the newborn period, peristalsis is irregular and completely unpredictable. Gastric emptying time may be prolonged in the newborn and premature, reaching adult values at about six months.[2] These factors affect the time to peak plasma concentration of the drug, but not necessarily the degree of absorption. The relatively achlorhydric situation in the first few days of life may partially explain the higher bioavailability in the newborn of several penicillins, which are basic, as well as the reduced absorption of acid compounds, such as phenobarbital, phenytoin, and nalidixic acid.[7] For individuals of all ages, decreased emptying of the stomach contents can occur without mechanical obstruction. Causes include immobilization and stress, and neurologic or metabolic disorders.[9] Similarly, in pathologic states, such as cardiac failure or hypovolemia, absorption will be reduced because of decreased splanchnic blood flow. Thus, bioavailability may also be decreased under these circumstances. Other factors that may influence intestinal drug absorption in the neonate include the gradual maturation of biliary function, the variable colonization of the intestine by bacterial flora, and the high level of β-glucuronidase activity in the newborn intestine.[8–10] The latter enzyme can break down glucuronidated compounds, thereby releasing the parent drug. During the first four days after birth, β-glucuronidase activity is about seven times that of the adult. It has been speculated that the higher capacity of β-glucuronidase to deconjugate bilirubin, over conjugation by the liver, may contribute to the hyperbilirubinemia often observed in neonates.[9] Similarly, the inactive metabolite of morphine, morphine glucuronide, may also be broken down to active morphine by the increased activity of β-glucuronidase, explaining the more potent respiratory depression that accompanies morphine use in the newborn compared with meperidine, which follows a different metabolic pathway. Beyond the newborn period, no functional differences are found between the healthy child and adult that would alter drug absorption from the gastrointestinal tract.

PARENTERAL

The absorption of drugs injected intramuscularly (IM) depends mainly on regional blood flow, which may be different for specific muscle groups.[11] Relative immobilization and decreased muscular activity may also be factors affecting the absorption rate of drugs. A different bioavailability thus can exist for drugs given either orally or intramuscularly. In the neonate, absorption of diazepam, gentamicin, and digoxin is reduced when injected IM in comparison with oral administration.[2] The unexpected decrease in absorption following IM administrations may be due to the physical and chemical properties of the drug itself, or to differences in the physiology of the neonate and the child as described above.

PERCUTANEOUS ABSORPTION

Drug absorption through the skin is also significantly higher in newborns and infants than in children and adults. This may be related to the relative thinness of the stratum corneum, and skin hydration.[2,12] The use of abrasive tapes and skin monitoring devices can further increase absorption via this route. Thus, toxic reactions have been shown to occur with some agents, including boric acid powders, naphthalene, and salicyclic acid.[2] Although percutaneous administration of drugs, such as nitroglycerin, has been used in adults, it has received little attention in the pediatric population.

RECTAL ABSORPTION

Venous blood from the rectum is drained by the superior, middle, and inferior rectal veins. Although some mixing occurs, most of the blood from the superior rectal vein drains into the liver (portal system), whereas the inferior and middle veins drain into the inferior vena cava (systemic circulation). From a pharmacokinetic standpoint, drugs administered in the lower two-thirds of the rectum bypass the liver, yielding a higher bioavailability of drugs normally metabolized in the liver (first-pass metabolism).[13] Drugs metabolized in this manner include most of the narcotics, barbiturate, methohexital, propranolol, and some of the benzodiazepines (midazolam and triazolam). If the metabolite, not the parent compound, is the active agent (e.g., chloral hydrate), then it would be preferable to administer the drug in the upper third of the rectum, since most of it will be drained by the superior rectal vein into the liver, where the drug will be metabolized, and the active compound released.

In addition to the anatomical and physiological factors that enhance drug absorption from the rectum, formulation also plays an important role. Absorption of drugs in an aqueous or alcoholic solution occurs more rapidly than drugs in suspension or emulsion. Although the total area of absorption in the rectum is much smaller than the stomach or small intestine, this route is nonetheless useful for the administration of many drugs.[14–16] Peak plasma concentrations similar to, or even higher than, other routes have been obtained for diazepam and theophylline.[13,14,16] Peak plasma concentrations associated with induction of sleep have been observed within 10–15 minutes of administering methohexital, 20–30 mg/kg via the rectum (Figure 6-1).[15] Thus, the rectal route can be a useful alternative, especially in the pediatric population, because of their distaste for oral medications and apprehension of parenteral medications. In addition, important therapeutic reasons may dictate rectal rather than oral administration, e.g., nausea and vomiting. The rectum can also be used for rapid suppression of convulsive attacks, when intravenous access may be difficult.[16]

TRANSFER VIA MOTHER

Drug delivery to the fetus and neonate via the placenta is an important mode of absorbing (transferring) drug into the systemic circulation. Because of ethical and experimental difficulties, a detailed analysis of the transfer of drugs across the placenta in humans has not been done. As with other modes, the passage of drugs across the placenta is influenced both by the physicochemical properties of the drug and the physiologic characteristics of the maternal placental–fetal unit. Physicochemical properties that influence such drug transfer include lipid solubility, extent of ionization, and molecular weight of the compound. Lipophilic drugs, such as diazepam and thiopental, are poorly ionized at physiologic pH and traverse the placenta very rapidly.[17] Skeletal–muscle relaxants, such as d-tubocurarine and succinylcholine, which contain a quaternary nitrogen, are highly ionized and thus traverse the placenta slowly.[18] When patients are exposed to such drugs for prolonged periods, however, significant concentrations have been observed in the fetus. Although salicylates are completely ionized at physiologic pH, they are able to cross the placenta, owing to their small molecular size.[17]

Protein binding also plays an important role in placental transfer. Only the fraction of drug not bound to plasma proteins is distributed out of the extravascular space. The higher the maternal protein binding, therefore, the lower the transfer of drugs to the fetus. In most instances, maternal serum protein binding is greater than that of fetal serum, thus providing a natural protection against drug transfer across the placenta. After the drug traverses the placenta, however, the fetus is exposed to higher active drug concentrations in relation to total plasma concentrations, since the plasma protein binding is decreased in the fetus. It is noteworthy that the binding of salicylate, bupivacaine, etidocaine, and diazepam to plasma is decreased in the mother at delivery, resulting in a higher free fraction available for transfer across the placenta.[18,19]

Because of the strategic position of the liver relative to placental and fetal circulation, uptake of drugs by the fetal liver is high. This serves as a buffer against the development of high systemic drug concentrations in the neonate. Studies have demonstrated, however, that widely distributed drugs, such as thiopental, halothane, and lidocaine, that have accumulated in the liver are redistributed to other tissues given enough time.[20] Thus, all drugs, including the anesthetics and analgesics used in obstetrics, are capable of crossing the placenta. Placental transfer is an important property of drugs used for treating conditions in the fetus (e.g., corticosteroids), but an undesirable feature for drugs given solely for maternal effect (e.g., $MgSO_4$). As a rule, the half-life of drugs acquired in utero is considerably longer. This may be an important factor in the clinical management of the newborn.

Another route of drug transfer to the newborn is via breast milk.[21] Although beneficial for the transfer of passive immunity, drugs taken by the mother also can be transferred during breast feeding, and depending upon the drug, may have deleterious effects on the infant.

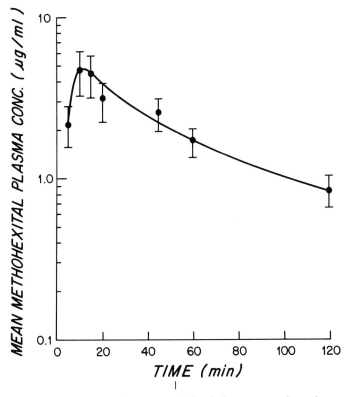

Figure 6-1. Mean plasma methohexital concentration–time curve after rectal administration of 25 mg/kg. The values represent mean ± SD. (Reproduced with pemission from Liu et al: *Anesthesiology*, 59:A450, 1983.)

DEVELOPMENTAL CHANGES IN BODY COMPOSITION

CHANGES IN BODY WATER

The total body water (TBW) at birth is around 85 percent in the premature, and about 78 percent in full-term infants. It decreases to about 60 percent at one year. During this time, the extra cellular water (ECW) decreases from about 50 percent in the premature and 45 percent in the full-term infant to 27 percent at one year. Intra cellular water (ICW), calculated as the difference between TBW and ECW, tends to increase in the first few months of life from about 34 percent to about 43 percent at three months. Between one and three years, there is a slight increase in all three components. From then on, there is a gradual reduction of all three components

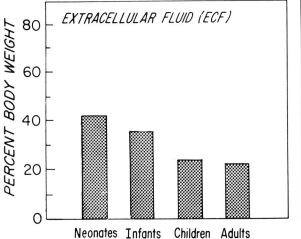

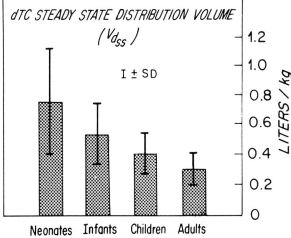

Figure 6-2. Values of ECF are compared to dTC Vd$_{ss}$. Note that the changes in ECF volume follow the same trend as the distribution volume for dTC. (Reproduced with permission from Fisher DM, et al: *Anesthesiology* 57:203–208, 1982.)

Table 6-1

Changes in Organ Weights with Age
(Percentage of Body Weight)

Organ System	Fetus	Full-term Newborn	Adult
Skeletal/Muscle	25.0	25.0	40.0
Skin	13.0	4.0	6.0
Skeleton	22.0	18.0	14.0
Heart	0.6	0.5	0.4
Liver	4.0	5.0	2.0
Kidneys	0.7	1.0	0.5
Brain	13.0	12.0	2.0

(Reproduced with permission from Widdowson, EM in *Scientific Foundations of Paediatrics, 2nd edition*, Baltimore, University Park Press, 1982.)

until adult values are reached in the early teens (50% of body weight for TBW and 20% for ECW).[22,23]

CHANGES IN BODY COMPOSITION

Along with the age-dependent changes in water content, changes in fat, muscle composition, and organ weight also occur (Table 6-1). The fat content is about 1 percent in mid-fetal life, increasing to 12 percent at birth.[23,24] It doubles by six months and reaches 30 percent of body weight at one year. During puberty, the fat content in boys decreases to 10–15 percent, while in girls it remains at 20–30 percent. Subsequently, in both sexes there is a gradual increase throughout life. Superimposed on all of these changes are the structural and functional changes occurring in the organs and tissues, and sometimes a disproportionate growth of some organs (Table 6-1).

CLINICAL IMPLICATIONS

The physiologic changes associated with maturation constitute a complex situation, with drugs localizing in different body regions, depending upon age. Although apparent volumes of distribution measured pharmacokinetically do not correspond to true body compartments, one would expect that age-related changes in body composition would be reflected in the measured distribution volumes. Most drugs distribute throughout the ECW before reaching their receptor sites. Thus, the size of the ECW influences the final drug concentration. This is particularly true for drugs that are minimally distributed in the tissues.[9] These drugs include some of the antipyretics, anticholinesterases, and muscle relaxants.[25] Fisher et al. have described the relationship between body water changes, occurring with age, and the steady state distribution volume of d-tubocurarine, a drug with limited tissue uptake (Figure 6-2).[26] In the neonatal period, because of the increased ECF volume, the distribution volume of d-tubocurarine is similarly increased. With age, as the ECF volume decreases, there is a proportionate decrease in the distribution volume of d-tubocurarine. Similar directional changes have been observed for other drugs with limited tissue uptake.[25] Thus, as a rule, to achieve a given plasma concentration for drugs distributed in the ECF, a higher dose for each kilogram of body weight must be administered in the

neonate and child in comparison with the adult. Otherwise, drug concentrations at the target organ will be inadequate. This rule assumes that target organ sensitivity does not change with age.

Observations with fentanyl also showed changes with age in the central and total volume of distribution.[27] There was an increase in total volume of distribution of drug in neonates and children compared with adults. Since fentanyl is distributed extensively in lipophilic tissues, and because fat and muscle content increase with age, these results are contrary to expectations.[23,27] These findings imply that, for a given dose, the younger brain is exposed to a more dilute concentration because of the increased volume of distribution. As a general rule, however, drugs that are lipophilic and highly bound to tissue, such as diazepam, morphine, and thiopental (fentanyl being an exception), the distribution volume will not be correlated with changes in ECW. This occurs because these drugs are strongly taken up by the tissues, and the contribution by ECW to the total distribution of drug is minimal.

DEVELOPMENTAL CHANGES IN THE METABOLIC CAPACITY

Metabolism and excretion together constitute the body's mechanism for eliminating drugs. Excretion or elimination is accomplished mainly through the bile and urine. Lipid-soluble molecules are not efficiently excreted by the bile or urine. They must first be transformed chemically into water-soluble molecules. Most drugs are biotransformed by the hepatic microsomal enzyme system or by the esterases present in plasma and various tissues before elimination. Increasing evidence shows that the lung and the kidneys also play a key role in the uptake and metabolism of substances, particularly those released endogenously.[28,29]

PATHWAYS IN DRUG BIOTRANSFORMATION

Most drugs are metabolized via two major pathways; phase I or degradative reactions (oxidation, reduction, and hydrolysis), and phase II or synthetic reactions (conjugation).[30] Most phase I reactions occur in the microsomal fraction of the liver. This group of enzymes is also collectively known as the cyctochrome p450 enzyme system, because the original discovery of it by Omura and Sato was made when they identified a sharp spectroscopic peak at 450 nanometers (nm) in liver homogenates that had been exposed to carbon monoxide. The contents of these homogenates were later identified as the important drug metabolizing enzymes of the liver. Degradation reactions include the conversion of pentobarbital or hexobarbital to the hydroxylated or keto derivative, aromatic hydroxylation of steroid hormones, and N-dealkylation of morphine and meperidine to normorphine and normeperidine.[9,30]

Drug metabolism can occur outside the liver microsomal system. Enzymes present in blood, plasma, and other tissues are able to hydrolyze amide and ester compounds. Examples of these include the local anesthetics and succinylcholine. Examples of drugs oxidized outside the microsomal system include theophylline, caffeine (xanthine oxidase), and ethyl alcohol (alcohol dehydrogenase).[9,29] The metabolites of phase I reactions, when compared with the parent compound, can be less active, equally active, or even more potent.

All phase II reactions are conjugation reactions and result in compounds with increased water solubility, thus facilitating excretion in the bile or urine. Examples of conjugation reactions include glucuronidation, methylation, acetylation, mercapturic acid formation, and sulfation. Examples of phase I and phase II reactions relevant to anesthesia are summarized in Table 6-2. Hepatic structural and functional abnormalities occur in a variety of disorders, including congestive heart failure, as well as during toxic, neoplastic, and inflammatory diseases. Phase I reactions are usually influenced by these abnormalities, and by coadministration of other drugs.[31] Conjugation, on the other hand, is less affected by the same factors. Some have suggested that, if there is a choice to be made, from a pharmacokinetic point of view, drugs metabolized by phase II reactions are preferable. This speculation, however, has not been validated clinically.

DRUG METABOLISM IN THE NEONATE

Most of the enzyme systems required for biotransformation are present at birth.[7,28,30,32] However, relative to adult values, both the concentration and activity of these enzyme systems are reduced. Quite unlike disease and pathologic states, conjugation or phase II reactions seem to be affected more by the immaturity of these systems than phase I reactions. For this reason, neonates cannot effectively conjugate bilirubin, chloramphenicol, sulfonamides, acetaminophen, and meprobamate.[33–36] This inability is more pronounced in the premature neonate; hence, the well-known syndromes of "grey baby" following chloramphenicol administration, and "yellow baby" due to poor conjugation of bilirubin. The glucuronide conjugation reaches adult values only after three years of age.[37,38] This enzyme system can be induced by drugs, however, such as phenobarbital, and has been applied clinically in the treatment of unconjugated hyperbilirubinemia.[39] The capacity for sulfate and glycine conjugation appears to compare well with adults.[32]

Among the phase I reactions, N-demethylation appears to be the most deficient step as in theophylline and caffeine degradation.[40,41] Hydroxylation reactions (phenobarbital, acetanilide, amobarbital, mepivacaine, lidocaine, nortriptyline) are also reduced, but not to the extent of theophylline and caffeine.[2,6] When evaluating drugs such as diazepam, lidocaine, and mepivacaine, dealkylation also is shown to be impaired.

The activity of plasma and blood enzymes is similarly depressed in the neonate[7,48] and represents another factor that may contribute to problems in the newborn when the mother has been given narcotics or local anesthetics during labor. The progressive increase in plasma enzyme activity parallels the increase of plasma proteins, both parameters achieving adult values at one year.[7] Thus, it is not surprising that almost all of the drugs studied in the neonatal period have prolonged elimination half-lives. The activity of the metabolizing enzymes in the newborn may be further depressed by the presence of other pathologic conditions, such as hypoxemia, cardiac failure, and poor nutritional status.[2] The activity of phase I reactions, as in phase II reactions, can be enhanced by maternal exposure to enzyme inducers, such as smoking and phenobarbitone, and it may explain why different and sometimes contrasting results have been obtained regarding maturation of different enzyme systems.

Table 6-2

Pathways in Drug Metabolism

Phase I	*Examples*
Oxidation Reactions	Thiopental, Methohexital
Aliphatic hydroxylation	Pentazocine, meperidine, glutethimide, doxapram, ketamine chlorpromazine
Aromatic	lidocaine, bupivacaine, mepivacaine, meperidine, glutethimide, fentanyl, propranolol
Expoxidation	Phenytoin
O-Dealkylation	Pancuronium, vecuronium, codeine, phenacetin, methoxyflurane
N-Dealkylation	Morphine, meperidine, fentanyl, diazepam, amide local anesthetics, ketamine, codeine, atropine, methadone
N-Oxidation	Meperidine, normeperidine, morphine, tetracaine
S-Oxidation	Chlorpromazine
Oxidative deamination	Amphetamine, epinephrine
Desulphuration	Thiopental
Dehalogenation	Halogenated anesthetics
Dehydrogenation	Ethanol
Reduction Reactions	
Azoreduction	Fazadinium
Nitroreduction	Nitrazepam, dantrolene
Carbonyl reduction	Prednisone
Alcohol dehydrogenase	Ethanol, chloral hydrate
Hydrolysis Reactions	
Ester hydrolysis	Ester local anesthetics, succinylcholine, acetyl-salicyclic acid, propanidid Amide local anesthetics
Conjugation Reactions (Phase II)	
Glucuronide	Oxazepam, lorazepam, morphine nalorphine, codeine, fentanyl, naloxone
Sulfate	Paracetanol, morphine, isoproterenol, cimetidine
Methylation	Norepinephrine
Acetylation	Procainamide
Amino Acid	Salicyclic acid
Mercapturic	Sulfbromothalein
Glutathione	Paracetamol

(Adapted from Tucker GT: Drug metabolism. *Br J Anaesth* 51:603–618, 1979.)

Table 6-3

Kinetics of Drugs in Neonates, Children, and Adults

	Plasma half-life (hr)		
Drug	Newborn	Infant/ Child	Adult
Morphine[43]	2.7	2.1–2.4	0.9–4.3
Mepivacaine[101]	8.7	—	3.2
Lidocaine[102]	3.2	—	1.8
Etidocaine[103]	6.4	—	2.6
Carbamazepine[104]	8.2–28.1	10.3–20.7	16.4–26.6
Theophylline[6]	30.2	3.7	5.8
d-Tubocurarine[26]	2.9	1.5	1.5
Digoxin[2]	69	18	15–70
Gentamicin[2]	51–110	15–46	87–173
Thiopental[44,105]	19.9	6.1	12.0

Single sets of numbers represent mean values; all others are the range reported in each study.

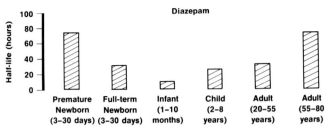

Figure 6-3. Changes in the elimination half-life with age. The elimination half-life is shortest in infants, and longest in neonates and the elderly. (Reproduced with permission. Rowland and Tozer, Clinical Pharmacokinetics. pp. 218–229, Lea and Febiger, Philadelphia, 1980. (Adapted from the data of Morselli, P.L., Spectrum Publications, N.Y., 1977, pp 311 and 456, and from the data of Klotz et al. J. Clin. Invest. 55:347, 1975).

DRUG METABOLISM IN THE INFANT AND CHILD

The initial phase of reduced metabolic clearance in the neonate is followed by a phase of marked increase in metabolic activity, mainly for phase I reactions in the infant and child.[2,7,28,32,34] The enhanced capacity of children to metabolize or clear drugs now has been confirmed in a number of studies (Table 6-3), (Figure 6-3). The mechanisms that regulate these activities in humans are not clear. One possibility is the relative size of the liver, which decreases from birth to puberty (Table 6-1).[24] In the neonate, the liver volume is 4 percent relative to body weight, but then the neonatal enzyme systems are immature. In contrast, the liver represents only 2 percent relative to body weight in the adult. From infancy to early childhood, the liver enzymes mature, but the volume of liver in relation to body weight remains at about 4 percent.[8,24] It has been suggested that it is the increased proportion of liver to body weight that causes the enhanced metabolic rate of children. None of these hypotheses have been proved, however, and probably several other factors are also involved.

The demonstrated decrease in half-lives of drugs suggests enhanced clearance in infants and children in comparison with either neonates or adults, particularly for drugs metabolized in the liver (Table 6-3, Figure 6-3). The change is rather striking in that the disposition of drugs goes from about 25 percent of the adult value in the neonate to two to six times the adult value in the child.[42] For example, it has been shown for the antiepileptic agents, phenobarbital and phenytoin, that usual adult doses (calculated as mg/kg) administered to children resulted in a lower serum concentration.[42] Children weighing 10–20 kilograms had the lowest concentration for a given dose. These changes could not be attributed to differences in distribution volume or enteral absorption. Thus, we may pass quickly from a situation of overdosing a neonate to a situation of underdosing an infant and child. The increased metabolic activity associated with childhood is first seen at about three months, peaks at about two to three years, and then gradually declines until reaching adult values after puberty.[2,6,9,28] An entirely different pharmacodynamic effect may thus be observed in the infant, the neonate, and the adult.

The capacity for enhanced metabolic clearance in children also has been observed for some anesthetic drugs, including morphine, thiopental, and muscle relaxants (Table 6-3).[43,44] The higher ED_{95} doses and the faster recovery from twitch paralysis in children compared with adults for pancuronium and metocurine can be explained on the basis of enhanced hepatic excretion or metabolic clearance of drug.[45] Similarly, for vecuronium, a muscle relaxant with high liver clearance, the ED_{95} dose and the recovery from twitch paralysis were consistently faster in the 2–10-year-olds, compared with the 11–17-year-olds.[46] On the other hand, the pharmacokinetic study of d-tubocurarine did not confirm this finding, probably because this drug is excreted unmetabolized by the kidney and therefore not subject to the influences of hepatic maturation.[26] The rapid recovery of motor function in the child compared with the adult following tetracaine spinal anesthesia, too, may be related to the enhanced kinetics in children.[47]

DEVELOPMENTAL CHANGES IN THE KIDNEY

Although many drugs and metabolites are excreted through the bile, the main route of excretion is the kidney, both for intact drugs and for drug metabolites produced at other sites. The healthy full-term infant has the same number of nephrons as an adult. Similar to the liver, the ratio of the kidney size to body mass is twofold higher in the newborn in comparison with the adult (Table 6-1).[24] However, the glomeruli and tubules are small, and the organ is anatomically and functionally immature.

GLOMERULAR FUNCTION IN NEONATES AND INFANTS

The glomerulus acts as a filter, retaining red cells and other formed elements with molecular weights larger than 70,000. The rate of glomerular filtration of a drug or metabolite (renal clearance) is dependent on the rate of blood flow through the glomeruli, the unbound fraction of drug, the area of the glomerulus, and the filtration pressure.[9] All of these factors, in turn, are influenced by age. Glomerular function in infants born before 34 weeks gestation is markedly depressed.[49,50] In utero, between 34–36 weeks gestation the

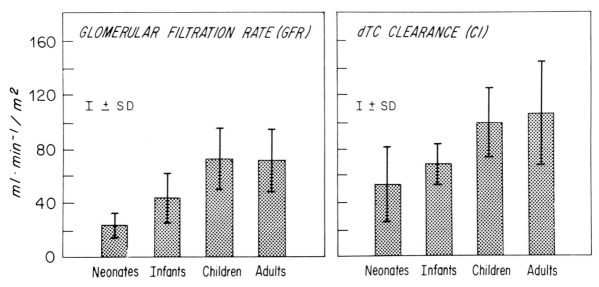

Figure 6-4. Known values for glomerular filtration are compared to dTC clearance. dTC clearance changes pari passu with maturation of renal function. (Reproduced with permission from Fisher DM, et al: *Anesthesiology* 57:203–208, 1982.)

glomeruli mature considerably. Thus, in infants born after this period, the postnatal development of glomerular and tubular function increases at the same rate as in normal infants.[50] Children born before the 34th to 36th week, however, develop full glomerular function much more slowly. Preterm infants therefore require special consideration, at least for the first month.[50] At birth, the glomerular filtration rate (GFR) is 2–4 ml/min in the full-term newborn. Preterm infants may have GFRs as low as 0.7–0.8 ml/min. As indicated, the GFR in children born after 34 weeks gestation increases rapidly to 8–20 ml/min after the first few days of life, compared with 2–3 ml/min in the premature.[49,51]

The increase in GFR with age is attributable to several factors, including increased cardiac output, changes in renal vascular resistance, which alter regional blood flow, and permeability changes in the glomerulus. Maturation of glomerular function is complete at about five to six months. Relative to anesthetic drugs the importance of the maturation of glomerular function relative to drug elimination has been shown for d-tubocurarine, which is almost exclusively dependent on the glomerular filtration for elimination (Figure 6-4). Additional drugs eliminated by glomerular filtration include the other long-acting muscle relaxants, the aminoglycoside antibiotics, the H_2-receptor blockers, and digoxin.

TUBULAR FUNCTION IN NEONATES AND INFANTS

The renal tubular system resorbs most of the protein-free glomerular filtrate. It also secretes several substances, including the xenobiotics (e.g., penicillin). Tubular function at birth is depressed in comparison with the adult as measured by the transport of glucose, phosphate, bicarbonate, and para-aminohippuric acid secretion. Maturation of the tubules lags slightly behind maturation of the glomeruli, reaching adult levels at about 35 weeks of life for full-term infants. Reasons for reduced tubular capacity include low blood flow to peritubular regions, immaturity of the energy supplying pro-

cess, and small mass of both the tubular working cells and the tubules themselves.[49–52] Passive reabsorption also may be reduced in the infant and newborn.[53] As in the case of the liver, kidney function can be induced in selected cases, producing some unexpected high rates of elimination.[52,56,57]

CLINICAL IMPLICATIONS

It is understandable that drugs or metabolites that depend on the kidney for their excretion are disposed of at very low rates in the newborn and young infant, in comparison with adults. Exceptions to this would include conditions referred to earlier that enhance kidney function in the neonate.[56,57] Impairment of renal drug excretion can have important therapeutic and toxicologic implications. The low clearance and long half-life of antibiotics, such as gentamicin, kanamycin, and digoxin, which are filtered by the glomerulus, or compounds like penicillin, digitoxin, and the sulfonamides, which are excreted by the tubules, are a good example of how renal function may modify the kinetics of several drugs, increasing the toxic effects to the newborn or the small child.[2] Thus, during the first few months of life, although the loading dose is increased to account for the increased volume of distribution of the drug, the dosing intervals also may have to be increased.

It is also important to remember that many pathologic states, such as heart failure, malnutrition, hypovolemia, respiratory distress syndrome, and hyperbilirubinemia, can modify renal function.[53–55] During these pathologic states the dosing interval should be increased, and whenever possible, blood levels should be monitored. Little information is available on renal drug excretion in older infants and children in comparison with neonates and adults. Peak renal capacity is reached at about two to three years, after which it appears to decrease at a rate of about 2.5 percent per year.[28] The exact cause of this phenomenon is unclear, but it is not clinically significant until later years, because of the tremendous reserve humans have in kidney function.

Table 6-4

Percent Plasma-Protein Binding of Various Drugs in
Newborn Infants, Adults, and Pregnant Women

Drug	Newborn Infants	Adults	Pregnant Women
Ampicillin	10	22	—
Atropine	31	39	—
Diazepam	84	96	—
Lidocaine	31	67	52
Morphine	31	42	—
Propranolol	57	85	80
d-Tubocurarine	31	43	41
Thiopental	87	93	—

(Adapted from Ehrnebo M, et al: *Eur J Clin Pharmacol* 3:189–193, 1971; Morselli, PL: *Clin Pharmacokinet* 1:189–193, 1976; Wood M, et al: *Clin Pharmacol Ther* 29:522–526, 1981.)

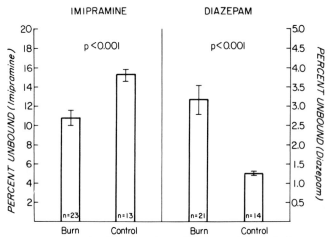

Figure 6-5. The free fraction of imipramine and diazepam in burned and healthy patients. The free fraction of imipramine from burn patients (left) is lower in comparison to healthy controls, whereas percent unbound diazepam in all samples from burn patients is higher than that of healthy controls. (Reproduced from Martyn JAJ, et al: Plasma protein binding of drugs after burn injury. *Clin Pharmacol Ther* 35:535–539, 1984 with permission.)

PLASMA PROTEINS

BINDING PROTEINS

Many drugs are highly bound to plasma proteins. The activity of such drugs is likely to depend more on the unbound than on the total drug concentration. Two major binding proteins have been identified in human plasma; albumin and alpha-acid glycoprotein (AAG).[58,59] AAG is a component of alpha-globulin. Other binding proteins in the globulin fraction include lipoprotein and hemoglobin. Drug molecules bind to proteins through weak van der Waals forces, and these are low affinity associations which are easily reversible. Albumin binds preferentially to acidic drugs.[58] Lipoprotein, AAG, and the globulins usually bind to basic drugs, although some basic drugs bind to albumin alone.[9,59] Drugs that bind predominantly to albumin include the antipyretics, antiepileptics, benzodiazepenes, and barbiturates, whereas drugs that bind to AAG include the neuroleptics, narcotics, muscle relaxants, local anesthetics, and β-blockers.

EFFECT OF AGE AND DISEASE

Albumin, AAG, and total protein concentrations increase with gestational age but still are low at birth. Qualitatively, too, the albumin and globulin are different, having a lower binding capacity in the neonate.[60] It is interesting to note that during delivery the total protein and albumin concentrations, as well as the binding capacity of some drugs, are decreased in the maternal blood in comparison with cord blood, a factor that could result in drug transfer from mother to fetus.[19,61] Thus, plasma binding of some drugs in newborn infants, adults, and pregnant mothers can be significantly different (Table 6-4).

Chronic disease states and any form of inflammation can cause changes in albumin and AAG concentrations.[59,62,63] In these situations albumin concentrations usually decrease, while AAG concentrations increase. Changes in the amounts of these proteins and their capacity to bind drugs may be striking and quite different during these times, causing changes in both pharmacokinetics and pharmacodynamics. The ability of the pediatric patient to respond similarly to the adult in terms of stress protein release has been verified in the burned patient (Figure 6-5). Using diazepam and imipramine as model drugs,

it has been shown that alterations in binding can be profound and can persist as long as the stress and inflammation are present.[62] Clinically significant alterations in binding also can occur due to competition between drugs or endogenous substances. Examples of these include interactions between phenytoin and valproic acid, or antibiotics and bilirubin.[63,64]

PHARMACODYNAMIC EFFECTS OF ALTERED BINDING

It is the concentration of free drug that reaches the target organ, which is generally assumed to be responsible for the effect. Alterations in free fractions (FF) are most likely to occur and to have greatest impact in drugs that are extensively bound. For a drug that is 99 percent bound (FF = 0.01), a decrease in binding to 98 percent results in a doubling of the FF to 0.02. A decrease in plasma binding due to age or disease will result in an increased distribution of drug to the extravascular tissues and increased drug availability at the target organ. That is, the apparent volume of distribution of the drug will increase. This may partly explain the marked respiratory depression observed in the neonate following morphine administration. Increased binding will give opposite results, causing a higher drug requirement for the same effect.[65,66] When alterations in binding occur, the therapeutic concentration range will need to be shifted to achieve the appropriate unbound fraction and effect. For a drug that is less extensively bound (for example, FF = 0.20), the same absolute change in FF as above (i.e., from 0.20 to 0.21) is inconsequential and causes undetectable changes in pharmacodynamics. In addition to changes in pharmacodynamics, alterations in binding also present difficulties in the interpretation of therapeutic plasma concentrations. Most clinical laboratories report total (free plus bound) drug concentrations. Thus, one has the added difficulty of determining whether the reported concentrations are therapeutic, toxic, or subtherapeutic.

PHARMACOKINETIC EFFECTS OF ALTERED BINDING

Depending on the drug, changes in binding can also alter distribution and elimination. One can, with caution, generalize about some of the kinetic effects of altered binding. For high extraction drugs (see below), changes in protein binding will have little effect on hepatic clearance.[67,68] For drugs with low hepatic extraction, changes in binding become important relative to clearance, especially for highly bound drugs. Decreased binding serves to increase the fraction available for clearance. In the absence of change in the unbound clearance, the total concentration will decrease, whereas the free concentration will remain the same.[69] With increased binding, the fraction available for pharmacologic effect will decrease, as will the fraction for clearance. Therefore, in the absence of change in the unbound clearance, the total concentration will increase, but the free concentration will remain the same. Thus, during chronic drug administration, if the clearance remains the same, changes in binding are not important.[69] The total concentration will be increased or decreased in the same direction as binding. Thus, the dose should not be changed. During an acute single dose, however, the FF may be quite important. An increased FF results in increased distribution to peripheral tissues, and clearance is not a factor, although this has not been well demonstrated clinically. Similarly, in the kidney, alterations in binding will have little effect on drugs actively secreted by the tubules. However, when a drug is excreted by glomerular filtration, since only free drug is filtered across the membrane, increased binding will result in decreased glomerular excretion of drug and vice versa.

DRUG-INTERACTION

Drug interaction is said to occur when the pharmacokinetics or pharmacodynamics of one drug are altered by another. Antagonism or potentiation due to drug interaction is a well-known phenomenon. In many cases this effect is due to pharmacokinetic rather than pharmacodynamic factors. The clinical problem of drug-drug interactions, however, has been vastly overestimated, and only a few are potentially dangerous.[70]

DRUG INTERACTION IN ABSORPTION AND DISTRIBUTION

Drug interaction in the gut usually is due to binding or chelation of one drug by the other, resulting in decreased absorption (e.g., antacid and tetracycline, antacid and cimetidine). Inhibition of gastric emptying by drugs also can affect peak plasma concentrations. However, potentiation due to competitive binding between drugs or between a drug and endogenous substances in the plasma or tissues has been known to occur. Many examples of potentiation have been reported in the literature, including the combination of warfarin and antipyretics, sulfonamides and bilirubin, and antipyretics and phenytoin. When a drug is displaced in this manner, the FF increases in the plasma and the volume of distribution of displaced drug will increase.[71] As indicated previously, however, since the FF increases, the total concentration will decrease with time, provided the free clearance does not change (see below).[72] If the displacement period is brief and elimination rapid, displacement should have little clinical significance. If displacement causes an increase in the free fraction for a prolonged period, however, toxic effects can ensue from combined agents, such as warfarin and chloral hydrate, and the many others enumerated above. Potentiation of one muscle relaxant by another is known to occur, and is not due to competitive binding or altered pharmacokinetics. Rather it is due to the different sites of action of muscle relaxants on the myoneural junction.[73]

DRUG INTERACTION-RENAL EFFECTS

Drugs can interfere with the excretion of other drugs from the kidney by causing alterations of the pH and GFR, or by competitively interfering with tubular secretion.[72] Probenicid can be used to decrease renal elimination of many drugs in order to increase their efficacy. This drug acts by inhibiting tubular secretion of weak acids. Examples of drugs enhanced by probenicid include the penicillins, the cephalosporins, and methotrexate. Certain anti-inflammatory drugs, such as indomethacin, decrease renal clearance of some drugs by inhibiting prostaglandin synthesis. Several other drugs affect the renal excretion; these include digoxin, cimetidine, quinidine, and furosemide. Increased elimination of drugs by the kidney can be induced by drugs or during treatment of pathologic states, such as burns and multiple trauma, which increase renal blood flow.[52,56,57,74]

DRUG INTERACTION-METABOLISM

Many drugs stimulate or inhibit the hepatic microsomal enzyme system, thereby altering blood levels and clinical effects. Increases in the body's drug metabolizing capacity occur mainly because of changes in the rate of synthesis of microsomal enzyme systems. For example, phenobarbital produces a reversible increase in liver weight, with an increase in the endoplasmic reticulum.[9,71] Potent enzyme inducers include the barbiturates, rifampin, and phenytoin. Many drugs can induce their own metabolism. Induction or inhibition can also occur due to environmental pollutants. As with the kidney, increased elimination of drugs dependent on flow rate for clearance occurs when blood flow increases to the liver. This is observed, for example, in hypermetabolic states (see below).[75]

Inhibition of drug metabolism can occur due to substrate competition, interference with drug transport, depletion of hepatic glycogen (starvation), and functional impairment due to hepatotoxicity.[76] Inhibition of drug metabolism often results in unexpected therapeutic or adverse effects, but in some instances it can be used to advantage in preventing accumulations of toxic metabolites. For example, cimetidine, which inhibits the cytochrome p450 enzyme system, has been used to prevent the formation of hepatotoxic oxidative metabolites following acetaminophen overdose.[77] It has also been used in animals to decrease the formation of oxidative metabolites following halothane administration.[78] Cimetidine affects only phase I reactions and spares phase II reactions.[77] Of the drugs used in anesthesia, lidocaine, diazepam, morphine, and fentanyl have been documented to interact with cimetidine.[79-82] Contrary to previous reports, recent studies indicate that ranitidine may also have similar effects to cimetidine, although not as prominent.[83]

Other drugs that have been shown to inhibit hepatic drug metabolism include disulfuram, propoxyphene, allopurinol, phenylbutazone, isoniazid, neuroleptics, and tricyclic antidepressants. β-blockers and vasodilator drugs may inhibit the elimination of hepatic flow-dependent drugs by decreasing hepatic blood flow as well as competitively inhibiting enzyme activity. Of the drugs used during anesthesia, it is important to remember the inhibitory effects on metabolism of the neuroleptics, cimetidine, and the β-blockers.[79–85] β-blockers, by their effect on hepatic blood flow, have been shown to affect the disposition of lidocaine.[82] Chlorpromazine and other phenothiazenes have been shown to have inhibitory effects on the metabolism of meperidine, the tricyclics, and phenytoin.[84,85] All of these interactions may be of clinical importance because of the narrow therapeutic index.

BASIC PRINCIPLES OF CLINICAL PHARMACOKINETICS

As indicated before, multiple factors can alter the intensity of the therapeutic or toxic effects of drugs in the pediatric patient. The quantitative study of the combined effect of all of these factors (e.g., absorption, distribution, biotransformation, and excretion) is called pharmacokinetics. Presentation of the pharmacokinetic properties of every drug used in anesthesia is beyond the scope of this chapter. However, the basic principles, definitions, and equations relevant to pharmacokinetic analysis will be reviewed. Precise description of drug kinetics requires the determination of drug concentrations, usually in plasma, and the use of complex mathematical models to describe kinetic processes. The relatively simple concepts obtained from these calculations, however, usually are sufficient for quantitative guidance during clinical use.

ONE-COMPARTMENT MODEL AND FIRST-ORDER KINETICS

The measurement of drug concentration over time forms the basis of all pharmacokinetic analyses. This relationship of drug concentration over time can be described in terms of drug distribution in one or more theoretical compartments. It is important to point out that these compartments do not represent specific anatomical entities, such as circulating volume, ECF volume, and so forth. Rather, they describe the behavior of different drugs in the body due to its own kinetic properties. The simplest model, the "one-compartment model," assumes that immediately after administration, the drug instantly attains the maximum distribution volume, reaching all areas of the body, including the plasma, extracellular fluid, peripheral tissues, or any combination of these. The one-compartment model can be represented schematically as in Figure 6-6A. The drug is injected into, distributed throughout, and then eliminated from one compartment. C is the concentration of drug in the compartment, V is the volume, and CV is the amount of drug in the compartment. Before the elimination process begins, CV is equal to the dose administered. This model assumes that the drug is completely absorbed, as occurs with intravenous administration, attains instantaneous equilibration, and then eliminated from the same compartment (Figure 6-6A).

As a result of the eliminating processes, the plasma concentration decreases gradually over time. The plot of concentration versus time gives a monoexponential curve, with declining concentration (Figure 6-6B). The line is extrapolated

at both ends, since one cannot physically or practically measure the concentration at time zero, (t_0), and drug concentrations are too low to be measured at the end of a test period.

Elimination from the body occurs as a first-order process, and is said to display linear kinetics. Described in terms of a chemical reaction, this means the rate of the reaction (drug clearance) is proportional to one of the reactants (the drug). That is, a constant *proportion* of the drug is excreted from the body for each unit of time, and the rate of change (elimination) is related to the magnitude of the variable. However, the *amount* of drug excreted for each unit of time declines from beginning to end of the test period.

When the decline is exponential, the ordinate can be replotted on a logarithmic axis, which converts the concentration–time curve to a straight line (Figure 6-6C). The slope (change in log plasma concentration over change in time) of a monoexponential curve has the same value at each point on the curve. Now the concentration at t_0 and the slope of the curve (K) can be more easily determined. The following differential equation is used to describe the events shown in Figures 6-6B and 6-6C (or the change in drug concentration with time),

$$\frac{dc}{dt} = -K \cdot C_t \qquad (1)$$

where dc/dt is the change in plasma concentration at time t. This interval, which is usually very small, is called the instantaneous slope. Since the concentration is decreasing, it has a negative sign. C_t is the concentration in plasma at time t, t is the time, usually in hours, and K is the proportionality constant. Thus, the change in concentration for each unit of time is equal to K times the concentration at time t. The proportionality constant, also called the rate constant, has reciprocal units of time (e.g., 1/hr).

The differential equation (1), describing the movement of drug in a one-compartment model (Figures 6-6B and 6-6C), can be integrated to give the following equation,

$$C_t = C_0 \cdot e^{-Kt} \qquad (2)$$

where C_t is the plasma concentration at time t, C_0 is the concentration at time 0 when equilibration is instantaneous and no elimination has taken place, and e is the base of the natural logarithms and is numerically equal to 2.718. A negative sign is used before K (proportionality constant) because the concentration is decreasing with time, t is the time, usually in hours.

None of the anesthetic drugs have a one-compartmental distribution, either in the pediatric or adult population, and all of the anesthetic drugs studied in children have first-order kinetics (see Nonlinear Kinetics, below).

ELIMINATION HALF-LIFE

Using equation (2) for a one-compartment model, one can calculate or predict the concentration of the drug at a given point in time. To do so, values must be obtained for C_0 and K. Measuring C_0 in the clinical situation is not practical. However, C_0 can be determined from the graph in Figure 6-6B by extrapolation, and K by drawing a tangent to the curve. Still, both equation (2) and Figure 6-6B are mathematically and graphically inconvenient. Plotting concentration versus time on a logarithmic scale, as in Figure 6-6C, transforms the curve to a straight line and simplifies the determination of C_0 and the slope (concentration/time = $\Delta y/\Delta x$). Alternatively, equation (2) can be transformed to natural logarithms. Taking natural logs,

$$\ln C_t = \ln (C_0 \cdot e^{-Kt})$$
$$= \ln C_0 + \ln e^{-Kt} \qquad (3)$$
$$= \ln C_0 - Kt$$

Similarly, equation (3) can also be written in $\log_{10}$. Since $\ln = \log \times 2.303$, equation (3) becomes

$$2.303 \log C_t = 2.303 \log C_0 - Kt \qquad (4)$$
$$\log C_t = \log C_0 - \frac{Kt}{2.303}$$

This equation describes the straight line logarithmic plot in Figure 6-6C.

The slope (K) characterizes the magnitude of the first-order process. The steeper the slope, the faster the elimination or disappearance of the drug from the central compartment.

The more commonly used measure of disappearance of drug is the half-life. The half-life ($T\frac{1}{2}$) is defined as that time required for the drug concentration to decrease by 50 percent. The half-life can be calculated easily from Figure 6-6B or 6-6C, as indicated. Since it is a first-order process, $T\frac{1}{2}$ is not dependent on the concentration, and therefore the point on the curve chosen for calculation is inconsequential. Thus, from Figures 6-6B and 6-6C, the time it takes for the concentration t to go from 50 to 25 is the same as it takes to go from 12.5 to 6.25. The elimination rate constant and half-life are related in the following manner. From equation (2) we know that

$$C_t = C_0 e^{-Kt}$$

Since the elimination half-life is also the time taken for the concentration and the amount of drug to decrease by half, it follows that

$$0.5 = e^{-K \cdot T_{1/2}}$$
$$\frac{1}{2} = \frac{1}{e^{K \cdot T_{1/2}}}$$
$$2 = e^{K \cdot T_{1/2}}$$
$$\ln 2 = K \cdot T_{1/2} \qquad (5)$$
$$T_{1/2} = \frac{0.693}{K}$$
$$T_{1/2} = \frac{\ln 2}{K} \qquad (6)$$

The concept of half-life is easily understood and useful in calculating dosing intervals. It is important to remember, however, that $T_{1/2}$ is a dependent variable, related to the two physiologically and pharmacologically important independent variables, *clearance* (Cl) and *volume of distribution* (Vd), in the following way,

$$T_{1/2} = \frac{\ln 2 \cdot Vd}{Cl}$$

such that changes in either clearance or distribution will change the half-life. This relationship is important since dur-

ing drug infusion or chronic dosing regimens, the steady-state plasma concentrations achieved are related *only* to clearance (a steady state is defined as input equaling output). After a single dose, however, the distribution may be important in defining the duration of the pharmacologic effect (e.g., thiopental). One should not be confused and equate $T_{1/2}$ with clearance (as is generally the case) *or* with duration of effect. As noted above, it is a dependent variable, and a simple function of the physiologically pertinent independent variables. The marked effects of age and maturity on $T_{1/2}$ were discussed above.

NONLINEAR KINETICS

For some drugs, the disposition follows a nonlinear, or zero-order, kinetics. Again, in terms of a chemical reaction, this implies that the rate of the reaction (clearance) is *independent* of the concentration of the reactants (drugs) and a function only of the amount of enzyme available for biotransformation. In other words, the amount (not proportion) of drug eliminated is constant. Nonlinear kinetics occurs because the enzymatic pathways involved in the metabolism become saturated with the drug. This dose-dependent maximum metabolizing capacity is described by the Michaelis–Menten equation,

$$\frac{dc}{dt} = \frac{Vm \cdot C}{Km + C} \qquad (7)$$

where, $\frac{dc}{dt}$ is the change in plasma concentration at time t; Vm is the theoretical maximum removal of drug; Km is the Michaelis–Menten constant, or that drug concentration at which elimination is half the maximum rate. When the enzyme system is saturated, small changes in dose will lead to greater serum concentrations than would be expected from dose versus serum concentration curves obtained prior to saturation.

Plotting serum concentration versus time on a linear graph gives a straight line (Figure 6-6D). In a logarithmic plot of these data, a curvilinear plot is obtained. Since a constant amount of drug is being removed, the decrease in concentration is slow, and the initial part of the plot is curved. At or below maximal velocity of enzymatic saturation, the disappearance follows first-order kinetics, and the concentration–time plot gives a curved line on an arithmetic scale (Figure 6-6D). The concept of nonlinear pharmacokinetics has been reviewed by Wagner.[86] Drugs that have been demonstrated to have zero-order kinetics in children include phenytoin and aspirin.[9] Alcohol and thiopental have been shown to have zero-order kinetics in adults.[87] There is no reason to believe that this should not be the same in children. To date, thiopental is the only anesthetic documented to have zero-order kinetics.[87]

PHARMACOKINETIC MODELS

The one-compartment model does not depict the true behavior of the majority of drugs.[88] For many intravenously administered drugs, the concentration–time plot results in an initial steep decline in the concentration followed by a more gradual decline. The two–compartment behavior can be represented graphically as in Figure 6-6E. The initial decline in concentration is due to the movement of drug (initial distribution phase) from high blood flow (brain, liver, kidney, heart) to low blood flow groups (muscle, fat, skin). This distribution phase is also called the α phase. As in all biologic (exponential) processes, it takes four to five half-lives for the distribution

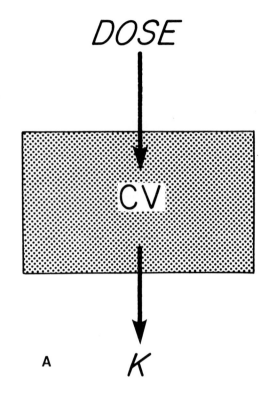

A

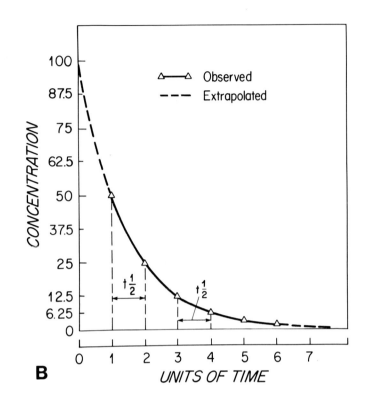

B

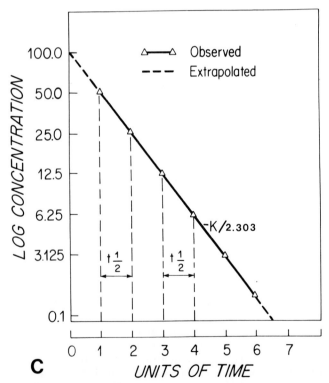

C

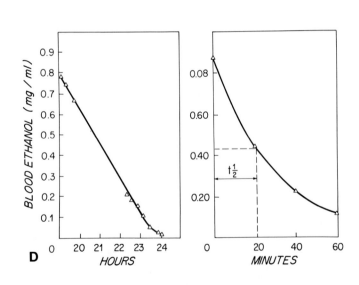

D

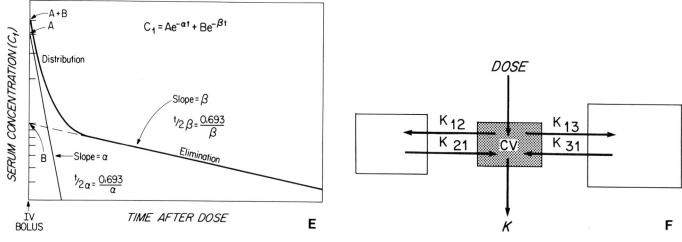

Figure 6-6. One-compartment model, showing that absorption (or injection), distribution, and elimination all occur in one compartment. (Fig. A) K characterizes the rate of elimination. The concentration of drug (C) in the compartment times the volume (V) of the compartment gives the amount of drug in the compartment. (Fig. B) One-compartment model concentration-time curve shows that ploting concentration on an arithmetic scale results in a monoexponential curve. The time required to decrease the concentration to 50 percent from any point is always constant (first-order process). (Fig. C) Concentration v time on a logarithmic scale. Plotting the concentration on a log scale converts the curve to a straight line. Extrapolation to t_0, or the concentration at time zero, is easier. K (slope) is the elimination rate constant. (Fig. D) Zero-order rate of elimination. Following a large dose of ethanol, the decline in plasma concentration is a straight line on an arithmetic scale. At lower concentrations 24 hours later, a change from zero-order to first-order kinetics is observed. (Adapted from Marshall and Fritz; *J Pharmacol Exp Ther* 109:431–443, 1953.) (Fig. E) Log plasma concentration v time in a two-compartment model; α and β are half-lives of the distribution and elimination phases, respectively. (Fig. F) Three-compartment model. One central and two peripheral compartments. The rate constants for intercompartmental transfer of drugs is shown. As in most instances, elimination occurs from the central compartment.

process to complete itself. During and after the distribution phase, the elimination or β phase begins. During this phase a pseudoequilibrium is reached between the plasma and other tissues. The biexponential behavior of the drug indicates that it is being distributed into two compartments. The drug enters the central compartment and then is distributed to a peripheral compartment. These compartments have no correlation with a specific anatomical entity; however, the central compartment usually corresponds to plasma, blood, extracellular fluid, and high blood flow organs. The peripheral compartment often consists of muscle, skin, and fat, and generally is larger than the central compartment.

In most situations it is extremely difficult to accurately evaluate the distribution phase in the central compartment. This is due to the fact that this process occurs so rapidly it is almost impossible to obtain blood samples frequently enough to document it. Immediately after injection, the drug has neither been distributed nor eliminated (see point A + B in Figure 6-6E). From this point on, three processes begin to occur simultaneously; (1) the drug is distributed from the central compartment to the peripheral compartment, by first-order kinetics, with a rate constant of K_{12}, (2) the drug can be diffused back into the central compartment at this time, as well as when the concentration in the central compartment decreases relative to the peripheral compartment by first-order kinetics at a rate constant of K_{21}, and (3) elimination commences from the central compartment at a rate of K_e.

Thus, in the two-compartment model, two distinct phases of decline can be seen on the plasma concentration–time curve (Figure 6-6E). The slower elimination phase has a slope of β. This can be extrapolated to meet the ordinate at B, which

would have been the drug concentration had equilibrium occurred in all tissues instantaneously. If extrapolated points from β are subtracted from the corresponding measured plasma values in the distribution phase and the residuals plotted, a straight line is obtained. This is called the feathering or residuals technique. The slope of this line is called α, and it intercepts the vertical axis at point A in Figure 6-6E. From this the $T_{1/2\alpha}$, or half-life of the distribution phase, can be calculated. $T_{1/2\alpha} = 0.693/\alpha$, where K is rate constant for the α phase. Similarly, the elimination rate constant is β and the half-life is equal to $0.693/\beta$. $T_{1/2}$ for α or β also can be derived from the graph by measuring the time taken for the concentrations to decrease by 50 percent.

The two-compartment model requires a biexponential equation for calculating drug elimination. The equation describing this curve is,

$$C_t = Ae^{-\alpha t} + Be^{-\beta t}$$

where C_t is the concentration at time t, A and B are the intercepts, α and β are the elimination rate constants of the initial distribution and subsequent elimination phases, respectively, e is the exponent (numerically equal to 2.718), and t is the time.

The pharmacokinetic model is only an aid to interpreting the data, and as has been previously noted, it is not physiologically based. A third exponent, called the P (π slope, is used when the drug behaves as if it distributes into three compartments (Figure 6-6F). Drug administration and elimination take place in the central compartment. In addition, this model has an intermediate compartment (P) as well as the peripheral compartment (B). Hence, each of the peripheral compartments has a different rate constant of disappearance (whether it is due to distribution or elimination), as shown in Figure 6-6F. Equation (7) describes this three-compartment model.

$$C_t = Ae^{-\alpha t} + Pe^{-\pi t} + Be^{-\beta t}$$

Where A is the intercept at the ordinate for the rapid distribution phase, α is the rate constant for the rapid distribution phase, P is the intercept for the slower intermediate phase, π is the rate constant for the intermediate phase, B is the intercept at time zero for the elimination phase, and β is the rate constant for the terminal elimination phase.

Drugs used in anesthesia, such as fentanyl, thiopental, and d-tubocurarine, have occasionally been described by a three-compartment model.[89-91] The presence of a third compartment suggests that a drug has been distributed to two sets of tissues, which have different capacities for retaining or binding the drug.[9] More complex models have been described but require extensive mathematical manipulation and possibly the use of several kinetic models. The fact that most drugs studied in children have shown distribution patterns consistent with a two-compartment model may be related to inadequate sampling times.

PHARMACOKINETIC PARAMETERS/VOLUME OF DISTRIBUTION

The distribution volume (V_d) of a drug is a measure of how the drug is distributed in the body. In the simplest one-compartment model the drug is administered intravenously and distributed instantaneously (Figure 6-6A). The concentration in the compartment at time zero is calculated as follows.

$$C_0 = \frac{Dose}{V_d} \qquad (8)$$

C_0, drug concentration at time zero, is calculated by extrapolation as described previously. If drug elimination has occurred, then equation (8) can be extended to calculate the amount of drug in the body,

$$C_t = \frac{amount\ of\ drug\ in\ body\ at\ time\ t}{V_d}$$

where C_t is the concentration of drug at any time. Restated in terms of the volume of distribution, we have

$$V_d = \frac{amount\ of\ drug\ in\ the\ body\ at\ time\ t}{C_t} \qquad (9)$$

When two or more compartments are present, one can calculate the volume of distribution for each of the compartments. In this case, the central compartment is called V_1, the peripheral compartments are V_2, V_3, and so forth. The total volume of distribution is usually denoted as V_d.

In the two-compartment model, the terms A, B, α, and β are hybrid coefficients. The magnitude of these coefficients depends on the combined effects of K_e, K_{21}, K_{12}, V_1, and V_2. These coefficients are used to calculate the pharmacokinetic parameters. For a comprehensive description of the mathematical steps and theory, the reader is referred to the works of Roland and Tozer, and Gibaldi.[92,93]

V_d can be calculated by many methods. For the two-compartment model, the area method is simple and useful. This method assumes that during the β phase changes in plasma concentration in the central compartment will reflect changes in other tissues. Here,

V_d (area) =

$$\frac{Dose}{\beta\left(\begin{array}{c} area\ under\ the\ serum\ concen- \\ tration\ curve\ from\ t = 0\ to\ t = \infty \end{array}\right)} = \frac{D}{\beta\left(\dfrac{A}{\alpha} + \dfrac{B}{\beta}\right)} \qquad (10)$$

and the volume of the central compartment is

$$V_1 = \frac{Dose}{A + B} \qquad (11)$$

The calculation of these coefficients has been discussed already. From these, V_2 (or the volume of the peripheral compartment) can be calculated quite simply as $V_d = V_1 + V_2$.

Another method commonly used to calculate V_d is the steady-state method. To achieve a steady state, one maintains the infusion long enough to ensure that the amount of drug lost by elimination equals the amount of drug infused, that is, the net transfer between the central and peripheral compartments is zero.

$$V_{d(ss)} = V_1 \frac{(K_{12} + K_{21})}{K_{21}} \qquad (12)$$

This calculation cannot be used for determining V_d after a single, bolus dose.[3,93]

The V_d is an estimate of the uptake of drug by tissues. The unit of measurement for V_d is liters/kilogram (l/kg) and values can vary widely. Drugs, such as antipyrine and muscle relaxants, do not distribute extensively, and have a V_d very close to plasma volume. Lipophilic drugs, such as the narcotics and diazepam, are extensively taken up by the tissues, and in such instances, the distribution volume can exceed one l/kg. Although this may seem impossible, bear in mind that this is a hypothetical volume, and just an expression of the ratio between plasma concentration and total drug in the body. It has no anatomical basis. Increased protein binding will decrease the V_d. The effect of age and protein binding on the distribution volume of drugs in children has been discussed earlier.

PHARMACOKINETIC PARAMETERS— CLEARANCE

Clearance is a measure of the efficiency of the eliminating process, and usually is considered to be removal of the drug from the central compartment. It is that volume of blood from which the drug is completely eliminated for each unit of time. The units are l/min/kg. The organs usually involved in clearance are the liver, kidney, gastrointestinal tract, and lung. For the one-compartment model clearance (Cl) is calculated as follows:

$$Cl = \frac{0.693 \cdot V_d}{T_{1/2\beta}} = \beta V_d =$$

$$\frac{Dose}{\begin{array}{c} Area\ under\ the\ serum\ concentration \\ curve\ for\ t = 0\ to\ t = \infty \end{array}}$$

As is demonstrated by this relationship, an increase in the V_d also can result in an increase in half-life without a change in clearance. Therefore, as previously indicated, knowledge of the slope or half-life, although easy to calculate, should not be equated to clearance since it is influenced by V_d. Consequently, in evaluating the ability of the body or particular organ to eliminate a certain drug, determining the clearance is always preferable to determining the half-life. It is also important to remember that the upper limit of clearance is dependent upon the plasma flow through all of the elimination organs.[28,94,95] However, clearance of drugs like procaine, atracurium, and succinylcholine may actually exceed flow, since the blood itself is an organ of elimination (due to circulating esterases).

Hepatic Clearance

Total body clearance is the sum clearance of all of the organs. Considering first a single organ, e.g., the liver, clearance can be expressed as the blood flow (Q) times the extraction ratio (E),

$$Cl_{(Hep)} = Q \cdot E_{(Hep)} \qquad (13)$$

$$E_{(Hep)} = Ca - Cv/Ca$$

where Ca and Cv are the hepatic and portal venous drug concentrations, and $E_{(Hep)}$ is the extraction ratio of the liver.

According to equation (13) hepatic blood flow and the activity of the hepatic excretion system both can influence drug elimination. When all of the drug presented to the liver is metabolized or excreted, E is equivalent to 1. In other words, the hepatic clearance of the drug is limited by blood flow only. Generally speaking, if the extraction is greater than 0.7, the capacity of the enzyme to metabolize the drug is high, and clearance is dependent only on blood flow. Such drugs are called high clearance or blood flow-limited drugs. Blood flow through the liver is highly variable, however, even in normal individuals (where it can increase four times the normal mean). Thus, these normal variations, together with alterations in blood flow that arise from pathological states, such as burns, hepatic disease, heart failure, or thyroid disease, and from physiological states, such as exercise, posture, age, or eating, can have a profound effect on hepatic clearance.[9,94,95] Drugs with a high extraction ratio therefore undergo extensive first-pass metabolism when administered orally, since after oral administration the drug passes through the portal circulation and liver prior to reaching the systemic circulation, and therefore systemic bioavailability will be decreased.[95] Some examples of drugs with high extraction ratios are the antiarrhythmics, β-receptor antagonists, opiate agonists and antagonists, tricyclics, and methohexital (Table 6-5). Drugs that alter liver blood flow, such as isoproterenol, nitroglycerin, and propranolol, can affect their own metabolism or that of other drugs.

If the extraction ratio is low (<0.2), liver enzyme activity is the main factor that limits excretion. Increasing or decreasing the blood flow will have little effect.[94,95] Thus, the clearance is said to be capacity- (enzyme-) limited, or flow insensitive.[28,96] Drugs in this category will undergo minimal first-pass metabolism when taken orally. Since elimination of drugs in this category is related to intrinsic enzyme activity, enzyme induction or inhibition will cause changes in clearance independent

Table 6-5

Hepatic and Renal Extraction Ratios of Selected Drugs

Low	High
Hepatic Extraction	
Amobartital	Indocyanine green
Antipyrine	Isoproterenol
Carbamazepine	Labetalol
Diazepam	Lidocaine
Mepivacaine	Lorcainide
Phenytoin	Meperidine
Procainamide	Methohexital
Theophylline	Metoprolol
Warfarin	Morphine
	Amytriptyline
	Oxprenolol
	Pentazocine
	Propranolol
	Verapamil
Renal Extraction	
Acetazolamide	Glucuronides
Chlorpropamide	Penicillins
Cimetidine	Sulfates
Digoxin	Glycine conjugates
Gentamicin	
Phenobarbital	
Sulfaxazole	
Tetracycline	

(Adapted from Stanski and Watkins,[97] Rane,[28] and George.[95])

of flow. Drugs in this category include the barbiturates, benzodiazepenes, methylxanthines, and anticoagulants. For the capacity-limited drug the matter is further complicated by the binding characteristics of the drug. When only the free fraction (FF) is removed, the extraction ratio is equal to, or less than, the unbound fraction in plasma. If both free and bound drug are removed, the extraction ratio can exceed the unbound fraction.[94–96] In the former group, if the FF increases, then the clearance will increase and vice versa. Drugs in this group include phenytoin, the benzodiazepines, and chlorpromazine. Those not affected by binding include theophylline, chloramphenicol, and paracetamol.[28,96]

Renal Clearance

Similar to the liver, the kidney also exhibits flow-dependent and capacity-limited drug excretion. If all of the drug presented to the renal tubules is actively secreted, the drug is said to have a high extraction ratio. Examples of these include the penicillins and metabolized glycine sulfates and glucuronide conjugates of many drugs (Tabel 6-5). Since only part of the renal plasma flow reaches the glomerulus, and only part of this is filtered, drugs excreted by glomerular filtration will have a low extraction ratio. Similar to the liver, increases and decreases in the FF will cause directly proportional changes in glomerular filtration.

IMPORTANCE AND LIMITATIONS OF PHARMACOKINETIC STUDIES

Pharmacokinetic and pharmacodynamic studies pose a number of technical difficulties. To perform accurate pharmacokinetic studies a sensitive assay, appropriate sampling time, and appropriate model are important. Even when these conditions are met, certain assumptions must be made, which can lead to inaccurate conclusions. If the assay is insensitive at low levels, for example, extrapolation to zero and calculation of the area under the curve will be inaccurate, resulting in determination of imprecise kinetic parameters. Inadequate sampling time can cause the same type of error. Other errors include those due to biologic variation and inappropriate choice of model, which may lead to false interpretations of the data. These aspects of pharmacokinetic studies should be considered before drawing conclusions from any pharmacokinetic analysis.[3,4,72,92,100]

The use of drugs in the pediatric age group is complicated by the continuous changes in the development of organs, body weight, composition, and response. Most pediatric drug regimens that are obtained by fractionating adult doses have proved unsatisfactory. The need for systematic, clinical pharmacokinetic and pharmacodynamic studies in children is tremendous. On the rare occasion, however, that such studies are performed, usually only a small group of children is involved, and the results broadly applied to all children. Because individual physiological states and pathologic conditions may affect disposition differently, in the same or opposite direction, drug disposition and response cannot be predicted on theoretical grounds; the effect of each disease state must be studied independently. These age-related variations in pharmacokinetics may be further confounded by differences in receptor sensitivity between adults and children. Finally, clinical pharmacokinetic studies are of limited value unless correlated to the degree and time course of the clinical effect. Such correlations can be examined only in prospective studies. However, pharmacokinetic studies alone will help us understand the disposition of drugs with age and disease so that drugs could be administered intelligently.

ACKNOWLEDGEMENTS

The author is indebted to Darryl R. Abernethy, M.D., Ph.D., for his review of the manuscript.

This was supported in part by grants from the Shriners Burns Institute and from the National Institutes of Health, GM37569 and GM21700.

REFERENCES

1. Curran WI, Beecher HK: Experimentation in children: A re-examination of legal and ethical principles. *JAMA* 10:77–83, 1969
2. Morselli PL, Franco-Morselli R, Bossi L: Clinical pharmacokinetics in newborns and infants. *Clin Pharmacokinet* 5:485–527, 1980
3. Greenblatt DJ, Koch-Weser J: Clinical pharmacokinetics. *N Engl J Med* 293:702–705, 964–970, 1975
4. Hug CC: Pharmacokinetics of drugs administered intravenously. *Anesth Analg* 57:704–723, 1978
5. Udkow G: Pediatric clinical pharmacology. *Am J Dis Child* 132:1025–1032, 1978
6. Rane A, Wilson JT: Clinical pharmacokinetics in infants and children. *Clin Pharmacokinet* 1:2–24, 1976
7. Morselli PL: Clinical pharmacokinetics in neonates. *Clin Pharmacokinet* 1:81–98, 1976
8. Yaffe SJ, Juchau MR: Perinatal pharmacology. *Ann Rev Pharmacol Toxicol* 14:219–238, 1974
9. Boreus LO: *Principles of Pediatric Pharmacology*. New York, Churchill Livingstone, 1982, pp 1–175
10. Long SS, Swenson RM: Development of anaerobic fecal bacteria. *J Pediatr* 91:298–301, 1977
11. Evans EF, Proctor JD, Frathein MJ, et al: Blood flow in muscle groups and drug absorption. *Clin Pharmacol Ther* 17:44–47, 1975
12. Morselli PI: Problems of drug administration in the neonatal period, In Duchenne-Marrulay, (ed): *Advances in Pharmacology and Therapeutics, vol 6, Clinical Pharmacology*. Oxford, Pergamon, 1978, pp 57–66
13. deBoer AG, Moolenaar F, Leede LGJ, et al: Rectal drug administration: Clinical pharmacokinetic considerations. *Clin Pharmacokinet* 7:285–311, 1982
14. Bolme P, Edlund PO, Erikksson M, et al: Pharmacokinetics of theophylline in young children: Comparison of rectal enema and suppositories. *Eur J Clin Pharmacol* 16:133–139, 1979
15. Liu LMP, Gaudreault P, Freidman PA, et al: Methohexitol plasma concentrations in children following rectal administration Anesthesiology 62:567–570, 1985
16. Agurell S, Berlin A, Fengren HG, et al: Plasma levels of diazepam after parenteral and rectal administration to children. *Epilepsia* 16:177–283, 1975
17. Mirkin BL: Perinatal pharmacology: Placental transfer, fetal localization and neonatal disposition of drug. *Anesthesiology* 43:156–170, 1975
18. Bochner F, Carruthers G, Kampnann J, et al: *Handbook of Clinical Pharmacology* (ed 2). Boston, Little, Brown, 1984
19. Nation RL: Drug kinetics in childbirth. *Clin Pharmacokinet* 5:340–364, 1980
20. Finster M, Pedersen H: Placental transfer and fetal uptake of drugs. *Br J Anaesth* 51:255–285, 1979
21. Wilson JT, Brown RD, Cherek DR, et al: Drug excretion in human breast milk: Principles, pharmacokinetics and projected consequences. *Clin Pharmacokinet* 5:1–66, 1980
22. Friis-Hansen B: Body water compartments in children: Changes during growth and related changes in body composition. *Pediatrics* 28:169–181, 1961
23. Friis-Hansen B: Body Composition during growth: In vivo measurements and biochemical data correlated to differential anatomical growth. *Pediatrics* 47:264–274, 1971
24. Widdowson EM: Changes in body composition during growth, in Davis JA, Dobbing J (eds): *Scientific Foundations of Paediatrics* (ed 2). Baltimore, University Park Press, 1982, pp 330–341
25. Roland M: Drug administration and regimens, in Melmon KF, Morrelli HF (eds): *Clinical Pharmacology: Basic Principles in Therapeutics*, (ed 2). New York, MacMillan, 1978, pp 40
26. Fisher DM, O'Keefe C, Stanski DR, et al: Pharmacokinetics and pharmacodynamics of d-tubocurarine in infants, children and adults. *Anesthesiology 57:203–208, 1982*
27. Johnson KL, Erickson JP, Holley FO, et al: Fentanyl pharmacokinetics in pediatric population. *Anesthesiology* 61:A441, 1984
28. Rane A: Drug metabolism at various ages—young, in Turner P (ed), *Clinical Pharmacology and Therapeutics*. MacMillan Journals, 1980, pp 98–107
29. Junod AF: State of the art: Metabolism, production, release of hormones, and mediators in the lung. *Am Rev Resp Dis* 112:93–124, 1975
30. Smith SE, Rawlins MD: *Variability in Human Drug Response*. London-Boston, Buttersworth, 1976

31. Greenblatt DJ, Shader RI, Abernethy DR: Current status of benzodiazepenses. *N Engl J Med* 309:354–388, 1984

32. Currin MR: Pharmacology of the neonate. *SA Med J* 56:101–105, 1979

33. Weiss CF, Glazko AG, Weston JK: Chloramphenicol in the newborn infant: A physiological explanation of its toxicity when given in excessive dose. *N Engl J Med* 262:787–794, 1960

34. Fichter EG, Curtis JA: Sulphonamide administration in newborn and premature infants. *Am J Dis Child* 90:596–597, 1955

35. Vest M, Streiff R: Studies on glucuronide formation in newborn infants and older children. Measurement of p-aminophenol glucuronide levels in the serum after an oral dose of acetanilid. *Am J Dis Child* 98:688–693, 1959

36. Yu WL, Aldrich RA: The glucuronide transferase system in the newborn infant. *Pediatr Clin North Am* 7:381–396, 1960

37. Miller RP, Roberts RJ, Fischer CJ: Acetaminophen elimination in neonates, children and adults. *Clin Pharmacol Ther* 19:284–294, 1976

38. Dutton GJ: Developmental aspects of drug conjugation with special reference to glucuronidation. *Ann Rev Pharmacol Toxicol* 18:17–35, 1978

39. Thomas CR: Routine phenobarbital for prevention of neonatal hyperbilirubinemia. *Obstet Gynecol* 47:304, 1976

40. Neims AH, Manchester DK: Drug disposition in the developing human, in Mirkin (Ed): *Clinical Pharmacology and Therapeutics: A Pediatric Perspective.* Chicago, Year Book Medical Publishers, 1978, pp 35–48

41. Aranda JV, Silar DS, Parson WD, et al: Pharmacokinetic aspects of theophylline in premature newborns. *N Engl J Med* 295:413–416, 1976

42. Svensmark O, Buchthal F: Diphenylhydantoin and phenobarbital. Serum levels in children. *Am J Dis Child* 108:82–87, 1964

43. Dahlstrom B, Bolme P, Feychting, et al: Morphine kinetics in children. *Clin Pharmacol Ther* 26:354–365, 1980

44. Sorbo S, Hudson RJ, Loomis JC: Pharmacokinetics of thiopental in pediatric surgical patients. *Anesthesiology* 61:666–670, 1984

45. Goudsouzian NG, Martyn JAJ, Liu LMP, et al: The dose–response effect of long-acting non-depolarizing neuromuscular blocking agents in children. *Can Anaesth Soc J* 31:246–250, 1984

46. Goudsouzian NG, Martyn JAJ, Liu LMP, et al: Safety and efficacy of vecuronium in adolescents and children. *Anesth Analg* 62:1083–1088, 1983

47. Dohi S, Naito H, Takahashi T: Age-related changes in blood pressure and duration of motor block in spinal anesthesia. *Anesthesiology* 50:319–323, 1979

48. Ecobichon DJ, Stephens DS: Perinatal developmental of human blood esterases. *Clin Pharmacol Ther* 14:11–17, 1973

49. Arant B: Developmental patterns of renal functional maturation compared in the human neonate. *J Pediatr* 92:705–712, 1978

50. Aperia A, Broberger O, Elinder G, et al: Postnatal development of renal function in preterm and full term infants. *Acta Pediatr Scand* 70:183–187, 1981

51. Leake RD, Trygstad CW: Glomerular filtration rate during the period of adaptation to extrauterine life. *Pediatr Res* 11:959–962, 1977

52. Hook JB, Hewitt WR: Development mechanisms for drug excretion. *Am J Med Sci* 62:497–502, 1977

53. Gladke E, Heinmann G: The rate of elimination functions in kidney and liver of young infants, in Morselli PL, Garantini S, Gereni F (Eds), *Basic and Therapeutic Aspects of Perinatal Pharmacology.* New York, Raven Press, 1972, pp 393–403

54. Guinard JP, Torrado A, Mazouni SM, et al: Respiratory distress syndrome. *J Pediatr* 88:845–850, 1976

55. Bromberger U, Aperia A: Renal function in infants with hyperbilirubinemia. *Acta Pediatr Scand* 68:75–79, 1979

56. Schwartz GJ, Heggi T, Spitzer A: Subtherapeutic dicloxacillin levels in a neonate. Possible mechanisms. *J Pediatr* 89:310–312, 1976

57. Frenzel J, Braunlich H, Schramm CD, et al: Effect on the maturation of kidney function in newborn infants of repeated administration of water and electrolytes. *Eur J Clin Pharmacol* 11:317–320, 1977

58. Koch-Weser J, Sellers EM: Binding of drugs to serum albumin. *N Engl J Med* 294:311–316, 526–531, 1976

59. Piafsky KM, Borga O: Plasma protein binding of basic drugs. *Clin Pharmacol Ther* 22:545–549, 1977

60. Kunz H, Michels H, Stickel HH: Differences in the binding of drugs to plasma proteins from newborn and adult man. *Eur J Clin Pharmacol* 11:469–472, 1977

61. Levy G, Procknal JA, Garrettson LK: Distribution of salicylate between neonatal and maternal serum at diffusion equilibrium. *Clin Pharmacol Ther* 18:210–214, 1975

62. Martyn JAJ, Abernethy DR, Greenblatt DJ: Plasma protein binding of drugs after burn injury. *Clin Pharmacol Ther* 35:535–539, 1984

63. Dahlquist R, Borga O, Rane A, et al: Decreased plasma protein binding of phenytoin in patients on valproic acid. *Br J Clin Pharmacol* 8:547–552, 1979

64. Silverman WA, Anderson DH, Blanc WA, et al: A difference in the mortality rate and incidence of kernicterus among premature infants allotted to two prophylactic antibiotic therapies. *Pediatrics* 18:614–625, 1956

65. Leibel WS, Martyn JAJ, Szyfelbein SK, et al: Elevated plasma binding cannot account for the burn related d-tubocurarine hyposensitivity. *Anesthesiology* 54:378–382, 1981

66. Martyn JAJ, Liu LMP, Szyfelbein SK, et al: Metocurine requirements and plasma concentrations in pediatric burn patients. *Br J Anaesth* 55:263–267, 1983

67. Wood AJJ: Drug disposition and pharmacokinetics in drugs, in Wood M, Wood AJJ (Eds): *Drugs and Anesthesia* (ed 1). Baltimore/London, Williams and Wilkins, 1982, pp 3–75

68. Gibaldi M, Nagashima R, Levy G: Relationship between drug concentration and amount of drug in the body. *J Pharm Sci* 58:193–197, 1969

69. Greenblatt DJ, Sellers EM, Koch-Weser J: Importance of protein binding for the interpretation of serum or plasma drug concentrations. *J Clin Pharmacol* 22:259–263, 1982

70. Koch-Weser J, Greenblatt DJ: Drug interactions in clinical perspective. *Eur J Clin Pharmacol* 11:405–408, 1977

71. Perucca E, Hebdige S, Frigo GM, et al: Interaction between phenytoin and valproic acid: Plasma protein binding and metabolic effects. *Clin Pharmacol Ther* 28:779–789, 1980

72. Gibaldi M: Pharmacokinetic variability–drug interaction, in *Biopharmaceutics and Clinical Pharmacokinetics* (ed 3). Philadelphia, Lea and Febiger, 1984, pp 257–285

73. Martyn JAJ, Leibel WS, Matteo RS: Competitive nonspecific binding does not explain the potentiating effect of muscle relaxant combinations. *Anesth Analg* 62:160–163, 1983

74. Martyn JAJ, Greenblatt DJ, Abernethy DR: Increased cimetidine clearance in burned patients. *JAMA* 253:1288–1291, 1985

75. Martyn JAJ, Snider MT, Szyfelbein SK, et al: Right ventricular dysfunction following burns. *Ann Surg* 191:330–335, 1980

76. Williams RL: Drug administration in hepatic disease. *N Engl J Med* 309:1616–1622, 1983

77. Abernethy DR, Greenblatt DJ, Diroll M, et al: Differential effect of cimetidine on drug oxidation (antipyrine and diazepam) v conjugation (acetaminophen and lorazepam): Prevention of acetaminophen toxicity by cimetidine. *J Pharmacol Exp Ther* 224:508–513, 1983

78. Wood M, Uetrecht J, Sweetman B, et al: Effect of cimetidine on the oxidative metabolism of halothane. *Anesthesiology* 61:A269, 1984

79. Borel JD, Bentley JB, Nenad RE, et al: Cimetidine alteration of fentanyl pharmacokinetics. *Anesth Analg* I.A.R.S. Meeting (abstract), New Orleans, 1982

80. Klotz U, Reimann I: Delayed clearance of diazepam due to cimetidine. N Engl J Med 302:1012–1014, 1980

81. Lam AM, Clement JL: Effect of cimetidine premedication on morphine induced ventilatory depression. *Can Anesth Soc J* 31:36–43, 1984

82. Ochs HR, Carsteus G, Greenblatt DJ: Reduction in lidocaine clearance during continuous infusion and by coadministration of propranolol. *N Engl J Med* 303:373–377, 1980

83. Osmond PV, Mashford ML, Harman PJ, et al: Decreased warfarin clearance after ranitidine and cimetidine. *Clin Pharmacol Ther* 35:338–341, 1984

84. Vestal RC: Inhibition of propranolol metabolism by chlorpromazine. *Clin Pharmacol Ther* 25:19–24, 1979

85. Stambaugh JE, Wainer IW: Drug interaction: Meperidine and chlorpromazine, a toxic combination. *J Clin Pharmacol* 21:140–146, 1981

86. Wagner JG: A modern view of pharmacokinetics. *J Pharmacokinet Biopharm* 1:363–401, 1973

87. Stanski DR, Mihm FG, Rosenthal MH, et al: Pharmacokinetics of high dose thiopental used for cerebral resuscitation. *Anesthesiology* 54:169–171, 1980

88. Riegelman S, Loo JCK, Rowland, M: Shortcomings in pharmacokinetic analysis by conceiving the body to exhibit properties of a single compartment. *J Pharm Sci* 57:117–123, 1968

89. Murphy MR, Olson WA, Hug CC: Pharmacokinetics of ^{3}H-fentanyl in the dog anesthetized with enflurane. *Anesthesiology* 50:13–19, 1979

90. Bischoff KB, Dedrick RL: Thiopental pharmacokinetics. *J Pharm Sci* 57:1346–1351, 1968

91. Matteo RS, Nishitateno R, Pua E, et al: Pharmacokinetics of d-tubocurarine in man: Effect of osmotic diuretics on urinary excretion. *Anesthesiology* 52:335–338, 1980

92. Rowland M, Tozer TN: *Clinical Pharmacokinetics: Concepts and Applications.* Philadelphia, Lea and Feibiger, 1980

93. Greenblatt DJ, Abernethy DR, Divoll M: Is volume of distribution at steady state a meaningful kinetic variable? *J Clin Pharmacol* 23:391–400, 1983

94. Nies AS, Shand DG, Wilkinson GR: Altered hepatic blood flow and drug disposition. *Clin Pharmacokinetics* 1:135–155, 1976

95. George CF: Drug kinetics and hepatic blood flow. *Clin Pharmacokinetics* 4:433–448, 1979

96. Maxwell GM: *Principles of Pediatric Pharmacology.* New York, Oxford University Press, 1980, pp 1–40

97. Stanski DB, Watkins WD: *Drug Disposition in Anesthesia.* New York, Grune & Stratton, 1982, pp 1–47

98. Riegelman S, Loo J, Rowland M: Concept of a volume of distribution and possible errors in the evaluation of this parameter. *J Pharm Sci* 57:128–133, 1968

99. Benet LZ, Ronfeld RA: Volume terms in pharmacokinetics. *J Pharm Sci* 58:639–641, 1969

100. Fell PJ, Stevens MT: Pharmacokinetics—uses and abuses. *Eur J Clin Pharmacol* 8:241–248, 1981

101. Moore RG, Thomas J, Triggs EJ, et al: The pharmacokinetics and metabolism of the anilide local anaesthetics in neonates. III. Mepivacaine. *Eur J Clin Pharmacol* 14:203–212, 1978

102. Mihaly GW, Phillips JA, Louis WJ, et al: Measurement of carbamazepine and its epoxide metabolite by high-performance liquid chromatography, and a comparison of assay techniques for the analysis of carbamazine. *Clin Chem* 23:2283–2287, 1978

103. Morgan D, McQuillan D, Thomas J: Pharmacokinetics and metabolism of anilide local anesthetics in neonates. II. Etidocaine *Eur J Clin Pharmacol* 13:365–371, 1978

104. Rane A, Bertilsson L, Palmer L: Disposition of placentally transferred carbamazepine (Tesretol) in the newborn. *Eur J Clin Pharmacol* 8:283–284, 1975

105. Christensen JH, Andreasen F, Jansen JA: Pharmacokinetics of thiopentol in caesarian section *Acta Anaesth Scand* 25:174–179, 1981

7

Practical Pharmacology of Anesthetic Agents, Narcotics, and Sedatives

Charles J. Coté

The pharmacodynamics and pharmacokinetics of most medications used in the pediatric patient, especially the neonate, are different from those used in the adult.[1-8] The reasons for this include altered protein binding, larger volume of distribution, smaller proportion of fat and muscle stores, and immature renal and hepatic function.[9-16] Each of these factors may alter the initial dose, and interval between doses, of a given drug necessary to achieve the desired clinical response, as well as delay its degradation or excretion. In addition, some medications may displace bilirubin from its protein binding sites, and may possibly predispose the infant to kernicterus.[17-19] This chapter will discuss basic pharmacologic principles, and anesthetic agents as they relate to their use in infants and children.

DISTRIBUTION

PROTEIN BINDING

The degree of protein binding is usually less in premature and full-term babies than in adults; this is due to lower total protein and albumin (Figure 7-1).[20] Most drugs that are highly protein-bound in the adult have less of an affinity for protein in the neonate, although some may have a higher degree of protein binding (Figure 7-2).[20-27] Lower protein binding may result in higher free plasma levels, thus providing more free drug for clinical action. Protein binding therefore may have considerable influence on the response to medications, especially those medications that are highly protein bound, e.g., diphenylhydantoin, salicylate, bupivacaine, barbiturates, antibiotics, theophylline, and diazepam. In addition, some medications, such as diphenylhydantoin, salicylate, sulfisoxazole, caffeine, and sodium benzoate, compete with bilirubin for

binding to albumin; if large amounts of bilirubin are displaced, kernicterus may result (Figure 7-3).[25,28,29] The propensity for kernicterus is worsened by hypoxia and acidosis, and since these metabolic derangements often occur in sick neonates coming to surgery, special care in the selection of drugs must be made for these patients.[25,29]

BODY COMPOSITION

Volume of Distribution

The premature and full-term baby have a much greater proportion of body water compared to the older child or adult (Figure 7-4).[14] Water-soluble medications will thus have a greater volume of distribution, suggesting the need for a higher initial (loading) dose, based on weight, in order to achieve the desired serum level when a water-soluble drug is administered.[30,31] The term neonate will therefore usually require a greater dosage; examples of this include digoxin, theophylline, most antibiotics, and succinylcholine.[24,32-35] The premature infant, on the other hand, is usually more sensitive to pharmacologic effects, and in general requires a lower blood level.[32-34] It is important, therefore, to carefully titrate all drugs administered to premature and term infants.

Fat and Muscle Content

Premature and full-term neonates have a smaller proportion of body fat and muscle mass; with growth the amount of these tissues increases (Figure 7-5).[1-8,14,16] Therefore, drugs which depend upon redistribution into muscle and fat will probably have a greater half-life, which may result in prolonged undesirable clinical effects, e.g., barbiturates and narcotics may cause prolonged sedation and respiratory depression.[1-3,16,23,36,37] The influence of the small muscle mass on muscle relaxant requirements is exemplified by curare;

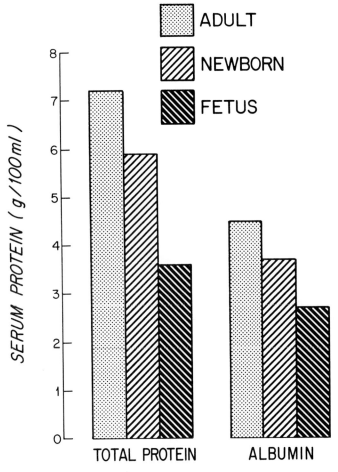

Figure 7-1. This figure presents the changes in total serum protein and albumin levels which occur during maturation. Note that both total protein and albumin are less in neonates compared to adults. This may result in altered pharmacokinetics and pharmacodynamics for drugs with a high degree of protein binding since less drug is protein bound; thus more is available for clinical effect. (Abstracted from Ehrnebo M et al: Eur J Clin Pharmacol 3:189–193, 1971.)

neuromuscular blockade is achieved at lower serum levels in infants, presumably in part because of the smaller muscle mass.[32]

METABOLISM AND EXCRETION

HEPATIC

Most hepatic enzymatic reactions involving drug metabolism convert the drug from a nonpolar state (lipid soluble) to a polar compound (water soluble). The ability to perform these reactions in general is reduced in the neonate. However, no categoric statement may be made for all hepatically metabolized medications; each medication must be considered individually.[3,11,38] As the infant matures, the ability to metabolize and conjugate drugs improves. Many other factors may also influence the rate of hepatic maturation and metabolism as well, e.g., sepsis, nutrition, or previous drug exposure.[38,39] Diazepam and thiopental have a markedly increased serum half-life in the infant compared to the adult (Figures 7-6 and

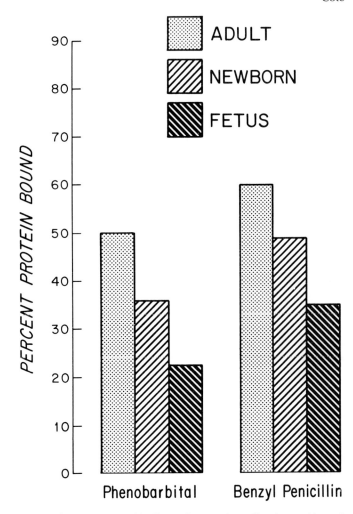

Figure 7-2. Protein binding of several medications: Altered protein binding may affect the clinical response to any medication; note the much lower protein binding of phenobarbital in the newborn and fetus compared to the adult. This decrease in protein binding in newborns may partially account for the prolonged pharmacologic effects of barbiturates in newborns since more free drug is able to be pharmacologically active. (Abstracted from Ehrnebo M, et al: Eur J Clin Pharmacol 3:189–193, 1971.)

7-7).[23,40] For diazepam this may be related in part to the higher protein binding as well as slower hepatic degradation.[40]

RENAL

The renal function of the neonate and premature infant is less efficient than the adult (Figure 7-8). This is related to the combination of incomplete glomerular development, low perfusion pressure, and inadequate osmotic load to produce full countercurrent effects.[41–46] Premature and full-term newborns will have immature glomerular filtration as well as tubular function; both will develop rapidly during the first few months of life. This development is hastened when the infant is exposed to a higher solute load (cow's milk v breast milk).[42,43] Healthy premature and full-term babies will have relatively normal renal drug clearance by three to four weeks of age. Complete maturation of glomerular filtration and tubular function, however, does not occur until 20 weeks of

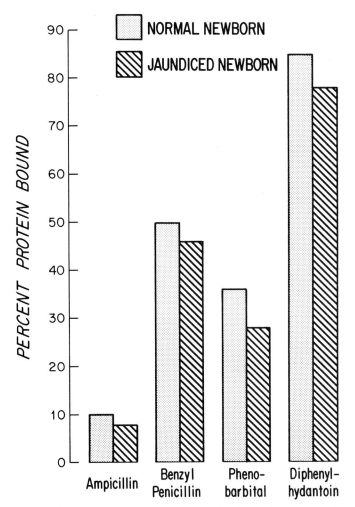

Figure 7-3. The effects of hyperbilirubinemia on protein binding: Note that in the presence of hyperbilirubinemia many drugs which are protein bound will compete with bilirubin for binding sites. This results in both elevated unbound bilirubin as well as increased unbound drug. This interaction may lead to an increased propensity for the development of kernicterus as well as more drug available for clinical effect. This is particularly important for drugs which are highly protein bound. (Abstracted from Ehrnebo M, et al: Eur J Clin Pharmacol 3:181–193, 1971.)

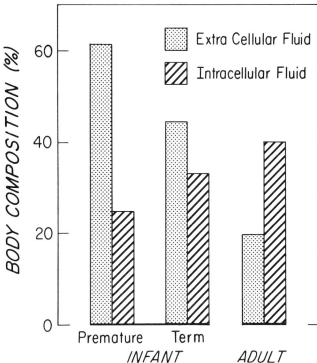

Figure 7-4. Changes in the intracellular and extracellular compartments which occur during maturation. Note the large proportion of extracellular water in premature and term infants. This large water compartment creates a larger volume of distribution for highly water soluble medications and may account for the high initial "loading" dose required for some medications to achieve a satisfactory clinical response. (Abstracted from data in Friis-Hansen B, Pediatrics 47:264–274, 1971.)

age, and achieves adult levels by two years of age (Figure 7-8).[44–46] For these reasons, drugs which are excreted primarily through glomerular filtration or tubular secretion (e.g. antibiotics, digoxin) will have a prolonged half-life in neonates (Figures 7-9 and 7-10).[47–49]

Often in the presence of renal failure a single administration of renally excreted drugs will achieve and maintain prolonged therapeutic drug levels if there is no alternate pathway of excretion. Thus, whenever administering a medication to a premature or full-term infant one must consider what role renal function will play in the termination of its action.

The pharmacokinetics and pharmacodynamics of curare exemplifies the complex interaction of increased volume of distribution, smaller muscle mass, and decreased rate of excretion due to immaturity of glomerular filtation. Fisher and co-workers found that the initial dose of curare to achieve neuromuscular blockade was similar in the infant or the adult.[32] Infants, however, achieved this blockade at lower serum concentrations than older children or adults, corresponding to the differences in muscle mass. The larger volume of distribution (total body water) accounts for the equivalent dose for each kilogram of body weight, and the reduced glomerular function in infants compared to older children or adults accounts for the longer duration of action.[32]

CENTRAL NERVOUS SYSTEM EFFECTS

Data from laboratory animals has demonstrated the lethal dose in 50 percent of animals (LD$_{50}$) for many medications to be significantly lower in the neonatal animal compared to the adult.[50,51] The sensitivity of the human newborn to most of the sedatives, hypnotics, and narcotics is clinically well known, and may in part be related to increased brain permeability for some medications, especially lipid soluble varieties (e.g., barbiturates, narcotics).[52,53] Several laboratory studies have demonstrated high brain concentrations in infant compared to adult animals for morphine and amobarbital. This may correlate with incomplete myelination, and thus reflect an immature blood–brain barrier, making it easier for lipid soluble drugs to enter the brain.[54–56] When considering the use of these med-

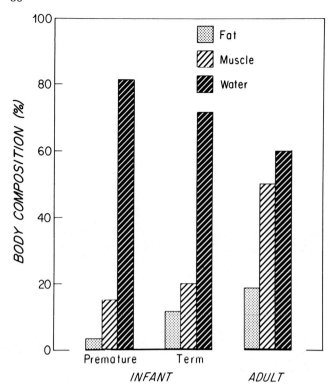

Figure 7-5. Changes in body content for fat, muscle, and water which occur with maturation. Note the markedly reduced fat and muscle content in premature and term infants. These factors may greatly influence the pharmacokinetics and pharmacodynamics of medications which redistribute into fat and muscle. (Abstracted from data in Friis-Hansen B: Pediatrics 47:264–274, 1971.)

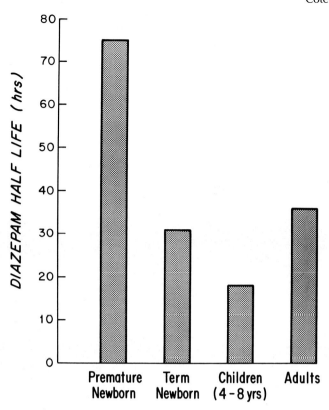

Figure 7-6. Effects of hepatic metabolism: Diazepam is excreted by means of hepatic mechanisms; note the markedly prolonged half-life in premature infants with undeveloped enzymatic function. (Abstracted from data in Mandelli et al: Clin Pharmacokinet 3:72–91, 1978.)

ications in children less than one year of age one must consider the potential risks and benefits. Dosage must be carefully calculated and therapeutic effects monitored, since prolonged effects or adverse clinical responses may occur.

PHARMACOLOGY OF INHALATIONAL AGENTS

The measure of anesthetic potency has traditionally been the minimum alveolar concentration (MAC), or the effective dose of 50 percent (ED_{50}), i.e., that expired concentration where 50 percent of patients do not move in response to a surgical stimuli. The anesthetic requirements of pediatric patients vary according to age. Early studies of inhalation agents revealed that young infants and teenagers had significantly greater halothane requirements than adults.[57,58] More recent studies of animal fetuses and human neonates have modified the interpretation of the earlier results, now demonstrating that the fetus (animal) has markedly reduced anesthetic requirements compared to the adult, and the human neonate aged 0–31 days has a lower MAC than infants aged 30–180 days (0.87 ± 0.03 v 1.20 ± 0.06 % halothane); the ED_{50} for the adult is 0.94 percent Figure 7-11.[59,60] The reasons for this apparently greater anesthetic requirement in infants are unclear, but may reflect an interaction of many factors such as residual elevated progesterone and/or endorphin

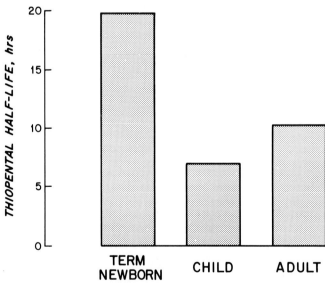

Figure 7-7. Effects of hepatic maturity on thiopental metabolism: Note the markedly prolonged serum half life for thiopental in the newborn compared to the adult. This may in part be related to immature hepatic metabolic pathways. (Abstracted from Christensen JH, et al: Acta Anaesth Scand 25:174–179, 1981, Ghoneim MM, et al: Br J Anaesth 50:1237–1241, 1978, and Sorbo S, et al: Anesthesiology 59:A449, 1983.)

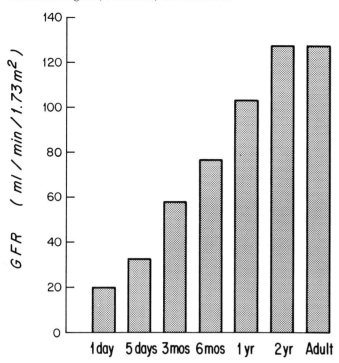

Figure 7-8. Changes in glomerular filtration rate (GFR) vs age. Note the rapid development of glomerular function during the first year of life. Abnormal as well as immature renal function may delay drug excretion. (Abstracted from data in chapters by C. Chantler in Clinical Pediatric Nephrology, Lippincott, 1976.)

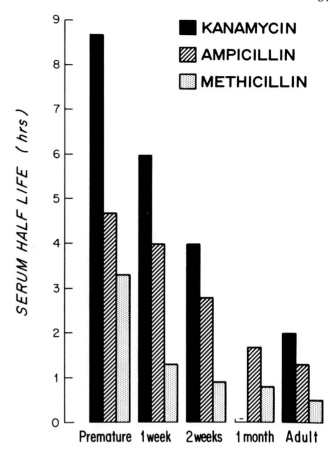

Figure 7-9. Serum half life for three antibiotics vs age. Note the inverse relationship between age and serum half life. This correlates well with maturing renal function. (Abstracted from data in Kaplan JM, et al: Ped Pharm Ther 84:571–577, 1974 and McCracken GH: Am J Dis Child 128:407–419, 1974.)

levels, as well as an immature central nervous system.[59,60] Thus, there is nearly a 30 percent greater anesthetic requirement for infants to attain the same depth of anesthesia. It must be emphasized that there is a smaller margin of safety between adequate anesthesia and severe cardiopulmonary depression in the infant and child compared to the adult. Studies in neonatal rats have confirmed that equianesthetic concentrations of halothane result in greater myocardial depression in neonatal compared to mature animals.[61] Because the cardiac output of neonates is markedly dependent on the heart rate, some of the myocardial depression of the potent inhalational agents may be reversed by the administration of vagolytic agents.[62]

A greater depth of anesthesia is required for airway manipulation than for superficial surgical procedures. For this reason another concept important for the pediatric anesthesiologist is MAC for endotracheal intubation (MAC_{EI}). Yakaitas et al. examined the end-tidal halothane concentration which would allow successful endotracheal intubation with no coughing or movement in 50 percent of pediatric patients aged 2 to 6 years, during or immediately after intubation.[63] Their data would indicate that MAC_{EI} is 1.33 percent for halothane. Thus, the anesthetic concentrations necessary for intubation are even closer to those levels which might result in severe cardiopulmonary depression.

The advent of neuromuscular blocking agents has greatly improved the safety of general anesthesia in infants, since lower concentrations of potent inhalational agents may be used while providing excellent surgical relaxation.

UPTAKE AND DISTRIBUTION

The uptake and distribution of inhalational agents is more rapid in infants and children than in adults (Figure 7-12). This may in part be related to their more rapid respiratory rate, increased cardiac index, and the distribution of a larger proportion of the cardiac output to vessel-rich organs. This results in a more rapid increase in the partial pressure of inhalational agents in mixed venous blood; this is one of the factors contributing to the rapid development of myocardial depression, and possibly of cardiac arrest in neonates when potent inhalational agents are used.[64–66]

Ventilation/perfusion mismatch, airway obstruction, and perhaps intracardiac defects, result in a slower rate of uptake and rise in alveolar concentration of the potent inhalational (soluble) agents. It takes longer to achieve an adequate plane of anesthesia for safe laryngoscopy and intubation in children with any of the above mentioned problems. This is an especially important concept when inducing anesthesia in a child with upper airway obstruction (epiglotitis, croup, subglottic stenosis, or bronchial foreign body) where safe, smooth control of the airway is vital.

Nitrous oxide is insoluble, compared to the potent inhalation agents, and therefore the effects of respiratory rate, increased cardiac index, distribution of cardiac output and

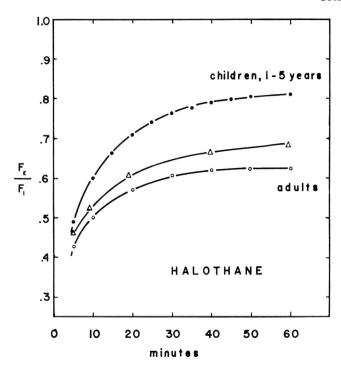

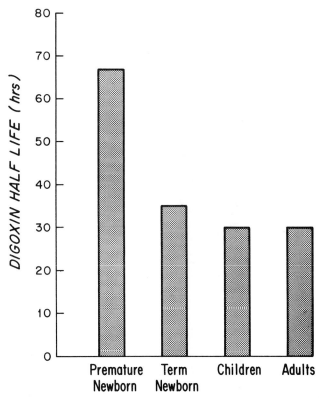

Figure 7-10. Effects of renal function on digoxin excretion: Note the markedly prolonged half-life of digoxin in premature infants. This correlates well with immature renal function. (Abstracted from data in Lang D et al: Pediatrics 59:902–906, 1977 and Wettrell G et al: Clin Pharmacokinet 2:17–31, 1977.)

Figure 7-12. This figure presents the uptake of halothane in children (upper curve) vs adults (two lower curves). Note the more rapid uptake in children which may reflect a more rapid respiratory rate, increased cardiac index, and greater blood flow to vessel rich organs. (Reproduced with permission from Salanitre E, et al: Anesthesiology 30:388–394, 1969.)

rate of increase of alveolar concentration are of negligible clinical import.

The rate of induction and awakening is also related in part to the type of anesthetic circuit utilized. A non-rebreathing system will produce a more rapid rise in alveolar anesthetic concentration than a similar concentration delivered by a rebreathing (circle) system. With a circle system, it is necessary to consider the volume of the anesthetic tubing, carbon dioxide absorber, and the humidifier, in relationship to the patient's lung volume. Thus, with a circle system (volume 3500 ml) any change in inspired concentration will take longer to equilibrate than a similar change made with a non-rebreathing circuit (volume 1200 ml). For this reason a more rapid induction and perhaps a better control of anesthetic depth may be achieved with a non-rebreathing system. This is an important concept for neonatal anesthesia where very small changes in anesthetic concentration rapidly equilibrate with the small lung volume. A non-rebreathing system also allows a more rapid elimination of potent inhalational agents. The above factors must each be considered when selecting an anesthetic circuit for use in infants and neonates. There is no ideal anesthetic circuit; the practitioner must know the advantages and disadvantages of each. (See Chapter 23.)

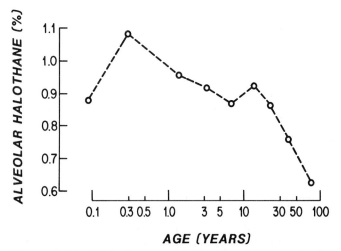

Figure 7-11. This figure presents the minimum alveolar concentration of halothane (MAC) vs patient age. Note the higher requirements in infants and teenagers. Neonates have lower requirements than infants. (Modified from Gregory GA, et al: Anesthesiology 30:488–491, 1969 and Lerman J, et al: Anesthesiology 59:421–424, 1983.)

HALOTHANE

GENERAL PROPERTIES

Halothane is the most commonly used potent inhalational agent for children because of its acceptance, ease and rapidity of induction, relative safety, and the rapid awakening it allows.

It is a relatively poor analgesic, and thus is frequently combined with nitrous oxide or a narcotic.[67] In high-risk patients halothane with oxygen allows delivery of a high inspired oxygen concentration, as well as an anesthetic agent which is rapidly eliminated at the conclusion of surgery. Halothane has weak neuromuscular blocking properties and will potentiate the action of non-depolarizing neuromuscular blocking agents.[68] It is also a potent bronchodilator; the mechanism of action seems to be mediated by beta adrenergic stimulation, which causes a buildup of cyclic AMP that in turn results in relaxation of bronchial smooth muscle.[69–72] Halothane is thus particularly useful for the management of asthmatic patients, since it depresses airway reflexes and causes smooth muscle relaxation. A major disadvantage is that halothane sensitizes the myocardium to the effects of catecholamines. Thus, the combination of halothane, high circulating catecholamines, and aminophylline may occasionally lead to serious arrhythmias.[73,74] A study of dogs anesthetized with halothane reported absence of arrhythmias at 1, 2, or 3 MAC with therapeutic levels of aminophylline (10–20 μg/ml); further carefully controlled human studies are needed in this area.[75]

CONTRAINDICATIONS

Hepatotoxicity

There is little evidence to suggest hepatotoxicity secondary to halothane in the pediatric age group.[76] There is a case report of a four year old who developed hepatic dysfunction several days after her fourth exposure to halothane.[77] This patient's serum was positive for antibodies to rat halothane-sensitized hepatocytes. Although there seems to be some evidence that this test has merit, further confirmation of this work by different investigators is needed.[78,79] Our fifteen years experience with 1,500 acutely burned children totaling over 6000 exposures to halothane, has not revealed a single case of proven "halothane hepatitis."[80] In addition, there are no data to suggest that patients with preexisting liver disease have an increased propensity to develop halothane hepatitis.[81] Several recent animal studies have found hypoxia to be a possible potentiating factor in halothane-mediated hepatic injury; thus there may be several mechanisms involved.[81–83] The true incidence of halothane hepatitis in children is unknown. If halothane hepatitis does exist in the pediatric age group the incidence is probably lower than it is in adults, around 1 in 30,000.[84,85] Overall, the proven efficacy, vast experience, safety, and ease of acceptance by a patient population that often requires a smooth mask induction to anesthesia, still make halothane the inhalational agent of choice for children. The pungent smell of isoflurane and enflurane make these agents less acceptable to awake patients.

Exogenous Catecholamines

Halothane has been found to sensitize the myocardium to arrhythmias secondary to exogenous catecholamines. The dose of epinephrine needed to cause this has been demonstrated to be 0.25–1.0 μg/kg subcutaneous in animals, but slightly higher (1.4–2.0 μg/kg subcutaneous) in adults.[86,87] Children seem to tolerate higher doses of epinephrine compared to adults (6–10 μg/kg); tachycardia and hypertension are more common side effects than arrhythmias.[88,89,90]

Increased intracranial pressure

Halothane markedly increases cerebral blood flow, and thus is contraindicated in most patients with increased intracranial pressure.[91,92] There are, however, occasions when it is almost impossible to secure an intravenous route for an alternate technique. The brief use of halothane in this situation cannot categorically be discarded. This problem will be discussed in greater detail in Chapter 17.

ENFLURANE

GENERAL PROPERTIES

Enflurane is another potent inhalational agent, related to ether. Several studies comparing its use with halothane found no significant advantage related to rapidity of induction or recovery, but did find a greater incidence of problems related to airway irritation.[93,94] Enflurane is a potent bronchodilator and may also be helpful in the management of the asthmatic patient.[71,95] Although it may prove to be a better choice for the asthmatic, since there is less myocardial sensitization to exogenous catecholamines, there have been no comparative studies in children demonstrating enflurane to have advantage over halothane for the treatment of bronchospasm.[86,95] Enflurane has slightly greater neuromuscular blocking properties compared to halothane.[96] There may be some therapeutic advantage to the combination of enflurane and succinylcholine, compared to halothane and succinylcholine, regarding the incidence of cardiac arrhythmias.[97]

Enflurane anesthesia may offer some advantage during cystometric evaluation of urodynamic function in children under anesthesia. One report found a latent period between bladder contraction and urethral sphincter relaxation in children anesthetized with enflurane, compared to halothane.[98] This may aid in the evaluation of coordination between sphincter and detrusor muscles.

CONTRAINDICATIONS

Hepatotoxicity

Hepatotoxicity in adults, but not in children, has been reported following enflurane anesthesia.[99]

Exogenous catecholamines

Enflurane is three times less sensitizing to the arrhythmogenic effects of exogenous catecholamines, and thus may be preferred over halothane when epinephrine is to be used.[86]

Increased Intracranial Pressure

Enflurane increases cerebral blood flow and is generally contraindicated in any patient with raised intracranial pressure or decreased cerebral compliance (see Chapter 17).[91,92,100]

Nephrotoxicity

There is some evidence in adults that the inorganic fluoride ion produced through enflurane metabolism may cause a defect in urine concentrating ability; this requires a very long enflurane anesthetic.[101] No such studies have been performed in children. Until further studies are obtained it is reasonable to avoid prolonged anesthetics with enflurane in children with abnormal renal function.

Seizure disorders

Enflurane in concentrations greater than 2.5 percent has been demonstrated to produce spike and wave electroencephalographic abnormalities. Seizure activity is increased with hypocarbia, and decreased with hypercarbia.[102] This pharmacologic response was used to help elicit and localize an epileptogenic focus prior to surgical excision.[103] Thus, enflurane should be used with caution in epileptic patients. On the other hand, there has been at least one clinical report of abolition of EEG abnormalities following the introduction of enflurane in a pediatric patient with a seizure disorder.[104]

ISOFLURANE

Isoflurane is a relatively new potent inhalational agent with a vapor pressure nearly identical to halothane and uptake characteristics similar to enflurane.[105,106] As yet there has been minimal published pediatric experience with this agent, though preliminary reports indicate that there is little advantage of this agent over halothane.[107,108] Isoflorane has respiratory depressant effects similar to halothane and enflurane.[106,107,109] Cardiovascular stability is one of the purported advantages of isoflurane; in *adult humans cardiac output is maintained by an increase in heart rate* and decrease in total peripheral resistance, which is also accompanied with a dose-related fall in systemic blood pressure.[105,106,110,111] In the hypovolemic patient there may be a precipitous fall in blood pressure secondary to vasodilation.[106] In a study of *healthy infants a fall in heart rate,* as well as blood pressure, was observed, which was similar to that observed with halothane.[107] Thus it would appear that in infants there is no significant cardiovascular advantage. Of more importance was the finding of marked production of secretions and laryngospasm; the former were eliminated with atropine, but laryngospasm frequently occurred (23%).

The properties of isoflurane that makes it attractive are the greater potentiation of neuromuscular blockade compared to halothane (but equivalent to enflurane), and less potentiation of cardiac arrthythmias in the presence of epinephrine.[105,106,112]

In order to take advantage of the above properties and circumvent the disadvantages of secretions and laryngospasm, an alternative would be to induce a patient with halothane, administer atropine, intubate the patient, and then switch to isoflurane for the remainder of the case. The disavantage here is that the child is exposed to two potent inhalational agents. Malignant hyperthermia has also been reported during isoflurane anesthesia; thus this double exposure of trigger agents may not be desirable.[113]

Another possible advantage of isoflurane is its use for neurosurgical procedures. Isoflurane produces smaller increments in cerebral blood flow (CBF) when compared to halothane or enflurane, and the reversal of this increased CBF by passive hyperventilation is more readily achieved.[92,106] There is also some evidence that cerebral metabolic rate for oxygen ($CMRO_2$) is reduced during isoflurane anesthesia by its direct effect on cortical electrical activity.[114] Thus at deeper planes of isoflurane anesthesia the reduction in electrical activity may provide some protective effect; this level of anesthesia may often be achieved with isoflurane while maintaining adequate cardiovascular stability.[105,106,115] Further studies are needed to examine the above mentioned effect on CBF and $CMRO_2$ in children before truly scientific recommendations may be made.

NITROUS OXIDE

GENERAL PROPERTIES

Nitrous oxide is a relatively potent analgesic but a weak anesthetic agent. For these reasons it is usually supplemented with a muscle relaxant, narcotic, barbiturate, or sedative. As with the potent inhalational agents there appears to be a lower requirement with increasing age.[116] A major advantage is its insolubility. In prolonged surgical procedures this property enables the patient to awaken more rapidly than with the more soluble potent inhalational agents. Other advantages include minimal myocardial and respiratory depression, no serious clinical interaction with exogenous catecholamines, and minimal effects on cerebral blood flow.[117]

CONTRAINDICATIONS

The major contraindications to the use of nitrous oxide are the need for a high inspired oxygen concentration or the presence of trapped air in a closed body space. The latter situation is particularly important in the pediatric patient. Nitrous oxide is 34 times more soluble than nitrogen, which is the major constituent of air in a closed space. Thus the entry of nitrous oxide is much more rapid than the exit of nitrogen.[118] This may lead to a rapid increase in the size of tension pneumothorax and bowel distension.[119] Thus with 75 percent nitrous oxide a two-fold increase of intestinal gas can be expected within *three hours,* and a pneumothorax can double in volume within *10 minutes.*[96] In the pediatric patient the increase in bowel size may be more rapid because of greater bowel perfusion compared to the adult.

Other areas of concern are the rapid increase of intracranial pressure following pneumoencephalography, the rupture of tympanic membranes previously infected, the rapid increase in the size of the pulmonary lobe in congenital lobar emphysema, and the possibility of pneumothorax in asthmatic patients with evidence of pulmonary blebs.[120–124] Other possible situations where nitrous oxide might be contraindicated include patients who have had intravitreal sulfur hexofluride injections, and patients with elevated pulmonary vascular resistance; further studies in these areas are needed.[125,126]

OXYGEN

The possible adverse effects of oxygen administration are of great concern to the pediatric anesthesiologist. Pulmonary oxygen toxicity is well documented, but it develops slowly. Of greater import, but less well documented, is the possibility of causing severe and perhaps irreparable damage to the immature neonatal retina resulting in retrolental fibroplasia (RLF).[127,128] Several cases of RLF have been reported in infants whose only known exposure to supplemental oxygen occurred in the operating room.[129,130] There are many other factors contributing to the development of RLF, since it has been reported in children with cyanotic congenital heart disease, infants who have not been exposed to exogenous oxygen, and even in stillborns.[131,132] Recently a possible relationship of the development of RLF to arterial carbon dioxide variations, as well as hypoxemia, have been suggested.[133,134]

The embryonal development of the retina involves the progressive increase in vascularization of retinal vessels in a nasal to temporal direction. Exposure to high levels of oxygen results in vasoconstriction of retinal vessels, the probable occlusion of these vessels by thrombi, the development of new vessels (neovascularization), the formation of arteriolar–venous anastomoses, vascularization of the vitreous, and in some cases fibrous degeneration and retraction of the scar, i.e., cicatrization and retinal detachment.[135] This sequence of events apparently does not occur once vascularization of the retina is complete (about 44 weeks gestation).[136,137]

The ample evidence implicating oxygen as a primary contributing factor to the development of RLF must be recognized; the anesthesiologist must therefore take *practical precautions* to protect the infant. This entails discussing with the surgeon the postponement of elective surgery on a neonate less than 44 weeks gestation to allow for further retinal maturation.[137] Obviously a life-threatening surgical problem must be corrected promptly. Once the decision has been made to proceed with surgery an ophthalmological assessment of possible preexisting RLF is desirable. Postoperative evaluation would help to delineate any retinal pathology related to operating room procedures. This type of evaluation also presumes experience by the ophthalmologist in diagnosing RLF; often a general anesthetic is required in order to perform a complete infant evaluation. Thus an ophthalmologic examination immediately prior to the scheduled surgical procedure will provide the necessary data, but in practical terms such an examination is difficult to coordinate and perform. It is only by careful pre- and postoperative assessment of the retina that some true understanding of the possible anesthetic implications can be made. To date there are no good epidemiologic studies examining this problem in general, nor has there been study of anesthetic risk factors.[138]

The intraoperative management of oxygen therapy must include careful monitoring of inspired oxygen concentration, as well as expired carbon dioxide concentration. An attempt to monitor arterial oxygen concentration and $PaCO_2$ by intermittent blood gas analysis should be made *where technically feasible*. A system capable of delivering a mixture of compressed air and oxygen is helpful in avoiding hyperoxia during nitrous oxide washout upon awakening from anesthesia, or in cases where nitrous oxide is contraindicated. Transcutaneous oxygen electrodes are variable in their function in the operating room, and are therefore most useful as trend indicators. Pulse oximetry may also prove useful for these patients. Every effort should be made to maintain the PaO_2 in the range of 60–80 torr, and the $PaCO_2$ 35–45 torr. A transport system equipped with an air/oxygen blender should also be available, in order to continue the careful titration of oxygen therapy from the operating room to the intensive care unit. While avoiding hyperoxia one must never lose sight of the importance of *avoiding hypoxia; hypoxia is life threatening whereas hyperoxia is not.* The death rate in premature babies markedly increased in both England and the United States during the years when oxygen use was greatly curtailed (1954–1958) (Figure 7-13).[139,140] We do not want to relearn this lesson in the operating room. Further study of this problem is clearly required, but

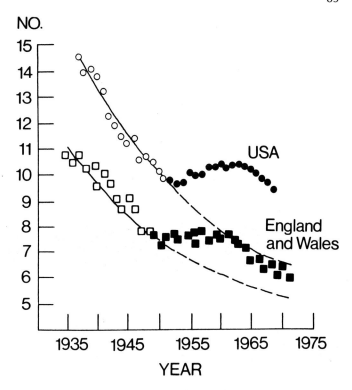

Figure 7-13. Mortality on the first day of life in the United States and in England and Wales, before (open circles and squares) and after (closed circles and squares) oxygen restriction. The general policy change toward restriction of oxygen use for premature infants took place somewhat earlier in Great Britain than in the United States. (Redrawn from Bolton and Cross, 1974; Reproduced with permission, Pediatrics 57:591–641, 1976. Copyright American Academy of Pediatrics, 1976.)

until such studies are completed anesthesiologists will be faced with a difficult dilemma. One cannot be faulted if RLF should occur, provided a reasonable and safe approach to oxygen administration and ventilation has been made, especially in view of the fact that the development of RLF may result from any disturbance in the neonatal oxygen supply, which in turn may be affected by any of 15 or more factors.[141]

INTRAVENOUS ANESTHETICS

The anesthetic effects of intravenous agents are primarily reflected by brain concentrations; thus to achieve anesthesia it is necessary to obtain an adequate cerebral blood level. Each drug administered will be rapidly redistributed from vessel-rich areas (brain, heart, kidneys) to muscle, and finally to vessel-poor areas (bone, fat).[142,143] The pharmacokinetics and pharmacodynamics of intravenous drugs may be altered by protein binding, the volume of distribution, body composition, metabolism, and excretion. Anesthesia may be altered if a constant cerebral blood level is not maintained. The changes in body composition and the blood–brain barrier, which occur during maturation, may greatly affect the duration of action of intravenous drugs, especially in neonates.[14,22,23,36,51–55]

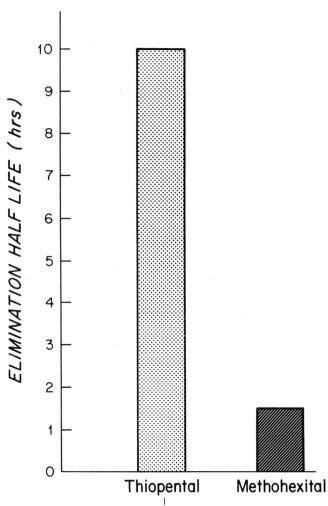

Figure 7-14. Difference in rate of excretion methohexital vs thiopental: Note the elimination half life of methohexital is one sixth that of thiopental. This results in more rapid elimination of methohexital and may help to hasten awakening. (Abstracted from Breimer DD: Br J Anaesth 48:643–649, 1976 and Ghoneim MM, et al, Br J Anaesth 50:1237–1241, 1978.)

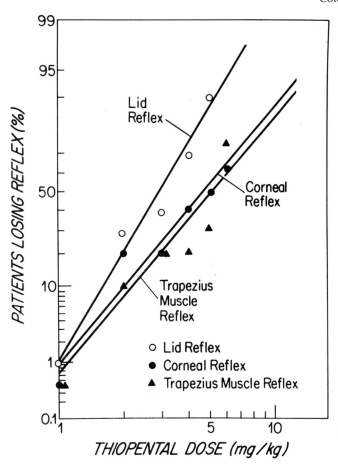

Figure 7-15. Dose response curve for loss of lid reflex, corneal reflex, and trapezius muscle response 60 seconds following intravenous thiopental in unpremedicated pediatric patients. (Reproduced with permission from Coté CJ, et al, Anesthesiology 55:703–705, 1981.)

BARBITURATES

METHOHEXITAL

Methohexital (Sodium Brevital) is a short-acting barbiturate for induction of anesthesia. Our experience with this medication, administered intravenously as a one percent solution (10 mg/ml), revealed a number of patients experiencing pain at the injection site, hiccough, apnea, and occasionally seizure-like activity.[144,145] Rectal methohexital, 20–30 mg/kg, on the other hand, is a very safe and atraumatic method of induction to anesthesia, with a low incidence of undesired side effects. It is an excellent technique for brief radiologic procedures such as computerized axial tomography (CAT scans), where often a single rectal administration 10% solution, (100 mg/ml given through a well-lubricated catheter) is sufficient for the 20–30 minutes required.[146] The absorption by this route is quite variable and may account for the occasional child with prolonged sedation.[147] We have used this technique and dosage safely in children from three months to six years of age. It is a useful adjunct to induction of anesthesia in older mentally handicapped children, or children who are frightened of the anesthesia mask or an intravenous needle. Methohexital should only be administered under the supervision of a physician trained in airway management to assure adequacy of ventilation. An electrocardiogram, blood pressure monitoring, and equipment for airway management and suction of secretions, should be readily available. A possible advantage for methohexital is that its rate of metabolism is much greater than thiopental; this suggests a more rapid recovery when high doses have been administered (Figure 7-14).[148–150]

THIOPENTAL

The induction of anesthesia with intravenous thiopental sodium (2.5%) is generally accomplished with a dose of 2–5 mg/kg, and then maintained with smaller incremental doses of 0.5–2.0 mg/kg as needed. Our studies, in *healthy unpremedicated children* ages 5–15, revealed that doses of 5–6 mg/kg were required to achieve an adequate induction to general anesthesia in the majority of patients (Figure 7-15).[151] It must be recalled that the termination of the clinical effect of thiopental is primarily dependent on redistribution rather than metabolism. Children, however, are able to metabolize thiopental twice as fast as adults.[152,153] Acute tolerance to thiopental has been well demonstrated in adults, and may also occur in children.[154] A total intravenous dose of 10 mg/kg is generally well-tolerated; however, it is common to have a prolonged period of sleep following surgery, with large doses administered for short procedures. Thiopental is a weak vasodilator and a direct myocardial depressant; both of these effects may result in significant systemic hypotension in the *hypovolemic* state, e.g. dehydration (prolonged fasting) or trauma. Studies in adult patients have found less myocardial depression with thiopental than with the potent inhalational agents. These studies, however, involved small induction doses followed by a slow infusion, which resulted in a gradual rise in arterial levels.[155] Another study of adults found equivalent decreases in blood pressure and increases in heart rate following bolus rather than incremental thiopental administration.[156] A 33 percent reduction in thiopental requirements for induction of anesthesia has been found in patients premedicated with 1.3 mg/kg hydroxyzine and 1.3 mg/kg meperidine.[157]

Thiopental in a solution of 10 percent (20–30 mg/kg) may also be used for induction of anesthesia by rectal instillation. The period of sedation may, however, be longer for thiopental than for methohexital due in part to the slower rate of metabolism.[120]

KETAMINE

Ketamine is a derivative of phencyclidine. Its action is related to central dissociation of the cerebral cortex, and it also causes cerebral excitation. The latter property may be responsible for precipitating seizures in susceptible patients.[158] Ketamine is an excellent analgesic and amnesic; the recommended dosage is 1–3 mg/kg IV or 5–10 mg/kg IM. The duration of action of a single IV dose is 5–8 minutes; further supplementary doses of 0.5–1.0 mg/kg are administered when clinically indicated. Atropine or other antisialogogue should usually accompany the initial dosage in order to diminish the production of copious secretions which occur with ketamine. Ketamine increases heart rate, cardiac index, and systemic blood pressure; it also raises pulmonary artery pressure, but has little effect on respiration.[159,160] The onset of anesthesia is about 30 seconds after an intravenous dose and this is usually heralded by horizontal or vertical nystagmus.[158,161] Studies separating equianesthetic doses of ketamine isomers revealed a lower incidence of side effects, more potent analgesia, and fewer cardiovascular effects with the dextro-ketamine isomer.[162] Acute tolerance to ketamine has been reported.[163]

Children require greater doses of ketamine (mg/kg) than adults because of more rapid degradation; however, there is a large patient-to-patient variability.[164]

The most common adverse reaction to ketamine is postoperative vomiting, which may occur in as many as one in three patients.[161] Intraoperative and postoperative dreaming and hallucinations occur more commonly in older than younger children.[161] The incidence of these latter adverse effects may be reduced when ketamine is supplemented with scopolamine or diazepam.[165] There is one clinical report of two children three years of age who had recurrent nightmares and abnormal behavior persisting for 10 months after a single ketamine administration.[166]

Indications

This is a useful agent for children who are mentally handicapped and unable to cooperate, or for the child who has come to the operating room many times who is frightened and combative. Ketamine can be useful for short-term procedures such as diagnostic spinal punctures, bone marrow aspiration, radiotherapy, angiography, and cardiac catheterization.[167] Other instances when it is of particular value are burn dressing changes, induction of anesthesia in hypovolemic patients, patients in which application of a face mask may prove hazardous such as epidermolysis bullosa, and in patients who require invasive monitoring prior to induction of general anesthesia.[166,168]

Contraindications

Ketamine produces marked increases in intracranial pressure as a result of cerebral vasodilation, and it increases cerebral metabolic rate; therefore, it is contraindicated in any patient with central nervous system pathology which might cause intracranial hypertension.[169,170] A 30 percent rise in intraocular pressure has also been found; thus ketamine may be potentially dangerous in the presence of a corneal laceration.[171]

In children with active upper respiratory tract infections copious secretions produced by ketamine may well exacerbate an already irritable airway and result in laryngospasm.[158,172] It also has been found to result in an incompetent gag reflex, and thus should not be administered as the only anesthetic agent to patients with a full stomach, hiatal hernia, or gastroesophageal reflux.[172]

Ketamine should not be utilized as the sole anesthetic agent in any surgical procedure where total control of the patient's position is necessary, since purposeless movements frequently occur during ketamine anesthesia. Ketamine may be inappropriate in any child with a history of psychiatric or seizure disorder because of its psychotropic and epileptogenic effects.[158]

Although the administration of ketamine seems simple, its side effects are potentially dangerous. *Ketamine must only be administered by physicians experienced with and thoroughly prepared to manage the compromised airway should an adverse reaction occur.* We urge that it not be utilized as a premedication unless given in the presence of continuous supervision by properly trained personnel. Ketamine is an excellent adjuvant to anesthesia, but should be reserved for specific cases and circumstances. A comprehensive review is available.[173]

DROPERIDOL

Droperidol is a centrally acting butyrophenone which alters synaptic transmission by causing a buildup of neurotransmitters; consequently it interferes with normal neurohumoral responses and produces a dissociative state of mind.[174] Because its action, like haloperidol, is primarily in the extrapyramidal areas of the brain, the side effects are extrapyramidal: muscle rigidity, visual disturbances, hallucinations, oculogyric crisis, and dysphoria. Droperidol causes a buildup of dopamine, and thus may be contraindicated in patients with endogenous depression or Parkinsonism.[175] There has been minimal experience in administering this drug to pediatric patients with metabolic defects or movement disorders that involve the extrapyramidal system. The inhibition of neurotransmitters by dopamine following a low dosage of droperidol may be used to advantage for the prevention of nausea and vomiting.[174,176] The classic adult response to droperidol is an outwardly calm patient who is feeling impending doom or depression but is unable to express this feeling.[177]

Its plasma half-life is about 130 minutes, duration of action is 6–12 hours, and some side effects may last as long as 24 hours.[174,178,179] The incidence of undesired side effects is reduced by combining droperidol with a narcotic, sedative, or barbiturate.[180,181] The duration of action of all these medications is less than that of droperidol, and therefore they may need to be supplemented in order to cover the full extent of droperidol's effects.

Droperidol is a weak alpha blocking agent that may cause significant hypotension in the hypovolemic patient, but has minimal cardiovascular effects in the normovolemic state.[182–184] It has been demonstrated to oppose epinephrine-induced arrhythmias.[185]

Respiratory effects of droperidol include a reduction in functional residual capacity (FRC), increased airway resistance, and, when accompanied by fentanyl, an increase in respiratory muscle tone. This may result in the need to use greater inflation pressures when no muscle relaxant is utilized, and may also be an important consideration for the patient whose closing volumes are close to functional residual capacity. Droperidol by itself has not been demonstrated to cause respiratory depression, although there may be considerable patient-to-patient variation.[184,186–191]

Droperidol has been used extensively for premedication as well as the primary anesthetic technique in some centers. There are a few reports of its use in neonates for general surgery as well as for pneumoencephalography.[192–194]

Advantages and Disadvantages

Alpha receptor blockade, the antiarrhythmia effect, sedative, and antiemetic properties of droperidol offer some advantage, especially for awake oral intubation when combined with narcotic and topical anesthetic.[195] The many side effects and prolonged duration of action may offer significant disadvantages. If it has been used with large doses of potent narcotics the threat of respiratory depression combined with the dissociative state it induces may result in airway obstruction, hypoxia, or even death. In addition, when used in patients with increased intracranial pressure or hypovolemia, the alpha blockade may result in a lowered systemic pressure and resultant reduction in cerebral perfusion pressure.[196] For these reasons high doses of droperidol should be limited to selected pediatric situations. Our primary use is in low doses for postoperative sedation in children in whom we wish to minimize postoperative movement.

NARCOTICS

MORPHINE

Morphine is one of the oldest narcotics, and probably the most frequently utilized in children. The usual dose of intravenous morphine is 0.1–0.2 mg/kg; a lower dose may be indicated in the critically ill. The analgesic response to morphine is the standard to which all others are compared. Most studies of morphine have been conducted in adults. Morphine is rapidly and completely absorbed in adults within 20 minutes of intramuscular injection and has a serum half-life of 2.9 ±

0.5 hours IV, and 4.5 ± 0.3 hours IM.[197] Morphine given intramuscularly attains a higher and more sustained level of analgesia than morphine given intravenously; this suggests rapid distribution, metabolism, and excretion.[198] There is a more rapid fall in the serum levels of younger adult patients, which correlates to some extent with the loss of analgesia, but no similar studies have been carried out in infants and children.[199] The major liability for pediatric patients is respiratory depression; it is interesting to note that the respiratory depressant effect of morphine does not correlate with plasma levels.[200,201]

The depression of ventilation is a result of both diminished tidal volume and ventilatory rate; there are also conflicting data regarding a parallel shift in the carbon dioxide response curve versus a change in slope as well as a shift in the carbon dioxide response. Studies in neonates have demonstrated an increased respiratory sensitivity to morphine compared to meperidine.[202] Studies in rats demonstrated a two to three fold greater brain uptake in neonatal rats compared to adult rats.[52,54] This may explain the lower LD_{50} of morphine in neonatal animals, which is 5 times lower than for adults.[2,50] This may also reflect, however, the fact that the synthetic narcotics cross the blood brain barrier easier than morphine. Since the infant has an immature blood brain barrier, a greater proportion of morphine may cross to the brain in the neonate compared to the adult.[50–52] This may account in part for the apparent increased sensitivity of the neonate to morphine compared to meperidine or fentanyl, which rapidly cross the adult or infant blood brain barrier.[203,204] Significant histamine release may follow an intravenous bolus of morphine, which may occasionally result in systemic hypotension.[205]

MEPERIDINE (DEMEROL)

Meperidine is another commonly used narcotic; its principal advantage compared to morphine is that there is less histamine release. This may be beneficial when dealing with the hypovolemic or asthmatic patient. The usual dose of meperidine is 1–2 mg/kg; reduced doses should be used in unstable patients. Most studies concerning uptake and distribution were performed on adults. Meperidine is rapidly absorbed after intramuscular injection, and has a serum half-life of 3.7 ± 1.6 hours when administered intravenously.[206] Since meperidine is commonly administered to the mother during labor and delivery, the neonatal response to this narcotic has been closely examined. The infant respiratory system appears to be less sensitive to meperidine than morphine.[202] The LD_{50} of the neonatal animal is only 20 percent lower than adult animal values corresponding with the human clinical response.[50] This information would seem to suggest that meperidine is safer than morphine when considering neonatal respiratory depression. This may, however, actually reflect the nearly equal ability of meperidine to cross the adult or infant blood–brain barrier. It is important to note that neurobehavioral alterations of the newborn related to meperidine may last *many* hours.[207] As with any narcotic, use in very young infants must be accompanied with careful observation for respiratory depression and airway obstruction.

FENTANYL (SUBLIMAZE)

Fentanyl is a potent narcotic analgesic commonly utilized in pediatrics. The initial popularity of this narcotic stemmed from its rapid onset and brief duration of action.[208] However, while the analgesic effect begins in minutes, and lasts for 30–45 minutes, the respiratory depressant effect begins within minutes and may last for *several hours*.[190] One adult study of low-dose fentanyl demonstrated a biphasic respiratory effect. The response to inspired carbon dioxide returned to normal two hours after the last dose, but fell to 55 percent of control at two and a half hours; the response to carbon dioxide again returned to normal at four hours.[189] Similar studies have not been carried out in infants or children. The implications, however, are clear; the possibility of respiratory depression must be anticipated even several hours after the last administered dose of fentanyl. Another study of adult patients found that with higher doses of fentanyl (25 μg/kg) and mild hyperventilation, respiratory depression could be found up to five hours later; there was a fairly good correlation between plasma levels and respiratory response.[209] Fentanyl is highly lipid-soluble, and rapidly crosses the blood-brain barrier. This may in part explain why the LD_{50} for fentanyl in neonatal animals is 90 percent of that found in adult animals; unlike morphine, the development of the blood-brain barrier has little effect on its entry into brain tissue.[204] Fentanyl half-life is 219 ± 10 minutes, primarily due to the marked affinity of this drug for muscle and fat. Thus, with low dose fentanyl, the termination of action is primarily a combination of redistribution and rapid clearance by the liver. High-dose fentanyl, on the other hand, will accumulate in muscle and fat and will therefore be released slowly, thus accounting for the prolonged respiratory depression when high doses are utilized. There is no evidence of dose-dependent kinetics, i.e., there is no tissue saturation in the clinically used ranges.[210] In some respects this narcotic is very similar to thiopental.[211–214] The usual initial dose is 1–3 μg/kg), to be supplemented as clinically indicated. The use of high-dose fentanyl/oxygen anesthesia (50 μg/kg) has been advocated for high risk operations on adults, but there is limited experience with this technique in children.[214] Continuous infusions of fentanyl have been utilized in some centers.[215,216]

Chest wall rigidity has been reported with many of the narcotic analgesics, but most often following fentanyl; the reason for this is not clear.[217–219] This can be minimized by slow administration. One recent report indicates that glottic rigidity may account for inability to ventilate by bag and mask following intravenous fentanyl.[220]

NEWER NARCOTICS

Alfentanyl, a fentanyl analog, has recently been introduced. Its main advantage appears to be much lower lipid solubility, and much smaller volume of distribution compared to fentanyl. Preliminary studies indicate that brain concentrations are seven to nine times less than fentanyl, the volume of distribution is four times less, and protein binding is greater. Compared to fentanyl more rapid elimination, and thus more rapid termination of its effects, should result. Pediatric applications of this medication may be promising.[221,222]

Butorphanol and nalbuphine are synthetic narcotic-agonist-antagonist analgesics. The claimed advantage of this family of drugs is adequate analgesia, with a ceiling on respiratory depression. No studies have been carried out in children.[223]

SEDATIVES

DIAZEPAM (VALIUM)

Diazepam is probably the most commonly utilized of the benzodiazepine group of sedatives. Diazepam is rapidly absorbed after oral administration, with peak plasma levels at 30 to 90 minutes; the absorption rate has been found to be more rapid in children.[224] Intramuscular administration is painful and results in irregular absorption; plasma levels are only 60 percent of those obtained with a similar oral dose.[225–227]

Diazepam is highly plasma-bound, with a serum half-life varying from 20 to 80 hours; the half-life is shorter in younger adults and children. This probably reflects a greater hepatic blood flow in younger patients compared to older patients.[228,229] The liver is the primary site of metabolism, and hepatic disease may decrease the rate of elimination.[187] Studies in neonates who received diazepam transplacentally from their mothers just prior to delivery have demonstrated prolonged drug effects and serum half-lives, probably as a result of immature hepatic excretory mechanisms (see Figure 7-6).[230–233]

Diazepam has been extensively used for premedication, as an adjunct to balanced anesthesia, for sedation during regional anesthesia, amnesia, and control of seizures. Generally 0.1–0.3 mg/kg (PO, IV or PR) is the recommended safe dosage.[225,226,232–234] We have found this medication particularly useful in the practice of pediatric anesthesia; however, its main disadvantage is that it is often painful when administered intravenously. This may be minimized by prior administration of intravenous lidocaine, and slow administration through a rapidly running IV. Its routine use in newborns or children under one year of age is not indicated because of the prolonged half-life.

CHLORAL HYDRATE

Chloral hydrate is one of the more commonly used sedatives. This drug does not have analgesic properties. The usual dose is 20–40 mg/kg (PO, PR). Its primary use in pediatrics is for sedation prior to noninvasive procedures or as a premedication. Its principal advantage is that it can be administered orally or rectally with excellent absorption and relatively rapid sedation; it also has minimal effects upon respiration. Its bitter taste is a disadvantage. Triclofos sodium is a more acceptable oral form, and may be administered in a dose of 40–70 mg/kg.[235] Like all oral premedicants the time of administration prior to surgery is important to obtain optimal results.

ANTIHISTAMINES

DIPHENHYDRAMINE HYDROCHLORIDE (BENADRYL)

Antihistamines are often used in pediatric anesthesia, both for their H_1 receptor inhibition and their sedative properties. Diphenhydramine hydrochloride is a commonly utilized antihistamine; it is rapidly absorbed and its effects last for three to six hours. The usual dose is 0.2–0.5 mg/kg (PO). It is often administered as a premedicant or as an in-hospital sedative. Caution is advised for patients with respiratory problems, since drying of secretions may make it difficult to expectorate.

CIMETIDINE

Cimetidine is a potent, highly hydrophilic, competitive inhibitor of H_2 mediated histamine reactions.[236,237] Its use in anesthesia is primarily to reduce gastric acidity prior to surgery.[238,240] In children it will reduce the volume of gastric acid and raise the pH above 2.5 when a single dose (7.5 mg/kg) is administered orally at least one hour prior to surgery.[241] Cimetidine appears to be ineffective if less than one hour or more than four hours has elapsed since receiving the drug. Our indications include a history of gastroesophageal reflux, hiatus hernia, bronchoscopy, or an anticipated difficult intubation which will require prolonged laryngoscopy.

ANTICHOLINERGICS

ATROPINE AND SCOPOLAMINE

Atropine (0.02 mg/kg) and scopolamine (0.01 mg/kg) have central nervous system effects, with the sedating effect of scopolamine being 5–15 times greater than atropine. Scopolamine is also a two to three times more potent antisialogogue.[242,243] Atropine and scopolamine decrease the ability to sweat, and thus may result in a slight rise in temperature. The normal response to cold stress is also altered, especially in the neonate.[244,245] Atropine and scopolamine appear to have equipotent cardiovascular accelerator properties; however, infants seem to require slightly greater doses for each kilogram than adults in order to achieve this response.[246,247] There are specific situations for which anticholinergics are appropriate; to diminish secretions preoperatively, to block laryngeal and vagal reflexes, to treat the bradycardia associated with succinylcholine, the muscarinic effects of neostigmine, the oculocardiac reflex, and the arrhythmias of the Wolf-Parkinson-White syndrome. Atropine is painful on intramuscular injection, and as a premedicant will not block laryngeal reflexes; it is much more effective for this purpose when given intravenously. There are some data suggesting that Down's syndrome children are more susceptible to the cardiac effects of atropine. Our clinical experience, and that of others, has not borne this out.[247–249] One must be aware, however, that Down's syndrome children frequently have narrow-angle glaucoma, and atropine must be cautiously administered in this situation.[248]

In our clinical practice we limit the use of scopolamine to those cases in which its sedative effect, combined with that of morphine, will be most advantageous, such as cardiac or hyperactive patients. It is also very useful as an adjuvant to ketamine anesthesia because of its antisialogogue and central sedative effects. The central sedative effects of both atropine and scopolamine may be reversed with physostigmine. We do not routinely administer anticholinergic medications as part of the premedication because it is painful, the optimal effect may not coincide with induction of anesthesia, and because the modern potent inhalational agents produce fewer secretions.

GLYCOPYRROLATE

Glycopyrrolate (0.005–0.01 mg/kg) is a synthetic quaternary ammonium compound with potent anticholinergic properties. It offers some advantage over atropine and scopolamine because minimal penetration of the blood–brain barrier occurs, and thus there are minimal central effects. Several studies have demonstrated glycopyrrolate to be superior to atropine because its anticholinergic effects last for three to four hours. There is minimal change in the heart rate after intravenous administration, and thus there is a lower incidence of cardiac arrhythmias.[250–254] In some children there appears to be the added advantage of a reduction in gastric volume and acidity.[255,256] This does not occur in adults in the usual clinical doses.[257]

REFERENCES

1. Cook DR: Paediatric anaesthesia: Pharmacological considerations. *Drugs* 12:212–221, 1976
2. Cook DR: Neonatal anesthetic pharmacology: A review. *Anesth Analg* 53:544–548, 1974
3. Yaffe SJ, Back N: Neonatal pharmacology, in Forbes GB (ed): *Recent Clinical Advances* Ped Clin NA 13:527–541, 1966. W.B. Saunders Co. Philadelphia
4. Morselli PL: Clinical pharmacokinetics in neonates. *Clin Pharmacokinet* 1:81–98, 1976
5. Rane A, Wilson JT: Clinical pharmacokinetics in infants and children. *Clin Pharmacokinet* 1:2–24, 1976
6. Currin MR: Pharmacology of the neonate. *S Afr Med J* 56:101–105, 1979
7. Udkow G: Pediatric clinical pharmacology. A practical review. *Am J Dis Child* 132:1025–1032, 1978
8. Levy G: Pharmacokinetics of fetal and neonatal exposure to drugs. *Obstet Gynecol* 58:S9–16, 1981
9. Rane A, Sjoqvist F: Drug metabolism in the human fetus and newborn infant, in Yaffe SJ (ed): *Pediatric Pharmacology.* Pedi Clin N A 19:37–49, 1972. Philadelphia, W.B. Saunders
10. Yaffe SJ, Juchau MR: Perinatal pharmacology. *Annu Rev Pharmacol Toxicol* 14:219–238, 1974
11. Mirkin BL: Perinatal pharmacology: Placental transfer, fetal localization, and neonatal disposition of drugs. *Anesthesiology* 43:156–170, 1975
12. Krasner J, Giacoia GP, Yaffe SJ: Drug–protein binding in the newborn infant. *Ann NY Acad Sci* 226:101–114, 1973
13. Krasner J: Drug–protein interaction, in Yaffe SJ (ed): *Pediatric Pharmacology.* Pedi Clin N A 19:51–63, 1972. Philadelphia, W.B. Saunders
14. Friis-Hansen B: Body composition during growth: In vivo measurements and biochemical data correlated to differential anatomical growth. *Pediatrics* 47:264–274, 1971
15. Brown AK, Zuelzer WW, Burnett HH: Studies on the neonatal development of the glucuronide conjugating system. *J Clin Invest* 37:332–340, 1958
16. Jusko WJ: Pharmacokinetic principles in pediatric pharmacology, in Yaffe SJ (ed): *Pediatric Pharmacology.* Pedi Clin N A 19:81–100, 1972. Philadelphia, W.B Saunders
17. Brodersen R: Bilirubin transport in the newborn infant, reviewed with relation to kernicterus. *J Pediatr* 96:349–356, 1980
18. Stern L: Drugs, the newborn infant, and the binding of bilirubin to albumin. *Pediatrics* 49:916–918, 1972
19. Silverman WA, Andersen DH, Blanc WA, et al: Difference in mortality rate and incidence of kernicterus among premature infants allotted to 2 prophylactic antibacterial regimens. *Pediatrics* 18:614–625, 1956
20. Ehrnebo M, Agurell S, Jalling B, et al: Age differences in drug binding by plasma proteins: Studies on human foetuses, neonates, and adults. *Eur J Clin Pharmacol* 3:189–193, 1971
21. Rane A, Lunde PK, Jalling B, et al: Plasma protein binding of diphenylhydantoin in normal and hyperbilirubinemic patients. *J Pediatr* 78:877–882, 1971

22. Kanto J, Erkkola R, Sellman R: Distribution and metabolism of diazepam in early and late human pregnancy. Postnatal metabolism of diazepam. *Acta Pharmacol Toxicol* 35:S49, 1974

23. Christensen JH, Andreasen F, Jansen JA: Pharmacokinetics of thiopental in caesarian section. *Acta Anaesthesiol Scand* 25:174–179, 1981

24. Aranda JV, Sitar DS, Parsons WD, et al: Pharmacokinetic aspects of theophylline in premature newborns. *N Engl J Med* 295:413–416, 1976

25. Odell GB: The dissociation of bilirubin from albumin and its clinical implications. *J Pediatr* 55:268–279, 1959

26. Thomas J, Climie CR, Mather LE: The maternal plasma levels and placental transfer of bupivacaine following epidural anesthesia. *Br J Anaesth* 41:1035–1040, 1969

27. Rane A, Lunde PKM, Jalling B, et al: Plasma protein binding of diphenylhydantoin in normal and hyperbilirubinemic infants. *J Pediatr* 78:877–882, 1971

28. Hamar C, Levy G: Serum protein binding of drugs and bilirubin in newborn infants and their mothers. *Clin Pharmacol Ther* 28:58–63, 1980

29. Brodersen R: Free bilirubin in blood plasma of the newborn. Effects of albumin, fatty acids, pH, displacing drugs, and phototherapy, in Stern L, Oh W, and Friis-Hansen B (eds): *Intensive Care in the Newborn II*. New York, Masson, 1978

30. Kaplan JM, McCracken GH, Horton LJ, et al: Pharmacologic studies in neonates given large dosages of ampicillin. *J Pediatr* 84:571–577, 1974

31. McCracken GH: Pharmacological basis for antimicrobial therapy in newborn infants. *Am J Dis Child* 128:407–419, 1974

32. Fisher DM, O'Keeffe C, Stanski DR, et al: Pharmacokinetics and pharmacodynamics of d-tubucurarine in infants, children, and adults. *Anesthesiology* 57:203–208, 1982

33. Pinsky WW, Jackobsen JR, Gillette PC, et al: Dosage of digoxin in premature infants. *J Pediatr* 94:639–642, 1979

34. Wettrell G, Andersson KE: Clinical pharmacokinetics of digoxin in infants. *Clin Pharmacokinet* 2:17–31, 1977

35. Cook DR: Muscle relaxants in infants and children. *Anesth Analg* 60:335–343, 1981

36. Krauer B, Draffan GH, Williams FM, et al: Elimination kinetics of amobarbital in mothers and their newborn infants. *Clin Pharmacol Ther* 14:442–447, 1973

37. Bovill JG, Sebel PS: Pharmacokinetics of high-dose fentanyl: A study in patients undergoing cardiac surgery. *Br J Anaesth* 52:795–801, 1980

38. Yaffe SJ, Krasner J, Catz CS: Variations in detoxication enzymes during mammalian development. *Ann NY Acad Sci* 151:887–899, 1968

39. Yaffe SJ, Levy G, Matsuzawa T, et al: Enhancement of glucuronide-conjugating capacity in a hyperbilirubinemic infant due to apparent enzyme induction by phenobarbital. *N Engl J Med* 275:1461–1466, 1966

40. Morselli PL, Mandelli M, Togononi G, et al: Drug interactions in the human fetus and in the newborn infant, in Morselli PL, Cohen (eds): *Drug Interactions*. New York, Raven Press, 1974, pp 259–270

41. West JR, Smith HW, Chasis H: Glomerular filtration rate, effective renal blood flow, and maximal tubular excretory capacity in infancy. *J Pediatr* 32:10–18, 1948

42. Chantler C: Newborn disorders, in Lieberman E (ed): *Clinical Pediatric Nephrology*. Philadelphia, J.B. Lippincott, 1976, pp 310–339

43. Chantler C: Evaluation of laboratory and other methods of measuring renal function, in Lieberman E (ed): *Clinical Pediatric Nephrology*. Philadelphia, J.B. Lippincott, 1976, pp 510–527

44. Guignard JP, Torrado A, DaCunha O, et al: Glomerular filtration rate in the first three weeks of life. *J Pediatr* 87:268–272, 1975

45. Leake RD, Trygstad CW, Oh W: Inulin clearance in the newborn infant: Relationship to gestational and postnatal age. *Pediatr Res* 10:759–762, 1976

46. Leake RD, Trygstad CW: Glomerular filtration rate during the period of adaptation to extrauterine life. *Pediatr Res* 11:959–962, 1977

47. Eichenwald HF, McCracken GH: Antimicrobial therapy in infants and children. *J Pediatr* 93:337–377, 1978

48. Ng PK, Coté J, Schiff D, et al: Renal clearance of digoxin in premature neonates. *Res Commun* Chem *Pathol Pharmacol* 34:207–216, 1981

49. Lang D, von Bernuth G: Serum concentrations and serum half-life of digoxin in premature and mature newborns. *Pediatrics* 59:902–906, 1977

50. Goldenthal EI: A compilation of LD_{50} values in newborn and adult animals. *Toxicol Appl Pharmacol* 18:185–207, 1971

51. Done AK: Developmental pharmacology. *Clin Pharmacol Ther* 5:432–479, 1964

52. Kupferberg H, Way E: Pharmacologic basis for the increased sensitivity of the newborn rat to morphine. *J Pharmacol Exp Ther* 141:105–112, 1963

53. Domek NS, Barlow CF, Roth LJ: An ontogentic study of phenobarbital-C^{14} in cat brain. *J Pharmacol Exp Ther* 130:285–293, 1960

54. Milthers K: The toxicity of morphine to fully grown and unweaned rats by constant intravenous infusion. *Acta Pharmacol Toxicol* 17:200–204, 1960

55. Ebert AG, Yim GK: Barbital sensitivity in the young rat. *Toxicol Appl Pharmacol* 3:182–187, 1961

56. Sanner JH, Woods LA: Comparative distribution of tritium labelled dihydromorphine between maternal and fetal rats. *J Pharmacol Exp Ther* 148:176–184, 1965

57. Nicodemus HF, Nassiri-Rahimi C, Bachman L, et al: Median effective doses (ED_{50}) of halothane in adults and children. *Anesthesiology* 31:344–348, 1969

58. Gregory GA, Eger EI, II, Munson ES: The relationship between age and halothane requirement in man. *Anesthesiology* 30:488–491, 1969

59. Gregory GA, Wade JG, Beihl DR, et al: Fetal anesthetic requirement (MAC) for halothane. *Anesth Analg* 62:9–14, 1983

60. Lerman J, Robinson S, Willis MM, et al: Anesthetic requirements for halothane in young children 0–1 month and 1–6 months of age. *Anesthesiology* 59:421–424, 1983

61. Cook DR, Brandom BW, Shiu G, et al: The inspired median effective dose, brain concentration at anesthesia, and cardiovascular index for halothane in young rats. *Anesth Analg* 60:182–185, 1981

62. Barash PG, Glanz S, Katz JD, et al: Ventricular function in children during halothane anesthesia: An echocardiographic evaluation. *Anesthesiology* 49:79–85, 1978

63. Yakaitis RW, Blitt CD, Angiulo JP: End-tidal halothane concentration for endotracheal intubation. *Anesthesiology* 47:386–388, 1977

64. Salanitre E, Rackow H: The pulmonary exchange of nitrous oxide and halothane in infants and children. *Anesthesiology* 30:388–394, 1969

65. Eger EI, II, Bahlman SH, Munson ES: The effect of age on the rate of increase of alveolar anesthetic concentration. *Anesthesiology* 35:365–372, 1971

66. Brandom BW, Brandom RB, Cook DR: Uptake and distribution of halothane in infants: In vivo measurements and computer simulations. *Anesth Analg* 62:404–410, 1983

67. Marshall BE, Wollman H: General anesthetics, in Gilman AG, Goodman LS, Gilman A (eds): *The Pharmacological Basis of Therapeutics*. New York, MacMillan, 1980, pp 276–299

68. Katz RL, Gissen AJ: Neuromuscular and electromyographic effects of halothane and its interaction with d-tubocurarine in man. *Anesthesiology* 28:564–567, 1967

69. Klide AM, Aviado DM: Mechanism for the reduction in pul-

monary resistance induced by halothane. *J Pharmacol Exp Ther* 158:28–35, 1967

70. Hickey RF, Graf PD, Nadel JA, et al: The effects of halothane and cyclopropane on total pulmonary resistance in the dog. *Anesthesiology* 31:334–343, 1969

71. Hirshman CA, Edelstein G, Peetz S, et al: Mechanism of action of inhalational anesthesia on airways. *Anesthesiology* 56:107–111, 1982

72. Hirshman CA. Airway reactivity in humans: Anesthetic implications. *Anesthesiology* 58:170–177, 1983

73. Roizen MF, Stevens WC: Multiform ventricular tachycardia due to the interaction of aminophylline and halothane. *Anesth Analg* 57:738–741, 1978

74. Koehntop DE, Liao J-C, Van Bergen FH: Effects of pharmacologic alterations of adrenergic mechanisms by cocaine, tropolone, aminophylline, and ketamine on epinephrine-induced arrhythmias during halothane–nitrous oxide anesthesia. *Anesthesiology* 46:83–93, 1977

75. Stirt JA, Berger JM, Ricker SM, et al: Aminophylline pharmacokinetics and cardiorespiratory effects during halothane anesthesia in experimental animals. *Anesth Analg* 59:186–191, 1980

76. Smith RM: Pediatric anesthesia in perspective. Sixteenth annual Baxter-Travenol lecture. *Anesth Analg* 57:634–646, 1978

77. Lewis RB, Blair M: Halothane hepatitis in a young child. *Br J Anaesth* 54:349–354, 1982

78. Vergani D, Mieli-Vergani G, Alberti A, et al: Antibodies to the surface of halothane-altered rabbit hepatocytes in patients with severe halothane-associated hepatitis. *N Engl J Med* 303:66–71, 1980

79. Dienstag JL: Halothane hepatitis: Allergy or idiosyncrasy? *N Engl J Med* 303:102–104, 1980

80. Szyfelbein SK: Personal communication.

81. Shingu K, Eger EI, II, Johnson BH: Hypoxia may be more important than reductive metabolism in halothane-induced hepatic injury. *Anesth Analg* 61:824–827, 1982

82. Van Dyke RA: Hepatic centrilobular necrosis in rats after exposure to halothane, enflurane, or isoflurane. *Anesth Analg* 61:812–819, 1982

83. Pohl LR, Gillette JR: A perspective on halothane-induced hepatotoxicity. *Anesth Analg* 61:809–811, 1982

84. Gall EA: Report of the pathology panel—National Halothane Study. *Anesthesiology* 29:233–248, 1968

85. Walzer, Sarita: Personal communication.

86. Johnston RR, Eger EI, II, Wilson C: A comparative interaction of epinephrine with enflurane, isoflurane, and halothane in man. *Anesth Analg* 55:709–712, 1976

87. Katz RL, Bigger JT, Jr: Cardiac arrhythmias during anesthesia and operation. *Anesthesiology* 33:193–213, 1970

88. Melgrave AP: The use of epinephrine in the presence of halothane in children. *Can Anaesth Soc J* 17:256–260, 1970

89. Karl HW, Swedlow DB, Lee KW, et al: Epinephrine–halothane interactions in children. *Anesthesiology* 58:142–145, 1983

90. Ueda W, Hirakawa M, Mae O: Appraisal of epinephrine administration to patients under halothane anesthesia for closure of cleft palate. *Anesthesiology* 58:574–576, 1983

91. Smith AL, Wollman H: Cerebral blood flow and metabolism: Effects of anesthetic drugs and techniques. *Anesthesiology* 36:378–400, 1972

92. Murphy FL, Kennell EM, Johnson RE, et al: The effects of enflurane, isoflurane, and halothane on cerebral blood flow and metabolism in man. Chicago, Abstracts of Scientific Papers, American Society of Anesthesiologists 1974, p. 61

93. Hoyal RHA, Prys-Roberts C, Simpson PJ: Enflurane in outpatient paediatric dental anesthesia: A comparison with Halothane. *Br J Anaesth* 52:219–221, 1980

94. Steward DJ: A trial of enflurane for paediatric out-patient anaesthesia. *Can Anaesth Soc J* 24:603–608, 1977

95. Hirshman CA, Bergman NA: Halothane and enflurane protect against bronchospasm in an asthma dog model. *Anesth Analg* 57:629–633, 1978

96. Fogdall RP, Miller RD: Neuromuscular effects of enflurane, alone and combined with d-tubocurarine, pancuronium, and succinylcholine, in man. *Anesthesiology* 42:173–178, 1975

97. Lindgren L, Saarnivaara L: Cardiovascular responses to enflurane induction followed by suxamethonium in children. *Br J Anaesth* 55:269–273, 1983

98. Koff SA, Solomon MH, Lane GA, et al: Urodynamic studies in anesthetized children. *J Urol* 123:61–63, 1980

99. Denlinger JK, Lecky JH, Nahrwold ML: Hepatocellular dysfunction without jaundice after enflurane anesthesia. *Anesthesiology* 41:86–87, 1974

100. Shapiro HM: Intracranial hypertension: Therapeutic and anesthetic considerations. *Anesthesiology* 43:445–471, 1975

101. Mazze RI, Calverley RK, Smith NT: Inorganic fluoride nephrotoxicity: Prolonged enflurane and halothane anesthesia in volunteers. *Anesthesiology* 46:265–271, 1977

102. Neigh JL, Garman JK, Harp JR: The electroencephalographic pattern during anesthesia with ethrane: Effects of depth of anesthesia, $PaCO_2$ and nitrous oxide. *Anesthesiology* 35:482–487, 1971

103. Flemming DC, Fitzpatrick J, Fariello RG, et al: Diagnostic activation of epileptogenic foci by enflurane. *Anesthesiology* 52:431–433, 1980

104. Gallagher TJ, Galindo A, Richey ET: Inhibition of seizure activity during enflurane anesthesia. *Anesth Analg* 57:130–132, 1978

105. Wade JG, Stevens WC: Isoflurane: An anesthetic for the eighties? *Anesth Analg* 60:666–682, 1981

106. Eger, EI, II: Isoflurane: A review. *Anesthesiology* 55:559–576, 1981

107. Friesen RH, Lichtor JL: Cardiovascular effects of inhalation induction with isoflurance in infants. *Anesth Analg* 62:411–414, 1983

108. Pandit UA, Leach AB, Steude GM: Induction and recovery characteristics of halothane and isoflurane anesthesia in children. *Anesthesiology* 59:A445, 1983

109. Dolan WM, Stevens WC, Eger EI, II, et al: The cardiovascular and respiratory effects of isoflurane-nitrous oxide anesthesia. *Can Anaesth Soc J* 21:557–568, 1974

110. Linde HW, Oh SO, Homi J, et al: Cardiovascular effects of isoflurane and halothane during controlled ventilation in older patients. *Anesth Analg* 54:701–704, 1975

111. Stevens WC, Cromwell TH, Halsey MJ, et al: The cardiovascular effects of a new inhalation anesthetic, forane, in human volunteers at constant arterial carbon dioxide tension. *Anesthesiology* 35:8–16, 1971

112. Vitez TS, Miller RD, Eger EI, II, et al: Comparison in vitro of isoflurane and halothane potentiation of d-tubocurarine and succinylcholine neuromuscular blockades. *Anesthesiology* 41:53–56, 1974

113. Joseph MM, Shah K, Viljoen JF: Malignant hyperthermia associated with isoflurane anesthesia. *Anesth Analg* 61:711–712, 1982

114. Newberg LA, Michenfelder JD: Cerebral protection by isoflurane during hypoxia or ischemia. *Anesthesiology* 59:29–35, 1983

115. Kissin I, Morgan PL, Smith LR: Comparison of isoflurane and halothane safety margins in rats. *Anesthesiology* 58:556–561, 1983

116. Koblin DD, Lurz FW, Eger EI, II: Age-dependent alterations in nitrous oxide requirement of mice. *Anesthesiology* 58:428–431, 1983

117. Henriksen HT, Jorgensen PB: The effect of nitrous oxide on intracranial pressure in patients with intracranial disorders. *Br J Anaesth* 45:486–492, 1973

118. Tenney SM, Carpenter FG, Rahn H: Gas transfers in a sulfur

hexafluride pneumoperitoneum. *J Appl Physiol* 6:201–208, 1953

119. Eger EI, II, Saidman LJ: Hazards of nitrous oxide anesthesia in bowel obstruction and pneumothorax. *Anesthesiology* 26:61–66, 1965

120. Saidman LJ, Eger EI, II: Change in cerebrospinal fluid pressure during pneumoencephalography under nitrous oxide anesthesia. *Anesthesiology* 26:67–72, 1965

121. Owens WD, Gustave F, Sclaroff A: Tympanic membrane rupture with nitrous oxide anesthesia. *Anesth Analg* 57:283–286, 1978

122. Perreault L, Normandin N, Plamondon L, et al: Middle ear pressure variations during nitrous oxide and oxygen anaesthesia. *Can Anaesth Soc J* 29:428–434, 1982

123. Perreault L, Normandin N, Plamandon L, et al: Tympanic membrane rupture after anesthesia with nitrous oxide. *Anesthesiology* 57:325–326, 1982

124. Coté CJ: The anesthetic management of congenital lobar emphysema. *Anesthesiology* 49:296–298, 1978

125. Wolf GL, Capuano C, Hartung J: Nitrous oxide increases intraocular pressure after intravitreal sulfur hexafluride injection. *Anesthesiology* 59:547–548, 1983

126. Schulte-Sasse U, Hess W, Tarnow J: Pulmonary vascular responses to nitrous oxide in patients with normal and high pulmonary vascular resistance. *Anesthesiology* 57:9–13, 1982

127. Winter PM, Smith G: The toxicity of oxygen. *Anesthesiology* 37:210–241, 1972

128. James LS, Lanman JT (eds): History of oxygen therapy and retrolental fibroplasia. *Pediatr* (suppl) 57:591–642, 1976

129. Betts EK, Downes JJ, Schaffer DB, et al: Retrolental fibroplasia and oxygen administration during general anesthesia. *Anesthesiology* 47:518–520, 1977

130. Merritt JC, Sprague DH, Merritt WE, et al: Retrolental fibroplasia: A multifactorial disease. *Anesth Analg 60:109–111, 1981*

131. Kalina RE, Hodson WA, Morgan BC: Retrolental fibroplasia in a cyanotic infant. *Pediatrics* 50:765–768, 1972

132. Adamkin DH, Shott RJ, Cook LN, et al: Nonhyperoxic retrolental fibroplasia. *Pediatrics* 60:828–830, 1977

133. Wolbarsht ML, George GS, Kylstra J, et al: Does carbon dioxide play a role in retrolental fibroplasia? *Pediatrics* 70:500–501, 1982

134. Phelps DL, Rosenbaum AL: Effects of marginal hypoxemia on recovery from oxygen-induced retinopathy in the kitten model. *Pediatrics* 73:1–6, 1984

135. Johnson L: Retrolental fibroplasia: A new look at an unsolved problem. *Hosp Pract* 16:109–121, 1981

136. Patz A: Retrolental fibroplasia. *Surv Ophthalmol* 14:1–29, 1969

137. Quinn GE, Betts EK, Diamond GR, et al: Neonatal age (human) at retinal maturation. *Anesthesiology* 55:S326, 1981

138. Phelps DL: Retinopathy of prematurity: An estimate of vision loss in the United States—1979. *Pediatrics* 67:924–925, 1981

139. Avery ME: Recent increase in mortality from hyaline membrane disease. *Pediatrics* 57:553–559, 1960

140. Bolton DPG, Cross KW: Further observations on cost of preventing retrolental fibroplasia. *Lancet* 1:445–448, 1974

141. Lucey JF, Dangman B: A reexamination of the role of oxygen in retrolental fibroplasia. *Pediatrics* 73:82–96, 1984

142. Saidman LJ: Uptake and distribution of intravenous agents: The thiopental model. *ASA Refresher Course Outlines, vol 3.* Philadelphia, W.B. Saunders, 1975, pp 141–151

143. Saidman LJ, Eger EI, II: Uptake and distribution of thiopental after oral, rectal, or intramuscular administration. *Clin Pharmacol Ther* 14:12–20, 1973

144. Liu LMP, Coté CJ, Goudsouzian NG, et al: Response to intravenous induction doses of methohexital in children. *Anesthesiology* 55:A330, 1981

145. Rockoff M, Goudsouzian NG: Seizures induced by methohexital. *Anesthesiology* 54:333–335, 1981

146. Liu LMP, Goudsouzian NG, Liu PL: Rectal methohexital premedication in children, a dose comparison study. *Anesthesiology* 53:343–345, 1980

147. Liu LMP, Gaudreault P, Friedman PA, et al: Methohexital plasma concentrations in children following rectal administration. *Anesthesiology* 62: 567–570, 1985

148. Breimer DD: Pharmacokinetics of methohexitone following intravenous infusion in humans. *Br J Anaesth* 48:643–649, 1976

149. Stanski DR, Watkins WD (ed): *Drug Disposition in Anesthesia.* New York, Grune & Stratton, 1982

150. Ghoneim MM, Van Hamme MJ: Pharmacokinetics of thiopentone: Effects of enflurane and nitrous oxide anaesthesia and surgery. *Br J Anaesth* 50:1237–1242, 1978

151. Coté CJ, Goudsouzian NG, Liu LMP, et al: The dose response of intravenous thiopental for the induction of general anesthesia in unpremedicated children. *Anesthesiology* 55:703–705, 1981

152. Burch PG, Stanski DR: The role of metabolism and protein binding in thiopental anesthesia. *Anesthesiology* 58:146–152, 1983

153. Sorbo S, Hudson RJ, Loomis JC: The pharmacokinetics of thiopental in pediatric surgical patients. *Anesthesiology* 61:666–670, 1984

154. Toner W, Howard PJ, McGowan WAW, et al: Another look at acute tolerance to thiopentane. *Br J Anaesth* 52:1005–1008, 1980

155. Becker KE, Jr, Tonnesen AS: Cardiovascular effects of plasma levels of thiopental necessary for anesthesia. *Anesthesiology* 49:197–200, 1978

156. Seltzer JL, Gerson JI, Allen FB: Comparison of the cardiovascular effects of bolus v. incremental administration of thiopentone. *Br J Anaesth* 52:527–529, 1980

157. Becker KE, Jr: Plasma levels of thiopental necessary for anesthesia. *Anesthesiology* 49:192–196, 1978

158. Wilson RD: Current status of ketamine. *ASA Refresher Courses, vol 1.* Philadelphia, W.B. Saunders, 1973, p 157–167

159. Virtue RW, Alanis JM, Mori M, et al: An anesthetic agent: 2-orthochlorophenyl, 2-methylamino cyclohexanone HCL (CI-581). *Anesthesiology* 28:823–833, 1967

160. Tweed WA, Minuck M, Mymin D: Circulatory responses to ketamine anesthesia. *Anesthesiology* 37:613–619, 1972

161. Hollister GR, Burn JMB: Side effects of ketamine in pediatric anesthesia. *Anesth Analg* 53:264–267, 1974

162. White PF, Ham J, Way WL, et al: Pharmacology of ketamine isomers in surgical patients. *Anesthesiology* 52:231–239, 1980

163. Byer DE, Gould AB, Jr: Development of tolerance to ketamine in an infant undergoing repeated anesthesia. *Anesthesiology* 54:255–256, 1981

164. Grant IS, Nimmo WS, McNicol LR, et al: Ketamine disposition in children and adults. *Br J Anaesth* 55:1107–1111, 1983

165. Jarem BJ, Walker JA, Parks DH, et al: Current practice in anesthesia for pediatric burns: 12 years' experience. *Anesth Rev* 10:16–23, 1978

166. Meyers EF, Charles P: Prolonged adverse reactions to ketamine in children. *Anesthesiology* 49:39–40, 1978

167. Corssen G, Groves EH, Gomez S, et al: Ketamine: its place for neurosurgical diagnostic procedures. *Anesth Analg* 48:181–188, 1969

168. LoVerme SR, Oropollo AT: Ketamine anesthesia in dermolytic bullous dermatosis (epidermolysis bullosa). *Anesth Analg* 56:398–401, 1977

169. Takeshita H, Okuda Y, Sari A: The effects of ketamine on cerebral circulation and metabolism in man. *Anesthesiology* 36:69–75, 1972

170. Crumrine RS, Pulsen FE, Weiss MH: Alterations in ventricular fluid pressure during ketamine anesthesia in hydrocephalic children. *Anesthesiology* 42:758–761, 1975

171. Yoshikawa K, Murai Y: The effect of ketamine on intraocular pressure in children. *Anesth Analg* 50:199–202, 1971

172. Carson IW, Moore J, Balmer JP, et al: Laryngeal competence with ketamine and other drugs. *Anesthesiology* 38:128–133, 1973

173. White PF, Way WL, Trevor AJ: Ketamine—its pharmacology and therapeutic uses. *Anesthesiology* 56:119–136, 1982

174. Edmonds-Seal J, Prys-Roberts C: Pharmacology of drugs used in neuroleptanalgesia. *Br J Anaesth* 42:207–216, 1970

175. Lassner J (chairman): Symposium on neuroleptanalgesia. *Acta Anaesth Scand* (suppl) 25:251–279, 1966

176. Abramowitz MD, Oh TH, Epstein BS, et al: The antiemetic effect of droperidol following outpatient strabismus surgery in children. *Anesthesiology* 59:579–583, 1983

177. Saarne A: Experiences with haloperidol (Haldol) as a premedicant. *Acta Anaesth Scand* 7:21–30, 1963

178. Korttila K, Linnoila M: Skills related to driving after intravenous diazepam, flunitrazepam or droperidol. *Br J Anaesth* 46:961–969, 1974

179. Cressman WA, Plostnieks J, Johnson PC: Absorption, metabolism, and excretion of droperidol by human subjects following intramuscular and intravenous administration. *Anesthesiology* 38:363–369, 1973

180. Norris W, Telfer ABM: Thalamol as a preoperative sedative. *Br J Anaesth* 40:517–521, 1968

181. Brown AS, Horton JM, MacRae WR: Anesthesia for neurosurgery: The use of haloperidol and phenoperidine with light general anaesthesia. *Anaesthesia* 18:143–150, 1963

182. Whitwam JG, Russell WJ: The acute cardiovascular changes and adrenergic blockade by droperidol in man. *Br J Anaesth* 43:581–591, 1971

183. Stanley TH, Bennett GM, Loeser EA, et al: Cardiovascular effects of diazepam and droperidol during morphine anesthesia. *Anesthesiology* 44:255–258, 1976

184. Stoelting RK, Gibbs PS, Creasser CW, et al: Hemodynamic and ventilatory responses to fentanyl, fentanyl–droperidol, and nitrous oxide in patients with acquired valvular heart disease. *Anesthesiology* 42:319–324, 1975

185. Long G, Dripps RD, Price HL: Measurement of anti-arrhythmic potency of drugs in man: Effects of dehydrobenzperidol. *Anesthesiology* 28:318–323, 1967

186. Kallos T, Wyche MQ, Garman JK: The effects of Innovar on functional residual capacity and total chest compliance in man. *Anesthesiology* 39:558–561, 1973

187. Kallos T, Smith TC: The respiratory effects of Innovar given for premedication. *Br J Anaesth* 41:303–306, 1969

188. Cottrell JE, Wolfson B, Siker ES: Changes in airway resistance following droperidol, hydroxyzine, and diazepam in normal volunteers. *Anesth Analg* 55:18–21, 1976

189. Becker LD, Paulson BA, Miller RD, et al: Biphasic respiratory depression after fentanyl–droperidol or fentanyl alone used to supplement nitrous oxide anesthesia. *Anesthesiology* 44:291–296, 1976

190. Harper MH, Hickey RF, Cromwell TH, et al: The magnitude and duration of respiratory depression produced by fentanyl and fentanyl plus droperidol in man. *J Pharmacol Exp Ther* 199:464–468, 1976

191. Prokocimer P, Delavault E, Rey F, et al: Effects of droperidol on respiratory drive in humans. *Anesthesiology* 59:113–116, 1983

192. Wolfson B, Kielar CM, Shenoy NR, et al: Analgesic "cocktails" for pneumoencephalography: Ketamine, diazepam, alphaprodine, and droperidol. *Anesth Analg* 52:779–783, 1973

193. Kay B: Neuroleptanesthesia for neonates and infants. *Anesth Analg* 52:970–973, 1973

194. McGarry PMF: A double blind study of diazepam, droperidol, and meperidine as premedication in children. *Can Anaesth Soc J* 17:157–165, 1970

195. Foldes FF: Neuroleptanalgesia for awake intubation and peroral endoscopies, in Oyama T (ed): *Neuroleptanesthesia. International Anesthesia Clinics, vol 11(3)*. Boston, Little, Brown, 1973, pp 93–102

196. Misfeldt BB, Jorgensen PB, Spotoft H, et al: The effects of droperidol and fentanyl on intracranial pressure and cerebral perfusion pressure in neurosurgical patients. *Br J Anaesth* 48:963–968, 1976

197. Stanski DR, Greenblatt DJ, Lowenstein E: Kinetics of intravenous and intramuscular morphine. *Clin Pharmacol Ther* 24:52–59, 1978

198. Brunk SF, Delle M: Morphine metabolism in man. *Clin Pharmacol Ther* 16:51–57, 1974

199. Berkowitz BA, Ngai SH, Yang JC, et al: The disposition of morphine in surgical patients. *Clin Pharmacol Ther* 17:629–635, 1975

200. Rigg JRA: Ventilatory effects and plasma concentration of morphine in man. *Br J Anaesth* 50:759–765, 1978

201. Weil JV, McCullough RE, Kline JS, et al: Diminished ventilatory response to hypoxia and hypercapnia after morphine in normal man. *N Engl J Med* 292:1103–1106, 1975

202. Way WL, Costley EC, Way EL: Respiratory sensitivity of the newborn infant to meperidine and morphine. *Clin Pharmacol Ther* 6:454–461, 1965

203. Meuldermans WEG, Hurkmans, RMA, Heykants JJP: Plasma protein binding and distribution of fentanyl, sufentanil, alfentanil, and lofentanil in blood. *Arch Int Pharmacodyn Ther* 257:4–19, 1982

204. McClain DA, Hug CC, Jr: Intravenous fentanyl kinetics. *Clin Pharm Ther* 28:106–114, 1980

205. Moss J, Rosow CE: Histamine release by narcotics and muscle relaxants in humans. *Anesthesiology* 59:330–339, 1983

206. Mather LE, Tucker GT, Pflug AE, et al: Meperidine kinetics in man: Intravenous injection in surgical patients and volunteers. *Clin Pharmacol Ther* 17:21–30, 1975

207. Brackbill Y, Kane J, Manniello RL, et al: Obstetric meperidine usage and assessment of neonatal status. *Anesthesiology* 40:116–120, 1974

208. Downes JJ, Kemp RA, Lambertsen CJ: The magnitude and duration of respiratory depression due to fentanyl and meperidine in man. *J Pharmacol Exp Ther* 158:416–420, 1967

209. Cartwright P, Prys-Roberts C, Gill K, et al: Ventilatory depression related to plasma fentanyl concentrations during and after anesthesia in humans. *Anesth Analg* 62:966–974, 1983

210. Murphy MR, Hug CC, Jr, McClain DA: Dose-independent pharmacokinetics of fentanyl. *Anesthesiology* 59:537–540, 1983

211. Murphy MR, Olson WA, Hug CC Jr: Pharmacokinetics of ^{3}H-fentanyl in the dog anesthetized with enflurane. *Anesthesiology* 50:13–19, 1979

212. Hug CC Jr, McClain DB: Ventilatory depression by fentanyl in anesthetized patients. *Anesthesiology* 53:S56, 1980

213. Stoeckel H, Hengstmann JH, Schuttler J: Pharmacokinetics of fentanyl as a possible explanation for recurrence of respiratory depression. *Br J Anaesth* 51:741–745, 1979

214. Stanley TH, Webster LR: Anesthetic requirements and cardiovascular effects of fentanyl–oxygen and fentanyl–diazepam–oxygen anesthesia in man. *Anesth Analg* 57:411–416, 1978

215. Pathak KS, Brown RH, Nash CL, Jr: Continuous opioid infusion for scoliosis fusion surgery. *Anesth Analg* 62:841–845, 1983

216. White PF, Dworsky WA, Horai Y, et al: Comparison of continuous infusion fentanyl or ketamide versus thiopental—determining the mean effective serum concentrations for outpatient surgery. *Anesthesiology* 59:564–569, 1983

217. Corssen G, Domino EF, Sweet RB: Neuroleptanalgesia and anesthesia. *Anesth Analg* 43:748–763, 1964

218. Sokoll MD, Hoyt JL, Gergis SD: Studies in muscle rigidity, nitrous oxide, and narcotic analgesic agents. *Anesth Analg* 51:16–20, 1972

219. Askgaard B, Nilsson T, Ibler M, et al: Muscle tone under fentanyl–nitrous oxide anaesthesia measured with a transducer apparatus in cholecystectomy incisions. *Acta Anaesthesiol Scand* 21:1–4, 1977

220. Scamman FL: Fentanyl-O_2-N_2O rigidity and pulmonary compliance. *Anesth Analg* 62:332–334, 1983

221. Bovill JG, Sebel PS, Blackburn CL, et al: The pharmacokinetics of alfentanil (R 39209): A new opioid analgesic. *Anesthesiology* 57:439–443, 1982

222. Stanski DR, Hug CC Jr: Alfentanil—a kinetically predictable narcotic analgesic. *Anesthesiology* 57:435–438, 1982

223. Gal TJ, DiFazio CA, Moscicki J: Analgesic and respiratory depressant activity of nalbuphine: A comparison with morphine. *Anesthesiology* 57:367–374, 1982

224. Garattini S, Marcucci F, Morselli PL, et al: The significance of measuring blood levels of benzodizepines, in Davies DS, Prichard BNC (eds): *Biological Effects of Drugs in Relation to Their Plasma Concentrations.* Baltimore, University Park Press, 1973, pp 211–225

225. Gamble JA, Dundee JW, Assaf RA: Plasma diazepam levels after single dose oral and intramuscular administration. *Anaesthesia* 30:164–169, 1975

226. Hillestad L, Hansen T, Melsom H, et al: Diazepam metabolism in normal man. I. Serum concentrations and clinical effects after intravenous, intramuscular, and oral administration. *Clin Pharmacol Ther* 16:479–484, 1974

227. Hillestad L, Hansen T, Melsom H, et al: Diazepam metabolism in normal man. II. Serum concentration and clinical effect after oral administration and cumulation. *Clin Pharmacol Ther* 16:485–489, 1974

228. Klotz U, Avant GR, Hoyumpa A, et al: The effects of age and liver disease on the disposition and elimination of diazepam in adult man. *J Clin Invest* 55:347–359, 1975

229. Morselli PL, Principi N, Tognoni G, et al: Diazepam elimination in premature and full term infants, and children. *J Perinat Med* 1:133–141, 1973

230. Morselli PL, Mandelli M, Tognoni G, et al: Drug interactions in the human fetus and in the newborn infant, in Morselli PL, Cohen SN (eds): *Drug Interactions.* New York, Raven Press, 1974, pp 259–270

231. Mandelli M, Tognoni G, Garattini S: Clinical pharmacokinetics of diazepam. *Clin Pharmacokinet* 3:72–91, 1978

232. Garattini S, Marcucci F, Morselli PL, et al: The significance of measuring blood levels of benzodiazepines in Davies DS, Prichard PNC (eds): *Biological Effects of Drugs in Relation to Their Plasma Concentrations.* Baltimore, University Park Press, 1973

233. Ghoneim MM, Korttila K: Pharmacokinetics of intravenous anaesthetics: Implications for clinical use. *Clin Pharmacokinet* 2:344–372, 1977

234. Mattila MAK, Ruoppi MK, Ahlstrom-Bengs, E, et al: Diazepam in rectal solution as premedication in children, with special reference to serum concentrations. *Br J Anaesth* 53:1269–1272, 1981

235. Lindgren L, Saarnivaara L, Himberg JJ: Comparison of oral triclofos, diazepam, and flunitrazepam as premedicants in children undergoing otolaryngological surgery. *Br J Anaesth* 52:283–290, 1980

236. Finkelstein W, Isselbacher KJ: Drug Therapy: Cimetidine. *N Engl J Med* 299:992–996, 1978

237. Manchikanti L, Kraus JW, Edds S: Cimetidine and related drugs in anesthesia. *Anesth Analg* 61:595–608, 1982

238. Maliniak K, Vakil AH: Pre-anesthetic cimetidine and gastric pH. *Anesth Analg* 58:309–313, 1979

239. Husemeyer RP, Davenport HT, Rajasekaran T: Cimetidine as a single oral dose for prophylaxis against Mendelson's syndrome. *Anaesthesia* 33:775–778, 1978

240. Kirkegaard P, Sorensen O, Kirkegaard P: Cimetidine in the prevention of acid aspiration during anesthesia. *Acta Anaesth Scand* 24:58–60, 1980

241. Goudsouzian NG, Coté CJ, Liu LMP, et al: The dose–response effects of oral cimetidine on gastric pH and volume in children. *Anesthesiology* 55:533–536, 1981

242. Ostfeld A, Jenkins R, Pasnav R: Dose response for autonomic and mental effects of atropine and hyoscine. *Fed Proc* 18:430, 1959

243. Wyant GM, Dobkin AB: Antisialogogue drugs in man: Comparison of atropine, scopolomine (1-hyoscine), and 1-hyoscyanine (Bellefoline). *Anaesthesia* 12:203–214, 1957

244. Eger EI, II: Atropine, scopolomine, and related compounds. *Anesthesiology* 23:365–383, 1962

245. Shutt LE, Bowes JB: Atropine and hyoscine. *Anaesthesia* 34:476–490, 1979

246. Gravenstein JS, Andersen TW, De Padua CB: Effects of atropine and scopolomine on the cardiovascular system in man. *Anesthesiology* 25:123–130, 1964

247. Dauchot P, Gravenstein JS: Effects of atropine on the electrocardiogram in different age groups. *Clin Pharmacol Ther* 12:274–280, 1971

248. Harris WS, Goodman RM: Hyper-reactivity to atropine in Down's syndrome. *N Engl J Med* 279:407–410, 1968

249. Kobel M, Creighton RE, Steward DJ: Anaesthetic consideration in Down's syndrome: Experience with 100 patients and a review of the literature. *Can Anaesth Soc J* 29:593–599, 1982

250. Mirakhur RK, Dundee JW, Clarke RS: Glycopyrrolate–neostigmine mixture for antagonism of neuromuscular block: Comparison with atropine–neostigmine mixture. *Br J Anaesth* 49:825–829, 1977

251. Wark HJ, Overton JH, Marian P: The safety of atropine premedication in children with Down's syndrome. *Anaesthesia* 38:871–874, 1983

252. Ostheimer GW: A comparison of glycopyrrolate and atropine during reversal of nondepolarizing neuromuscular block with neostigmine. *Anesth Analg* 56:182–186, 1977

253. Mirakhur RK: Intravenous administration of glycopyrronium: Effects on cardiac rate and rhythm. *Anaesthesia* 34:458–462, 1979

254. Oduro KA: Glycopyrrolate methobromide. 2. Comparison with atropine sulphate in anaesthesia. *Can Anaesth Soc J* 22:466–473, 1975

255. Warran P, Radford P, Manford MLM: Glycopyrrolate in children. *Br J Anaesth* 53:1273–1276, 1981

256. Salem MR, Wong AY, Mani M, et al: Premedicant drugs and gastric juice pH and volume in pediatric patients. *Anesthesiology* 44:216–219, 1976

257. Stoelting RK: Responses to atropine, glycopyrrolate, and riopan of gastric fluid pH and volume in adult patients. *Anesthesiology* 48:367–369, 1978

8

Preanesthetic Medication and Induction of Anesthesia

Letty M.P. Liu
John F. Ryan

PREMEDICATION

The preanesthetic visit marks the commencement of the anesthetic management of a patient. After obtaining a complete history, performing a physical examination, and evaluating the results of pertinent laboratory tests, the anesthesiologist prepares the patient for anesthesia. Eliminating or minimizing the anxiety of the patient, and providing conditions that lead to a smooth, atraumatic induction of anesthesia, are two major objectives of the preoperative visit. These goals may be accomplished by establishing rapport with the patient and/or by the administration of drugs.

The efficacy of premedication for children is controversial. Although numerous articles have been published on the subject, there are no data to support or refute the contention that children derive psychological benefit from premedicant drugs, or that one premedication regimen is superior to another. The decision whether or not to administer drugs should be made according to the needs of each individual patient. Some important factors that should be considered are the child's expectations, physical status, age, weight, anxiety level, cooperative ability, prior anesthetic history, the presence of pain, the proposed surgical procedure, and the parents' attitudes.

This chapter focuses on the preanesthetic preparation of the child, with emphasis on the use of premedicant drugs.

PSYCHOLOGICAL PREPARATION OF THE CHILD

Preoperative psychological preparation of the child and family can reduce emotional trauma associated with the surgical experience, as well as provide conditions that will lead to a smooth, atraumatic induction of anesthesia. Establishing rapport with the patient is often more effective in calming the child than utilizing pharmacologic agents to allay anxiety. This may be difficult in only one preoperative visit, especially if the child is not mature enough to talk and understand why he or she requires anesthesia. A more detailed discussion on the psychological preparation of the child is found in Chapter 4.

PHARMACOLOGIC PREPARATION OF THE CHILD

Monitoring a child's attitude and behavior is very important. A child who clings to his or her parents, avoids eye contact, and will not talk is probably very anxious. This child will probably benefit from tranquilization or sedation prior to the induction of anesthesia. The very self-assured, cocky child who "knows it all" may also require heavy preanesthetic medication. These children are frequently extremely frightened and are trying to mask their true emotions. They will often decompensate just when their cooperation is required.

The reasons for administering preanesthetic medication are (1) to allay anxiety, (2) to facilitate the induction of anesthesia, (3) to decrease autonomic (vagal) reflexes, and (4) to reduce airway secretions.

Age, emotional maturity, personality, and past history are important determinants of whether or not a child should be given premedicant drugs prior to anesthesia. Infants under six months of age do not appear to be affected by short periods of separation from their parents. They are usually willing to accept a nurse as a mother substitute. In addition, many of these infants appear to like the smell of halothane and respond to it by sucking. As a result, preanesthetic medication for these babies is generally limited to drugs that modify their physiological responses to anesthesia. Drugs that produce sedation are not usually administered prior to the arrival of the baby in the operating room. Of major concern is the cardiovascular and respiratory depression that can result from sedation. Infants tend to have more difficulty than older children maintaining a patent airway when heavily sedated. This is due in part to the poor head control of young infants, and to the size of the tongue, which is large in relation to the size of the pharynx.

As children mature, they become increasingly aware of their surroundings. Considerable anxiety may be provoked if they are placed in an unfamiliar environment, especially if the situation appears threatening. Hospitalized children often become anxious when they recognize unusual situations (e.g., the operating room) yet are unable to comprehend the reason they are there. Preschool-age children seem to have more difficulty than other children adjusting to new situations because they are generally too young to understand explanations. Even if their parents are with them, these children may be apprehensive, especially if they detect that their parents are anxious.

Children between six months and six years of age generally cling to their parents. Separating a child in this age group from the parents can be extremely stressful for both. Children of this age are generally happier if their parents are present when anesthesia is induced, or if they are allowed to fall asleep in their parents' arms in a nonthreatening environment before entering the operating room. We have found that premedication for children of this age group is usually most effective if it produces sleep. This allows anesthesia to be induced without having to wrestle with an anxious child who may be partially sedated.

Children older than six years, as well as some younger ones who go to preschool or kindergarten, are generally a little more willing to accept short periods of separation from their parents. They are a little more independent than other children because of their school experience. Their increased ability to communicate with adults, and their better understanding of reality, enables them to handle their feelings and fears better. Their sense of curiosity and interest in new things can be utilized to elicit their cooperation. Many children of this age trust adults and are easily convinced to accept a mask induction of anesthesia. In these cases, preoperative sedation is not necessary and may interfere with the ability of the child to cooperate.

As children grow older they become more aware of their bodies. This often leads the fear of mutilation. Some children fear being "put to sleep" and never coming back, like a pet they once knew that was "put to sleep." It is extremely important to reassure these children that they will not be "put to sleep" but that they will nap for a short time and that the anesthesiologist is someone who can be trusted to take good care of them while the surgeon is correcting their problem.

Adolescents have unique problems that must be considered. Although teens appear quite independent and self-confident, their self-esteem and body image are easily altered. Volatile aggressive and irrational behavior is not uncommon for these children, even under normal circumstances. In a moment the teenager's mood can change from that of an intelligent mature adult to that of a very young child who needs much support and reassurance. Changes taking place in their bodies are frequently the cause of their anxieties; these patients continually compare their physical development with their peers', and this makes them extremely anxious when they have a physical problem. Their anxieties include the fear that their medical problem might not be corrected, waking up in the middle of the operation, never waking up from anesthesia, and waking up handicapped. Coping with a disability or illness is often very difficult for patients of this age. These children like to feel that they are in control of their situation and frequently dislike being sedated. They generally like to know exactly what will transpire during the course of anesthesia and appreciate an honest answer. Although most teenagers are quite cooperative and do not require preanesthetic sedation, the very anxious or rambunctious patient will generally benefit from drugs that produce sedation.

Since Waters classic paper in 1938[1] on preanesthetic medication of children, numerous articles on this subject have appeared in the literature. Despite the efforts of all subsequent investigators, there is still no single drug or combination of drugs that is ideal for all children. This is due in part to the similar effects produced by many of the drugs used for premedication, and to the varying effects that can result from a specific drug in different children and in the same child under different conditions. Age, weight, drug history, disease state, physical status, anesthetic drugs, anesthetic technique, operative procedure, and the time of drug administration are a few factors that alter the effects of drugs in children.

ROUTES OF ADMINISTRATION

In children preanesthetic drugs are most frequently administered via the oral, rectal, or intramuscular routes. Since there is no ideal premedication for all children, the decision of what drugs to use, how much to give, and how drugs should be administered, must be individualized. In general, needles are very unpopular with children and contribute to the unpleasantness of their hospital experience. Whenever possible, needles should be avoided because they produce pain and generally cause children to become upset. There are, however, some children who will benefit from intramuscular premedication. These include children who are extremely apprehensive, uncooperative and rambunctious, and those who require narcotics for pain.

Although the absorption of drugs may be less certain after oral or rectal administration than after intravenous injection, adequate effects may be achieved when certain drugs are given by these routes.[2,3] In general, the child, parents, and nursing personnel are all much happier if medication can be given without the pain of an injection.

HYPNOTICS

The major goal of premedication is to reduce the anxiety of patients so that a smooth induction of anesthesia may be achieved. Many of the drugs used for premedication will make patients drowsy, and in this way reduce their anxiety level. These drugs include the barbiturates, nonbarbiturate sedatives, and antihistamines.

Barbiturates

Pentobarbital and secobarbital are two short-acting barbituric acid derivitives that are frequently used in the preanesthetic period to sedate children and to relieve their anxiety. They produce minimal respiratory and circulatory depression, and rarely cause nausea and vomiting when administered orally or intramuscularly in doses of 3–5 mg/kg to healthy children, 1.5–2.0 hours prior to anesthesia. Since pain often persists at the injection site after intramuscular pentobarbital, this route of administration should be avoided.[4]

Ultrashort acting barbiturates have been administered rectally to young children for many years. These drugs, when administered in large doses, will produce sleep in the majority of children. Sodium thiopental was the first of these drugs to be used rectally for preanesthetic sedation and hypnosis. A suppository of approximately 44 mg/kg will produce sleep in 42 percent of children, and adequate sedation in 79 percent. Elimination of this drug from plasma at this dose takes between 24 and 48 hours.[5]

Methohexital is another ultrashort-acting barbiturate which is used rectally as a premedicant. It has a shorter elimination half-life than thiopental.[5–8] For almost two decades, methohexital has been the most frequently used drug for premedication of pediatric anesthesia patients in our hospital. Rectal administration (1) eliminates the pain associated with parenteral drug administration, (2) decreases separation anxiety of both the child and parents, since the drug is administered in the presence of the parents and the child allowed to fall asleep before being taken away from them, (3) provides conditions conducive to a smooth induction of anesthesia, and (4) decreases anesthetic gas pollution in the anesthetic induction area because an inhalation induction of anesthesia is more easily accomplished in a sleeping child.

The usual dose of rectally administered methohexital ranges from 20–30 mg/kg. The drug is prepared by dissolving 500 mg of methohexital sodium crystals in 5 ml of sterile water to make a 10 percent solution. The calculated dose of this solution is drawn into a 5 ml syringe and the tip of a lubricated 10–14 French catheter is attached to the tip of the syringe. If 1–2 ml of air are drawn into the syringe and positioned between the drug solution and the plunger, all the drug may be emptied into the patient's rectum. The number of patients that fall asleep in 15 minutes is not significantly different (87% v 93%) when the dose is increased from 20 to 30 mg/kg.[9] The mean sleep induction time is 6.7 minutes in children who receive 30 mg/kg, compared to 7.8 minutes in those who received 20 mg/kg. These doses do not produce clinically significant cardiovascular or respiratory depression in healthy children.[9] Higher doses may be administered to patients who have a higher-than-normal tolerance to the drug (e.g., patients on phenobarbital, dilantin, and other drugs that induce the production of hepatic enzymes), and to patients who require an intravenous line before receiving additional drugs (e.g., CAT scan patients who require intravenous Renografin for their study).

The disadvantages of rectal methohexital are[9,10]

• An average of 7 minutes are required for sleep to occur
• The systemic bioavailability is unpredictable
• Some patients will not sleep after receiving the drug
• Sleep may be prolonged in some children following a short anesthetic
• The presence of an anesthesiologist or someone skilled in resuscitating children is required from the time the drug is administered until the patient recovers from the drug effect
• There is a high incidence of defecation (13%)
• Some children will strenuously object to any rectal intervention while awake

Contraindications to the use of rectal methohexital include hypersensitivity to the drug, temporal lobe epilepsy, and porphyria.[11–13]

Table 8-1

Comparison of the Sedative Effect of Pentobarbital, triclofos and methohexital*

Condition of Patient	Pentobarbital 4 mg/kg (IM)	Triclofos 70 mg/kg (PO)	Methohexital 20 mg/kg (rectal)
Asleep	15 (36.6%)	12 (37.5%)	25 (83.3%)
Well Sedated, Cooperative	19 (46.3%)	16 (50%)	4 (13.3%)
Agitated, Crying	7 (17.1%)	4 (12.5%)	1 (3.3%)
Total Number Of Patients	41 (100%)	32 (100%)	30 (100%)

* Data from Jasinska MT, Goudsouzian NG, Ryan JF: Oral premedication for pediatric patients. American Society of Anesthesiologists Annual Meeting. Abstract of Scientific Papers, 1974, pp 353–354.

Nonbarbiturate Sedatives

Chloral hydrate and triclofos are two orally administered nonbarbiturate drugs that have been used in children for preanesthetic sedation. These drugs are relatively long acting and are converted to trichloroethanol, which has a plasma half-life of eight hours.[14] Chloral hydrate, which is frequently used by pediatricians but rarely by anesthesiologists, is irritating to the skin as well as to mucous membranes. It has an unpleasant taste and is a gastrointestinal tract irritant. The average dose ranges from 10–30 mg/kg PO. It is generally administered 1.5–2.0 hours prior to anesthesia.

Triclofos per se produces little gastrointestinal tract irritation. Some irritation, however, is produced because a small amount is converted to chloral hydrate in the stomach. A dose of 70 mg/kg, 1.5–2.0 hours prior to anesthesia, has been utilized for premedication of children. Very little or no respiratory or cardiovascular depression is produced at this dose.

The effects of commonly used doses of pentobarbital, triclofos, and methohexital for preanesthetic medication were compared in 103 patients (Table 8-1).[15] There was no difference in the number of patients that were adequately sedated or asleep after receiving pentobarbital (4 mg/kg IM) or trichofos (70 mg/kg PO). There was a significantly greater number of patients, however, that fell asleep after 20 mg/kg of rectal methohexital.

Antihistamines

Drugs in this class are rarely used in infants and young children, but are used occasionally in older children, especially hyperkinetic individuals. The most widely used drug in this class is hydroxyzine (Atarax, Roerig, New York, NY). Doses of 0.5–1.0 mg/kg of body weight may be given either orally or intramuscularly. The drug produces minimal respiratory and circulatory changes, and is used mainly for its ataractic properties.[16,17] Additional benefits may be derived from its antiemetic, antihistaminic, and antispasmodic effects.

TRANQUILIZERS

This group of drugs includes the phenothiazines, benzodiazepines and butyrophenones. While the major effect of these drugs is to allay anxiety, the major side effect is sedation.

Phenothiazines

Promethazine (Phenergan, Wyeth Laboratories, Philadelphia, PA) is the most commonly used drug in this class for preanesthetic medication of children. In addition to its sedative properties, it has antiemetic, antihistaminic, anti-motion sickness, and anticholinergic effects. It is frequently given with narcotics one hour prior to anesthesia to prevent and control nausea and vomiting. The recommended dose is 0.5–1.0 mg/kg of body weight.

Benzodiazepines

Several benzodiazepine derivatives have been recommended for preanesthetic medication. These drugs are used to allay anxiety and to diminish a patient's recall of perioperative events. At low doses they produce minimal drowsiness and depression of the cardiovascular or respiratory system. Nausea and vomiting are rarely a problem. The major disadvantage of these drugs is that they are long acting.

Diazepam (Valium, Roche Laboratories, Nutley, NJ) is presently the most widely used drug in this class. Although it can be administered by several methods, the intravenous route is the most effective, followed by the oral and intramuscular routes respectively.[18-20] After intramuscular injection, the systemic bioavailability of the drug is variable.[19] This is also true after rectal administration.[21,22] Diazepam is rarely used as a premedicant for infants. In older children, the average oral dose ranges from 0.4–0.5 mg/kg of body weight. Other benzodiazepine derivitives that have been used for premedication in children include lorazepam (Ativan, Wyeth Laboratories, Philadelphia, PA) and flunitrazepam.[23-25]

Butyrophenones

Droperidol (Inapsine, Janssen, Piscataway, NJ) is the most commonly used drug for preanesthetic medication in this class of major tranquilizers. In addition to its ataractic and soporific properties, this drug has an antiemetic effect. It potentiates the effect of other central nervous system depressants, and produces mild alpha adrenergic blockade. While the onset of action after intravenous or intramuscular administration is 3–10 minutes, the peak effect may not be apparent until 30 minutes have elapsed. This drug is rarely used in infants and young children. In older children, the recommended dose for premedication ranges from 0.10–0.15 mg/kg. In some patients this dose will induce anesthesia. Sedation and ataraxia after this dose generally lasts for 2–4 hours, but could last for up to 12 hours. When droperidol is administered in combination with other drugs, such as fentanyl and other central nervous system depressants, the dose of droperidol should be reduced. All children that receive droperidol should be monitored closely. If hypotension develops, hypovolemia should be considered in the differential diagnosis. Other side effects of the drug include restlessness, extrapyramidal symptoms, and hypertension.

OPIOIDS

Drugs in this class have been used for many years for preanesthetic medication of children. They are especially useful in providing analgesia and in sedating patients who suffer from preoperative pain. The major disadvantages of these drugs include nausea, vomiting, and respiratory depression. Hypotension, bile duct spasm, dysphoria, and hallucinations, are other undesirable side effects.

Morphine sulfate is probably the most frequently administered narcotic. In addition to providing analgesia, it can also produce significant respiratory depression. The incidence of both preoperative and postoperative vomiting is increased by this drug.[26,27] Morphine is not generally administered as a premedicant drug to infants; they seem to be more sensitive to its respiratory depressant effects, even though age has little effect on morphine pharmacokinetics.[28,29] The recommended intramuscular dose for preanesthetic medication is 0.1–0.2 mg/kg, one hour prior to the induction of anesthesia.

Meperidine is another narcotic analgesic that is commonly used in children. Its actions and disadvantages are similar to morphine. At equianalgesic doses, meperidine produces less sedation, smooth muscle spasm, depression of the cough reflex, and respiratory depression, than morphine.[28] The onset of action of meperidine is slightly faster than morphine, and the duration of action is slightly shorter. The usual dose for preanesthetic medication of children is 1–2 mg/kg of body weight, 30–90 minutes prior to the induction of anesthesia. Both morphine and meperidine are contraindicated in patients that are allergic to these drugs, and in those on monoamine oxidase inhibitors.[30]

KETAMINE

Occasionally one encounters a very apprehensive or combative child who is difficult to reason with. In these cases, intramuscular ketamine (4–5 mg/kg) will produce sedation within 3–4 minutes. A dose of 10 mg/kg will usually produce surgical anesthesia which lasts from 12–25 minutes. When this drug is used for premedication, vital signs should be monitored closely and resuscitative equipment should be readily available.

ANTICHOLINERGIC DRUGS

These drugs are utilized to decrease secretions and to block the vagal effect on the heart. They may also produce sedation and amnesia, and decrease gastric volume and acidity. Some undesirable effects of these drugs include tachycardia, dry mouth, skin erythema, and hyperthermia.

Since most modern anesthetics do not stimulate secretions as ether does, the need for a drying agent is not essential. Although an anticholinergic drug may be desirable in some children (e.g., patients who drool constantly, those receiving ketamine as the sole anesthetic drug, and those with a history of anesthetic problems due to excessive secretions), the discomfort of a dry mouth can cause some patients to complain bitterly before the operation, and in some cases afterwards as well. The routine use of an anticholinergic agent for the sole purpose of drying secretions is probably unwarranted these days. An anticholinergic agent is useful, however, if the purpose is to prevent bradycardia which can result from airway manipulation (e.g., laryngoscopy and intubation), surgical manipulation (e.g., retracting the vicera or extraoccular muscles), or the administration of anesthetic adjuvants (e.g., succinylcholine).[31-35]

Anticholinergic drugs are frequently administered intramuscularly by a nurse before the child leaves the room for the operating suite. Since the peak vagolytic effect of the drug has often passed by the time anesthesia is induced, it is more effective to give the drug just before it is required. By this time a patent intravenous line is often available, and the drug may be administered intravenously. Although anticholinergic drugs may be given either orally, intramuscularly, or intravenously, the intravenous route is probably the most reliable route of administration.[36]

The most common anticholinergic drugs used for premedication of children are atropine, scopolamine, and glycopyrrolate (Robinul, A.H. Robins Company, Richmond, VA). The dose of both atropine and scopolamine is the same (0.02 mg/kg IM or IV). A dose of 0.1 mg IM or IV is generally the lowest given, unless the child is a very tiny preterm infant. The maximum single dose is generally 0.6 mg/kg. Atropine blocks the vagus more effectively than scopolamine, whereas scopolamine is a better sedative, antisialogogue, and amnesic.

Glycopyrrolate is a synthetic quaternary ammonium compound which does not cross the blood–brain barrier. Thus, it does not produce the restlessness and confusion that can be seen after atropine and scopolamine. It is twice as potent as atropine in decreasing the volume of secretions, lasts three times longer, and is effective against the bradycardic effects of both neostigmine and pyridostigmine.[37–41] The recommended dose of glycopyrrolate (0.01 mg/kg) is approximately half the dose of atropine. Thus, for every mg of neostigmine, approximately 0.2 mg of glycopyrrolate is administered.

OTHER DRUGS

Other drugs that are given to children prior to the induction of anesthesia include steroids, insulin, antibiotics, and cimetidine.

Steroids

It is advisable to give patients on chronic corticosteroid therapy, and those that have been off steroids for less than six months, a dose of corticosteroids prior to anesthesia to prevent symptoms of adrenal–cortical insufficiency. Children should receive 1.5–2.0 mg/kg of hydrocortizone or an equivalent dose of dexamethasone intramuscularly approximately one hour prior to the induction of anesthesia, or, intravenously as soon as an intravenous line is established.

Insulin

Optimal management of the diabetic patient undergoing anesthesia entails avoiding hypoglycemia, ketoacidosis, and a hyperosmolar state. Several protocols have been advocated to control the diabetic patient.[42] Prolonged starvation should be avoided. Diabetic children are often given an intravenous solution containing five percent dextrose early in the morning at a rate equal to their hourly maintenance requirement. Once the solution is started, insulin is added to the IV solution, or half of the child's usual morning insulin requirement is administered subcutaneously. Blood glucose, urine glucose, and acetone determinations should be made at frequent intervals during the perianesthetic period, and insulin or sugar given as needed.

Antibiotics

This class of drugs is frequently administered preoperatively to prevent or reduce infection in surgical patients.[43] Antibiotics are frequently given to children with structural heart disease 30–60 minutes prior to the start of anesthesia and surgery. The preoperative doses recommended by the American Heart Association are presented in table 16-3. (Chapter 16)

Antacids

Pulmonary aspiration of gastric contents in anesthetized patients was first described in 1946 by Mendelson.[44] It has been estimated that 26 percent of the anesthetic-related deaths are due to inhalation of gastric contents.[45] If a child aspirates a volume greater than 0.4 ml/kg of gastric juice, and the pH of the fluid is less than 2.5, the child has a high risk of developing pulmonary acid aspiration syndrome (Mendelson's syndrome).[46,47] Certain children (e.g., those with a hiatus hernia) are more prone to gastric reflux and aspiration. Preanesthetic administration of drugs which reduce gastric volume and acidity will reduce the risk of pulmonary acid aspiration syndrome.[46–48] The most frequently used drug in this category for children is cimetidine, a histamine H_2 receptor antagonist. The recommended dose for children is 7.5 mg/kg, 1–3 hours prior to the induction of anesthesia.[46] Other drugs that decrease gastric volume and/or acidity are sodium citrate, metoclopramide, and ranitidine.[49–51]

INDUCTION OF ANESTHESIA

The period during the induction of anesthesia can be one of the busiest times for the anesthesiologist, and it can be an extremely stressful period for the anesthesiologist, child, and observers in the anesthesia induction area. Changes can occur quickly at this time, and danger may be only an instant away. The incidence of critical events is high. These events (e.g., airway obstruction, hypotension and bradycardia), can lead to morbidity and mortality if unrecognized and allowed to persist. We found that 34 percent of the infants under one year of age experienced critical incidents during the anesthetic period (LMP Liu, unpublished data). Critical incidents occurred in 22 percent of patients during the induction of anesthesia, more than any other anesthetic period. Identification of potential problems and their causes during the induction period can reduce the incidence of critical events. Appropriate anesthetic equipment must be readily available and in perfect working condition, necessary drugs must be prepared, and patients must be in optimal condition before receiving anesthesia. In addition to correcting fluid, electrolyte and metabolic imbalances, the child must be prepared psychologically for anesthesia and surgery (see chapter 4). It is the responsibility of the anesthesiologist to provide conditions that will lead to a smooth induction of anesthesia. This section will focus on techniques of inducing anesthesia in children.

In the majority of children, anesthesia is induced either by inhalation or intravenous administration of anesthetic agents. In some children, the intramuscular and rectal routes have been utilized, and in selected patients hypnosis can be a useful method of inducing anesthesia.

During the induction of anesthesia, heart sounds, heart rate, blood pressure, the electrocardiogram, and respirations should be monitored so that any deleterious changes in these parameters can be promptly detected and corrected. In patients who are extremely ill, monitoring of additional parameters may be required (see chapter 23).

INHALATION

A common method of inducing anesthesia in children is to place an anesthetic mask over the nose and mouth and have them breath a potent inhalation anesthetic (e.g., halothane or enflurane). This method is generally tolerated by cooperative children even though they may not like the smell of the anesthetic gas. Many small infants also tolerate this method well. They appear to enjoy the scent of halothane and will start sucking as soon as the gas is administered. Initially 100 percent oxygen at a low flow rate is administered. The flow is increased slowly, and nitrous oxide is gradually added to the oxygen. Following several breaths of the nitrous oxide–oxygen mixture, the potent inhalation agent is gradually added to the mixture. Increasing the inspired concentration of the potent anesthetic by 0.5 percent every 3–4 breaths will generally lead to a smooth induction of anesthesia. Increasing the concentration more rapidly can be irritating, and may cause patients to cough. A slower rate of increase will prolong induction time, and will make the patient vulnerable to all the problems that could arise during a prolonged excitement period.

Some children may object to having a mask placed over their face and will feel that they are being suffocated. These individuals may feel better if the mask is held a few inches away from their faces. If this is objectionable, removing the mask from the elbow and holding the elbow (or anesthetic delivery hose) between two fingers and just above the child's face may be acceptable. The anesthetist can cup his or her hand around the orifice of the elbow to concentrate the flow of gases in the area under the palm of his or her hand. As the patient gets drowsy, the anesthesiologist can move the hand closer to the child's face. Once the child is amnesic, the anesthetic mask can be attached to the elbow and applied to the child's face.

The odor of the anesthetic may be very objectionable to some children. If patients are instructed to breath through their mouth instead of their nose they may find the odor less obnoxious. A small amount of a fruit scented liquid* applied to the inside of the mask will help to conceal the smell of the anesthetic drug. Too much liquid applied to the mask may result in too strong a scent for the child. One must be careful not to spill the liquid on the anesthesia equipment or the operating table because the scent will be present for hours. Patients may select a scent prior to the induction of anesthesia or during the preanesthetic visit. An alternative to liquid scents is flavored Chapstick (A.H. Robins Co., Richmond, VA). Patients can be presented with the various tubes of Chapstick prior to the induction of anesthesia and allowed to paint the inside of the anesthetic mask with the flavor they wish to breath while they fall asleep.

During the induction of anesthesia, noise in the room should be kept to a minimum. The anesthesiologist can tell the child a non-frightening story, or talk in a quiet soothing voice about things that the child likes. This will help direct the child's thoughts away from fear, the smell of the anesthetic gases, the anesthetic equipment, and the events in the anesthesia induction area.

A few children will be very cooperative until the scent of the anesthetic drug is perceived. This change in attitude can usually be circumvented if the inhalation induction time can be shortened. We have had success using a modification of the single breath halothane induction technique.[52,53] After the anesthetic circuit is filled (with 4–5% halothane or ethrane, in either 5 l of oxygen or a 3:2 l mixture of nitrous oxide and oxygen) the child is instructed to ①take a deep breath of room air, ②expire maximally, and ③hold his or her breath at the end of expira-

* Lorann Oils, Lansing Michigan.

tion. While he or she is breath holding, the anesthetic mask is gently placed on his face without gripping his lower jaw. He is then instructed to take a deep breath through his mouth and then to breath normally. This technique will usually induce anesthesia within 1 minute whether or not the child breath holds or breathes normally after the initial breath of anesthetic gas (Liu LMP. Unpublished data). If a patient fails to exhale completely, or takes a small breath of room air before breathing the anesthetic gas mixture, anesthesia will still be induced within two minutes if the child's second breath is a deep inhalation of the anesthetic mixture, or if the child breathes normally into the mask. Contrary to the opinion of some individuals, hypoxic mixtures of anesthetic gases have no place in pediatric anesthesia. These mixtures may decrease the anesthetic induction time, but they are potentially hazardous and unnecessary.

INTRAVENOUS INDUCTION

If an intravenous line is available, or if it can be started without undue trauma to the child, anesthesia may be induced via this route. In children with a full stomach an intravenous induction is preferred to other methods. Anesthesia can be induced rapidly, and the airway protected from aspiration of gastric contents by rapid insertion of an endotracheal tube. These children should receive oxygen prior to the induction of anesthesia in order to assure adequate oxygenation during the "rapid-sequence" induction of anesthesia. Cricoid pressure (Sellick's maneuver) should be applied before the child shows signs of drowsiness.[54] To prevent potential aspiration of gastric contents, pressure should be maintained until the endotracheal tube is in place and the cuff is inflated (if a cuffed tube is used).

Thiopental is the most frequently used drug for inducing anesthesia via the intravenous route. It is an ultrashort-acting barbiturate that will produce sedation within one minute after administration. The recommended dose ranges from 2–6 mg/kg.[55–58] For healthy unpremedicated children, a dose of 5–6 mg/kg should be used.[58] Less drug will be required by debilitated and severely ill patients and those that have been premedicated.

Thiamylal is an ultrashort-acting thiobarbiturate that is very similar to thiopental. Like thiopental, a 2.5 percent solution is recommended for intravenous administration. The recommended anesthestic induction dose is similar to thiopental.

Methohexital is an ultrashort-acting oxybarbiturate that is used intravenously in a 1 percent solution. Recovery from intravenous anesthesia after this drug is more rapid than after thiopental.[59] Pharmacokinetic studies indicate that methohexital is cleared more rapidly than thiopental, and that it has a shorter elimination half-life than thiopental.[60] The recommended dose for children ranges from 1.0–2.5 mg/kg.[56,60–62] In unpremedicated children the recommended induction dose is 2.0–2.5 mg/kg IV.[62] At higher doses skeletal muscle hyperactivity and hiccups are common. Pain is more common at the intravenous injection site after methohexital than after thiopental.

INTRAMUSCULAR

There will be occasions where a well planned induction of anesthesia goes awry and the anesthesiologist is confronted with a child who suddenly looses his composure, or one who is upset and uncooperative. In these situations, the administration of drugs intramuscularly may be the least traumatic way to induce anesthesia, especially if venous access is a problem. In infants and very small children, intramuscular methohexital (10 mg/kg of body weight of a 5% solution) will produce sleep in the majority of patients within 1–2 minutes. In older patients, ketamine can be a useful drug. An initial dose of 5–10 mg/kg IM is generally required for anesthesia. The cardiovascular stimulating properties of the drug are particularly appealing, particularly in situations where hypotension is a potential problem. In infants the effect of ketamine can be very unpredictable . Some may require extremely large doses, while others will be anesthetized after receiving low doses of the drug. Ketamine may also be dangerous in children with airway problems. Although respiration is stimulated in most patients, severe respiratory depression may sometimes also result. The increase in airway secretions after ketamine administration may produce laryngospasm. The administration of anticholinergic drugs will eliminate this side effect. The high incidence of hallucinations in children following the administration of ketamine is another disadvantage.

Ketamine and methohexital are rapidly absorbed after intramuscular administration and anesthesia is produced rapidly. The induction of anesthesia, however, might be delayed in situations where there is poor tissue perfusion. While a speedy induction of anesthesia and simplicity in administering the induction drug are the appealing characteristics of an intramuscular induction of anesthesia, the disadvantages include injection pain and the possibility of sterile abscess formation.

RECTAL

There is clearly a spectrum from drowsiness to light sleep to anesthesia, and in general the dose of the rectally administered drug should be higher when the situation calls for anesthesia rather than sedation. Earlier in this chapter we described the use of methohexital as a premedicant–induction agent. Ketamine (5–10 mg/kg) can also be administered rectally to produce anesthesia.[63] For certain procedures (i.e., computerized tomography, dressing changes, drainage of abscesses), rectally administered ketamine may be the sole anesthetic.

Rectal drug administration is certainly an advantage in an extremely frightened child who does not want a needle or a mask induction of anesthesia, but who does not object to rectal thermometers. It may also be utilized effectively in mentally retarded patients. Other advantages of this method of inducing anesthesia include ease of drug administration, easy repetition of the dose if sleep does not ensue, and elimination of the anxiety produced by separating the child from parents when the child is awake. Disadvantages include failure of inducing anesthesia in a small percentage of patients due to poor bioavailability of the drug, defecation, and delayed recovery from anesthesia in short cases due to the variability of absorption of rectal drugs.[10,63]

HYPNOSIS

Hypnosis may be successfully employed in pediatric as well as adult anesthesia patients. To utilize hypnosis as the sole anesthetic technique requires expertise. There are many common misconceptions about hypnosis, even among professionals. Nevertheless, the competent anesthesiologist uses any and every opportunity to employ therapeutic suggestions to help the patient, even though the formal trance state may not be induced. Carefully worded suggestions reassuringly spoken will direct the patient's attention to the positive aspects of events. Phrases such as "you will feel very comfortable and relaxed as you concentrate on your breathing," spoken slowly and rhythmically with meaningful pauses and emphasis on key words, will instill confidence in the child and abets the induction of chemical hypnosis. To the child the anesthesiologist is not only an adult but an authority figure, which further assists the aura of the doctor as a hypnotist. In this instance, words are exceedingly powerful tools that can have a profound influence on the mental attitude of the patient toward his or her therapeutic regimen and illness.

REFERENCES

1. Water RM: Pain relief in children. *Am J Surg* 39:470–475, 1938
2. Orme M: Drug absorption in the gut. *Br J Anaesth* 56:59–67, 1984
3. DeBoer AG, DeLeede LGJ, Breimer DD: Drug absorption by sublingual and rectal routes. *Br J Anaesth* 56:69–82, 1984
4. Dundee JW, Nair SG, Assaf RAE, et al: Pentobarbitone premedication for anaesthesia. *Anaesthesia* 31:1025–1031, 1976
5. Hudson RJ, Stanski DR, Burch PG: Pharmacokinetics of methohexital and thiopental in surgical patients. *Anesthesiology* 59:215–219, 1983
6. Breimer DD: Pharmacokinetics of methohexitone following intravenous infusion in humans. *Br J Anaesth* 48:643–649, 1976
7. Morgan DJ, Blackman GL, Paull JD, et al: Pharmacokinetic and plasma binding of thiopental. I: Studies in surgical patients. *Anesthesiology* 54:468–473, 1981
8. Jung D, Mayersohn M, Perrier D, et al: Thiopental disposition in lean and obese patients undergoing surgery. *Anesthesiology* 56:269–274, 1982
9. Liu LMP, Goudsouzian NG, Liu PL: Rectal methohexital premedication in children, a dose–comparison study. *Anesthesiology* 53:343–345, 1980
10. Liu LMP, Gaudreault P, Friedman PA, et al: Methohexital plasma concentrations in children following rectal administration. *Anesthesiology* 62:567–570, 1985
11. Rockoff MA, Goudsouzian NG: Seizures induced by methohexital. *Anesthesiology* 54:333–335, 1981
12. Liu LMP, Liu PL, Moss J: Severe histamine-mediated reaction to rectally administered methohexital. *Anesthesiology* 61:95–97, 1984
13. Parikh RK, Moore MR: Anaesthetics in porphyria: Intravenous induction agents. *Br J Anaesth* 47:907, 1975
14. Sellers EM, Lang M, Kock-Weser J, et al: Interaction of chloral hydrate and ethanol in man. I. Metabolism. *Clin Pharmacol Ther* 13:37–49, 1972
15. Jasinska MT, Goudsouzian NG, Ryan JF: Oral premedication for pediatric patients. Abstract of Scientific Papers, American Society of Anesthesiologist Annual Meeting, 1974, pp 353–354
16. Lauria JI, Markello R, King BD: Circulatory and respiratory effects of hydroxyzine in volunteers and geriatric patients. *Anesth Analg* 47:378–382, 1968
17. Anderson TW, Gravenstein JS: Cardiovascular effects of sedative doses of pentobarbital and hydroxyzine. *Anesthesiology* 27:272–278, 1966
18. Gamble JAS, Mackay JS, Dundee JW: Plasma levels of diazepam. *Br J Anaesth* 45:1085, 1973
19. Hillestad L, Hansen T, Melsom H, et al: Diazepam metabolism in normal man. I. Serum concentrations and clinical effects after intravenous, intramuscular and oral administration. *Clin Pharmacol Ther* 16:479–484, 1974

20. Kanto J: Plasma levels of diazepam after oral and intramuscular administration. *Br J Anaesth* 46:817, 1974

21. Lindahl S, Olsson AK, Thomson D: Rectal premedication in children. Use of diazepam, morphine and hyscine. *Anaesthesia* 36:376–379, 1981

22. Mattila MA, Ruoppi MK, Ahlstrom-Bengs E, et al: Diazepam in rectal solution as premedication in children, with special reference to serum concentrations. *Br J Anaesth* 53:1269–1272, 1981

23. Richardson FJ, Manford ML: Comparison of flunitrazepam and diazepam for oral premedication in older children. *Br J Anaesth* 51:313–317, 1979

24. Lindgren L, Saarnivaara L, Himberg JJ: Comparison of oral triclofos, diazepam and flunitrazepam as premedicants in children undergoing otolaryngological surgery. *Br J Anaesth* 52(3):283–290, 1980

25. Burtles R, Astley B: Lorazepam in children. A double-blind trial comparing lorazepam, diazepam, trimeprazine and placebo. *Br J Anaesth* 55:275–279, 1983

26. Booker PD, Chapman DH: Premedication in children undergoing day-care surgery. *Br J Anaesth* 51:1083–1087, 1979

27. Smith BL. Manford MLM: Postoperative vomiting after paediatric adenotonsillectomy. *Br J Anaesth* 46:373–378, 1974

28. Way WL, Costley EC, Way EL: Respiratory sensitivity of the newborn infant to meperidine and morphine. *Clin Pharmacol Ther* 6:454–461, 1965

29. Dahlstrom B, Bolme P, Feychting H, et al: Morphine kinetics in children. *Clin Pharmacol Ther* 26(3):354–365, 1979

30. Evan-Prosser CDG: The use of pethidine and morphine in the presence of monoamine oxidase inhibitors. *Br J Anaesth* 40:279–282, 1968

31. Lipton EL, Steinschneider A, Richmond JB: Autonomic function in the neonate. VIII. Cardiopulmonary Observations. *Pediatrics* 33:212, 1964

32. Sagarminaga J, Wynands JE: Atropine and the electrical activity of the heart during induction of anesthesia in children. *Can Anaesth Soc J* 10:328–342, 1963

33. Mirakhur RK, Jones CJ, Dundee JW, Archer DB: IM or IV atropine or glycopyrrolate for the prevention of oculocardiac reflex in children undergoing squint surgery. *Br J Anaesth* 54(10):1059–1063, 1982

34. Friesen RH, Lichtor JL: Cardiovascular depression during halothane anesthesia in infants: Study of three induction techniques. *Anesth Analg* 61(1):42–45, 1982

35. Friesen RH, Lichtor JL: Cardiovascular effects of inhalation induction with isoflurane in infants. *Anesth Analg* 62(4):411–414, 1983

36. Burghem L, Bergman U, Schildt B, Sorbo B: Plasma atropine concentrations determined by radioimmunoassay after a single-dose IV and IM administration. *Br J Anaesth* 52:597–601, 1980

37. Mirakhur RK, Jones CJ: Atropine and glycopyrrolate: Changes in cardiac rate and rhythm in conscious and anesthetized children. *Anesth Intensive Care* 10:328–332, 1982

38. Wyant GM, Kao E: Glycopyrrolate methobromide. I. Effect on salivary secretion. *Can Anaesth Soc J* 21:230–241, 1974

39. Mirakhur RK, Jones CJ: Atropine and glycopyrrolate: Changes in cardiac rate and rhythm in conscious and anaesthetised children. *Anaesth Intensive Care* 10(4):328–332, 1982

40. Warran P, Radford P, Manford ML: Glycopyrrolate in children. *Br J Anaesth* 53:1273–1276, 1981

41. Mirakhur RK, Briggs LP, Clarke RS, et al: Comparison of atropine and glycopyrrolate in a mixture with pyridostigmine for the antagonism of neuromuscular block. *Br J Anaesth* 53:1315–1320, 1981

42. Walts LF, Miller J, Davidson M, Brown J: Perioperative management of diabetes mellitus. *Anesthesiology* 55:104–109, 1981

43. Kaplan EL, Anthony BF, Bisno A, et al: Prevention of bacterial endocarditis. *Circulation* 56:139A–143A, 1977

44. Mendelson CL: The aspiration of stomach contents into the lungs during obstetric anesthesia. *Am J Obstet Gynecol* 52:191–205, 1946

45. Graff TD, Phillips OC, Benson DW, Kelley E: Baltimore anesthesia study committee: Factors in pediatric anesthesia mortality. *Anesth Analg* 43:407–414, 1964

46. Goudsouzian NG, Coté CJ, Liu LMP, Dedrick DF: The dose–response effects of oral cimetidine on gastric pH and volume in children. *Anesthesiology* 55(5):533–536, 1981

47. Coté CJ, Goudsouzian NG, Liu LMP, et al: Assessment of risk factors related to the acid aspiration syndrome in pediatric patients—Gastric pH and residual volume. *Anesthesiology* 56:70–72, 1982

48. Tryba M, Yildiz F, Kuhn K, et al: Rectal and oral cimetidine for prophylaxis of aspiration pneumonitis in paediatric anaesthesia. *Acta Anaesthesiol Scand* 27:328–330, 1983

49. Manchikanti L, Marrero TC, Roush JR: Preanesthetic cimetidine and metoclopramide for acid aspiration prophylaxis in elective surgery. *Anesthesiology* 61:48–54, 1984

50. Morison DH, Dunn GL, Fargas-Babjak AM, et al: A double-blind comparison of cimetidine and ranitidine as prophylaxis against acid aspiration syndrome. *Anesth Analg* 61:988–992, 1982

51. Durrant JM, Strunin L: Comparative trial of the effect of ranitidine and cimetidine on gastric secretion in fasting patients at induction of anaesthesia. *Can Anaesth Soc J* 29:446–451, 1982

52. Ruffle JM, Latta WB, Snider MT: Single breath halothane oxygen induction in man. *Anesthesiology* 57:A416, 1982

53. Ruffle JM, Snider MT: Onset of hypnosis with halothane induction using single breath, triple breath and conventional techniques. *Anesthesiology* 61:A498, 1984

54. Sellick BA: Cricoid pressure to control regurgitation of stomach contents during induction of anesthesia. *Lancet* 2:404–406, 1961

55. Steward DJ: *Manual of Pediatric Anesthesia—The Hospital for Sick Children.* New York, Churchill-Livingston, 1979, p 281

56. Smith RM: *Anesthesia for Infants and Children.* St. Louis, C.V. Mosby, 1980, p 667

57. Brown TCK, Fisk GC: *Anesthesia for Children.* Oxford, Blackwell Scientific Publications, 1979, p 30

58. Coté CJ, Goudsouzian NG, Liu LMP, et al: The dose–response of intravenous thiopental for the induction of general anesthesia in unpremedicated children. *Anesthesiology* 55:703–705, 1981

59. Korttilla K, Linnoila M, Ertama P et al: Recovery and simulated driving after intravenous anesthesia with thiopental, methohexital, propanidid, or alphadione. *Anesthesiology* 43:291–299, 1975

60. Gray TC, Utting JE, Nunn JF: *General Anaesthesia* (ed 4). London, Butterworth, 1980, p 1526

61. Gregory GA: *Pediatric Anesthesia.* New York, Churchill-Livingstone, 1983, p 329

62. Liu LMP, Coté CJ, Goudsouzian NG et al: Response to intravenous induction doses of methohexital in children. *Anesthesiology* 55:A330, 1981

63. Idvall J, Holasek J, Stenberg P: Rectal ketamine for induction of anaesthesia in children. *Anaesthesia* 38(1):60–64, 1983

9

Muscle Relaxants in Children

Nishan G. Goudsouzian

This chapter will review basic principles in evaluating the myoneural junction of the child, practical pharmacology of muscle relaxants in relation to age, and present practice in the use of muscle relaxants in infants and children.

The response of the older child to muscle relaxants is practically similar to that of the adult; however, the small infant occasionally demonstrates a different response [e.g., resistance to the action of succinylcholine (SCh), and a sensitivity to the action of nondepolarizing muscle relaxants[1]]. This response has been attributed to the immaturity of the myoneural junction of the newborn infant, and has led to the misconception that the infant's neuromuscular system in the first few months of life reacts in a manner similar to that of the myasthenic patient. The diverse conclusions reached by various authors have depended a great deal upon the methodologies used to investigate these questions.[2]

MONITORING NEUROMUSCULAR FUNCTION

The standard method for evaluating neuromuscular function in adults is to measure evoked responses.[3] This method is advantageous in that it does not require the cooperation of the patient and therefore can be carried out in the unconscious individual. The resultant activation of the muscle fibers can be evaluated either electrically (electromyogram [EMG]) or mechanically (twitch). For EMG measurement, the compound muscle action potential is recorded by surface or needle electrodes applied to any muscle, but usually to the adductor policis brevis, the abductor digiti minimi, or the first

dorsal interosseous muscle of the hand. Although the EMG is one of the better ways of recording muscle activity, it has had the practical drawbacks of being difficult to record, expensive, and easily affected by extraneous electrical activity which makes its routine use in the operating room impractical. With the introduction of newer prototypes of EMG equipment, most of these difficulties have now been overcome.

Tension measurements are more easily achieved in the operating room using the force of contraction of the adductor pollicis. This muscle is the only one supplied by the ulnar nerve acting on the thumb, and measurements therefore approach the single-muscle precision of the experimental nerve–muscle preparation.[3] The evoked tension of the adductor pollicis in response to the stimulation of the ulnar nerve by needle or surface electrodes can be recorded by a standard force displacement transducer (Figure 9-1). To achieve reproducibility, and to ensure full activation of all nerve and muscle fibers stimulated, the stimuli used should be supramaximal in intensity, square wave in nature, and no longer than 0.2. msec.

Despite the fact that evoked tension measurements are relatively easy to perform, they have been used infrequently in infants and children.[2,4,5] Most of the earlier studies evaluated the response of children to relaxants in terms of clinical factors such as the optimal conditions for endotracheal intubation, surgical relaxation, requirement of a repeat dose, or the dose which allows control of respiration.[6,7] These studies give valuable information on the clinical use of the drug, but are scientifically inconsistent because of differing methodology. The definition of "adequate relaxation" can vary amongst anesthesiologists and surgeons, and from institution to institution.

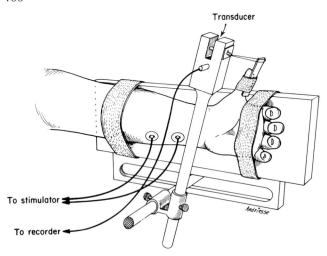

Figure 9-1. The arrangement used for studying evoked tensions in infants and children. In the clinical setting, and in the absence of recording apparatus, feeling the twitch response is adequate.

FREQUENCY OF STIMULATION

Clinically, three frequency groups of stimulation are used (Figure 9-2).

1. Single twitch rates of stimulation, i.e., 0.1–0.25 Hz.
2. Train-of-four, 2 Hz for 2 seconds.
3. Tetanic rates of 50 Hz.

Single twitch rates are useful whenever there is a control response. By comparing the percentage of change of twitch tension before and after the relaxant drug, one can obtain a percentage value that will indicate the degree of paralysis. Single stimuli detect relatively high degrees of muscle relaxation. Depression of the twitch response can only be observed if more than three-fourths of the postsynaptic receptors are blocked.[8] One must be aware that higher doses of relaxants are required to depress the twitch height at 0.1 Hz than at 0.25 Hz.[9]

The *train-of-four* is a simple qualitative technique for measurement of nondepolarizing neuromuscular blockade (Figure 9-2). It consists of four supramaximal stimuli applied to the ulnar nerve at a frequency of 2 Hz. The ratio of the amplitude of the fourth twitch to the first is used for assessment of neuromuscular blockade. The main advantage of the train-of-four over single twitch is that it does not require a control response. Also, it can be repeated every 10 seconds, allowing rapid changes in neuromuscular blockade to be closely monitored.[3]

The theory of the train-of-four technique is grounded in the fact that a rate of 2 Hz is rapid enough to produce depletion of the immediately available stores of acetylcholine, yet slow enough to prevent transmitter facilitation. Four stimuli were chosen because it was found that during partial non-depolarizing neuromuscular blockade the fourth response was depressed at its maximum; thereafter the twitch height leveled off.[10] In infants and children, the train-of-four correlates directly with the twitch height, and is a more sensitive indicator of neuromuscular blockade than single twitch height at 0.25 Hz[2] (Figure 9-3).

In children anesthetized with halothane all the compo-

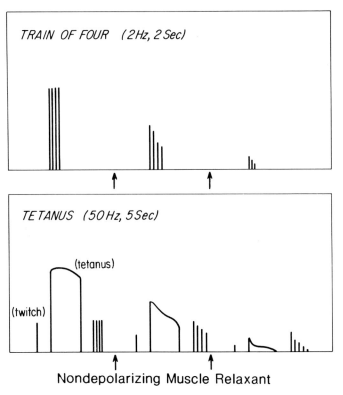

Nondepolarizing Muscle Relaxant

Figure 9-2. Idealized recording of the effect of nondepolarizing muscle relaxants on the train-of-four and tetanic contractions. Note in the upper figure the four equal twitches prior to the administration of nondepolarizing muscle relaxant. After curare the fourth twitch is less in amplitude than the first (train-of-four); the last sequence indicates greater neuromuscular blockade, since only three of the four twitches are observed. The lower figure demonstrates the corresponding single twitch/tetanus observations at a lower amplification. Note the marked fade and post-tetanic facilitation after the second dose of muscle relaxant.

nents of the train-of-four are practically equal in size (100%), whereas in infants less than one month the fourth evoked response in the train is lower (95%).[11] The change to the higher value in the important first month of development indicates the probable maturation of the myoneural junction. Premature infants (less than 32 weeks of developmental age) have lower train-of-four values (83 ± 2%) than more mature neonates[12] (Figure 9-4).

Adults with a train-of-four value above 75 percent sustain head lift for three seconds or more, while tidal volume, vital capacity, inspiratory flow, and peak expiratory flow, are not significantly altered.[13]

During *tetanic* stimulation, there is an increased mobilization and enhanced synthesis of acetylcholine. However, this increase is limited. If the duration of stimulation is too long, or the frequency of stimulation too high, *fade* will occur. In infants and children anesthetized with halothane, the percent of fade during tetanic stimulation for five seconds at 20 Hz is five percent, and at 50 Hz is nine percent.[11] These values are comparable to those in the adult.[14] If the duration of stimulation is prolonged, a higher degree of fade may be seen. In small infants, more than a 50 percent decrement in the height of tetanus has been seen during 15 seconds of tetanic stimu-

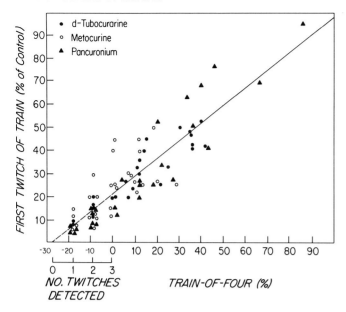

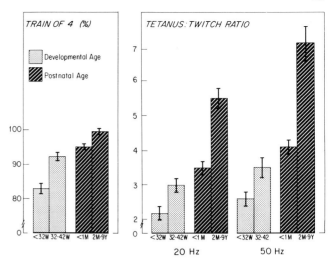

Figure 9-3. Correlates between the train-of-four values and the twitch height. Note that at about 20 percent of control twitch height the fourth contraction during train-of-four stimulation disappears.

Figure 9-4. The train-of-four values and tetanus; twitch ratios of critically ill infants less than 42 weeks developmental age in the neonatal intensive care unit, and infants and children anesthetized with halothane. Note the evidence of maturation of the myoneural junction in the older children (Reproduced with permission from Goudsouzian et al: *Br J Anaesth*, 1981).

lation; this decrement is more marked in premature infants.[15,16]

Increasing the rate of stimulation from 20 Hz to 50 Hz to 100 Hz increases the degree of fade from 5 percent to 9 percent to 17 percent respectively during a five second tetanic stimulation.[11] With fast sweep electromyogram, infants less than 12 weeks showed more marked fade than older children and adults; this difference was greater at high frequencies (50 Hz).[17] When tetanic stimulation is used, therefore, the duration as well as the frequency should be noted.

The integrity of the myoneural junction can also be analyzed by evaluation of *post-tetanic facilitation* (PTF). The increased synthesis of acetylcholine, which occurs during tetanic stimulation, continues for a short interval after discontinuation of tetanic stimulation. Normally this increased production of acetylcholine will not cause PTF because all the muscle fibers are normally excited by each stimulus. In the presence of non-depolarizing (competitive) neuromuscular blockade, however, this increased post-tetanic acetylcholine release will stimulate a larger number of muscle fibers, thus producing PTF.[14]

In infants and children, following tetanus of five seconds at 20 Hz, the PTF is 10 percent; it increases to 18 percent when the tetanic stimulation is increased to 50 Hz. When the rate of stimulation reaches the non-physiological range of 100 Hz, however, post-tetanic exhaustion occurs, i.e., the post-tetanic twitch is lower than the pre-tetanic one, indicating the depletion of acetylcholine reserves.

The *tetanus–twitch* ratio is a derived measure used for evaluation of the myoneural junction. In infants less than a month of age, this ratio is 4:1; in children older than a month, it increases to 6:1, indicating maturation of the myoneural junction or the muscle itself at about that time (Figure 9-4). This ratio is lower in patients who have received relaxants and increases after the reversal of neuromuscular blockade.

Maturation of both the myoneural junction and muscle

appears to occur after birth. Physiological studies in animals indicate maturation of neuromuscular transmission in the first two months of extrauterine life. Growing animals have shown an increase in tension generating sites, a muscular mechanism that can explain the increase in tetanus–twitch ratios.[18] A diminution in quantum content of acetylcholine has also been observed in young rat diaphragms as evidenced by a decrease in quantum content of the first end-plate potential of the train-of-four.[19] This diminution can lead to a decrease in the amount of acetylcholine release after the discontinuation of tetanic stimulation. The latter sequence occurring in the myoneural junction can explain the lower values of train-of-four and post-tetanic facilitation observed in the newborn infant.

For the anesthesiologist, twitch rates and the train-of-four ratios are the most practical. If twitch rates are used, the rate of stimulation should be noted. Slow rates of stimulation (0.1–0.15 Hz) are more helpful because the necessary levels of clinical neuromuscular blockade can be identified without the necessity of abolishing the twitch response.[9] The main drawback of the single twitch rate of stimulation is the necessity of obtaining a control twitch tension for quantitative assessment of neuromuscular blockade. The main advantage of the train-of-four is that there is no need for a control response since the ratio of the fourth twitch to the first is the quantitated parameter.

In the clinical situation where recording instruments are not available, the number of contractions during a train-of-four are counted. When the twitch height at 0.1 Hz is about 21 percent of the control value, only three contractions are detected during train-of-four stimulation. At 14 percent of control height, two contractions are detected, and at 7 percent of control height, one contraction is detected (Figure 9-3).[20] In children, where the hand is frequently covered by surgical drapes, palpating the number of contractions is a satisfactory alternative. The number of contractions during train-of-four stimulation thus provides a practical assessment of neuromuscular blockade.

Tetanic rates of stimulation are useful in difficult situations. By calculating the rate of fade, PTF, and the tetanus–twitch ratio, one can reach reasonable conclusions of the state of muscular relaxation. The main drawback in using tetanic stimulation, however, is that it cannot be repeated frequently.

NEUROMUSCULAR BLOCKING AGENTS

DEPOLARIZING MUSCLE RELAXANTS

Succinylcholine

Succinylcholine (SCh) is the only depolarizing muscle relaxant which is frequently used in infants and children. Infants in general have been found to be more resistant than adults to the neuromuscular effects of SCh.[21,22] Stead noted in 1955 that apnea after 0.8 mg/kg IV of SCh lasted for only 50 seconds in neonates, a much shorter duration than that observed in adults.[1]

Investigations on the effect of a single dose of SCh showed that the neuromuscular blockade achieved by 1 mg/kg IV in infants was equal to that produced by 0.5 mg/kg IV in older children.[4] SCh is rapidly distributed in the extracellular fluid space because of its small molecular size.[23] In general, the extracellular space and body surface area are related throughout childhood; thus it is not suprising to find a correlation between the dose of SCh for each square meter of surface area and the neuromuscular response.

The infant less than six months of age has about half the pseudocholinesterase activity of the older child or adult; however, this low level of pseudocholinesterase does not seem to affect the duration of action of a single dose of SCh in infants.[24] Rather, redistribution of SCh from a relatively small muscle mass into a relatively large extracellular volume appears rapidly to terminate the action of SCh.[23]

The effects of continuous IV infusion of SCh are also different in infants and children anesthetized with halothane. Although both groups develop tachyphylaxis and phase II block after comparable mean doses of SCh (tachyphylaxis after 3.0–3.6 mg/kg and phase II block after 4.1–5.3 mg/kg), some infants are extremely resistant to the neuromuscular effect of SCh, requiring three to four times the dose required by most children to maintain the same degree of neuromuscular blockade.[21] These resistant infants were from five days to four months old, and recovered much faster from the neuromuscular effects of SCh than older infants and children. The higher requirements of these infants can be only partly explained by the larger extracellular volume. It appears that the relatively immature myoneural junction of the infant may explain its different behavior.

SCh has been administered intralingually. With this technique, apnea was noted to occur after 75 seconds from the time of administration,[26] and a high incidence of arrhythmias was observed, even with concomitant use of atropine.

SCh is very effective when administered intramuscularly (IM); however, a three to four minute interval is required to achieve complete relaxation.[5] An IM dose of 2 mg/kg does not achieve satisfactory relaxation in all patients. A higher dose (3 mg/kg IM) produces a mean twitch depression of 85 percent,

whereas 4 mg/kg IM produces profound relaxation in all patients; the effects of such a large dose, however, may last up to 20 min.[5] In infants under six months of age a dose of 5 mg/kg is required to achieve profound relaxation. Again, recovery from the neuromuscular effects of IM SCh is faster in infants than in children.[27] On occasion after such a large IM dose, phase II block (as evidenced by train-of-four less than 50%) is seen. This appearance of phase II block is not considered clinically important, since it is not associated with prolonged neuromuscular blockade.

The administration of SCh in one or two injection sites, or at two or five percent concentration, does not affect the onset or the duration of action.[28] Changes in heart rate (usually mild, transient increases) are frequently seen after the administration of SCh. Of more concern is occasional bradycardia; these fluctuations of heart rate appear to be more common in children anesthetized with halothane than enflurane.[30] The maximum change occurs in 45–60 seconds after SCh, at a time when laryngoscopy is typically performed; laryngoscopy accentuates the vagal response to SCh. After IM SCh, changes in the pulse rate may also be seen, usually mild bradycardia, except with the concomitant use of 0.03 mg/kg atropine, when mild increases in heart rate occur.[31]

Arrhythmias frequently occur after the IV administration of SCh. The incidence after a single IV dose has varied between 40–60 percent, depending on the anesthetic agent used.[32] Most of the arrhythmias occurring after IV SCh are only detected through continuous electrocardiographic recording. The arrhythmias are usually transient, and predominantly vagal in origin; hence their blockade by anticholinergic agents. Cardiac irregularities are occasionally due to ventricular irritability. Prior administration of *IV* atropine markedly decreases, but does not completely abolish, the incidence of these arrhythmias.[32] Administration of IM atropine with the preoperative medication does not offer any special protection. As in adults, the incidence and the severity of these irregularities in heart rate increase after a second dose; and usually are not seen after IM SCh.[26]

An elevation in serum potassium occurs after the IV administration of SCh to normal children; however, these changes are too small to have significant effect.[33] A life-threatening arrhythmia related to hyperkalemia may occur after the IV administration of SCh in patients with burns, tetanus, paraplegia, encephalitis, crush injury, or neuromuscular disease.[34–39] In these situations the whole muscle membrane becomes permeable; thus the prolonged depolarization caused by SCh may induce a massive efflux of potassium, with possible cardiac arrest.[40]

Although it is stated that dangerous hyperkalemia is associated with burns greater than 20 percent of surface area, it would be prudent not to use SCh in any patient with ungrafted wounds. We avoid the use of SCh for at least one year following the healing of a major burn injury.

Myoglobinemia, a sensitive indicator of muscle injury, occurs in 40 percent of children anesthetized with halothane who have received SCh.[41] This effect is seen only in three percent of adults and does not occur with intramuscular SCh. In a recent study a rise in serum myoglobin concentration has been seen in all children, whether they received 1 or 2 mg of SCh IV.[42] Gallamine did avert fasciculations in these patients, but did not decrease the incidence of myoglobinemia. Eight percent of the patients achieved sufficiently high levels of myoglobin to cause myoglobinuria.

Fasciculations are not seen in children under three years of age. They do occur in older children, but are less intense than in adults; the rise in intragastric pressure is minimal.[43] Intraocular pressure rises after SCh administration in children whether or not they fasciculate; this is due to contraction of the extraocular muscles.[44] The intraocular pressure usually begins to rise within 60 seconds, peaks in two to three minutes, and then returns to baseline in five to seven minutes. It is advisable, therefore, to wait for at least seven minutes before performing tonometry in children who have received intravenous SCh. In general, SCh is contraindicated in patients with penetrating ocular wounds, glaucoma, or retinal detachment.

Clinical uses of SCh. Succinylcholine is the muscle relaxant with the most rapid onset and the shortest duration available for clinical use. It is most commonly used to facilitate intubation. In infants under a year of age, a dose of 2 mg/kg IV would be appropriate because of their large extracellular volume. In older children 1 mg/kg IV will suffice in most situations. These doses will produce apnea for approximately three minutes. To decrease the incidence of arrhythmias, it is preferable to pretreat with atropine, in a dose of 0.01 mg/kg IV.

In emergency situations with the possibility of a "full stomach," a rapid sequence induction with thiopental and SCh is an appropriate technique. In children under three years, because of the absence of fasciculation and consequent insignificant rise of intragastric pressure, there is no need to pretreat with nondepolarizing muscle relaxants. In general pretreatment is not necessary since cricoid pressure (Sellick maneuver) can effectively block the consequences of a mild rise of intragastric pressure.[43]

In situations where an IV is difficult to secure, SCh may be given intramuscularly. In these situations, 4 mg/kg IM in children,[5] or 5 mg/kg in infants,[27] provides the most satisfactory intubating conditions.

SCh may also be given as a continuous IV infusion for surgical relaxation. In this situation, however, when the dose exceeds 3 mg/kg IV, tachyphylaxis occurs; after 4 mg/kg IV, phase II block occurs. Therefore, if these doses have been administered, and additional SCh is necessary, then monitoring of the twitch response and train-of-four is strongly advised.

NONDEPOLARIZING MUSCLE RELAXANTS

Intermediate Acting Relaxants

Atracurium and vecuronium, the recently introduced intermediate acting agents have been satisfactorily evaluated in children[46–52] and have been used in infants also.[48,49,51] Although both have an intermediate duration of action, their chemical composition and mode of elimination are completely different. Atracurium is a bisquaternary compound which undergoes spontaneous decomposition to inactive metabolites at physiologic pH (Hofmann elimination), and undergoes enzymatic hydrolysis independent of plasma cholinesterase. On the other hand, vecuronium is a demethylated derivative of pancuronium and is partly excreted in bile.

With clinical doses, these two drugs have the specific advantage over the existing nondepolarizers of not causing cardiovascular changes. Large doses of atracurium, if given rapidly, may cause a slight to moderate amount of histamine

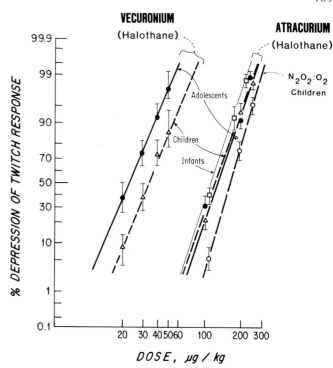

Figure 9-5. Cumulative dose–response curves for vecuronium and atracurium in adolescents, children, and infants. (The data are compiled from references 46–48.)

release, which can result in a slight diminution in blood pressure and a rash. These effects are very transient and disappear spontaneously.[53] They can be prevented by administering the drug slowly (60–75 s). Atracurium is a less potent stimulator of histamine release than is d-tubocurarine or metocurine.[53] At doses about three times those necessary for muscle relaxation (ED_{95}), stimulation of histamine release by atracurium is a third that of d-tubocurarine, and half that of metocurine. Our clinical experience with children under 10 years of age is that these histamine-related phenomena are not usually seen, even with large doses.

Vecuronium does not produce any histamine related side effects. A slight drawback with vecuronium, however, is that it is provided in powder form and has to be dissolved before administration.

With atracurium we found that the dose–response curves of infants older than a month, of children, and of adolescents, were practically superimposed[46,52] (Figure 9-5). A dose of 0.4 mg/kg IV in the presence of halothane will provide satisfactory conditions for intubation in all children. This dose will abolish the twitch response within two minutes, at which time tracheal intubation can be satisfactorily accomplished. After this dose the twitch height recovers to 5 percent of control in 20–25 minutes from 5–25 percent in another 10 minutes, and from 25–95 percent of control in an additional 20–25 minutes.

Since atracurium is hydrolyzed in plasma, it is noncumulative. It can therefore be readily administered via continuous infusion, the average requirement during N_2O/O_2 narcotic anesthesia being 8–10 µg/kg/min.[50] In the presence of halothane and enflurane the effective infusion rate decreases by about a third, and after prolonged enflurane anesthesia by about half that of N_2O/O_2 anesthesia.

Vecuronium is slightly more potent than pancuronium. The effective dose of the drug is comparable in infants, children, and adults.[47] Adolescents appear to require a slightly larger dose,[47] though for practical purposes the difference between these groups is rather insignificant. Interestingly, in small infants the duration of action of vecuronium is longer than in children, the 90 percent recovery of the twitch height from 0.07 mg/kg in infants being 73 minutes and in children 35 minutes.[49] The longer duration of action may be due to the larger distribution volume in infants, or to slow clearance, which is probably due to the relative immaturity of the infant's liver.

Because these two new agents have a relatively short duration of action, it is necessary to use a neuromuscular monitor in evaluating children to whom they are administered, since relaxation may change from a satisfactory to an unsatisfactory state very quickly, generally in less than 10 minutes.

LONG ACTING NONDEPOLARIZING RELAXANTS

d-Tubocurarine (dTc) and pancuronium are the most commonly administered of the long acting nondepolarizing muscle relaxants used in infants and children; metocurine is less commonly used. Gallamine is only occasionally employed in children. The tachycardia induced by gallamine may offer an advantage or disadvantage depending on the clinical situation.

d-Tubocurarine

Early studies of the use of curare in infants less than one month of age showed marked sensitivity based upon clinical indicators of adequate operating conditions and control of ventilation.[1,6] Further studies using electromyography confirmed these early clinical observations.[54] More recent studies in halothane-anesthetized children, using twitch response of the thumb adductor, demonstrated marked variation in the response of infants under two months of age. The dose that caused 95 percent depression of the twitch (ED$_{95}$) varied between 0.16–0.64 mg/kg IV in infants less than 10 days; whereas the range of the ED$_{95}$ in older children was 0.23–0.46 mg/kg IV.[2] Bennet et al. reevaluated the clinical requirement of dTc of neonates and found that in the newborn 0.25 mg/kg IV of dTc is needed, while a 28 day old infant required 0.5 mg/kg IV.[56]

Conclusions in the literature regarding whether the neonate is more sensitive to dTc than the older child are confusing. Closer examination shows the judgments reached depend on the method of inquiry. When clinical evaluations were used as the indicator, small infants required less relaxant. When the evoked response of the muscles of the hand was evaluated, infants required amounts of relaxant equivalent to older children.[2] There are several possible explanations for these findings. First is that the respiratory muscles are more sensitive to dTc than the peripheral muscles. However, this has not been proven in the peripheral muscles in the newborn human. In fact, the central muscles, including the diaphragm, are more developed than the peripheral muscles in the neonate.[57] In addition, the ratio of fast to slow muscles, as determined by histochemical techniques, is much greater in the respiratory musculature of the newborn than the six-month old.[58] What must be investigated is whether the maturational stage or the type of muscle studied has any correlation with the human response to muscle relaxants.

Pharmacokinetic Studies

Pharmacokinetic and pharmacodynamic studies have demonstrated that the plasma dTc concentration at which 50 percent depression of the twitch height occurs is lower in neonates and infants than in children and adults, whereas the steady state distribution volume is greater in neonates than in infants, children, or adults.[59,60] The product of the two, i.e., the quantity of drug present at a steady state to produce 50 percent paralysis, was practically the same in all the age groups. These data indicate that during nitrous oxide–halothane anesthesia, neonates and infants are paralyzed at lower plasma curare concentrations. This effect is counterbalanced, however, by the larger volume of distribution in infants and hence the requirements (mg/kg) of the infant for dTc is practically the same as that of the older child or young adult. In addition, neonates demonstrate a wide variability in their response to the effect of muscle relaxants; it has been observed that in some infants three times the average plasma level of dTc is required to achieve the same degree of relaxation.[61] The reason for this marked variation is not clear. It may in part be related to a nonhomogeneous group of patients in whom the myoneural junction was at different stages of development. In addition, surgery in newborns is often performed urgently; in this situation associated metabolic disorders may affect the distribution of body fluids and consequently the distribution of muscle relaxants.

dTc clearance in infants and children is similar to that of young adults. Because of the neonates' larger distribution volume, however, a smaller fraction of dTc is eliminated every minute. This longer elimination half-life may result in a slower rate of recovery from neuromuscular blockade.[60]

In general, several factors make the newborn more vulnerable to the action of muscle relaxants: (1) immaturity of the neuromuscular system, as evidenced by the lower values of train-of-four, post-tetanic facilitation, and tetanus–twitch ratios and the marked fade during prolonged tetanic stimulation; (2) longer elimination half-life of relaxants; (3) the respiratory system of the newborn, which works on a higher demand with less reserve due to greater oxygen consumption for each kilogram of body weight (hence, small doses of relaxants, which might not affect the respiratory exchange of the older child, might adversely affect the newborn); (4) the closing volume of the neonate, which is within the tidal volume, i.e., some airways close at the end of expiration.[62] Therefore, if respiration is impaired even to a mild degree due to residual muscle paralysis, more alveoli will collapse. This may result in dangerous hypoxemia and acidosis, which might potentiate and prolong the action of muscle relaxants, thus creating a vicious cycle.

Metocurine

Metocurine iodide is a methyl derivative of dTc, and is twice as potent. It causes less histamine release than does dTc, and therefore minimal changes in cardiovascular parameters.

The dose–response curve of metocurine is parallel to that of dTc, with a potency ratio of about 2:1 (Figure 9-6). In clinical studies, metocurine at a dose of 0.5 mg/kg IV in infants and children did not significantly alter the blood pressure or heart rate.[63] The return of tetanic fade and post-tetanic facilitation after this large dose was 38 minutes in the presence of halothane anesthesia, and 19 minutes with thiopental N_2O/O_2 anesthesia.

Burned children for several reasons are resistant to the action of metocurine (or any other nondepolarizing muscle relaxant) and may require two to four times the usual dose to achieve neuromuscular blockade.[64]

Pancuronium

Pancuronium bromide is a bisquaternary ammonium steroid compound with nondepolarizing neuromuscular blocking properties. Pancuronium has some advantages over dTc, since it frequently causes tachycardia (increased cardiac output) and has minimal histamine releasing properties. The systolic blood pressure thus tends to rise after its administration, whereas with dTc it tends to fall or remain at preoperative levels.[65]

Pancuronium at a dose of 0.1 mg/kg IV offers satisfactory conditions for endotracheal intubation in 90 percent of infants and children; in 10 percent conditions remain less than ideal.[7] Increasing the dose to 0.15 mg/kg IV provides satisfactory intubating conditions in all children. At this high dose, the conditions for antagonism (reversal) are not optimal even after 40 minutes. The clinical duration of action of a smaller dose 0.08 mg/kg IV of pancuronium in the presence of halothane is approximately 40 minutes in children.[66]

There is no significant difference between the dose–response curves of infants and children, though there is wide individual variation.[67] The dose–response curve of pancuronium is slightly steeper than that of dTc or metocurine; this may be due to less protein binding. At clinically effective doses, pancuronium is five times more potent than dTc.[68]

Pancuronium has become a popular drug in the neonatal intensive care unit to achieve muscular relaxation because of its cardiovascular stabilizing properties.[69] It is usually administered in increments of 0.1 mg/kg every hour for prolonged periods. Oxygenation is often improved, while peak transpulmonary pressure is decreased; this therapy may diminish the incidence of pneumothorax.[69,70] Pancuronium may also reduce the incidence of increases in intracranial pressure.[70] Despite large cumulative doses of pancuronium, adequate reversal can be achieved with the usual doses of atropine and neostigmine, even though these patients are often receiving aminoglycoside antibiotics.[12]

CLINICAL CONSIDERATIONS IN THE USE OF NONDEPOLARIZING MUSCLE RELAXANTS

The choice of a nondepolarizing muscle relaxant will depend on the clinical situation. If the technique chosen is N_2O/O_2 and muscle relaxant, then dTc may be preferred, since it may lower blood pressure under conditions of light anesthesia. With halothane anesthesia, pancuronium may be preferred since its vagolytic effects lead to tachycardia and a rise in blood pressure counteracting the myocardial depressant effects of halothane. If no change in heart rate or peripheral vascular resistance is indicated, then metocurine may be the relaxant of choice. In this respect, the recently developed short to intermediate acting relaxants offer a specific advantage, since at the usual clinical doses they do not cause significant changes in heart rate and blood pressure.

The effective doses that will cause 95 percent depression of the twitch height (ED_{95}) in the presence of halothane are 0.3 mg/kg IV of dTc tubocurarine, 0.15 mg/kg IV of metocurine,

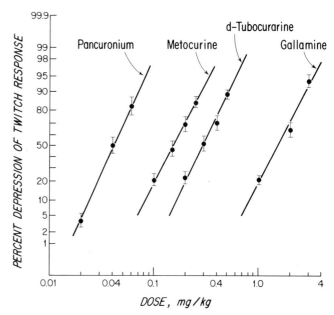

Figure 9-6. Cumulative dose–response curves for pancuronium, metocurine, and d-tubocurarine, in infants and children during N_2O/O_2 narcotic anesthesia (Reproduced from Goudsouzian NG, et al: The dose response effect of long acting nondepolarizing neuromuscular blocking agents in children. *Can Anaesth Soc J* 31:246–250, 1984. With permission.)

and 0.06 mg/kg IV of pancuronium; these doses are about a third higher in the absence of halothane. These doses provide satisfactory muscle relaxation in the intubated child; the expected mean duration of action is about 25 minutes for dTc and metocurine and 15 minutes for pancuronium. If the child is to be intubated, these halothane, supplemented doses are multiplied by 2.5 (0.8 mg/kg IV for dTc, 0.5 mg/kg IV for metocurine, or 0.13 mg/kg IV for pancuronium) to ensure satisfactory intubating conditions. Following these intubation doses, the twitch height will recover to 5 percent of control in 54 minutes (mean) and to 25 percent of control in a total of 83 minutes (mean).[20] This technique is suitable for prolonged surgical procedures.

In the neonate, endotracheal intubation often is performed with the infant awake. After the endotracheal tube is secured, a dose of 0.25 mg/kg IV dTc may be given; the equivalent IV dose of metocurine is 0.125 mg/kg, and 0.05 mg/kg of pancuronium. Slightly smaller doses are chosen initially in neonates because of their wide variation in response. Therefore, additional doses should be carefully titrated. In the premature infant or the sick neonate a smaller initial dose of relaxant is recommended.

Because recovery from the action of muscle relaxants occurs very rapidly in children, early supplementation with additional relaxant or potent inhalational agent is necessary to prevent interruption of satisfactory surgical anesthesia. For prolonged surgical procedures, the long acting relaxants seem desirable. With the recent introduction of atracurium and vecuronium, however, the pediatric anesthesiologist will have more flexibility than previously, especially in the management of those surgical procedures which tend to be of short duration (e.g., herniorrhaphies, tonsillectomies). One intubating dose of these agents is usually sufficient for the entire surgical procedure; occasionally a supplementary dose will be required. Since these agents have a relatively short duration of action, the conditions of relaxation can change from satisfactory to unsatisfactory very quickly, generally in less than 10 minutes. It is necessary, therefore, to use a neuromuscular monitor in evaluating patients to whom these relaxants are administered.

ANTAGONISM OF MUSCLE RELAXANTS

In children, especially in infants, the oxygen consumption for each kilogram of body weight is higher than in adults. Therefore, a slight diminution in respiratory muscle power may lead to hypoxemia and CO_2 retention, leading in turn to acidosis, with further potentiation of the action of the relaxant. Consequently, it is very important in pediatric patients that all neuromuscular function return to normal levels at the end of the surgical procedure.

The clinical evaluation of the adequacy of antagonism of neuromuscular blockade in infants and children is more difficult than in adults. Of course, neither grip strength nor voluntary head lifting can be expected from small children. Rather, it is important with infants to observe the clinical conditions preoperatively (muscle tone, depth of respiration, vigor of crying), and then to aim for a return to that level in the post-reversal period. An exception to this is the child who will be ventilated postoperatively; here antagonism of muscle relaxation may not be indicated. Evaluation may be modified if a narcotic has been given near termination of surgery.

Useful clinical signs of antagonism are the ability to flex the arms and lift the legs.[71] In addition, return of abdominal muscle tone is a helpful sign. Inspiratory force may be measured, a force greater than 25 cm of water being taken as a satisfactory sign of adequate antagonism.[72] A crying vital capacity of more than 15 ml/kg is also considered an adequate sign of recovery of respiratory reserve.[73] The train-of-four is an invaluable aid. The force of contraction can be easily felt in infants—four equal contractions indicate adequate antagonism. Alternatively, tetanic stimulation without fade at 50 Hz for five seconds may be used.

It is frequently stated that the required dose for reversal of nondepolarizing muscle relaxants is higher in children.[23] Consequently, the frequently quoted doses for reversal have been 0.02 mg/kg of atropine and 0.06–0.07 mg/kg of neostigmine. However, a recent study indicated that the requirement of neostigmine may be surprisingly less in children than in adults—a dose of 0.02 mg/kg neostigmine was found to be satisfactory.[74] One should be aware that during this recent investigation, a twitch height of at least 10 percent of the control value was maintained throughout. Consequently, the clinical anesthesiologist might decide to start with the smaller dose (0.02 mg/kg) and then repeat the dose if there is doubt about the adequacy of reversal.

Edrophonium has the theoretical advantage of an onset of action two or three minutes faster than neostigmine. Whether this difference is of any practical significance is a matter of opinion. The dose required for children is higher than for adults, at least 0.3 mg/kg being needed.[75–76] Because heart rate changes seem to occur earlier with edrophonium, its administration should be delayed until the full effect of atropine has occurred.

The question arises whether the neuromuscular effects of muscle relaxants should be reversed in all patients, even if a prolonged time has elapsed since the administration of the last dose. This has previously been true primarily because the techniques of evaluation of muscle relaxants have been inadequate. Since the advent of reliable neuromuscular monitors and their use in conjunction with clinical observations and measurements of respiratory adequacy, however, one can be far more certain that in some cases reversal will not be required. This is especially true with the recently developed relaxants, particularly for atracurium, which is hydrolyzed in plasma. In infants, but not in children, the excretion of vecuronium might be delayed, necessitating the prophylactic use of reversing agents. If there is any doubt, the clinician should err on the side of reversal.

Hypothermia potentiates the action of muscle relaxants and delays their excretion. This can create a special problem at the end of a surgical procedure. The effort to raise body temperature by increasing oxygen consumption will augment the load on the respiratory system. If the respiratory muscles are unable to match this increased load, hypoxemia and CO_2 retention will occur, leading to acidosis, again potentiating the action of the relaxant. If at the end of a surgical procedure the infant's temperature is less than 35°C, the infant should be warmed by external means. Once the temperature is above 35°C, reversal then may be attempted if appropriate.

Antibiotics enhance the neuromuscular blocking properties of muscle relaxants.[77] In general, aminoglycoside derivatives (e.g., gentamicin, tobramycin, neomycin) have the greatest effect. The antibiotics that have neuromuscular blocking properties may be classified into three groups according to their mode of action:

1. Drugs inhibiting synthesis of the bacterial cell wall. Penicillin is the best known example of this group. Drugs of this type are the safest of the antibiotics in terms of producing neuromuscular blockade. Penicillin blockade, if it occurs, may be reversed by calcium, but is unaffected by neostigmine.

2. Drugs affecting the permeability of the cell membrane. Polymycins and colistin are examples of this group. They cause a blockade of complex origin which is not reversed by calcium or neostigmine but responds to 3–4, aminopyridine.

3. Agents inhibiting protein synthesis. There are two groups of such agents. The first consists of tetracycline and oxytetracycline, compounds which have weak and clinically insignificant neuromuscular blocking properties that can be reversed with calcium. The second group is clinically the more important and includes the aminoglycosides (streptomycin, neomycin, kanamycin, gentamicin, lincomycin and clindamycin). These drugs decrease acetylcholine release and inhibit the cholinergic receptor (postsynaptic blocking action). Their effect is antagonized by calcium.

The usual recommended single dose of cefazoline, gentamicin, or tobramycin lack any clinical or subclinical relaxant potentiating neuromuscular effects.[78] However, this does not exclude the possibility that large concentrations of antibiotics, especially in the presence of other potentiating factors, may contribute to neuromuscular paralysis.

Clinically it is extremely difficult to diagnose antibiotic-induced neuromuscular blockade. It is usually a diagnosis of exclusion. In our experience, we have not found significant difficulty in reversing the neuromuscular effects of pancuronium in critically ill neonates who have been receiving pancuronium for a prolonged duration in addition to receiving gentamicin and ampicillin.[12] In the infants we studied, however, hypocalcemia had been corrected and blood calcium levels were higher than 7.5 mg/dl prior to "reversal." A reasonable approach in the clinical situation, when confronted with an infant who does not seem to be adequately reversed with the usual doses of atropine and neostigmine, would be to administer calcium chloride (3 mg/kg) slowly, and then repeat to a total dose of 30 mg/kg over one hour. This should be done only with continuous cardiac monitoring.

REFERENCES

1. Stead AL: The response of the newborn infant to muscle relaxants. *Br J Anaesth* 27:124–130, 1955
2. Goudsouzian NG, Donlon JV, Savarese JJ, et al: Reevaluation of d-tubocurarine dosage and duration in the pediatric age group. *Anesthesiology* 43:416–425, 1975
3. Ali HH, Savarese JJ: Monitoring of neuromuscular function. *Anesthesiology* 45:216–249, 1976
4. Cook DR, Fischer CG: Neuromuscular blocking effects of succinylcholine in infants and children. *Anesthesiology* 42:662–665, 1975
5. Liu LMP, DeCook T, Goudsouzian NG, et al: Dose response to intramuscular succinylcholine in children. *Anesthesiology* 55:599–602, 1981
6. Bush GH, Stead AL: The use of d-tubocurarine in neonatal anesthesia. *Br J Anaesth* 34:721–728, 1962
7. Bennett EJ, Daugherty MJ, Bowyer DE, et al: Pancuronium bromide: Experiences in 100 pediatric patients. *Anesth Analg* 50:798–807, 1971
8. Waud BE, Waud DR: The margin of safety of neuromuscular transmission in the muscle of the diaphragm. *Anesthesiology* 37:417–422, 1972
9. Ali HH, Savarese JJ: Stimulus frequency and dose–response curve to d-tubocurarine in man. *Anesthesiology* 52:36–39, 1980
10. Ali HH, Utting JE, Gray TC: Quantitative assessment of residual antidepolarizing block (pt II). *Br J Anaesth* 43:478–485, 1971
11. Goudsouzian NG: Maturation of neuromuscular transmission in the infant. *Br J Anaesth* 52:205–214, 1980
12. Goudsouzian NG, Crone RK, Todres ID: Recovery from pancuronium blockade in the neonatal intensive care unit. *Br J Anaesth* 53:1303–1309, 1981
13. Ali HH, Wilson RS, Savarese JJ, et al: The effect of tubocurarine on indirectly elicited train-of-four muscle response and respiratory measurements in humans. *Br J Anaesth* 47:570–574, 1975
14. Stanec A, Heyduc J, Stanec G, et al: Tetanic fade and post-tetanic tension in the absence of neuromuscular blocking agents in anesthetized man. *Anesth Analg* 57:102–107, 1978
15. Churchill-Davidson HC, Wise RP: Neuromuscular transmission in the newborn infant. *Anesthesiology* 24:271–278, 1963
16. Koenigsberger MR, Patten B, Lovelace RE: Studies of neuromuscular function in the newborn: A comparison of myoneural function in the full term and the premature infant. *Neuropediatrics* 4:350–361, 1973
17. Crumrine RS, Yodlowski EH: Assessment of neuromuscular function in infants. *Anesthesiology* 54:29–32, 1981
18. Close R: Dynamic properties of fast and slow skeletal muscles of the rat during development. *J Physiol* 173:74–95, 1964
19. Kelly SS, Roberts DV: The effect of age on the safety factor in neuromuscular transmission in the isolated diaphragm of the rat. *Br J Anaesth* 49:217–222, 1977
20. Goudsouzian NG, Liu LMP, Coté CJ: Comparison of equipotent doses of nondepolarizing muscle relaxants in children. *Anesth Analg* 60:862–866, 1981

21. Goudsouzian NG, Liu LMP: The neuromuscular response of infants to continuous infusion of succinylcholine. *Anesthesiology* 60:97–101, 1984
22. Cook DR, Fischer CG. Characteristics of succinylcholine neuromuscular blockade in infants and children. *Anesth Analg* 57:63–68, 1978.
23. Cook DR: Muscle relaxants in infants and children. *Anesth Analg* 60:335–343, 1981
24. Zsigmond EK, Downs JR: Plasma cholinesterase activity in newborns and infants. *Can Anaesth Soc J* 18:278–285, 1971
25. DeCook TH, Goudsouzian NG: Tachyphylaxis and phase II block development during infusion of succinylcholine in children. *Anesth Analg* 59:639–643, 1980
26. Mazze RI, Dunbar RW: Intralingual succinylcholine administration in children: An alternative to intravenous and intramuscular routes? *Anesth Analg* 47:605–615, 1968
27. Liu LMP, Goudsouzian NG: Neuromuscular effect of intramuscular succinylcholine in infants. *Anesthesiology* 57:A413, 1982
28. Sutherland GA, Bevan JC, Bevan DR: Neuromuscular blockade in infants following intramuscular succinylcholine in two or five percent concentration. *Can Anaesth Soc J* 30:342–346, 1983
29. Craythorne NWB, Turndorf H, Dripps RD: Changes in pulse rate and rhythm associated with the use of succinylcholine in anesthetized children. *Anesthesiology* 21:465–470, 1960
30. Lerman J, Robinson S, Willis MM, et al: Succinylcholine-induced heart rate changes in children during isoflurane and halothane anesthesia. *Anesthesiology* 59:A443, 1983
31. Hannallah RS, Oh TH, McGill WA, et al: Changes in heart rate and rhythm following intramuscular injection of succinylcholine and atropine in anesthetized infants. *Anesthesiology* 59:A444, 1983
32. Goudsouzian NG: Turbe del ritmo cardiaco durante intubazione tracheale nei bambini. *Acta Anesth Ital* 32:293–299, 1981
33. Kenally JP, Bush GH: Changes in serum potassium after suxamethonium in children. *Anesth Intensive Care* 2:147–150, 1974
34. McCaughey TJ: Hazards of anaesthesia for the burned child. *Can Anaesth Soc J* 9:220, 1962
35. Cooperman LH: Succinylcholine-induced hyperkalemia in neuromuscular disease. *JAMA* 213:1867–1871, 1970
36. Cowgill DB, Mostello LA, Shapiro HM: Encephalitis and a hyperkalemic response to succinylcholine. *Anesthesiology* 40:409–411, 1974
37. Roth F, Wuthrich H: The clinical importance of hyperkalemia following suxamethonium administration. *Br J Anaesth* 41:311–316, 1969
38. Smith RB, Grenvic A: Cardiac arrest following succinylcholine in patients with central nervous system injuries. *Anesthesiology* 33:558–560, 1970
39. Mazze RI, Escue HM, Houston JB: Hyperkalemia and cardiovascular collapse following administration of succinylcholine to the traumatized patient. *Anesthesiology* 31:540–547, 1969
40. Gronert GA, Theye RA: Pathophysiology of hyperkalemia induced by succinylcholine. *Anesthesiology* 43:89–99, 1975
41. Ryan JF, Kagen LJ, Hyman AI: Myoglobinemia after a single dose of succinylcholine. *N Engl J Med* 285:824–827, 1971
42. Harrington JF, Ford DJ, Striker TW: Myoglobinemia and myoglobinuria after succinylcholine in children. *Anesthesiology* 59:A439, 1983
43. Salem MR, Wong AY, Lin YH: The effect of suxamethonium on the intragastric pressure in infants and children. *Br J Anaesth* 44:166–169, 1972
44. Craythorne NWB, Rottenstein HS, Dripps RD: The effect of succinylcholine on intraocular pressure in adults, infants and children during general anesthesia. *Anesthesiology* 21:59–66, 1960
45. McGoldrick KE: Anesthesia for ophthalmic surgery, in Smith RM (Ed): *Anesthesia for Infants and Children.* St. Louis, C.V. Mosby, 1980, pp 477–487
46. Goudsouzian NG, Liu LMP, et al: Safety and efficacy of

atracurium in adolescents and children anesthetized with halothane. *Anesthesiology* 59:459–462, 1983

47. Goudsouzian NG, Martyn JAJ, Liu LMP, et al: Safety and efficacy of vecuronium in adolescents and children. *Anesth Analg* 60:1083–1088, 1983

48. Goudsouzian NG, Liu LMP, Gionfriddo M, et al: Atracurium in infants and children. *Anesthesiology* 62:75–79, 1985

49. Fisher DM, Miller RD: Neuromuscular effects of vecuronium (ORG NC45) in infants and children during N_2O, halothane anesthesia. *Anesthesiology* 58:519–523, 1983

50. Cook DR, Brandom BW, Woelfel SK, et al: Atracurium infusion in children during fentanyl, halothane and isoflurane anesthesia. *Anesth Analg* 63:201, 1984

51. Brandom BW, Woelflel SK, Cook DR, et al: Clinical pharmacology of atracurium in infants. *Anesth Analg* 63:309–312, 1984

52. Goudsouzian NG, Gionfriddo M: Muscle relaxants and children. *Semin Anesth* 3:50–58, 1984

53. Basta SO, Savarese JS, Ali HH, et al: Histamine releasing potencies of atracurium, dimethyl d-tubocurarine and tubocurarine. *Br J Anaesth* 55:139S, 1983

54. Churchill-Davidson HC, Wise RP: The response of the newborn infant to muscle relaxants. *Can Anaesth Soc J* 11:1–6, 1964

55. Long G, Bachman L: Neuromuscular blockade by d-tubocurarine in children. *Anesthesiology* 28:723–729, 1967

56. Bennett EJ, Ignacio A, Patel K, et al: Tubocurarine and the neonate. *Br J Anaesth* 48:687–689, 1976

57. Crelin ES: *Functional Anatomy of the Newborn.* New Haven, Conn, Yale University Press, 1973

58. Keens TG, Bryan AC, Levison H, et al: Developmental pattern of muscle fiber types in human ventilatory muscles. *J Appl Physiol* 44:909–913, 1978

59. O'Keeffe C, Gregory GA, Stanski DR, et al: d-Tubocurarine: Pharmacodynamics and kinetics in children. *Anesthesiology* 51:S270, 1977

60. Fisher DM, O'Keeffe C, Stanski DR, et al: Pharmacokinetics and pharmacodynamics of d-tubocurarine in infants, children and adults. *Anesthesiology* 57:203–208, 1982

61. Matteo RS, Lieberman IG, Salanitre E, et al: d-Tubocurarine concentration and neuromuscular blockade in the neonate. *Anesthesiology* 53:S281, 1980

62. Mansell A, Bryan L, Levison H: Airway closure in children. *J Appl Physiol* 33:711–714, 1972

63. Goudsouzian NG, Liu LMP, Savarese JJ: Metocurine in infants and children: Neuromuscular and clinical effects. *Anesthesiology* 49:266–269, 1978

64. Martyn JAJ, Goudsouzian NG, Matteo RS, et al: Metocurine requirements and plasma concentration in burned paediatric patients. *Br J Anaesth* 55:263–268, 1983

65. Nightingale DA, Bush GH: A clinical comparison between tubocurarine and pancuronium in children. *Br J Anaesth* 45:63–70, 1973

66. Yamamoto T, Baba H, Shiratsuchi T: Clinical experience with pancuronium bromide in infants and children. *Anesth Analg* 51:919–924, 1972

67. Goudsouzian NG, Ryan JF, Savarese JJ: The neuromuscular effects of pancuronium in infants and children. *Anesthesiology* 41:95–98, 1974

68. Goudsouzian NG, Martyn JAJ, Liu LMP, et al: The dose response effect of long acting nondepolarizing neuromuscular blocking agents in children. *Can Anaesth Soc J* 31:246–250, 1984

69. Stark AR, Bascom R, Frantz ID: Muscle relaxation in mechanically ventilated infants. *J Pediatr* 94:439–443, 1979

70. Finer NN, Tomney PM: Controlled evaluation of muscle relaxation in the ventilated neonate. *Pediatrics* 67:641–646, 1981

71. Mason LJ, Betts EK: Leg lift and maximum inspiratory force, clinical signs of neuromuscular blockade reversal in neonates and infants. *Anesthesiology* 52:441–442, 1980

72. Belani KG, Gilmour IJ, McComb RC, et al: Physical ventilatory weaning parameters in neonates and infants. *Anesthesiology* 51:S330, 1979

73. Shimada Y, Yoshiya I, Tanaka K, et al: Crying vital capacity and maximal inspiratory pressure as clinical indicators of readiness for weaning of infants less than a year of age. *Anesthesiology* 51:456–459, 1979

74. Fisher DM, Cronnelly R, Miller RD, et al: The neuromuscular pharmacology of neostigmine in infants and children. *Anesthesiology* 59:220–225, 1983

75. Fisher DM, Cronnelly R, Sharma M, et al: Clinical pharmacology of edrophonium in infants and children. *Anesthesiology* 61:428–433, 1984

76. Fisher DM, Cronnelly R, Miller RE: Dose–response relationship for edrophonium in anesthetized children. *Anesthesiology* 59:A282, 1983

77. Sokoll MD, Gergis SD: Antibiotics and neuromuscular function. *Anesthesiology* 55:148–159, 1981

78. Lippmann M, Yang E, Au E, et al: Neuromuscular blocking effects of tobramycin, gentamicin and cefazolin. *Anesth Analg* 61:200–201, 1982

10

Perioperative Fluid Management

Letty M.P. Liu

The management of fluid and electrolyte balance in anesthesia patients is a primary responsibility of the anesthesiologist. As children get older, physiologic as well as anatomic changes take place. Consideration of these changes is important because it provides the basis of a rational approach to fluid management. Following a review of some of the important maturational changes that affect fluid balance, guidelines for fluid administration in children will be discussed.

DEVELOPMENTAL CONSIDERATIONS

BODY COMPOSITION

Physiological differences between patients of various ages become apparent when the composition of total body mass is examined. Total body mass may be considered in terms of body solids and body water (Figure 10-1). Body water is contained in two compartments, the intracellular fluid compartment (ICF) and the extracellular fluid compartment (ECF). This latter compartment is divided into two parts, the plasma volume (PV) and the interstitial fluid volume (ISF), by a capillary membrane that prevents proteins, which are high in concentration in the plasma, from entering the interstitial fluid. In the normal patient, the osmolality of the ECF (PV and ISF) and the ICF are similar (290–310 mOsm); the electrolyte composition, however, differs. The ECF contains approximately 154 mEq/l of anions and a similar concentration of cations, whereas the ICF has 200 mEq/l of each of these ions. The ECF contains large quantities of sodium and chloride ions, a substantial amount of bicarbonate ions, and a small number of potassium, calcium, and magnesium ions. In contrast, the ICF has a high concentration of potassium ions, a significant quantity of magnesium ions, and very few sodium

and bicarbonate ions. The major result of these differences in electrolyte concentration is a large sodium gradient in one direction across the cell membrane (ECF to ICF), and a large potassium gradient in the other direction (ICF to ECF).

Rapid changes in the composition of body mass take place during gestation and continue at a slower rate throughout the neonatal period. With growth, an inverse relationship exists between the percentage of total body fat and total body water (Figure 10-2). Fat, which represents a very low percentage of the body weight of the fetus younger than 30 weeks gestation, increases to about 16 percent of body weight by term, and to about 23 percent by the end of the first year of life.[1] Conversely, body water decreases with age,[2] accounting for about 94 percent of weight of a 10 week old fetus, 75 percent of the weight of a full-term newborn, 65 percent of the weight of a 12 month old child, and 55–60 percent of the weight of an adult. The ECF, which represents about 40 percent of the neonate's body weight, decreases to about 20 percent in the adult. The ICF, on the other hand, increases from approximately 35 percent of body weight to about 40 percent by the end of the first year of life.

RENAL FUNCTION

At birth, renal function is still immature. The glomerular filtration rate of the newborn is 25–30 percent of an adult's, and the newborn can not excrete or conserve sodium as well as an adult.[3-6] This reduced ability of the young infant to conserve sodium can result in hyponatremia if fluids without sodium are administered to replace fluid losses. The neonate can neither concentrate nor dilute urine as well as an adult.[7-9] However, the newborn is better able to clear free water and increase urine volume when challenged with a large fluid load over a short period of time than he or she is able to concentrate

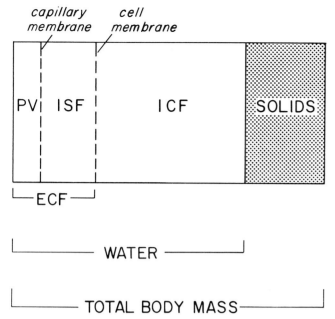

Figure 10-1. Composition of total body mass in terms of body solids and body water. Total body water is contained in the intracellular fluid compartment (ICF) and the extracellular fluid compartment (ECF). This latter compartment is comprised of the plasma volume (PV) and the interstitial fluid volume (ISF).

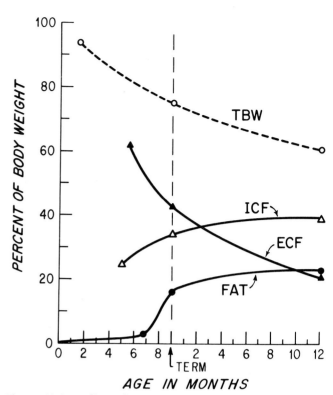

Figure 10-2. Effect of age on the relative distribution of total body water (TBW), intracellular fluid compartment (ICF), extracellular fluid compartment (ECF), and fat to total body mass.

urine when volume depleted. Consequently, the healthy newborn will tolerate a moderate fluid overload better than moderate dehydration.

Renal function matures rapidly during the first few weeks after birth. By the end of the first month, renal function is 80–90 percent mature, and by eight to nine months of age maturation is nearly complete.

CARDIOVASCULAR SYSTEM

The newborn's cardiovascular system does not usually present a problem for the anesthesiologist, provided the baby is well oxygenated and has an adequate circulating blood volume. If congenital cardiac anomalies are present, however, or if the transition from intrauterine to extrauterine circulation does not take place, the rate, amount, and composition of fluid administered may be crucial in averting heart failure. The administration of large volumes of fluid to the neonate has been correlated with the development of symptoms of congestive heart failure, as well as a delay in ductal closure.[10,11]

CALORIC EXPENDITURE

During intrauterine life, the fetus gradually increases in weight. However, after birth the newborn generally loses weight for about three to five days. This is related to the low oral intake of the baby. As intake improves, caloric, fluid, and electrolyte balances become positive, and the body weight gradually increases.[12]

The basal caloric expenditure of a full term newborn in a neutral thermal environment is about 32 Cal/kg/d during the first few hours of life.[13] As the child becomes more active, caloric expenditure increases. This increase is very rapid

during the first week. With maturation, caloric expenditures continue to rise, but at a slower rate.

The caloric expenditure of hospitalized patients was estimated by Holliday and Segar from data obtained from patients of different weights and states of activity (Figure 10-3).[14] Patients weighing up to 10 kg expend 100 Cal/kg/d; those weighing between 10 and 20 kg expend 100 Cal, plus 50 Cal for each kg above 10 kg; those weighing over 20 kg expend 1500 Cal, plus 20 Cal for each kg above 20 kg.

Certain conditions will markedly alter the caloric expenditure of patients. If the ambient air temperature is low, full term and preterm babies will increase heat production in order to maintain their body temperature. This response is proportional to the degree of cold stress, and may result in a metabolic rate which is 2.5 times the basal metabolic rate.[13] A high ambient air temperature in the operating room, warm anesthetic gases, radiant warmers, warming blankets and warm isolettes will reduce cold stress. If patients become hypothermic, caloric expenditures will decrease by approximately 12 percent for each degree centigrade drop in temperature from normal. With fever, caloric expenditures will increase approximately 12 percent for each degree centigrade rise in temperature above the normal. In other hypermetabolic states, e.g., hyperthyroidism, caloric expenditures may increase 25–75 percent above normal, whereas in other hypometabolic states, e.g., hypothyroidism, expenditures may decrease 10–25 percent.[15]

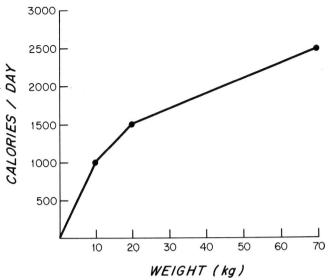

Figure 10-3. Computed daily caloric requirements of average hospitalized patients in relation to body weight. (Holliday MA, Segar WE. The maintenance need for water in parenteral fluid therapy. *Pediatrics* 19:823–832, 1957. Copyright American Academy of Pediatrics 1959. With permission.)

WATER REQUIREMENT

Formulas used to determine maintenance fluid requirements are based on body weight, surface area, or estimated metabolic rate. Since a healthy 70 kg adult requires about 2500 ml each day (35 ml/kg/d), and a healthy infant 100 ml/kg/d, a patient's maintenance requirements can not be accurately calculated using a formula based solely on weight. Formulas based on surface area will also be inaccurate. Calculation of maintenance fluid requirements should probably be based on metabolic rate.

Under normal circumstances, 100 ml of water is required for every 100 calories expended (Table 10-1). This includes water lost as urine, through respiration, and through the skin. Loss through the gastrointestinal tract is generally negligible except in certain situations such as vomiting, diarrhea, bowel obstruction, enemas, and surgical manipulation of the bowel.

Due to the developmental characteristics of the skin and the large surface area to body weight ratio of the newborn, water loss through the skin can be significant. As gestational age decreases, insensible water loss through the skin in-

Table 10-1

Normal Maintenance Water Losses

	Water (ml/100 Cal)
Output	
Urine	70
Insensible Loss	
Skin	30
Respiratory Tract	15
"Hidden Intake"	
(from burning 100 calories)	−15
Total	100

Table 10-2

Hourly Maintenance Fluid Requirements

Weight (kg)	ml/hr
<10	4
10–20	40 + 2 ml for each kg above 10 kg
>20	60 + 1 ml for each kg above 20 kg

creases.[16–18] If a high ambient air temperature is required to maintain thermal balance, water loss through the skin may increase. The degree of water loss will depend on the humidity of the ambient air; saturation of this air will decrease loss.

The daily fluid requirement of the average hospitalized patient can be estimated by combining the data on water lost from burning 100 Calories with the results generated by Holiday and Segar on the metabolic expenditures of these patients. Children weighing below 10 kg require 100 ml/kg/d; those weighing 10–20 kg require 1000 ml, plus 50 ml/kg for every kg above 10 kg; and those heavier than 20 kg require 1500 ml, plus 20 ml/kg for each kg above 20 kg. The hourly requirement for fluid maintenance may be calculated by dividing the daily fluid requirement by 24, or by using the guidelines in Table 10-2.

For example, the hourly requirement for fluid maintenance for a healthy 27 kg child may be calculated as follows:

	Calculation	Total (ml)
4 ml/kg for the first 10 kg	4 × 10 =	40
2 ml/kg for each kg between 10 and 20 kg	2 × 10 =	20
1 ml/kg for each kg above 20 kg	1 × 7 =	7
Hourly fluid requirement		67

FLUID COMPOSITION

In addition to determining the rate at which fluid should be administered, the anesthesiologist is also responsible for selecting the appropriate fluid. Neonates should be given intravenous fluids which contain sodium, because their kidney lacks the ability to retain sodium even when hyponatremia exists.[5] Sodium requirements have been related to age. Full-term neonates required 20 mEq/l of sodium, whereas neonates born before 36 weeks of gestation required 40 mEq/l to maintain sodium balance.[6] Although older children and adults can tolerate salt-free fluids somewhat better than infants, older patients should not be given this type of fluid exclusively. These patients need some salt in their intravenous fluid, since normal fluid losses contain electrolytes. Thus, to avoid water intoxication and hyponatremia, an electrolyte-free solution (e.g., 5% dextrose in water) should be used discriminantly.

Ideally, one calorie should be provided for every calorie expended. If a glucose solution is used to achieve this goal, a 25 percent solution will be necessary in order not to exceed a

Table 10-3

Relation of Physical Findings With the
Severity of Dehydration

Physical Findings	Dehydration (%)
Poor tissue turgor, dry mouth	5
Sunken fontanellae, tachycardia, oliguria	10
Sunken eyeballs, hypotension	15
Coma	20

child's water requirement. A solution of this strength is unfortunately very hypertonic and can sclerose peripheral veins. Since body fat stores are generally adequate to meet caloric needs in most patients on short-term intravenous fluid therapy, caloric expenditures do not need to be replaced entirely. Short-term fluid therapy should provide enough calories to spare protein and prevent ketosis. This amounts to about 20–25 calories for every 100 calories required. Since each gram of glucose provides about four calories, the administration of five grams of glucose for every 100 calories expended should satisfy caloric needs. In patients who have very little or no fat stores, however, such as premature infants and debilitated patients, vigorous efforts should be made to fully replace caloric expenditures. A five percent dextrose solution is generally sufficient to maintain a normal blood sugar in a healthy child undergoing anesthesia. Although neonates who receive intravenous fluid therapy preoperatively are frequently given a more concentrated (10%) sugar solution because they depend on carbohydrates and free fatty acids for fuel during the first days of life, they rarely need this hyperosmolar solution to maintain a normal blood sugar during anesthesia.

In addition to sugar, intravenous fluids should contain reasonable quantities of electrolytes so that the kidney will not have to excrete or conserve large amounts of these substances in order to maintain electrolyte balance. The following guide may be used to replace maintenance losses of electrolytes for every 100 Calories expended:

Sodium—2.5 mEq
Potassium—2.5 mEq
Chloride—5.0 mEq

A quarter-strength saline solution may be used to replace maintenance fluid losses. If urine output is adequate (0.5 ml/kg/hr), potassium (16–20 mEq/l) should be added to the intravenous solution.

PREOPERATIVE FLUID MANAGEMENT

Fluid management of the pediatric patient undergoing anesthesia should commence at the time of the preanesthetic visit. In addition to taking a thorough history and performing a physical examination, all laboratory data should be evaluated and additional studies ordered if indicated. Abnormal findings such as dehydration, electrolyte imbalance, and severe anemia should be corrected prior to the induction of anesthesia.

DEHYDRATION

The state of hydration of a child can be evaluated in two ways. If the child became ill acutely and his or her weight prior to the acute illness is known, the amount of water the child has lost or gained can be determined by obtaining the difference between his or her present weight and the pre-illness weight. If the child's weight is unknown, or if he or she is chronically ill, hydration may be estimated by using the criteria presented in Table 10-3. The rapidity at which fluids and electrolytes can be replaced depends upon the severity of dehydration and electrolyte imbalance. Approximately 10 ml of fluid for each kilogram of body weight will be required to replace each percent dehydration.

ELECTROLYTE IMBALANCES

When there is a disproportionate loss of water to salt, the osmolality of body fluids increases and hypernatremia results. This situation can be caused by fever, diarrhea, or vomiting. When the serum sodium reaches 165 mEq/l, symptoms related to changes in the central nervous system are likely to occur. Unlike other tissues of the body where the equilibration of water and salts occurs almost instantaneously, the brain has a six to eight hour lag when it comes to sodium achieving a new equilibrium.[19] Water, on the other hand, moves almost instantaneously across tissues. The result is the removal of water from the interstitial compartment of the brain and a decrease in cerebral spinal fluid pressure. Thus, hypernatremia should be corrected slowly with five percent dextrose in a quarter-strength saline over a period of at least 24 hours. Rapid correction with electrolyte-free solutions should be avoided to prevent the development of cerebral edema and seizures.[20]

The administration of inappropriate quantities of salt-poor water can result in hyponatremia (serum sodium level of 130 mEq/l). Patients are rarely symptomatic if their serum sodium concentration is above 120 mEq/l. Below this concentration, seizures or coma secondary to cerebral edema may occur. If a patient is symptomatic, treatment should begin immediately. Three percent sodium chloride (1–10 ml/kg) should be given slowly until the patient becomes asymptomatic. Once this occurs, the three percent sodium chloride solution should be stopped and normal saline administered until the serum sodium concentration becomes normal.

Severe acidosis, hypoaldosteronism, renal failure, and the overzealous administration of potassium are situations that can all lead to hyperkalemia. Corrective therapy should be instituted without delay when the serum potassium rises above 6.0 mEq/l. Potassium administration should cease immediately. The electrocardiogram should be continuously monitored and initial treatment directed at reversing cardiac manifestations of hyperkalemia. Sodium bicarbonate (1–2 mEq/kg), calcium chloride (5 mg/kg), and hyperventilation will provide an initial effect while waiting for longer acting drugs such as insulin (1 unit/kg) in glucose (1 g/kg of 20% or 50% dextrose) to shift potassium intracellularly. The reduction in the concentration of total body potassium may be accomplished by administering an ion exchange resin, e.g., Kayexalate (sodium polystyrene sulfonate) (1–2 g/kg/day) rectally or orally in four divided doses. One gram for each kilogram of body weight of this drug should lower the serum potassium by 1 mEq/l.

Overzealous treatment of hyperkalemia can lead to hypokalemia. More often, however, this condition is a result of chronic diuretic therapy, vomiting, diarrhea, bowel obstruction, and inappropriate fluid administration. A serum potassium of less than 3.0 mEq/l should be corrected prior to starting anesthesia. Unless urgent correction is required, potassium deficit should be corrected over 8–12 hours. If rapid correction is mandatory, potassium may be administered at a rate of up to 1 mEq/kg/hr, provided that the electrocardiogram and urine output are closely monitored and frequent determinations of serum potassium are made. If hypokalemia is associated with hypochloremia, correction of the chloride deficit may be necessary before the potassium deficit can be corrected.

Hypochloremia may be caused by vomiting, bowel obstruction, and chronic diuretic therapy. This condition may be corrected with normal saline (0.9% NaCl) administered over a 24 hour period.

The following formula can be used to correct electrolyte deficits,

$$Wt \times (C^+_D - C^+_M) \times 0.3 = mEq \text{ required}$$

where, Wt is weight in kilograms, C^+_D is serum concentration desired, and C^+_M is serum concentration measured. For example, if the measured serum potassium of a 10 kg child is 2.5 mEq/l and the desired level is 4.0 mEq/l, the deficit would be 4.5 mEq.

$$10 \times (4.0 \text{ mEq/l} - 2.5 \text{ mEq/l}) \times 0.3 = 4.5 \text{ mEq}$$

Metabolic acidosis may result from diarrhea, hypovolemia, hypoxia, hypoglycemia, diabetic ketoacidosis, renal failure, and hypothermia. A base deficit of 10 mEq/l or greater warrants urgent correction of both the acidosis and the underlying cause of acidosis. A dose of 1–2 mEq/kg of sodium bicarbonate may be administered while determining the amount of drug required to correct the acidosis. The following formula may be used to calculate the bicarbonate requirement,

$$Wt \times \text{base deficit} \times 0.3 = mEq \text{ of bicarbonate required}$$

After half of the calculated dose of bicarbonate is administered, the acid–base status of the patient should be reassessed and therapy adjusted accordingly.

FASTING

Guidelines for writing preoperative fasting orders (NPO) for children who do not require intravenous therapy prior to surgery are presented in Table 10-4. Solid food (including milk) should be withheld after midnight of the day prior to surgery from children scheduled for elective surgical procedures. Since water turnover is higher in younger children than older children and adults, babies and young children should be awakened and offered clear fluids prior to fasting. If surgery is delayed for several hours, an intravenous infusion should be started to avert dehydration and starvation hypoglycemia.

INTRAOPERATIVE FLUID MANAGEMENT

Intravenous fluid therapy during the intraoperative period is generally aimed at replacing previous fluid deficits as well as intraoperative losses of fluids, electrolytes, and blood.

Table 10-4

Fasting Period (hours) Prior to Anesthesia

Age	Milk and Solids	Clear Fluid
Neonate	4	2
1–5 mo	4	4
6–36 mo	6	6
36 mo and older	8	8

During anesthetic procedures involving minimal blood loss, most pediatric patients will maintain fluid and electrolyte balance if an initial 250 ml bottle of five percent dextrose in lactated Ringer's solution is followed with solutions of lactated Ringer's solution without sugar. Caution should be exercised, however, when administering five percent dextrose in lactated Ringer's solution is used only to replace ongoing caloric and maintenance fluid losses. All patients undergoing prolonged surgical procedures should have serum glucose and electrolytes measured periodically, and the composition of intravenous solution should be changed accordingly.
cations may be avoided if a five percent dextrose in lactated Ringer's solution is used only to replace ongoing caloric and fluid losses. All patients undergoing prolonged surgical procedures should have serum glucose and electrolytes measured periodically and the composition of intravenous solution should be changed accordingly.

REPLACEMENT OF DEFICIT AND MAINTENANCE FLUIDS

If one assumes that the normal healthy child is in water and electrolyte balance following the last oral feeding, an estimate of the fluid deficit incurred during the fasting period may be made by multiplying the patient's hourly maintenance fluid requirement by the number of hours elapsed since the last feeding. In a normal healthy child who has a small fluid deficit, the calculated deficit is generally replaced during the first three hours of anesthesia.

In addition to replacing the patient's preoperative fluid deficit, ongoing maintenance fluid losses should also be replaced during anesthesia. During the first hour of surgery, the amount of fluid administered should replace half of the patient's fluid deficit as well as his or her maintenance fluid loss during that hour. During the second hour, fluid is given to replace one fourth of the preanesthetic deficit, in addition to the maintenance fluid loss during that hour. The same amount of fluid should be administered during the third hour of anesthesia. Subsequently, only ongoing fluid losses are replaced.

REPLACEMENT OF "THIRD SPACE" FLUID LOSS

Replacement of the preoperative fluid deficit and ongoing maintenance fluid losses may be inadequate to maintain water and electrolyte balance during many surgical procedures. A substantial amount of fluid may be lost from the effective circulating blood volume into the interstitial fluid volume as a result of surgical manipulation of tissues. The volume of transudated fluid which is lost will vary according to the degree of surgical trauma.[21] Unfortunately, the magnitude of fluid lost into the "third space" is difficult to measure, and can only be estimated at present. In major abdominal surgical procedures, this loss can represent as much as 15 ml/kg/hr. In less traumatic procedures, such as an inguinal hernia repair, transudated fluid loss may amount to only 1 ml/kg/hr. If this transudated fluid loss is not replaced, the patient may become hypotensive. Since the fluid lost into the third space is due to capillary leakage into tissues, the electrolyte and protein concentration of this fluid is similar to plasma. Balanced salt solutions, such as lactated Ringer's solution, are effective and inexpensive solutions which can replace this loss. If the serum protein concentration is low, albumin (5%) may be used.

REPLACEMENT OF BLOOD LOSS

The replacement of intraoperative blood loss is discussed in Chapter 11.

POSTOPERATIVE FLUID MANAGEMENT

During the immediate postoperative period, intravenous fluids are generally administered to replace maintenance fluid loss and ongoing third space fluid loss. Five percent dextrose in 0.2 percent saline, with 20 mEq/l of potassium added, generally satisfies fluid requirements, since the amount of third space loss is generally minimal during the recovery period. Additional fluid and electrolytes may have to be administered if there is fluid loss through gastric drainage, draining fistuli, pleural effusions, peritoneal drains, chest tubes, postoperative bleeding, fever, etc. The volume of fluid loss in these circumstances can be substantial. For example, a neonate with a nasogastric tube in place can lose as much as 125 ml/kg/d (normally 20–40 ml/kg/d) of gastric juice.[22] After certain surgical procedures (e.g., gastroschisis repair) additional fluid and electrolytes may be required to replace the large volume of fluid lost to the third space, which can be expected to continue for several hours or days postoperatively.[23] Following other procedures (e.g., cardiac or neurosurgical procedures) fluid and salt restriction may be indicated. In any case, the composition of the intravenous fluid, as well as the rate of fluid administration, must be adjusted according to the needs of the individual patient.

FLUID ADMINISTRATION DEVICES

In order to prevent accidental volume overload, the amount of intravenous fluid available to a child at any one time should not exceed the child's calculated hourly requirement. A useful device is a volumetric chamber. With this, the amount of fluid available for infusion can be limited; a micro-drip infusion set will limit the rate of fluids administered, and a fluid infusion pump can be utilized to regulate the rate of administration of fluids more precisely. Although these pumps can be very useful, they are a hinderance in certain circumstances. If intravenous drugs are required urgently, as is often the case during the induction of anesthesia, they are often easier to administer if the rate of administration of the intravenous fluid is adjusted by hand. When the upper limit of infusion of a pump is less than that required to keep up with fluid losses (e.g., cases involving rapid blood loss), pumps should not be used. An infusion pump is also inappropriate

when the lower limit of infusion is higher than the child's fluid requirement.

MONITORING

Although the guidelines for fluid administration presented in this chapter are useful, each patient must be managed individually. Careful monitoring, therefore, plays an integral role in fluid management. The following parameters should be routinely monitored during all anesthetic procedures: heart sounds, heart rate, breath sounds, blood pressure, the electrocardiogram, body temperature, and skin color. A change in the color of the skin may be the first sign of impending hypoxia or hypotension due to depletion of the circulating blood volume. A drop in blood pressure, a decrease in the intensity of heart sounds, or an increase in heart rate are other indicators of hypovolemia. A change in breath sounds may signify fluid overload and impending pulmonary edema. Alterations in the electrocardiogram may denote acid–base or electrolyte imbalance. A change in body temperature may require the warming or cooling of intravenous fluids.

Patients with severe cardiac or renal disease, and those having surgical procedures involving large fluid shifts and/or blood loss, may require additional monitoring. An indwelling arterial line and a central venous or pulmonary artery catheter may be necessary in order to measure pressure directly. It may also be helpful to monitor blood gases, electrolytes, osmolality, proteins, ionized calcium, and glucose, and to follow urine output, specific gravity, and electrolyte levels.

REFERENCES

1. Sinclair JC, Driscoll JM, Jr., Heird WC, et al: Supportive management of the sick neonate: Parenteral calories, water and electrolytes, in Behrman RE (Ed): *The Newborn. Ped Clin North Am* 17:863–893, 1970
2. Friis-Hansen B: Body water compartments in children: Changes during growth and related changes in body composition. *Pediatrics* 28:169–181, 1961
3. Guignard JP, Torrado A, Gautier E: Glomerular filtration rate in the first three weeks of life. *J Pediatr* 87:268–272, 1975
4. Aperia A, Broberger O, Herin P, et al: A comparative study on the response to an oral NaCl and NaHCO₃ load in newborn pre-term and full-term infants. *Pediatr Res* 11:1109–1111, 1977
5. Bennett EJ, Daughety MJ, Jenkins MT: Fluid requirements for neonatal anesthesia and operation. Anesthesiology 32:343–350, 1970
6. Aperia A, Broberger O, Thodenius D, et al: Renal control of sodium and fluid balance in newborn infants during intravenous maintenance therapy. *Acta Paediatr Scand* 64:725–731, 1975
7. Jahrig K, Zollner H, Margies D: Osmolar clearance and clearance of total electrolytes newborn infants. *Biol Neonate* 20:93–100, 1972
8. Leake RD, Zakauddin S, Trygstad CW, et al: The effects of large volume intravenous fluid infusion in neonatal renal function. *J Pediatr* 89:968–972, 1976
9. Edelman CM, Jr, Barnett HL, Troupkoui V: Renal concentrating mechanisms in newborn infants. Effect of dietary protein and water content, role of urea, and responsiveness to antidiuretic hormone. *J Clin Invest* 39:1062–1069, 1960
10. Stevenson JG: Fluid administration in the association of patent ductus complicating respiratory distress syndrome. *J Pediatr* 90:257–261, 1977
11. Bell EF, Warburton D, Stonestreet BS, et al: Effect of fluid administration on the development of symptomatic patent

ductus arteriosus and congenital heart failure in premature infants. *N Engl J Med* 302:598–604, 1980

12. Wilkinson AW, Stevens LH, Hughes EA: Metabolic changes in the newborn. *Lancet* 1:983–987, 1962
13. Brueck K: Temperature regulation in the newborn infant. *Biol Neonate* 3:65–119, 1961
14. Holliday MA, Segar WE: The maintenance need for water in parenteral fluid therapy. *Pediatrics* 19:823–832, 1957
15. Winter RW: *Principles of Pediatric Fluid Therapy.* North Chicago, Abbot Laboratories, 1970
16. Fanaroff AA, Wald M, Gruber HS, et al: Insensible water loss in low birthweight infants. *Pediatrics* 50:236–245, 1972
17. Hammarlund K, Sedin G: Transepidermal water loss in newborn infants III. Relation to gestational age. *Acta Paediatr Scand* 68:795–801, 1979

18. Wu PYK, Hodgman JE: Insensible water loss in preterm infants: Changes with postnatal development and non-ionizing radiant energy. *Pediatrics* 54:704–712, 1974
19. Bakay L: Studies in sodium exchange. *Neurology* 10:564–571, 1960
20. Finberg L: Hypernatremic (hypertonic) dehydration in infants. *N Engl J Med* 289:196–198, 1973
21. Shires T, Williams J, Brown F: Acute changes in extracellular fluids associated with major surgical procedures. *Ann Surg* 154:803–810, 1961
22. Bennett EJ. Fluid balance in the newborn. *Anesthesiology* 43:210–224, 1975
23. Mollitt DL, Ballantine TVN, Grosfeld JL, et al: A critical assessment of fluid requirements in gastroschisis. *J Pediatr Surg* 13:217–219, 1978

11

Blood Replacement and Blood Product Management

Charles J. Coté

With the advent of modern reconstructive and oncologic surgery the number of pediatric patients sustaining major operative blood loss has significantly increased. Little information has been gathered as to when to expect coagulation defects in the pediatric age group; there are, however, data on adult patients which, in our experience, appear to reflect the events in children. Recent advances in blood banking techniques, component therapy, and blood salvage have also altered the problems associated with massive blood replacement.

BLOOD VOLUME ESTIMATION

An estimation of circulating blood volume (BV) should be made prior to induction. The BV of a premature infant (90–100 ml/kg) constitutes a greater portion of body weight than that of the full-term newborn (80–90 ml/kg). Infants between three months and one year will have a circulating BV of 70–80 ml/kg. In general, the majority of older children have an estimated BV (EBV) of 70 ml/kg. Consideration must also be given to body habitus, if a child is extremely obese one would estimate the BV to be 60–65 ml/kg. It is from this estimate, and knowledge of the initial hematocrit, that a calculation of the maximal allowable blood loss (MABL), prior to the requirement for red cell transfusion, is made. Since no untoward effects are expected at a hematocrit of 30, most anesthesiologists have designated 30 to be the minimum acceptable. However, we prefer to allow a healthy child to have a post-operative hematocrit of 20–25% if further losses are unlikely, rather than expose that child to the dangers of a blood transfusion.

There are three commonly accepted methods for estimating the MABL:[1-3] the first uses an approximation of cir-

culating red cell mass, the second a modified logarithmic equation, and the third a simple proportion. Any method is acceptable and the numbers calculated are not significantly different clinically.[1-3] The most straightforward method is to estimate the MABL by simple proportion.[1]

$$\frac{\text{Estimated blood volume (EBV)} \times (\text{patient hematocrit} - 30)}{\text{patient hematocrit}} = \text{MABL}$$

For example, a ten-kilogram child would have an EBV of 10 kg × 70 ml/kg, equaling 700 ml. If the patient's hematocrit were 42, the MABL would be:

$$\frac{700 \times (42 - 30)}{42} = \frac{700 \times 12}{42} = 200 \text{ ml} = \text{MABL}$$

The next factor to consider after knowing the EBV and MABL is the fluid deficit and maintenance (see Chapter 10). Thus, initial volume replacement is directed toward replacement of the deficit and maintenance fluids, followed by blood loss replacement. According to the work of Shires et al., each milliliter of blood lost should be replaced by 2–3 milliliters of balanced salt solution; another alternative is to replace blood lost milliliter for milliliter with five percent albumin.[4,5] The latter type of replacement is expensive and there is no clear evidence that colloid is superior to crystalloid. Work in adult patients has shown large differences in colloid osmotic pressure and total volume of fluid necessary to maintain cardiac output and cardiac filling pressures, but there was no difference in the volume of shunted blood (Qs/Qt) or the development of pulmonary edema when either five percent albumin or balanced salt solution was used intraoperatively.[6] These data were gathered in patients with significant cardiovascular disease, and suggest that even fewer clinically important changes would occur in normal healthy pediatric patients, although no such studies have as yet been published.

Returning to the previous example of a 10-kg child with a 700-ml blood volume and 200-ml MABL, replacement of blood loss up to that point could be made in two ways; either 400–600 milliliters of balanced salt solution or 200 milliliters of five percent albumin. If blood loss will continue beyond the MABL, either during surgery or into the recovery period, replacement of lost red cells beyond the MABL should be matched with red cells. If one unit of blood has been started it is reasonable to give the patient an excess transfusion of five to ten percent rather than risk the need for another transfusion with a second unit postoperatively.[7] Since little data have been gathered in children, one mode of replacement therapy cannot be stated as absolutely superior to another, i.e., whole blood, citrated packed red blood cells (PRBCs), or frozen packed red blood cells.

In our experience there seems to be little danger in allowing the MABL to be replaced entirely with balanced salt solutions, provided that one is dealing with a healthy child, and postoperative oozing will not exceed the MABL. Balanced salt solutions are inexpensive and will spare valuable blood component products. If replacement of lost red blood cells is necessary, it is simple to calculate the volume of PRBCs needed to return the hemoglobin to an acceptable value.[7] If one estimates the hematocrit of PRBCs to be 75, then for each 10 milliliters infused, 7.5 milliliters will be red blood cells.

In the previous example, if the blood loss was 300 milliliters (exceeding the MABL by 100 milliliters) then replacement of lost RBCs must be carried out. If one desired to increase the hematocrit up to 30, then the calculation would be:

$$\frac{\text{blood volume to be replaced (100 ml)} \times \text{desired hematocrit (30)}}{\text{Hematocrit in PRBC (75)}} = \frac{100 \times 30}{75} = 40 \text{ ml}$$

Simplifying this, approximately half a milliliter of PRBC for each milliliter of blood loss beyond the MABL usually raises the hematocrit above 30. In these calculations it is important to know the average hematocrit of PRBCs for your institution.

COMPONENT THERAPY

When caring for the pediatric patient, the anesthesiologist must think in terms of *percent of blood volume* rather than units of blood. For example, one unit of blood represents 10 percent of the blood volume of a 70-kg adult, but it represents 100 percent of the blood volume of a 7-kg child. This then allows one to order the appropriate volume of blood or blood components. Many blood banks now split units of blood into "quad" packs, so that multiple transfusions can be given to an infant from a single unit.[8] The Massachusetts General Hospital uses predominantly frozen PRBCs in pediatric patients. Frozen PRBCs offer theoretical advantages in that there is less chance for transmission of viral disease, HL-A, and blood group sensitization, better preservation of 2,3-diphosphoglycerate, and no elevation of potassium or citrate.

BLOOD

Blood may be transfused into the patient in several forms, fresh whole blood, citrated whole blood, citrated PRBCs, or frozen PRBCs (Table 11-1).[9–12] The advantages and disadvantages of each become evident when one considers their specific properties, which will be discussed in the section below concerning massive transfusion.

FRESH FROZEN PLASMA

Fresh frozen plasma (FFP) contains all clotting factors except platelets, and usually requires 30 to 45 minutes to thaw and crossmatch. However, it is only when the plasma has been administered within six hours of thawing that it contains all clotting factors at normal concentrations; after six hours labile Factors V and VIII begin to diminish.[13] In addition, some blood banks harvest Factor VIII prior to freezing the plasma so that FFP may not contain the full complement of Factor VIII; this must be noted on the plasma container. FFP contains proportionally more citrate than whole blood, and therefore may present the problem of citrate toxicity if rapidly administered. The major surgical indication for FFP is in association with massive blood transfusion, von Willbrand's disease, and occasionally hemophilia A. Frequently FFP is given without clear hematologic indication; by understanding massive transfusion the indications for FFP will be better defined.

PLATELETS

Platelet therapy by the anesthesiologist is commonplace due to the frequency of drug-induced thrombocytopenia (cancer chemotherapy), and more aggressive surgical procedures with associated massive blood loss.[14,15] In general, there are two categories of patients: those whose platelet count has fallen gradually secondary to disease or therapeutic intervention, and those whose platelet count has fallen rapidly because of massive blood loss and subsequent transfusion (dilutional thrombocytopenia).

The patient whose platelet count has fallen gradually to the $10,000-20,000/\text{mm}^3$ range does not usually require additional platelets unless there are overt signs of clinical bleeding or a surgical procedure is imminent. The patient whose platelet count has fallen rapidly secondary to massive transfusion may require a significantly higher platelet count for hemostasis ($50,000-75,000/\text{mm}^3$) and in this situation it is the anesthesiologist's responsibility to determine the number of platelet packs to be administered.[14,15]

Two further considerations in both of these situations are that (1) the platelet is essential to hemostasis associated with the vascular injury of surgery and thus is necessary for the control of surgical bleeding (Figure 11-1), and (2) there are many frequently used medications, e.g., aspirin, that cause abnormal platelet function which may then lead to problems with surgical hemostasis.[16–18]

There are no clear cut guidelines regarding platelet counts and clinical bleeding; each patient must be individually assessed. If the thrombocytopenia relates to drug therapy,

Table 11-1

Differences in Composition of Major Blood Products

	Normal whole blood (in vivo)	Citrated whole blood (2 wk old) ACD/CPD	Citrated packed red blood cells*	Frozen packed red blood cells	FFP
PH	7.4	6.6–6.9	6.6–6.9	6.6–7.2	6.6–6.9
pCO$_2$	35–45	180–210	180–210	0–10	180–210
Base deficit (mEq/l)	0	9–15	9–15	?	9–15
Potassium (mEq/l)	3.5–5.0	18–26	18–26 mEq/l	1–2 mEq/l	4–8
Citrate	None	++++	++	None	++++
Factors V and VIII	Normal	20–50%	20–50%	None	85–100%
Fibrinogen	Normal	Normal	Normal	None	Normal
Platelets	240,000–400,000	None	None	None	None
2–3 DPG	Normal	3% of normal	3% of normal	Nearly normal	—
Hematocrit	35–45	35–45	60–70	50–95	—
Temperature	37°C	4–6°C	4–6°C	4–6°C	Cold

(Modified from Miller RD: Refresher Courses in Anesthesiology 1:101, 1973)
*Citrated whole blood and citrated PRBCs have the same chemical composition, but citrated PRBCs have considerably less plasma volume.

fewer platelets will be required than if the thrombocytopenia is secondary to an immunologic abnormality. Similarly, the patient with ongoing consumption of platelets, as in disseminated intravascular coagulopathy, will have much higher platelet requirements than a patient with dilutional thrombocytopenia from massive blood replacement. Some patients with massive trauma and associated multiple transfusions may develop a thrombocytopathy where platelets are present in adequate numbers but their function is impaired. The most expeditious way to assess platelet function is to perform a bleeding time (Ivy).[19,20]

One unit of platelets will usually increase the platelet count by 7,000–11,000/mm^3 for each square meter of body surface area.[21] Standard transfusions for the pediatric patient are 0.1–0.3 units/kg of body weight; this usually produces an increment of 20,000–70,000/mm^3.[15,18,21] If one is dealing with dilutional thrombocytopenia with ongoing losses, a larger transfusion of platelets may be required to boost the platelet count above 65,000/mm^3. The anesthesiologist should anticipate the need for platelets so that excessive surgical bleeding does not occur. The decision to administer platelets must not be made lightly. The more frequently platelets are administered, the greater will be the antibody production, and this may lead to a shortened half-life for future transfused platelets.[14,15,18]

In addition, three further points should be made. First, not all hospitals have platelets readily available; thus, unless the need is anticipated prior to surgery, platelets may not be available when required. Second, for patients who are thrombocytopenic before surgery, it is recommended that platelets be infused just prior to the surgical procedure to ensure the highest levels during the time of peak demand. Third, platelets should only be filtered by the special large-pore filter provided by the blood bank; micropore filters may adsorb large numbers of platelets and therefore diminish the effectiveness of a platelet transfusion.[22]

OTHER COMPONENTS

Cryoprecipitate; Factor VIII concentrate; Factor IX concentrate

Cryoprecipitate is a concentrated plasma protein fraction which contains 20–50 percent of the Factor VIII of the original plasma.[21] It also contains large quantities of Factor XIII and fibrinogen. Its principal use is in the treatment of classic hemophilia A, and some patients are now on self-transfusion programs at home.[23] It must be emphasized that these patients have many problems related to their disease,

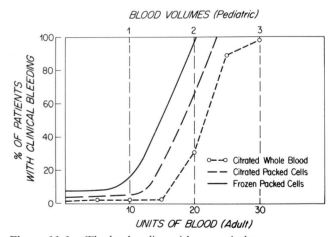

Figure 11-1. The broken line with open circles represents an adult study of citrated whole blood; bleeding in most cases was secondary to dilutional thrombocytopenia. Other lines represent postulated points of clotting factor deficiency if solely citrated packed cells or frozen cells are transfused. (Modified and reproduced with permission from Miller RD, Transfusion therapy and associated problems. ASA Refresher Courses in Anesthesiology 1:107, 1973.)

Table 11-2

Sources of Replacement for Factors VIII and IX

Factor VIII
  Plasma (fresh, fresh-frozen, or lyophylized)
  Cryoprecipitate*
  Concentrates**
    Abbott (antihemophilic factor—human)
    Armour (Factorate)
    Cutter (Koate)
    Hyland (Hemofil)
Factor IX
  Plasma (fresh to 21 days, fresh-frozen, lyophilized)
  Concentrates***
    Cutter (Konyne)
    Hyland (Proplex)

(Reproduced with permission from Abildgaard CF: Current concepts in the management of hemophilia. *Sem Hematol* 12:224, 1975.)
*Average bag contains approximately 100 units.
**Usual vial contains 250–300 units.
***Usual vial contains 500 units.

including splenomegaly, abnormal liver function, joint disease related to hemarthrosis, and the possibility of the hepatitis and acquired immune deficiency syndrome (AIDS) carrier state.[24] Careful planning of any surgical procedure must entail close communication with the patient's hematologist in order to ensure optimal therapy.

In general, for hemophiliac patients replacement is aimed at increasing the deficient factors. This is determined by measuring the content of the missing factors in the patient's plasma, and knowing the concentrations in plasma cryoprecipitate, or factor concentrate. The activity of one milliliter of normal plasma is defined as one unit. Each unit of Factor VIII/kg will result in an increase of Factor VIII of approximately two percent, whereas the in vivo response to Factor IX is less and ranges from 0.5–1.0 percent for each unit/kg.[25] Sources of replacement therapy and dosage are reproduced in Table 11-2 and 11-3. It should be noted that these are guidelines, and consultation with the patient's hematologist is essential, especially if there are complicating factors such as Factor VIII or Factor IX inhibitors that would greatly increase the factor replacement requirements.

Patients with hemophilia B, or Factor IX deficiency, are generally treated with commercially available concentrates which contain prothrombin and Factors VII, IX, and X. These concentrates carry a significant risk of hepatitis and AIDS, thus judicious use must be planned with the attending hematologist; for minor surgical procedures an attempt is often made to manage the bleeding with fresh frozen plasma rather than the commercially available pooled concentrates.

MASSIVE BLOOD TRANSFUSION

Massive blood transfusion may be defined as that situation in which the patient's entire blood volume will be replaced one or more times. As previously emphasized, when dealing with children, the anesthesiologist must think in terms of percent of blood volumes lost rather than units of blood lost. In addition, it is important to appreciate the composition of each blood component (fresh whole blood, fresh frozen plasma, stored

Table 11-3

Suggested Doses of Factor VIII and Factor IX for Replacement Therapy in Hemophilia

Type of Bleed	Dose
Early minimal bleed (usually spontaneous) with no known trauma and few objective signs	10 units/kg (single dose usually sufficient)
Moderate bleed (fully developed hemarthrosis, known trauma, etc.)	20–25 units/kg (repeat dose may be required at 12–24 hr)
Severe bleed (head injury, major wound, etc.)	40–50 units/kg (repeat doses of 20–25 units/kg at 12 hr intervals until hemorrhage is controlled or wound is healed)

(Reproduced with permission from Abildgaard CF: Current concepts in the management of hemophilia. *Semin Hematol* 12:226, 1975.)

citrated whole blood, citrated PRBCs frozen PRBCs) in order to anticipate problems, and at what stage of transfusion these problems might arise (see Table 11-1).

The use of these various blood components may seriously affect coagulation, electrolyte and calcium balance, acid–base balance, body temperature, oxygen–hemoglobin dissociation, and hematocrit.

COAGULOPATHY

The coagulopathy of massive blood transfusion is primarily related to dilution of either clotting factors or platelets. The point at which clotting factor deficiency sufficient to produce coagulopathy occurs is dependent both on the volume of blood lost and the type of blood component transfused. Dilutional thrombocytopenia sufficient to cause clinical bleeding depends on the starting platelet count and the volume of blood lost.

Factor Deficiency

A study of Vietnam trauma patients found that the onset of clinical bleeding occurred after about 15 units of whole blood had been transfused (Figure 11-1). The incidence of coagulopathy was unrelated to abnormal prothrombin time (PT) or partial thromboplastin time (PTT), but was highly correlated with a platelet count of less than $65,000/mm^3$.[26] If we consider the average male to weigh 70 kilogram, he will have a blood volume of five liters (10 units) of blood. In order to relate the data in Figure 11-1 to children, assume each 10 units of whole blood in the adult to be equivalent to one blood volume. One would thus anticipate some children to develop coagulopathy after 1.5 blood volumes lost, but the majority of children would develop clinical bleeding after 2.0–2.5 blood volumes lost. *This only applies if replacement is with citrated whole blood*, and the coagulopathy would be due to thrombocytopenia, not clotting factor deficiency.

The normal coagulation sequence is presented in Figure 11-2. The PT measures the adequacy of Factors VII, X, V, prothrombin and fibrinogen (the extrinsic system). The PTT assesses the adequacy of Factors XII, XI, IX, VIII, X, V, prothrombin and fibrinogen (intrinsic system).

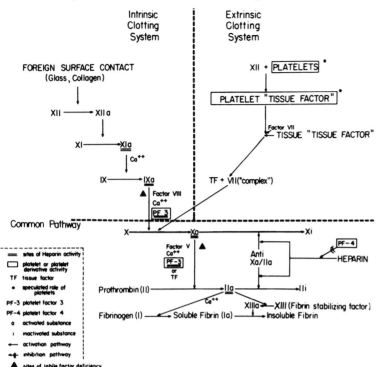

Figure 11-2. Normal coagulation cascade with sites of platelet action. Note that labile cofactors VIII and V are the most readily diluted during massive transfusion with citrated blood products. All clotting factors are diluted during frozen blood transfusion. (Reproduced and modified with permission from Barrer MJ, Ellison N: Platelet function. Anesthesiology 46:205, 1977.)

Banked citrated whole blood has all blood components, but a reduced concentration of Factors V and VIII (20–50% of normal) (Table 11-1). In order for coagulopathy secondary to a factor deficiency to develop, Factor VIII must drop to less than 30 percent of normal, and Factor V to less than 20 percent of normal.[9] For this to occur, a two to three blood-volume exchange with citrated whole blood is necessary. The first coagulation test to be altered is the PTT, because Factor VIII would be diluted to less than 30 percent. If, however, replacement is being made with citrated PRBCs, with minimal plasma present, dilution of Factors V and VIII will occur much earlier than with whole blood (Figure 11-1). If frozen PRBCs are used, in which there are no clotting factors present, clotting factor dilutional coagulopathy may result sooner than with citrated PRBCs. Thus clotting factor deficiency is unlikely when replacement is made with whole blood, but very likely when replaced with PRBCs. Our current clinical practice is to transfuse FFP in a volume of at least 20–30 percent for each blood volume, when blood losses exceed certain volumes and have been replaced with a specific component (see Table 11-4), i.e. the indications for and timing of FFP transfusion depend on which blood product has been transfused.

Thrombocytopenia (Dilutional)

A platelet count will give the number of circulating platelets (normal = 150,000–350,000 mm³), but only a bleeding time will determine if platelet function is normal.[18–20] For a patient with acute blood loss a platelet count in excess of 50,000–75,000/mm³ is adequate, whereas for one with a

Table 11-4

Minimal Fresh Frozen Plasma (FFP) Recommendations According to The Type of Blood Replaced and Volume Lost

Type blood replaced	Juncture FFP indicated	Volume FFP to be transfused
Citrated whole blood	1.5–3.0 blood volumes and each blood volume thereafter	20–30% of each blood volume lost
Citrated packed cells	1–2 blood volumes and each blood volume thereafter	20–30% of each blood volume lost
Frozen packed cells	0.75–1.50 blood volumes and each blood volume thereafter	20–30% of each blood volume lost

chronic deficiency the platelet count may be sufficient when greater than 10,000–15,000/mm³, the reason for this difference is unknown.[26–28]

Adult and pediatric studies of acute dilutional thrombocytopenia found a high correlation of clinical bleeding with a platelet count of 65,000/mm³ or less.[26,27,29,30] Figure 11-3 represents the calculated reduction in platelet count compared with the observed fall in platelet count. The observed fall is probably different from the calculated reduction because of increased platelet release from the bone marrow, lungs, and lymphatic tissue. The important point is that the platelet count usually did not fall to dangerous levels until 20–25 units in adults, or two blood volumes in children, were lost.[26] Our observations in pediatric patients who lost one to five blood volumes correlate well with the adult studies. Clinical bleeding did not occur in children whose platelet count remained above 50,000/mm³ despite blood losses as great as five blood volumes (Figure 11-3).[30] The starting platelet count thus was very important. For example, if a patient started with 600,000/mm³ platelets, dilutional thrombocytopenia did not occur until four or more blood volumes were lost. If, however, the starting platelet count was 100,000/mm³, then dilutional thrombocytopenia occurred after one blood volume was lost. There is some evidence that platelets do not function normally after massive trauma. Thus, a thrombocytopathy may exist as well as thrombocytopenia; however, we did not observe this in our study of pediatric patients.[9,30]

It is, therefore, important to obtain basic clotting studies, especially a platelet count, prior to elective surgery, so that adequate blood bank stores are reserved for anticipated need. If coagulopathy appears earlier than expected (Figure 11-1), i.e., before one blood volume loss, search for other causes of bleeding, such as increased arterial or venous pressure in the surgical field, or consider the possibility of disseminated intravascular coagulopathy.

In summary, the coagulopathy associated with massive blood transfusion using whole blood is usually secondary to dilutional thrombocytopenia. However, other factors such as thrombocytopathy must also be considered during such situations. In addition, with the increased use of component therapy, especially citrated PRBCs and frozen PRBCs, there is a greater tendency for dilution of other clotting factors which

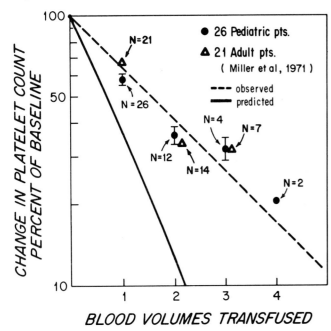

Figure 11-3. Percent of change in platelet count versus blood volumes transfused in adults and children.[29,30] The broken line represents observed values, whereas the solid line represents calculated values. This difference suggests mobilization of platelets during massive transfusion. The baseline platelet count is invaluable in estimating potential platelet needs in relation to blood volumes transfused. A low initial count suggests the need for early exogenous platelet transfusion, whereas a high initial platelet count indicates that exogenous platelets may not be required until several blood volumes have been lost. (Reproduced with permission from Coté CJ, Liu LMP, Szyfelbein SK, et al. Changes in serial platelet counts following massive blood transfusions in pediatric patients. *Anesthesiology*, 62:197–201, 1985.)

are not present in frozen blood, or only present in small quantities in citrated packed cells. Thus, when any form of PRBCs is transfused in large quantity, the use of fresh frozen plasma must be considered early, i.e., at one blood volume.

HYPERKALEMIA

Hyperkalemia has been described as a problem of massive transfusion. However, it is only a problem when whole blood is given rapidly.[9–11] Whole blood may have a plasma potassium level as high as 26 mEq/l, the degree of potassium elevation being related to the shelf age. This hyperkalemia reflects leakage of intracellular potassium into the extracellular space. Hyperkalemia may occur in adults who receive greater than 120 milliliters of citrated whole blood per minute.[31] If one relates this to patient weight,

$$120 \text{ ml} = 1/4 \text{ unit of blood}$$
$$= 1/40 \text{ blood volume}$$
$$= 1.5–2.0 \text{ ml/kg/min}$$

or 10 percent of the blood volume in four minutes. The need to relate the size of the patient to the speed of blood replacement rarely occurs clinically in adults, but is important to

consider in an infant. Referring to Table 11-1, it is clear that this would only be a problem with old whole blood, and would not occur with citrated PRBCs because of the small volume of plasma. Frozen PRBCs have a low potassium content and one study documented hypokalemia after the administration of large volumes of frozen PRBCs.[32] In our experience with burned patients, who often lose one to two blood volumes, and whose blood is completely replaced with FFP and frozen PRBCs, hypokalemia has not been a problem.

When the rate of infusion of citrated whole blood exceeds 1.5–2.0 ml/kg/min, the EKG must be closely monitored. Should ventricular arrhythmias occur with peaked T waves, appropriate treatment for hyperkalemia is instituted pending measurement of the serum potassium level. Recently a death was reported following neonatal exchange transfusion with whole blood which was less than 48 hours old; a study of the fresh whole blood used for exchange transfusion at that institution revealed 30 percent of units to have a potassium level greater than nine mEq/l, and 21 percent to have a potassium level greater than 11 mEq/l.[33] This complication occurred with relatively fresh blood. Thus it would be advantageous to administer frozen PRBCs or citrated PRBCs to avoid hyperkalemia in neonates requiring massive blood transfusion. *If whole blood is to be used in a neonate it is advised that the potassium level be measured prior to administration.*

HYPOCALCEMIA

Hypocalcemia has been reported with massive blood transfusion of whole blood; this is related to the binding of ionized calcium with sodium citrate.[34–39] Clinically, it is rare for hypocalcemia to occur unless the rate of transfusion is very rapid; Bunker demonstrated in adults that this rate must be one unit of whole blood over 3–4 minutes.[34] Stulz et al found no improvement in the ventricular function curve (i.e., no increase in CO) and a low ionized calcium when citrated whole blood was administered at 1.5 ml/kg/min: when a similar volume and rate of heparinized blood was administered there was an increase in cardiac output and no change in ionized calcium.[39] These findings correlate well with Bunker's data, and thus one would expect hypocalcemia of clinical importance to occur when the rate of infusion of citrated whole blood exceeds. 1.5–2.0 ml/kg/min.

The rate of infusion of citrated whole blood that produces hypocalcemia and hyperkalemia are nearly identical, while the cardiac electrophysiologic effects produced by hypocalcemia and hyperkalemia are opposite. It is important to note the EKG abnormalities, especially widening of the QRS complex, prolonged Q–T interval, and flattening or peaking of the T wave.[9] The treatment for both hypocalcemia and hyperkalemia is infusion of calcium. Calcium chloride (5 mg/kg) or calcium gluconate (15 mg/kg) should be administered if hypotension occurs which cannot be explained on the basis of hypovolemia. If the patient is hemodynamically stable then smaller doses of calcium will correct ionized hypocalcemia without producing wide fluctuations [CA++]. The problem of hypocalcemia following large volumes of citrated PRBCs or frozen PRBCs has not been examined, but it is unlikely that clinically significant hypocalcemia would result with either.

Fresh frozen plasma contains relatively more citrate than whole blood and thus milliliter for milliliter is potentially more hazardous than citrated whole blood. Therefore caution is urged when FFP is to be infused, especially if the patient already has a low ionized calcium level.[40] Figure 11-4 graphically presents the changes in ionized calcium which occurred in a 12-kg child during FFP transfusion. Maximal change in ionized calcium (1.24–0.48 mM/l) occurred at four minutes. The effects of hypocalcemia on the heart may be increased if FFP is administered through a central venous catheter; therefore, it probably should be given peripherally. Calcium administration should be carried out *during* rapid transfusion of FFP (more than 1.0 ml/kg/min) in order to minimize this dangerous but transient citrate toxicity. An intravenous preparation of calcium should always be available whenever major blood loss is anticipated.

ACID-BASE STATUS

A patient requiring massive transfusion usually falls into one of two categories:

1. The patient has sustained severe trauma and is in a state of shock.
2. The patient is undergoing major surgery which will result in massive blood loss, but will never be in a state of shock.

In the first situation, severe metabolic acidosis may result because of low cardiac output and diminished oxygen delivery. In this circumstance correction of the acidosis with sodium bicarbonate is part of the resuscitation, along with blood volume replacement. In the operating room, the second category usually predominates; replacement of the blood loss is more controlled. Even with repeated massive blood loss, metabolic acidosis is not usually a problem provided severe hypovolemia is avoided.[41,42] The major source of acid in whole blood is carbon dioxide, which is readily eliminated via the lungs (Table 11-1). The natural buffers in blood (hemoglobin and bicarbonate) rapidly counteract any residual lactic acid. Less is known about the effects of massive transfusion with frozen blood. Depending on the method of preparation, the pH of frozen blood may vary from 6.5 to 7.2 with minimal carbon dioxide content. The volume of acid is small and should be readily buffered.

Sodium bicarbonate therapy must therefore be governed by actual measurement of acid–base status, since metabolic acidosis does not occur with massive transfusion unless accompanied by severe hypovolemia, low cardiac output, or hypoxemia. Routine administration of alkali may have deleterious effects on oxygen–hemoglobin dissociation.

HYPOTHERMIA

Hypothermia is a significant problem associated with major blood loss and its replacement. Hypothermia causes a shift to the left in the oxygen–hemoglobin dissociation curve, which may have adverse effects on oxygen delivery. Referring to Table 11-1, all banked blood products have a temperature of 4–6°C, and therefore must be warmed prior to infusion. This is generally accomplished by use of a blood warmer. However, prolonged warming or overheating (greater than 42°C) may result in red cell hemolysis. Furthermore, unless care is taken to warm all other replacement solutions prior to massive infusion, hypothermia will develop. With a core temperature drop to 28°C, there is a potential for refractory ventricular tachycardia.[43] This mandates that every effort be made to keep the patient warm. Warming the blood and all

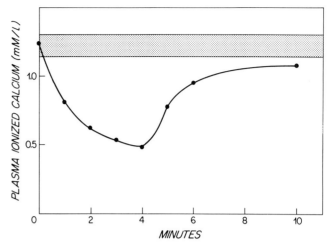

Figure 11-4. Changes in arterial ionized calcium in a 12-kg child during fresh frozen plasma infusion of 1.5 ml/kg/min for 5 minutes via infusion pump. Note the dangerous though transient fall in ionized calcium whose nadir was at four minutes.

other intravenous infusions, warming the operating room, using a warming blanket, radiant warmers, plastic wrap around extremities, and inserting a heated humidifier in the anesthesia circuit will all help to maintain body heat. The last method is particularly effective in children.

OXYGEN-HEMOGLOBIN DISSOCIATION

Oxygen binding to hemoglobin is primarily dependent on temperature, acid–base status, and 2,3-diphosphoglycerate (2,3-DPG). Figure 11-5 illustrates these effects on the oxygen–hemoglobin dissociation curve. Maintenance of optimum temperature is equally important in the recovery period when the patient's oxygen demands increase as a result of shivering and increased metabolism. Citrate is rapidly metabolized to bicarbonate, and thus causes a metabolic alkalosis several hours after massive transfusion.[34] If exogenous bicarbonate therapy is superimposed on this endogenous metabolic alkalosis, a significant effect on the dissociation of oxygen and hemoglobin could result. It is therefore necessary to determine the acid–base status *before* administering sodium bicarbonate to avoid intensifying the left shift caused by hypothermia and metabolized citrate. Citrated whole blood and FFP will therefore have the greatest effect on the oxygen–hemoglobin dissociation curve because of the large volume of citrate contained in these blood products. Citrated packed cells have little citrate and therefore minimal effects; frozen packed cells are citrate free.

Oxygen binding to hemoglobin is affected by 2,3-DPG; a low 2,3-DPG level results in less oxygen delivery to tissue secondary to increased affinity of oxygen for hemoglobin.[44,45] Citrated whole blood or citrated PRBCs rapidly lose 2,3-DPG, but frozen blood maintains it at nearly normal levels (Table 11-1).

Each type of blood component has slightly different effects on the oxygen–hemoglobin dissociation curve; the point at which these factors are clinically important has yet to be fully evaluated in the pediatric patient. Frozen blood would appear to have significant advantages because 2,3-DPG levels are

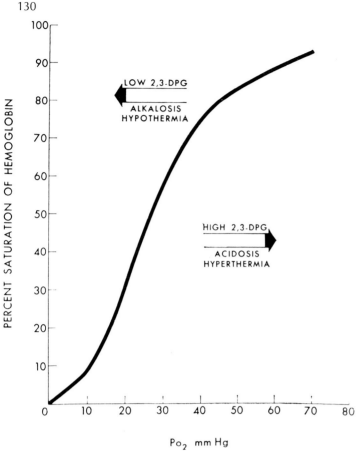

Figure 11-5. Oxygen–hemoglobin dissociation curve with alterations that can shift the curve to the right or left. A leftward shift indicates a low P_{50} or increased affinity of hemoglobin for oxygen; thus less oxygen is released to tissues. (Reproduced with permission from Miller RD: Transfusion therapy and associated problems. ASA Refresher Courses in Anesthesiology 1:102, 1973.)

preserved and it is citrate free (Table 11-5). For most patients any shift in the oxygen–hemoglobin dissociation curve is readily corrected by compensatory mechanisms, e.g., increased cardiac output or vasodilation. However, when there is compromise of a vascular bed, e.g., cardiac or cerebral, then severe shifts in the oxygen–hemoglobin dissociation curve may result in tissue ischemia.[46,47]

Table 11-5

The Effect of Blood-Stored Products on the Oxygen–Hemoglobin Dissociation Curve

	Temperature	2–3 DPG	Acid load
Fresh frozen plasma	←	0	→
Citrated whole blood	←← ←←	←← ←←	→ →
Citrated packed cells	←←	←←	→
Frozen packed cells	←←	0	→

← = left shift; → = right shift.

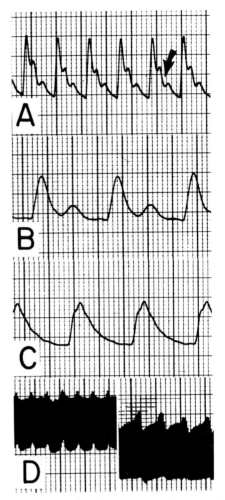

Figure 11-6. Changes in the contour of an arterial tracing with hypovolemia. In the normal tracing (A) note the sharp upswing of arterial pulse wave and position of the dicrotic notch. A slightly slower recording speed was used for (A) than for (B) and (C). In (B) there is movement of the dicrotic notch and widening of the pulse wave. In (C) we see a further widening of the pulse wave and loss of the dicrotic notch. An exaggerated ("picket fence") respiratory variation of pulse wave is shown in (D) (right tracing compared to left). *Caution:* Factors other than hypovolemia, such as hypothermia, deep anesthesia, vasodilator therapy, or damped tracing (clot, air bubble) may produce artifactual changes in the shape of the arterial wave form.

PULMONARY EFFECTS OF MASSIVE TRANSFUSION

The effects of massive blood transfusion on pulmonary function have been of great concern. There is laboratory evidence that embolism of fibrinous debris contained in blood products may be detrimental; however this has not been confirmed clinically.[48,49] On the other hand, laboratory studies have demonstrated that large quantities of fibrinous material are removed by micropore filtration.[50–52] If large transfusions are expected, it is our practice to use a micropore filter with all blood products except platelets, which should be filtered with a large pore filter for reasons previously described.

MISCELLANEOUS COMPLICATIONS OF MASSIVE TRANSFUSION

There are many other problems associated with massive transfusion relating to volume as well as rate of administration. Transmission of malaria and viral diseases such as hepatitis, cytomegalovirus, and Epstein-Barr virus, may occur, although donor screening and the increased use of frozen blood has decreased the incidence of these complications.[53]

The recent epidemic of AIDS has many implications for the use of blood products. This represents an infectious agent transmitted through blood transfusion.[54] Although this risk is very small, it emphasizes the importance of careful consideration before any blood product is administered.[55] It would be prudent to document in the anesthesia record the indications for transfusion of any blood product. A rare but fatal complication of transfusion is sickling of transfused blood in a neonate; most blood banks now routinely perform sickle screening on all donor blood.[56]

MONITORING DURING MASSIVE BLOOD TRANSFUSION

If massive blood loss can be anticipated prior to surgery, then adequate monitoring should be in place *before* surgery begins, so that all baseline information may be gathered.

If the patient arrives in the operating room in shock (e.g., the trauma patient), one must be careful to separate hypovolemia from other causes of shock (e.g., tension pneumothorax, cardiac tamponade). Invasive monitoring inserted during resuscitation will help with the differentiation. Our philosophy is one of aggressive invasive monitoring to provide maximal data for evaluation and management of the critically hypovolemic child.

1. Routine monitoring, including EKG, blood pressure cuff, stethoscope and temperature.
2. A urinary catheter allows accurate measurement of urine output and assessment of organ perfusion and intravascular volume status.
3. An arterial catheter enables heartbeat to heartbeat blood pressure monitoring and repeat determinations of oxygenation, ventilation, acid–base status, and hematocrit. The adequacy of the circulating blood volume may be inferred by the shape of the arterial wave form, loss of the dicrotic notch, or exaggerated respiratory variation (Figure 11-6).
4. A central venous line (CVP) may provide useful information, and its ease and safety of insertion has been demonstrated for children of all sizes.[57] It is our clinical impression that in healthy anesthetized, supine patients a very small change in CVP (2–3 torr) may represent a change of as much as 10–15 percent of the patient's blood volume. In most pediatric patients right-sided pressures correlate well with left-sided pressures, and thus the CVP is an accurate indicator of cardiac filling pressures of both ventricles.
5. The pulmonary artery flow directed catheter will provide more direct measurement of left-sided cardiac filling pressures, and is a useful monitor in any patient where pulmonary or cardiac pathology might lead to confusion in interpretation of central venous pressure. This catheter may also be inserted in newborns.[58]

Monitors and the data they generate are helpful but one must not rely on "numbers". *It serves no purpose to have sophisticated monitoring if the data provided cannot be interpreted and related to clinical events. The final monitor is ultimately the anesthesiologist's judgment.*

DISSEMINATED INTRAVASCULAR COAGULOPATHY

Disseminated intravascular coagulopathy (DIC) is frequently associated with shock. When dealing with massive blood loss, it is crucial that DIC be differentiated from dilutional coagulopathy. This can be difficult, since both are associated with pathologic oozing of blood in the surgical field. Each may result in prolongation of the partial thromboplastin time (PTT), prothrombin time (PT), and thrombocytopenia. With massive replacement using whole blood or packed cells and *adequate* fresh frozen plasma, the fibrinogen level should remain normal; with DIC it may be decreased. However, it is important to appreciate that replacement with packed cells, albumin, and crystalloid also leads to a reduction in fibrinogen. The most helpful test for DIC is to document a significant increase in fibrin split products.[59] The most effective treatment for DIC is to eliminate the cause, such as correcting shock, acidosis, or sepsis; heparin therapy remains controversial.

ACKNOWLEDGMENT

Supported in part by Shriner's Burns Institute Grant 15866.

REFERENCES

1. Kallos T, Smith TC: Replacement for intraoperative blood loss. *Anesthesiology* 41:293–295, 1974
2. Furman EB, Roman DG, Lemmer LAS, et al: Specific therapy in water, electrolyte, and blood-volume replacement during pediatric surgery. *Anesthesiology* 42:187–193, 1975
3. Bourke DL, Smith TC: Estimating allowable hemodilution. *Anesthesiology* 41:609–612, 1974
4. Shires T, Williams J, Brown F: Acute changes in extracellular fluids associated with major surgical procedures. *Ann Surg* 154:803–810, 1961
5. Shires T, Cohn D, Carrico J, et al: Fluid therapy in hemorrhagic shock. *Arch Surg* 88:688–693, 1964
6. Virgilio RW, Rice CL, Smith DE, et al: Crystalloid vs. colloid resuscitation: Is one better? A randomized clinical study. *Surgery* 85:129–139, 1979
7. Furman EB: Intraoperative fluid therapy, in EB Furman (ed): The Anesthesiologist's Role in Pediatric Acute Care. *Int Anesthesiol Clin* 13:133–147, Little Brown Co., 1975
8. Kakaiya RM, Morrison FS, Rawson JE, et al: Pedi-pack transfusion in a newborn intensive care unit. *Transfusion* 19:19–24, 1979
9. Miller RD: Transfusion therapy and associated problems. *Refresher Courses in Anesthesiology* 1:101–113, 1973
10. Miller RD: Complications of massive blood transfusions. *Anesthesiology* 39:82–93, 1973
11. Collins JA: Problems associated with the massive transfusion of stored blood. *Surgery* 75:274–295, 1974
12. Umlas J, Gootblatt S: The use of frozen blood in neonatal exchange transfusion. *Transfusion* 16:636–640, 1976

13. Urbaniak SJ, Cash JD: Blood replacement therapy. *Br Med Bull* 33:273–282, 1977

14. Becker GA, Aster RH: Platelet transfusion therapy. *Med Clin North Am* 56:81–94, 1972

15. Van Eys J, Thomas D, Olivos B: Platelet use in pediatric oncology: A review of 393 transfusions. *Transfusion* 18:169–173, 1978

16. Deykin D: Emerging concepts of platelet function. *New Engl J Med* 290:144–151, 1974

17. Weiss HJ: Antiplatelet drugs—a new pharmacologic approach to the prevention of thrombosis. *Am Heart J* 92:86–102, 1976

18. Barrer MJ, Ellison N: Platelet function. *Anesthesiology* 46:202–211, 1977

19. Levine PH: Platelet function tests: Predictive value. *N Engl J Med* 292:1346–1347, 1975

20. Harker LA, Slichter SJ: The bleeding time as a screening test for evaluation of platelet function. *N Engl J Med* 287:155–159, 1972

21. Myhre BA (ed): *Blood Component Therapy—A Physician's Handbook.* American Association of Blood Banks, 1977

22. Marshall BE, Wurzel HA, Neufeld GR, et al: Effects of Fenwal 4C2423 transfusion microfilter on microaggregates and other constituents of stored blood. *Transfusion* 18:38–45, 1978

23. Levine PH: Efficacy of self therapy in hemophilia: A study of 72 patients with hemophilia A & B. *N Engl J Med* 291:1381–1384, 1974

24. Levine PH, McVerry BA, Segelman AE, et al: Comprehensive health care clinic for hemophiliacs. *Arch Int Med* 136:792–794, 1976

25. Abildgaard CF: Current concepts in the management of hemophilia. *Semin Hematol* 12:223–232, 1975

26. Miller RD, Robbins TO, Tong MJ, et al: Coagulation defects associated with massive blood transfusions. *Ann Surg* 174:794–801, 1971

27. Counts RB, Haisch C, Simon TL, et al: Hemostasis in massively transfused trauma patients. *Ann Surg* 190:91–99, 1979

28. Schiffer CA: Some aspects of recent advances in the use of blood cell components. *Br J Haematol* 39:289–294, 1978

29. Lim RC Jr, Olcott C IV, Robinson AJ, et al: Platelet response and coagulation changes following massive blood replacement. *J Trauma* 13:577–582, 1973

30. Coté CJ, Liu LMP, Szyfelbein SK, et al: Changes in serial platelet counts following massive blood transfusion in pediatric patients. *Anesthesiology* 62:197–201, 1985

31. Marshall M: Potassium intoxication from blood and plasma transfusions. *Anesthesia* 17:145–148, 1962

32. Rao TLK, Mathru M, Salem MR, et al: Serum potassium levels following transfusion of frozen erythrocytes. *Anesthesiology* 52:170–172, 1980

33. Scanlon JW, Krakaur R: Hyperkalemia following exchange transfusion. *J Pediatr* 96:108–110, 1980

34. Bunker JP: Metabolic effects of blood transfusion. *Anesthesiology* 27:446–455, 1966

35. Denlinger JK, Nahrwold ML, Gibbs PS, et al: Hypocalcemia during rapid blood transfusion in anaesthetized man. *Br J Anaesth* 38:995–1000, 1976

36. Hinkle JE, Cooperman LH: Serum ionized calcium changes following citrated blood transfusion in anaesthetized man. *Br J Anaesth* 43:1108–1112, 1971

37. Das JB, Eraklis AJ, Filler RM, et al: Serum ionic calcium: Changes with large volume blood transfusions in the infant. *J Pediatr Surg* 6:333–338, 1971

38. Scheidegger D, Drop LJ: The relationship between duration of Q–T interval and plasma ionized calcium concentration: Experiments with acute steady-state $[Ca^{++}]$ changes in the dog. *Anesthesiology* 51:143–148, 1979

39. Stulz PM, Scheidegger D, Drop LJ, et al: Ventricular pump performance during hypocalcemia: Clinical and experimental studies. *J Thorac Cardiovasc Surg* 78:183–194, 1979

40. Szyfelbein SK, Drop LJ, Martyn JA, et al: Persistent ionized hypocalcemia in patients during resuscitation and recovery phases of body burns. *Crit Care Med* 9:454–458, 1981

41. Miller RD, Tong MJ, Robbins TO: Effects of massive transfusion of blood on acid–base balance. *JAMA* 216:1762–1765, 1971

42. Collins JA, Simmons RL, James PM, et al: Acid–base status of seriously wounded combat casualties. II. Resuscitation with stored blood. *Ann Surg* 173:6–18, 1971

43. Boyan CP: Cold or warmed blood for massive transfusions. *Ann Surg* 160:282–286, 1964

44. Bunn HF, Jandl JH: Control of hemoglobin function within the red cell. *N Engl J Med* 282:1414–1421, 1970

45. Wagner PD: The oxyhemoglobin dissociation curve and pulmonary gas exchange. *Semin Hematol* 11:405–421, 1974

46. Sheldon GF: Diphosphoglycerate in massive transfusion and erythropoiesis. *Crit Care Med* 7:407–411, 1979

47. Woodson RD: Physiological significance of oxygen dissociation curve shifts. *Crit Care Med* 7:368–373, 1979

48. McNamara JJ, Burran EL, Larson E, et al: Effect of debris in stored blood on pulmonary microvasculature. *Ann Thorac Surg* 14:133–139, 1972

49. Connel RS, Swank RL: Pulmonary microembolism after blood transfusion: An electron microscopic study. *Ann Surg* 177:40–50, 1973

50. Aukburg SJ, Marshall BE, Wurzel HA, et al: Evaluation of the Swank IL-201 transfusion filter. *Anesth Analg* 57:463–469, 1978

51. Cullen DJ, Ferrara L: Comparative evaluation of blood filters: A study in vitro. *Anesthesiology* 41:568–575, 1974

52. Marshall BE, Wurzel HA, Neufeld GR, et al: Effects of Intersept micropore filtration of blood on microaggregates and other constituents. *Anesthesiology* 44:525–534, 1976

53. Lang DJ, Valeri CR: Hazards of blood transfusion. *Adv Pediatr* 24:311–338, 1977

54. Curran JW, Lawrence DN, Jaffe H, et al: Acquired Immunodeficiency Syndrome (AIDS) associated with transfusions. *N Engl J Med* 310:69–75, 1984

55. Bove JR: Transfusion-associated AIDS—a cause for concern. *N Engl J Med* 310:115–116, 1984

56. Murphy RJ, Malhotra C, Sweet AY: Death following an exchange transfusion with hemoglobin SC blood. *J Pediatr* 96:110–112, 1980

57. Coté CJ, Jobes DR, Schwartz AJ, et al: Two approaches to cannulation of a child's internal jugular vein. *Anesthesiology* 50:371–373, 1979

58. Todres ID, Crone RK, Rogers MC, et al: Swan-Ganz catheterization in the critically ill newborn. *Crit Care Med* 7:330–334, 1970

59. Ellison N: Diagnosis and management of bleeding disorders. *Anesthesiology* 47:171–180, 1977

12

Controlled Hypotension, Hemodilution, and Autotransfusion

Charles J. Coté

This chapter will consider three techniques for intraoperative blood salvage. These techniques should only be attempted by the anesthesiologist who has a thorough working knowledge of the physiologic consequences and pharmacology of the drugs to be used, as well as the ability to evaluate the risks and benefits of their use.

CONTROLLED HYPOTENSION

Controlled hypotension, the intentional reduction of systemic perfusion pressure, has been used for many years to reduce intraoperative blood loss and/or to provide a relatively "bloodless" operating field.[1] The use of controlled hypotension in the anesthetic and surgical management of children with a variety of problems has been well documented.[1-8] This section reviews the physiology, pharmacology, and general principles of controlled hypotension, its benefits, risks, and application to the pediatric patient.

PHYSIOLOGY

Central Nervous System

All anesthetic agents affect the cerebral metabolic rate for oxygen consumption ($CMRO_2$). However, the degree of decreased metabolic demand is unpredictable at best, and cannot be depended on for cerebral protection during hypotension. Therefore, one of the most important considerations of any hypotensive technique is the effect it will have on cerebral blood flow (CBF). Adult studies demonstrate that there is little change in cerebral metabolism when mean arterial pressure (MAP) is maintained above 55 torr.[9] There are no comparable data for pediatric patients, but the experience with children on cardiac bypass would suggest that children will

tolerate pressures below this level on an age-related basis, i.e., neonates will tolerate a lower pressure than small children, who in turn will tolerate a lower mean pressure better than adults. There has been clear documentation in adults of brain ischemia when a mean perfusion pressure of 55 torr is combined with hypocarbia; however, there have been no similar studies carried out in children.[10] Therefore, maintenance of a normal $PaCO_2$ is a vitally important concept; the relationship of CBF to $PaCO_2$ is well described in Chapter 17. We maintain mean arterial perfusion pressure at 55 torr, and keep the $PaCO_2$ at 35–45 torr.

During induced hypotension CBF decreases from baseline with all vasodilating agents, although the extent of altered CBF varies with each agent and the degree of induced hypotension.[11,12] Studies attempting to find the ideal vasodilator agent have demonstrated significant differences in cerebral metabolites and regional distribution of CBF between trimethaphan and sodium nitroprusside. Sodium nitroprusside appears to maintain a more homogeneous distribution of CBF than trimethaphan, and for this reason may prove to be more useful.[13,14] On the other hand, nitroprusside has been found to have more profound effects on the blood–brain barrier compared to trimethapan; the clinical implications of this observation are unclear.[15] Data for nitroglycerin have yet to be reported.

The use of vasodilating agents in the presence of increased intracranial pressure (ICP) is controversial; all hypotensive agents have been found to increase ICP under these conditions. Both increased flow and increased capacitance of the cerebral blood vessels have been implicated; the key to safe administration of vasodilators in this circumstance is careful monitoring of cerebral perfusion pressure (MAP − ICP = CPP), and maintaining the CPP above 50 torr. Should such a circumstance arise, either measurement of ICP or direct visualization of brain tissue would be most helpful.

Hypotension may also affect spinal cord blood flow.[16] Studies using radiolabeled microspheres and xenon 133 washout have demonstrated that autoregulation occurs between 50–150 torr mean systemic pressure. These studies suggest that there is little compromise of spinal cord blood flow, provided mean systemic pressure does not fall below 50 torr. These experiments, however, were performed in laboratory animals, not in humans.[17,18]

Myocardium

Coronary blood flow has been found to autoregulate with metabolic demand, and to be dependent on diastolic filling pressure. All vasodilators appear to improve left ventricular function by reducing afterload.[19,21] For children who have a normal coronary circulation, trimethaphan, nitroprusside, or nitroglycerine appear to be equally well tolerated.

Renal System

Renal blood flow autoregulates between a mean blood pressure of 80–180 torr; however, general anesthesia has been found to have profound effects on autoregulation depending upon the anesthetic agent.[22] Sodium nitroprusside has been demonstrated to maintain and perhaps increase renal blood flow during induced hypotension compared to trimethaphan, which may decrease renal blood flow.[20,23] Both drugs result in transient reduction in creatinine clearance and sodium reabsorption.[24–26] No studies comparing the effect of nitroglycerin on renal blood flow have been reported. Sodium nitroprusside may be the agent of choice for maintaining renal blood flow. Measuring urinary output is a simple method of monitoring the adequacy of renal perfusion and function.

Pulmonary System

An increase in physiologic dead space and intrapulmonary shunting during induced hypotension has been reported in adults.[26–27] This does not seem to occur in children, possibly due to less gravitational pooling of blood in the lungs.[6] It is important, therefore, to measure arterial blood gases in order to assess this possibility.

Hepatic System

The portal circulation is influenced by catecholamines, $PaCO_2$, circulating blood volume, and anesthetic agents.[28] The liver is oxygenated by the arterial circulation, but receives the majority of its blood flow through the portal circulation; thus changes in portal blood flow may have profound effects on total hepatic blood flow. In dogs reduction of both hepatic arterial and portal flow occurred during sodium nitroprusside-induced hypotension, but hepatic oxygenation was preserved by increases in arterial flow during periods of insufficient portal flow.[29] A prospective study of adults using either deep halothane anesthesia or nitroprusside-induced hypotension detected no postoperative abnormalities in hepatic function for either group.[30] It appears, then, that adequate hepatic oxygenation is maintained during induced hypotension, provided $PaCO_2$ is normal and an adequate circulating blood volume maintained.

Skin and Muscle

Blood flow redistribution to skin and muscle may be an undesirable side effect of hypotensive anesthesia, especially during a reconstructive plastic surgical procedure. There is at least one animal study reporting this effect with trimethaphan but not with sodium nitroprusside; no reports comparing nitroglycerin have been published.[21]

Hormonal Responses

Catecholamine levels, plasma renin activity, and angiotensin II increase following sodium nitroprusside, but not after trimethaphan; these differences may result from the ganglionic blockade produced by trimethaphan.[31,32] The clinical significance of these differences has yet to be proven.

PHARMACOLOGY

Pentolinium (Ansolysen)

Pentolinium is a potent ganglionic blocking drug utilized to induce controlled hypotension.[33] When first introduced, its principal advantages were stated as (1) slow onset (peak effect at 30 minutes), (2) long duration of action (1–4 hours), (3) minimal tachycardia and tachyphylaxis, (4) maintenance of a relatively stable blood pressure, and (5) ease of administration (no separate IV required).[34–36] Pentolinium-induced hypotension is posture dependent; the use of the reverse Trendelenburg position is often required. In children, tachycardia may be a problem because the increased heart rate increases cardiac output, tending to offset the hypotensive effect of the drug.[35] The same qualities which were formerly considered advantages are now considered by some as disadvantages, i.e., its onset of action is slow, its duration of action is long, and in children it results in tachycardia. The recommended starting dose is 0.1–0.3 mg/kg given as an intravenous bolus. Pentolinium may produce markedly dilated pupils, which is a consequence of the ganglionic blockade.

Trimethaphan (Arfonad)

Trimethaphan is a ganglionic blocking drug which also has direct vasodilator properties. Its advantages over pentolinium are a more rapid onset of action (minutes), and because its duration of action is much shorter (minutes), it can be conveniently titrated by constant IV infusion. Disadvantages include tachycardia, tachyphylaxis, histamine release, inhibition of pseudocholinesterase hydrolysis of succinylcholine, potentiation of non-depolarizing neuromuscular blockade, and, in children, resistance to hypotension secondary to tachycardia.[35–37] Trimethaphan may be contraindicated in asthmatic patients because of its histamine releasing properties. In high doses this medication produces markedly dilated pupils, a situation which could be confused with an intracerebral catastrophe. The usual starting dose is 25–100 μgm/kg/min, which may be gradually increased as clinically indicated.

Cardiovascular Effects. Trimethaphan appears to have an unpredictable response because its major effect is on sympathetic tone, which is quite variable from one patient to another.[38] Cardiac work is decreased because of reduced afterload. Coronary blood flow may be reduced precipitously because of the sharp fall in diastolic pressure, and this is potentially dangerous in patients with a compromised coronary circulation.[21]

Renal Circulation. Renal blood flow is markedly diminished by trimethaphan, with resultant increase in renal vascular resistance.[21] This may be an important consideration for patients with abnormal renal function.

Pulmonary Circulation. Pulmonary blood flow is usually diminished because of redistribution of blood into the peripheral circulation. Studies in adults have demonstrated an increase in the dead space to tidal volume (V_D/V_T) ratio; however, similar studies in children did not confirm this alteration.[6,27,39]

Cerebral Circulation. It appears that trimethaphan produces a profound reduction in cerebral blood flow, with possible redistribution away from cortical areas.[13,14] In addition, if there is reduced cerebral compliance because of an intracranial lesion, the vasodilation produced by trimethaphan may result in a sudden rise in intracranial pressure.[11]

Skin and Muscle. There is evidence indicating an undesirable redistribution of blood flow to skin and muscle by trimethaphan.[13]

Sodium Nitroprusside

Sodium nitroprusside has a very rapid onset of action (seconds), brief duration of action (minutes), and minimal side effects when used in the recommended dose range.[40] This agent is extremely potent and is *most safely administered by an infusion pump through a separate intravenous site.* Its principal mechanism of action is direct vascular smooth muscle relaxation, primarily causing arteriolar dilation, as well as some venodilation.

Cardiovascular Effects. Sodium nitroprusside improves cardiovascular hemodynamics by rapidly reducing afterload, reducing myocardial oxygen consumption, and maintaining coronary blood flow.[6,41] However, there is a tendency to develop tachycardia, especially in children. Central toxicity (poisoning of the cytochrome oxidase system) appears to precede direct cardiac toxicity.[42]

Pulmonary Circulation. Sodium nitroprusside reduces pulmonary artery pressure by both a reduction in venous return and direct dilation of pulmonary vessels.[43]

Renal Circulation. Extensive studies in animals have demonstrated a gradual increase in renal blood flow secondary to a fall in renovascular resistance.[20,21] This is in contrast to the effect of trimethaphan, which increases renovascular resistance. Both agents reduce renal blood flow at hypotensive levels.

Hepatic Circulation. A study of controlled hypotension in dogs found that concentrations of sodium nitroprusside, which reduce systemic arterial pressure by 40 percent, do not lead to hepatic hypoxemia.[29]

Cerebral Circulation. Sodium nitroprusside decreases cerebral perfusion pressure and increases intracranial pressure; this is believed to be secondary to cerebral vasodilation.[11] Cerebral autoregulation and metabolic homeostasis are less affected by sodium nitroprusside than by trimethaphan.[12,13] In addition, one animal study demonstrated a more homogeneous perfusion of the cerebral microcirculation with sodium nitroprusside.[14] These studies suggest that sodium nitroprus-

side may offer an advantage concerning cerebral perfusion and metabolism.

Dosage. It is recommended to commence sodium nitroprusside infusion at 0.5–1.0 μgm/kg/min, and gradually increase the dose as needed.[44] A satisfactory reduction of systemic perfusion pressure can usually be obtained well below the recommended maximum of 10 μgm/kg/min. Three responses to sodium nitroprusside infusion may herald impending cyanide toxicity:

1. Greater than 10 μgm/kg/min required for response
2. Tachyphylaxis developing within 30–60 minutes
3. Immediate resistance to the drug[45]

If any of these occur, sodium nitroprusside should be discontinued and the patient investigated for possible cyanide toxicity. There have been several pediatric anesthetic-related deaths due both to cyanide toxicity and its treatment.[46–48]

Toxicity. The diagnosis of cyanide toxicity is characterized by the unexplained development of metabolic acidosis, elevated blood lactate, and an elevated, mixed venous oxygen content.[40] The nitroprusside radical interacts with the sulphydryl groups of erythrocytes causing the release of cyanide. Nitroprusside contains five cyanide molecules, and as the cyanide is released it is converted to nontoxic thiocyanate by the rhodanase enzyme system contained in the liver, and is then excreted by the kidney.[34] If the amount of cyanide released overwhelms the capacity of the rhodanase system, cyanide toxicity (binding to the cytochrome electron transport system) results; this in turn produces a change to anaerobic metabolism, metabolic acidosis, and eventually death.[40,46–49]

Treatment of cyanide poisoning is directed toward reversal of the binding of cyanide to the cytochrome enzymes. This can be accomplished by producing methemoglobinemia with amylnitrate. Methemoglobin has a greater affinity for cyanide than the cytochrome system. Thus, the reaction is pushed in the direction of forming cyanomethemoglobin. The breakdown of cyanomethemoglobin is promoted by administering thiosulfate, which reacts with the cyanide to form nontoxic thiocyanate, which is then excreted by the kidneys.[42,45,49–55]

It is important to emphasize, however, that this treatment is not without hazard. As Posner states, "Overzealous treatment may merely convert a cytotoxic hypoxia to an anemic hypoxia."[50]

Recently there have been some data to suggest that hydroxycobalamin (vitamin B_{12}) may prevent toxicity by formation of cyanocobalamin.[50] There are few human studies of this therapy. In addition, prophylactic infusion of sodium thiosulfate may prove to be helpful in reducing toxicity by promoting the production of thiocyanate.[55] The first step in treatment of toxicity is the *intermittent* administration of amylnitrate (through inhalation), until sodium nitrite can be given intravenously. The second step is sodium nitrite given as a three percent solution [300 mg/ml, 0.2 ml/kg, not to exceed 10 ml (3 gm)]. Immediately after the above, sodium thiosulfate in a dosage of 175 mg/kg, not to exceed 12.5 gm, should be administered. Oxygen (100%) should be delivered continuously. A cyanide poisoning kit is available.*

The best management for cyanide toxicity is to prevent it. Sodium nitroprusside is a safe medication provided one is

---

* Eli Lilly Company, Indianapolis, Indiana.

careful to remain well within the guidelines that have been established by various investigators.[51-54] For children this is a maximum of 50 μgm/kg/min for *30 minutes* and about 8–10 μgm/kg/min for *3 hours*, with frequent blood gas analysis.[44,54]

Nitroglycerin

Nitroglycerin is a recently introduced agent for induction of controlled hypotension. Extensive experience has not been reported in children. The main advantage of nitroglycerin is a relatively rapid onset of action (minutes), lack of tachyphylaxis and toxicity, and brief duration of action (minutes). Its primary mode of action is to dilate both resistance and capacitance vessels.[56]

Cardiovascular Effects. Nitroglycerin has been demonstrated to be a more potent coronary artery dilator than sodium nitroprusside, and to increase myocardial blood flow.[57,58]

Pulmonary Effects. Nitroglycerin reduces pulmonary artery pressures by both a direct effect and reducing venous return.

Cerebral Effects. Nitroglycerin reduces cerebral perfusion pressure, dilates cerebral blood vessels and, in the presence of reduced cerebral compliance, may increase intracranial pressure.[59]

Dosage. Commence infusion at the rate of 1 μgm/kg/min and increase the dose until the desired response is obtained. No toxicities or deaths have been reported with nitroglycerin. Further pediatric investigation is warranted.

GENERAL CONCEPTS

Before using controlled hypotension, it is important to understand the rationale for using this technique. If used to reduce surgical blood loss, the preparation and monitoring of the patient is different from a procedure where the main objective for lowering the perfusion pressure is to improve operating conditions (e.g., microsurgical techniques). In the former case direct assessment of circulating blood pressure and volume with the use of an arterial line and central venous or flow-directed pulmonary artery catheter would be exceedingly important, whereas in the latter case only a direct means of measuring blood pressure (arterial line) would be acceptable.

Premedication

Premedication of the patient scheduled for hypotensive anesthesia may include a drug with vasodilating properties such as morphine, chlorpromazine, or droperidol. This will help to reduce anxiety as well as facilitate the hypotensive technique.[60]

Anesthesia

If anesthesia is supplemented by one of the potent inhalational agents a smaller amount of hypotensive agent will be necessary.[61] The best method for administration of the vasodilating agent is by infusion pump, preferably one that infuses in a constant rather than a pulsatile mode, so as to achieve the smoothest reduction in blood pressure. It is also important to use a *separate intravenous site* so as to minimize accidental bolus infusion of the vasodilator during changes in fluid requirements, or during the administration of other medications.

Monitoring

The anesthesiologist should carefully monitor these baseline parameters: hematocrit, blood sugar, arterial blood gases and acid–base status, mean systemic pressure ($\overline{BP}$), and central venous pressure (CVP) or pulmonary artery occlusion pressure (PAOP) where indicated. When the desired $\overline{BP}$ has been attained, a new baseline CVP or PAOP should be measured and maintained at this lower level throughout the procedure. In order to use any hypotensive technique safely it is mandatory that the patient remain *normovolemic* at all times; this means strict correction of even a 1- or 2-torr change in CVP or PAOP. A small change of cardiac filling pressures in a healthy, supine, anesthetized patient may represent a significant reduction in circulating blood volume. In healthy patients right-sided filling pressures nearly parallel left-sided filling pressures; thus in children the CVP is an excellent parameter to follow, and a pulmonary artery catheter is rarely indicated. Another common and in some respects more useful indicator of volume status is urine output. Even during hypotensive anesthesia the kidneys should produce 0.5–1.0 ml/kg/hr. Frequently the failure to detect urine output is due to obstruction or kinking of the urinary catheter. If the catheter is patent then an intravenous fluid challenge should be considered. Urine output is one of the best indicators of organ perfusion and function; for this reason it is perhaps the most useful of monitors during hypotensive anesthesia.

Once hypotension has been induced, the $\overline{BP}$ can be slowly raised until it is obvious that bleeding has increased; with this method it is sometimes only necessary to reduce the pressure 10–20 percent from baseline in order to achieve the desired clinical response.

Position

The position of the patient is very important; it is most desirable to make the operative field the highest point of the patient's body so as to take advantage of gravitational forces.[60,62] Care must also be taken to minimize any possible impedance to venous drainage when positioning the patient, since this may contribute to blood loss. If the head is the surgical site, then $\overline{BP}$ must be calibrated at head level so as to maintain adequate cerebral perfusion pressure.

Laboratory Parameters

As previously mentioned, certain laboratory parameters must also be carefully followed. Adequate levels of hemoglobin must be maintained in order to have sufficient oxygen-carrying capacity. Studies have indicated that at normal blood pressures a hemoglobin of 5 gm/100 ml is well tolerated in laboratory animals, but ischemia may occur with a lower hemoglobin.[63] Preliminary studies, in children undergoing spinal fusion (Harrington rod) with combined hemodilution and hypotension, suggest that children tolerate this combination well.[64] For additional safety, however, until further studies are performed, we would suggest keeping the hemoglobin level at 8 gm % or higher during controlled hypotension.

Arterial blood gases must also be carefully evaluated on a 30–60 minute basis, in order to be immediately aware of any change in oxygenation, ventilation, or perfusion. It is exceedingly important that an adequate PaO_2 be maintained at all times; the use of an in-line oxygen analyzer will signal failure of oxygen delivery by the circuit, but only arterial blood gas analysis or pulse oximetry will demonstrate that oxygen is being delivered to vital organs. In addition, examination of the $PaCO_2$ is mandatory during any hypotensive anesthetic technique, since cerebral perfusion is directly proportional to $PaCO_2$.[65,66] For this reason the patient should be kept normocarbic; *the combination of hypocarbia and hypotension should be avoided.* Controlled ventilation is desirable because it maintains a constant $PaCO_2$. The metabolic components of acid–base equilibrium must also be carefully followed; the development of acidosis will reflect inadequate oxygen delivery or toxicity from the hypotensive agent (e.g., sodium nitroprusside).[40]

Although we do not advocate the use of propranolol, blood sugar should be measured serially if propranolol is part of the chosen hypotensive technique. Propranolol inhibits glycogenolysis and may cause severe unsuspected hypoglycemia.[6,67]

Benefits

Hypotensive anesthesia facilitates surgical technique in difficult procedures, such as cerebral aneurysm and arteriovenous malformation, middle ear surgery, or plastic reconstructive surgery. The technique also produces a marked diminution of blood loss for a variety of procedures (e.g., orthopedic reconstruction or burn wound debridement).[3,4,6–8,29,68,69]

Contraindications

The risks of hypotensive anesthesia are significant. Any systemic disease compromising function of a major organ is a relative contraindication to the use of controlled hypotension. The majority of complications reported, however, relate to the inexperience of the practitioner, unfamiliarity with the drugs involved, inattention to details such as blood volume status, pH, $PaCO_2$, blood sugar, and perhaps inappropriate patient selection.[6,46,47,70] If the patient is healthy, and meticulous attention is paid to all the parameters previously detailed, the benefits of improved surgical technique, shorter surgical time, and decreased blood transfusion usually outweigh the potential risks. We caution that this technique should be attempted only after attaining a clear understanding of its physiology and pharmacology, and after gaining experience by working with colleagues intimately familiar with controlled hypotension.

A major pediatric indication for this technique at the present time is during Harrington rod insertion for spinal fusion. There is concern for the effect of combining lower perfusion pressure, anemia, traction on the spinal cord, and the effects of these on spinal cord blood flow. Larger series of studies in major centers are required before this application of controlled hypotension is generally advised.

HEMODILUTION

Intentional *isovolemic* hemodilution is an important adjunct to the anesthesiologist's armamentarium, because it reserves a quantity of the patient's own fresh whole blood, which can be returned at the end of the surgical procedure. For a Jehovah's Witness, this technique often conforms to religious guidelines.[71] Hemodilution is usually applied to those procedures where blood loss is expected to exceed half of the patient's blood volume.

PHYSIOLOGY

Blood Viscosity

One of the major effects of hemodilution is a marked reduction in blood viscosity. This is primarily due to the reduction in red cell mass, but also in part to dilution of the plasma.[72,73] The reduced viscosity improves blood flow through capillary beds.

Cardiac Output

There is increased venous return with isovolemic hemodilution, and an increase in cardiac output which seems to be related to increased stroke volume.[73–75] However, in our experience and that of others it is not unusual to have little or no increase in cardiac output in children under anesthesia.[64]

Tissue Oxygenation

The delivery of oxygen to tissues during acute anemia may be maintained by three compensatory mechanisms: increased flow, increased extraction, and changes in the oxygen–hemoglobin dissociation curve.[76,77] During acute normovolemic hemodilution there is a definite improvement in blood flow distribution with a lowered hematocrit. This improved blood flow is the major compensatory mechanism maintaining oxygen delivery. Increased oxygen extraction only occurs when there is an inadequate circulating blood volume or when the hematocrit falls below 20; if the hematocrit falls below 15 myocardial ischemia may develop as demonstrated by impaired subendocardial perfusion.[63,68,78,79] There is also a right shift in the oxygen–hemoglobin dissociation curve secondary to increased erythrocyte 2,3-DPG; this improves oxygen release to tissues. This compensatory mechanism occurs primarily during chronic anemia, and becomes important when the hematocrit falls below 20.[71,80]

Lung Water

The volume of pulmonary water has been demonstrated to increase with hemodilution, and this amount is quantitatively greater with crystalloid than colloid replacement. However, there was no clinical difference as measured by arterial blood gases.[81–83] There appears to be no clinical advantage of colloid over crystalloid hemodilution, although the cost of the latter is much less.

TECHNIQUE

The most common method of hemodilution in pediatrics is to allow blood to run directly from an arterial line into sterile acid-citrate-dextrose (ACD) or citrate-phosphate-dextrose (CPD) blood collection bags. The bag must be agitated often but gently to assure even distribution of the anticoagulant. Each unit must be weighed to determine precisely the volume that has been removed. This volume should be calculated preoperatively, and usually amounts to 30–40 percent of the estimated blood volume of the child; any one of three formulae presented in Chapter 11 may be used. Most often the blood removed will reduce the hematocrit to the 20–25 percent range. Care must be taken to replace the blood removed with either five percent albumin milliliter for milliliter, or two or three milliliters of Ringer's lactate solution for each milliliter of blood removed. It is preferable to hemodilute prior to the surgical incision, though this can also be performed during the initial phases of surgery.

Blood losses after initial hemodilution are replaced with either banked whole blood, packed red blood cells and crystalloid, or packed red blood cells and five percent albumin. The central concern is to maintain a normal circulating blood volume and assure hemostasis. Once surgical blood loss has ceased, or if apparent coagulopathy secondary to dilution of clotting factors or platelets has developed, reinfusion of the autologous blood may be made. It may be administered one unit at a time, or may be saved and reinfused at the end of the procedure. In order to use this technique most effectively the anesthesiologist must be intimately familiar with the differences in composition of the various blood components utilized (see Chapter 11, Table 11-1). If whole blood is used for replacement, coagulopathy most commonly will be secondary to thrombocytopenia, and will not usually develop until 1.5–3.0 blood volumes have been lost. If packed cells or frozen packed cells are used, coagulopathy secondary to dilution of clotting factors will develop first, probably after 1–2 blood volumes have been lost. Thus blood removed at the beginning of the procedure acts as a ready source of fresh plasma and platelets; however, it is important to remember that a small-pore filter (20 microns) would trap many of the platelets that a large-pore filter (120 microns) would allow to pass. The time at which the patient's blood is best reinfused must be determined according to the type of blood replaced, the volume lost, and the total clinical picture.

INDICATIONS

Hemodilution may be indicated in any procedure where blood loss is expected to exceed half the blood volume.

CONTRAINDICATIONS

Hemodilution is contraindicated in sickle cell disease, septicemia, or compromised function of any major organ which may be significantly affected by changes in perfusion and oxygenation.

COMPLICATIONS

The major complications of hemodilution relate to blood volume status, hemoglobin content, and coagulopathy. The anesthesiologist must pay meticulous attention to blood volume replacement. As long as normovolemia is maintained, the hematocrit kept above 15, and clotting factors are maintained, there should be no problems with organ perfusion or oxygenation.

ADVANTAGES

Hemodilution provides a ready source of fresh whole blood rich in platelets and clotting factors. There is no problem with hepatitis or cross match, and there is a net saving in loss of red cell mass, since the surgical losses occur with a hemocrit of 15–20 as compared to 30–45 otherwise.

AUTOTRANSFUSION
(INTRAOPERATIVE BLOOD SCAVENGING)

Blood scavenging techniques have been applied to major vascular, cardiac, and multiple trauma situations for many years.[84–88] Initially blood saved from the patient was anticoagulated and reinfused with equipment used for cardiopulmonary bypass. The main disadvantage of this technique was the reinfusion of cellular debris, partially clotted blood, and the possibility of air embolization.[88] In recent years a new technique that includes a method for the washing of scavenged blood has demonstrated significant advantages over previous procedures.[89,90] The most important among them is that by washing the salvaged blood the patient receives primarily red blood cells suspended in saline; cellular debris, excess citrate or heparin, free hemoglobin, and clotted blood are almost completely removed prior to reinfusion. Thus the blood returned to the patient is very similar to frozen packed red cells; it is usually of high hematocrit value and nearly free of clotting factors.

The use of intraoperative blood salvage has to this point had little application to the pediatric patient.[91] At present, the equipment available is designed for adult-sized patients, limiting its use to larger pediatric patients. We have found it a useful adjunct to minimizing blood transfusions in scoliosis surgery and, if a patient has been able to donate blood prior to elective surgery, it may prevent the use of homologous blood. At present the equipment is expensive; however, if at least three units of blood are reinfused, there is a net saving to the patient. The development of pediatric-sized equipment will make this technique more widely utilized and more cost effective for pediatric surgery.

INDICATIONS

The indications for intraoperative blood salvage include major vascular or reconstructive procedures where there is potential for massive blood loss, in patients with very rare blood types, and multiple trauma without fecal contamination.

CONTRADICATIONS

The chief contraindications are surgery on malignant lesions, contamination secondary to bowel trauma or abscess, and sickle cell disease.

ADVANTAGES

In utilizing autotransfusion one is returning the patient's own blood; thus there is no risk of hepatitis or transfusion reaction. This is an additional source of blood that does not stress the blood bank, and this technique reduces the overall intraoperative blood loss. Washing the salvaged blood has significant advantage over other methods of intraoperative blood salvage.

REFERENCES

1. Leigh JM: The history of controlled hypotension. *Br J Anaesth* 47:745–749, 1975
2. Anderson SM: Controlled hypotension with Arfronad in paediatric surgery. *Br Med J* 2:103–104, 1955
3. Salem MR, Toyama T, Wong AY, et al: Haemodynamic responses to induced arterial hypotension in children. *Br J Anaesth* 50:489–494, 1978
4. Diaz JH, Lockhart CH: Hypotensive anaesthesia for craniectomy in infancy. *Br J Anaesth* 51:233–235, 1979
5. McNeil TW, DeWald RL, Ken NK, et al: Controlled hypotensive anesthesia in scoliosis surgery. *J Bone Joint Surg* 56A:1167–1172, 1979

6. Salem MR, Wong AY, Bennett EJ, et al: Deliberate hypotension in infants and children. *Anesth Analg* 53:975–981, 1974

7. Viguera MG, Terry RN: Induced hypotension for extensive surgery in an infant. *Anesthesiology* 27:701–702, 1966

8. Szyfelbein SK, Ryan JF: Use of controlled hypotension for primary surgical excision in an extensively burned child. *Anesthesiology* 41:501–503, 1974

9. Smith AL, Wollman H: Cerebral blood flow and metabolism: Effects of anesthetic drugs and techniques. *Anesthesiology* 36:378–400, 1972

10. Harp JR, Wollman H: Cerebral metabolic effects of hyperventilation and deliberate hypotension. *Br J Anaesth* 45:256–262, 1973

11. Turner JM, Powell D, Gibson RM, et al: Intracranial pressure changes in neurosurgical patients during hypotension induced with sodium nitroprusside or trimethaphan. *Br J Anaesth* 49:419–425, 1977

12. Stoyka WW, Schutz H: The cerebral response to sodium nitroprusside and trimethaphan controlled hypotension. *Can Anaesth Soc J* 22:275–283, 1975

13. Michenfelder JD, Theye RA: Canine systemic and cerebral effects of hypotension induced by hemorrhage, trimethaphan, halothane, or nitroprusside. *Anesthesiology* 46:188–195, 1977

14. Maekawa T, McDowall DG, Okuda Y: Brain-surface oxygen tension and cerebral cortical blood flow during hemorrhage and drug-induced hypotension in the cat. *Anesthesiology* 51:313–320, 1979

15. Ishikawa T, Funatsu M, Okamoto K, et al: Blood–brain barrier function following drug-induced hypotension in the dog. *Anesthesiology* 59:526–531, 1983

16. Grundy BL, Nash CL, Jr, Brown RH: Deliberate hypotension for spinal fusion: Prospective randomized study with evoked potential monitoring. *Can Anaesth Soc J* 29:452–462, 1982

17. Fahmy NR, Mossad B, Milad M: Effect of blood pressure on spinal cord blood flow in dogs. *Anesthesiology* 51 [Suppl]:S79, 1979

18. Jacobs HK, Lieponis JV, Bunch WH, et al: The influence of halothane and nitroprusside on canine spinal cord hemodynamics. *Spine* 7:35–40, 1982

19. Fahmy NR: Nitroglycerin as a hypotensive drug during general anesthesia. *Anesthesiology* 49:17–20, 1978

20. Page IH, Corcoran AC, Dustan HP, et al: Cardiovascular actions of sodium nitroprusside in animals and hypertensive patients. *Circulation* 11:188–198, 1955

21. Wang HH, Liu LMP, Katz RL: A comparison of the cardiovascular effects of sodium nitroprusside and trimethaphan. *Anesthesiology* 46:40–48, 1977

22. Larson CP, Jr, Mazze RI, Cooperman LH, et al: Effects of anesthetics on cerebral, renal, and splanchnic circulations: Recent developments. *Anesthesiology* 41:169–181, 1974

23. Leighton KM, Bruce C, MacLeod BA: Sodium nitroprusside-induced hypotension and renal blood flow. *Can Anaesth Soc J* 24:637–640, 1977

24. Behnia R, Sigueira EG, Brunner EA: Sodium nitroprusside-induced hypotension: Effect on renal function. *Anesth Analg* 57:521–526, 1978

25. Behnia R, Martin A, Koushanpour E, et al: Trimethaphan-induced hypotension: Effect on renal function. *Can Anaesth Soc J* 29:581–586, 1982

26. Askrog VF, Pender JW, Eckenhoff JE: Changes in physiological dead space during deliberate hypotension. *Anesthesiology* 25:744–751, 1964

27. Casthely PA, Lear S, Cottrell JE, et al: Intrapulmonary shunting during induced hypotension. *Anesth Analg* 61:231–235, 1982

28. Strunin L: Organ perfusion during controlled hypotension. *Br J Anaesth* 47:793–798, 1975

29. Gelman S, Ernst EA: Hepatic circulation during sodium nitroprusside infusion in the dog. *Anesthesiology* 49:182–187, 1978

30. Thompson GE, Miller RD, Stevens WC, et al: Hypotensive anesthesia for total hip arthroplasty: A study of blood loss and organ function (brain, heart, liver, kidney). *Anesthesiology* 48:91–96, 1978

31. Knight PR, Lane GA, Hensinger RN, et al: Catecholamine and renin–angiotensin response during hypotensive anesthesia induced by sodium nitroprusside or trimethaphan camsylate. *Anesthesiology* 59:248–253, 1983

32. Zubrow AB, Daniel SS, Stark RI, et al: Plasma renin, catecholamine, and vasopressin during nitroprusside-induced hypotension in ewes. *Anesthesiology* 58:245–247, 1983

33. Enderby GE: Pentolinium tartrate in controlled hypotension. *Lancet* 2:1097–1098, 1954

34. Fahmy NR, Laver MB: Hemodynamic response to ganglionic blockade with pentolinium during N_2O–halothane anesthesia in man. *Anesthesiology* 44:6–15, 1976

35. Salem MR: Therapeutic uses of ganglionic blocking drugs, in Ivankovich AD (ed): *Nitroprusside and Other Short-acting Hypotensive Agents. International Anesthesiology Clinics 16.* Boston, Little, Brown, 1978, pp 171–200

36. Klowden AJ, Ivankovich AD, Miletich DJ: Ganglionic blocking drugs: general considerations and metabolism, in Ivankovich AD (ed): *Nitroprusside and Other Short-acting Hypotensive Agents. International Anesthesiology Clinics 16.* Boston, Little, Brown, 1978, pp 113–150

37. Sklar GS, Lanks KW: Effects of trimethaphan and sodium nitroprusside on hydrolysis of succinylcholine in vitro. *Anesthesiology* 47:31–33, 1977

38. Miletich DJ, Ivankovich AD: Cardiovascular effects of ganglionic blocking drugs, in Ivankovich AD (ed): *Nitroprusside and Other Short-acting Hypotensive Agents. International Anesthesiology Clinics 16.* Boston, Little, Brown, 1978, pp 151–170

39. Eckenhoff JE, Enderby GE, Larson A, et al: Pulmonary gas exchange during deliberate hypotension. *Br J Anaesth* 35:750–759, 1963

40. Tinker JH, Michenfelder JD: Sodium nitroprusside: Pharmacology, toxicology, and therapeutics. *Anesthesiology* 45:340–354, 1976

41. Chatterjee K, Parmley WW, Ganz W, et al: Hemodynamic and metabolic responses to vasodilator therapy in acute myocardial infarction. *Circulation* 48:1183–1193, 1973

42. Tinker JH, Michenfelder JD: Cardiac cyanide toxicity induced by nitroprusside in the dog: Potential for reversal. *Anesthesiology* 49:109–116, 1978

43. Wildsmith JAW, Marshall RL, Jenkinson JL, et al: Haemodynamic effects of sodium nitroprusside during nitrous oxide/halothane anaesthesia. *Br J Anaesth* 45:71–74, 1973

44. Bennett NR, Abbott TR: The use of sodium nitroprusside in children. *Anaesthesia* 32:456–463, 1977

45. Ivankovich AD, Miletich DJ, Tinker JH: Sodium nitroprusside: Metabolism and general considerations, in Ivankovich AD (ed): *Nitroprusside and Other Short-acting Hypotensive Agents, International Anesthesiology Clinics 16.* Boston, Little, Brown. 1978, pp 1–29

46. Davies DW, Kadar D, Steward DJ, et al: A sudden death associated with the use of sodium nitroprusside for induction of hypotension during anaesthesia. *Can Anaesth Soc J* 22:547–552, 1975

47. Pershau RA, Modell JH, Bright RW, et al: Suspected sodium nitroprusside-induced cyanide intoxication. *Anesth Analg* 56:533–537, 1977

48. Berlin CM, Jr: The treatment of cyanide poisoning in children. *Pediatrics* 46:793–796, 1970

49. Palmer RF, Lasseter KC: Drug therapy: Sodium nitroprusside. *N Engl J Med* 292:294–297, 1975

50. Posner MA, Tobey RE, McElroy H: Hydroxocobalamin therapy in cyanide intoxication in guinea pigs. *Anesthesiology* 44:157–160, 1976

51. Vesey CJ, Cole PV, Simpson PJ: Cyanide and thiocyanate concentrations following sodium nitroprusside infusion in man. *Br J Anaesth* 48:651–660, 1976

52. Michenfelder JD, Tinker JH: Cyanide toxicity and thiosulfate protection during chronic administration of sodium nitroprusside in the dog: Correlation with a human case. *Anesthesiology* 47:441–448, 1977

53. Michenfelder JD: Cyanide release from sodium nitroprusside in the dog. *Anesthesiology* 46:196–201, 1977

54. Aitken D, West D, Smith F, et al: Cyanide toxicity following nitroprusside induced hypotension. *Can Anaesth Soc J* 24: 651–660, 1977

55. Ivankovich AD, Braverman B, Shulman M, et al: Prevention of nitroprusside toxicity with thiosulfate in dogs. *Anesth Analg* 61:120–126, 1982

56. Mason DT, Zelis R, Amsterdam EA: Actions of the nitrites on the peripheral circulation and myocardial oxygen consumption: Significance in the relief of angina pectoris. *Chest* 59:296–305, 1971

57. Goldstein RE, Michaelis LL, Morrow AG, et al: Coronary collateral function in patients without occlusive coronary artery disease. *Circulation* 51:118–125, 1975

58. Chiariello M, Gold HK, Leinbach RC, et al: Comparison between the effects of nitroprusside and nitroglycerin on ischemic injury during acute myocardial infarction. *Circulation* 54:766–773, 1976

59. Rogers MC, Hamburger C, Owen K, et al: Intracranial pressure in the cat during nitroglycerin-induced hypotension. *Anesthesiology* 51:227–229, 1979

60. Edwards MV, Jr, Flemming DC: Deliberate hypotension. *Surg Clin North Am* 55:929–945, 1975
    sia. Surg Clin North Am Philadelphia, W.B. Saunders, 1975

61. Bedford RF: Increasing halothane concentrations reduce nitroprusside dose requirement. *Anesth Analg* 57:457–462, 1978

62. Adams AP: Techniques of vascular control for deliberate hypotension during anaesthesia. *Br J Anaesth* 47:777–792, 1975

63. Graham BH, Wilkinson PL, Brown C: Anemia, anesthesia, and distribution of myocardial blood flow. *Anesthesiology* 51 [Suppl]:S92, 1979

64. Oberts BJ, Furman ED, Plews JL: The effect of combining hemodilution and hypotension on oxygen delivery to the tissues. Abstract, Anesthesiology Section, American Academy of Pediatrics, April 1978

65. Kety SS, Schmidt CF: The effects of active and passive hyperventilation on cerebral blood flow, cerebral oxygen consumption, cardiac output, and blood pressure of normal young men. *J Clin Invest* 25:107–119, 1946

66. Kety SS, Schmidt CF: The effects of altered arterial tensions of carbon dioxide and oxygen on cerebral blood flow and cerebral oxygen consumption of normal young men. *J Clin Invest* 27:484–492, 1948

67. Merin RG: Anesthestic management problems posed by therapeutic advances. III. Beta-adrenergic blocking drugs. *Anesth Analg* 51:617–624, 1972

68. Eckenhoff JE: Deliberate hypotension. *Anesthesiology* 48:87–88, 1978

69. Stoelting RK, Viegas O, Campbell RL: Sodium nitroprusside-produced hypotension during anesthesia and operation in the head-up position. *Anesth Analg* 56:391–394, 1977

70. Lindop MJ: Complications and morbidity of controlled hypotension. *Br J Anaesth* 47:799–803, 1975

71. Messmer K: Hemodilution. *Surg Clin North Am* 55:659–678, 1975

72. Murray JF, Escobar E, Rapaport E: Effects of blood viscosity on hemodynamic responses in acute normovolemic anemia. *Am J Physiol* 216:638–642, 1969

73. Guyton AC, Richardson TQ: Effect of hematocrit on venous return. *Circ Res* 9:157–164, 1961

74. Messmer K, Sunder-Plassman L, Kloevekorn WP, et al: Circulatory significance of hemodilution: Rheological changes and limitations. *Adv Microcirc* 4:1–2, 1972

75. Hagl S, Bornikoel K, Mayr N, et al: Cardiac performance during limited hemodilution. *Bibl Haematologica* 41:152–172, 1975

76. Schmid-Schonbein H: Blood rheology and the distribution of blood flow within the nutrient capillaries. *Bibl Haematologica* 41:1–15, 1975

77. Neuhof H, Wolf H: Oxygen uptake during hemodilution. *Bibl Haematologica* 41:66–75, 1975

78. Kessler M, Messmer K: Tissue oxygenation during hemodilution. *Bibl Haematologica* 41:16–33, 1975

79. Buckberg G, Brazier J: Coronary blood flow and cardiac function during hemodilution. *Bibl Haematologica* 41:173–189, 1975

80. Sunder-Plassmann L, Kessler M, Jesch F, et al: Acute normovolemic hemodilution. Changes in tissue oxygenation supply and hemoglobin-oxygen affinity. *Bibl Haematologica* 41:44–53, 1975

81. Cooper JD, Maeda M, Lowenstein E: Lung water accumulation with acute hemodilution in dogs. *J Thorac Cardiovasc Surg* 69:957–965, 1975

82. Laks H, O'Conner NE, Anderson W, et al: Crystalloid versus colloid hemodilution in man. *Surg Gynecol Obstet* 142:506–512, 1976

83. Lowenstein E, Cooper JD, Erdman AJ III, et al: Lung and heart water accumulation associated with hemodilution. *Bibl Haematologica* 41:190–202, 1975

84. Rakower SR, Worth MH, Jr, Lackner H: Massive intraoperative autotransfusion of blood. *Surg Gynecol Obstet* 137:633–636, 1973

85. Brener BJ, Raines JK, Darling RC: Intraoperative autotransfusion in abdominal aortic resections. *Arch Surg* 107:78–84, 1973

86. Due TL, Johnson JM, Wood M, et al: Intraoperative autotransfusion in the management of massive hemorrhage. *Am J Surg* 130:652–658, 1975

87. Glover JL, Smith R, Yaw P, et al: Intraoperative autotransfusion: An under utilized technique. *Surgery* 80:474–479, 1976

88. Stillman RM, Wrezlewicz WW, Stanczewski B, et al: The haematological hazards of autotransfusion. *Br J Surg* 63: 651–654, 1976

89. Gilcher RO, Orr M: Intraoperative autotransfusion. Haemonetics Proceedings of the Advanced Component Seminar, Haemonetics Research Institute, 1976

90. Mattox KL: Comparsion of techniques of autotransfusion. *Surgery* 84:700–702, 1978

91. Csencsitz TA, Flynn JC: Intraoperative blood salvage in spinal deformity surgery in children. *J Fla Med Assoc* 66:39–41, 1979

13

Neonatal Emergencies

I. David Todres
Susan Firestone

Anesthesia for newborns presents unique concerns that make it necessary to consider them apart from older children. A detailed description of the maturing newborn organ systems is given in Chapter 2. Therefore, this section will focus on the special problems of the newborn undergoing surgery (Table 13-1). Normal serum, urine, and CSF chemistries of the newborn are compared to the adult in Table 13-2.

THERMAL INSTABILITY

Heat loss in the newborn infant is a significant cause of morbidity. The newborn loses heat readily by radiation, convection, and evaporation (see Chapter 3). To limit this loss the infant must be transported to the operating room in a temperature-controlled incubator that maintains a neutral thermal environment. In the operating room the ambient temperature must be kept even warmer for the low-birth-weight infant than the full-term neonate. What is felt to be uncomfortably warm by the personnel in the operating room is probably just satisfactory for the infant. In addition, overhead heating lamps and radiant warmers will help to maintain the infant's temperature. Children who weigh less than 10 kg will benefit from the use of a heating blanket, and warming of inspired anesthetic gases will help maintain the infant's temperature.[1]

It is imperative to monitor temperature to prevent hypothermia and avoid accidental hyperthermia. Temperature may be monitored via the skin (abdominal wall, axilla), or a rectal or esophageal probe which measures core temperature. The normal range is 36.5–37.2°C. Care should be taken with the rectal probe to avoid perforation of the rectum.

There are several periods during surgery when the potential for heat loss is significant. Latent heat of vaporization can have serious cooling effects on the infant when large areas of the body are "prepped" for surgery. Rapid infusion of large quantities of cold blood or lavage of the abdominal cavity or bladder with cold fluids are common causes of severe hypothermia. Efforts towards maintaining temperature stability must continue during transport of the infant from the operating room to the recovery room or intensive care unit.

AIRWAY AND BREATHING MECHANICS

The infantile larynx can present difficulties at the time of intubation. The tongue is relatively large and the glottic opening may be obscured by the omega-shaped epiglottis (see Chapter 5). The larynx is situated anteriorly and the narrow diameter of the cricoid ring limits the diameter of the endotracheal tube to be inserted. This may produce high airway resistance and increase the work of breathing. Diaphragmatic movement may be impaired by abdominal distension, surgical packs, or retractors in the abdomen. Abdominal decompression (i.e., emptying the stomach) should be routinely employed, since even oral feedings have been shown to have significant effects on oxygenation.[2] In addition, the highly compliant chest limits the effectiveness of breathing, which may be further compromised by the hands of the surgical assistant resting on the chest wall. These effects are compounded by the diminished proportion of the muscle fiber, which carries out sustained respiratory effort in the newborn compared with the older child.[3] For these reasons totally spontaneous respiration under anesthesia is disadvan-

Table 13-1

Special Concerns of the Neonate Undergoing Surgery

- Thermal instability
- Airway and breathing mechanics
- Blood volume and circulatory problems
- Metabolic and electrolyte balance
- Renal function
- Liver function and jaundice
- Coagulation deficits
- Susceptibility to sepsis
- Associated medical conditions
- Nutrition

tageous for the newborn, and the anesthesiologist should control the infant's breathing.

BLOOD VOLUME AND CIRCULATION

Adequate perfusion must be present at all times. The anesthesiologist should anticipate hypovolemia in the newborn when the underlying condition suggests hemorrhage (intracranial, intra-abdominal), or fluid and electrolyte loss (intestinal obstruction with vomiting and fluid loss within the bowel). The blood volume of the full-term newborn is 85 ml/kg, while the low-birth-weight infant is 95 ml/kg.[4,5] Appreciation of the small blood volume in the neonate is necessary, since intraoperative blood and fluid loss (third space), although relatively small, can have significant effects on hemodynamic stability. The infant may lose 15 percent of its blood volume, leading to reduced stroke volume and cardiac output, yet develop little change in heart rate or blood pressure. It is essential, therefore, to measure these losses and replace them before a significant deficit occurs. Secure, guaranteed access to the circulation, as well as a means to deliver small and measured quantities of blood, must be established prior to surgery.

In addition to maintaining adequate perfusion, it is necessary to ensure adequate oxygen transport. This necessitates effective gas exchange and a hematocrit of greater than 40 percent. Polycythemia (a central venous hematocrit above 70 percent) may have serious effects in the newborn. The increased blood viscosity can lead to renal vein thrombosis in some infants; others have cerebral symptoms (e.g. convulsions). Polycythemia is commonly seen in SGA infants together with hypoglycemia. Management includes a partial exchange transfusion with colloid solutions (5% albumin) to bring the hematocrit down to 60 percent.[6]

A significant feature of the newborn cardiovascular system is its dependancy on heart rate for an adequate cardiac output.[7] Stroke volume is relatively fixed, and any bradycardia significantly reduces cardiac output (see Chapter 15). *Unexplained bradycardia should be considered to be due to hypoxemia,* which can develop with alarming rapidity in the neonate. The anesthesiologist must also be alert to the avoidance of reflex bradycardia associated with passage of nasogastric tubes, oral airways, endotracheal tubes, and surgical manipulations. For these reasons, it is advisable to consider treating the neonate with atropine to block these vagal reflexes.

Table 13-2

Normal Levels of Biochemical Tests in the Newborn

	Newborn	Adult
Blood gases		
PaO_2	75–85 torr	95–100 torr
$PaCO_2$	33–36 torr	36–44 torr
pH	7.30–7.35	7.36–7.44
Bicarbonate	19–21 mEq/l	24–30 mEq/l
Electrolytes		
Sodium	135–145 mEq/l	135–145 mEq/l
Potassium	3.5–5.0 mEq/l	3.5–5.5 mEq/l
Chloride	95–110 mEq/l	95–110 mEq/l
Total calcium	8.0–9.5 mg%	8.5–10.5 mg%
Ionized calcium	1.14–1.30 mM/l	1.14–1.30 mM/l
Magnesium	1.5–2.2 mEq/l	1.5–2.0 mEq/l
Phosphate	4–6 mg%	3.0–4.5 mg%
Osmolality	275–295 mOsm/l	285–295 mOsm/l
BUN	5–20 mg%	8–25 mg%
Creatinine	0.5–1.0 mg%	0.6–1.5 mg%
Glucose	>40mg%	70–100 mg%
Total protein	4.5–6.0 gm%	6.0–8.4 gm%
Albumin	3.2–4.5 gm%	3.5–5.0 gm%
CSF		
Glucose	35–65 mg%	50–75 mg%
Protein	40–120 mg%	14–45 mg%
Urine		
Osmolality	75–300 mOsm/l	50–1200 mOsm/l
Sodium	20–40 mEq/l	80–200 mEq/l
Potassium	10–40 mEq/l	35–100 mEq/l

METABOLIC, FLUID AND ELECTROLYTE BALANCE

SODIUM

Sodium requirements for the full-term infant are 2–3 mEq/kg/24 hr after the first 24 hours of life. However, in the low-birth-weight infant large renal losses of sodium occur, and the infant may require 6–8 mEq/kg/24 hr.[8] Hyponatremia (<125 mEq/l) may lead to lethargy and seizures (Table 13-3).

Hypernatremia may occur when the infant is given excess sodium bicarbonate, or after salt solutions and colloid administration. Infants under phototherapy and infrared radiant warmers lose excessive amounts of water (insensible water loss) and may develop hypernatremia.[9,10]

POTASSIUM

Potassium administration is usually required after the first day of life, provided urine output is adequate. The infant requires 2–3 mEq/kg/24 hr. Normal serum potassium is

Table 13-3

Causes of Neonatal Hyponatremia

- Shortly after birth the level may reflect a low serum sodium in the mother.
- Excessive administration of fluids without sodium
- Diuretic therapy or loss from diarrhea
- Inappropriate ADH secretion
- Adrenal insufficiency due to congenital adrenal hypoplasia (rare)

3.5–5.5 mEq/l. Hypokalemia develops from inadequate intake or diuretic therapy. Hyperkalemia is potentially life threatening; potassium levels may be spuriously elevated if determined from a "capillary" sample that is hemolysed. Hyperkalemia will result from administration of excess amounts of potassium, renal failure, or "old" whole blood.[11]

CALCIUM

Ideally, ionized calcium should be monitored and maintained within the normal range. If ionized calcium measurements are not available, then total calcium levels should be maintained at about 7.5 mg/100ml with exogenous calcium therapy. Hypocalcemia is commonly seen in stressed preterm infants, SGA infants, perinatal asphyxia, infants of diabetic mothers, renal failure, and following exchange transfusion with citrated whole blood or infusions of fresh frozen plasma where the citrate chelates calcium (Chapter 11).[12]

FLUID BALANCE

In evaluating the infant's state of hydration prior to undergoing surgery the following are monitored:

- Weight change.
- Urine output—at least one ml/kg/hr.
- Urine specific gravity—this should be between 1.005 and 1.015. Albuminuria and glycosuria may interfere with evaluation of urine specific gravity.
- Urine and plasma osmolality. Urine osmolality is usually between 75–300 mOsm/l. The newborn has much less ability to concentrate its urine than the adult.

If the above parameters indicate a fluid deficit, additional fluids should be administered. In addition to maintenance fluids, 10–20 ml/kg of balanced salt solution is recommended initially. Further amounts will depend upon the clinical response (weight, urine output, and hemodynamic status). The constitution of the fluid, i.e. the amounts of sodium, potassium, calcium, should be titrated according to need.

ACID–BASE BALANCE

Acid–base balance should be stabilized as close to normal as possible prior to surgery. The underlying cause for a deviation from normal should be sought and actively treated. Rapid sodium bicarbonate administration in the preterm infant for the correction of metabolic acidosis may precipitate intraventricular hemorrhage.[13] For this reason the neonatal preparation of sodium bicarbonate (4.2% = 0.5 mEq/ml) is recommended.

Table 13-4

Causes of Hypoglycemia in Neonates

Low glycogen stores
   Preterm and SGA infant
   Perinatal asphyxia
Hyperinsulinemia
   Infants of diabetic mothers
   Sudden discontinuation of intravenous dextrose solutions
   Beckwith-Wiedemann syndrome
Others (rare)
   Galactosemia
   Glycogen storage disease

Respiratory acidosis must be corrected by increasing alveolar ventilation, and identifying and treating the underlying cause.

GLUCOSE

The anesthesiologist must constantly consider the glucose needs of the newborn undergoing surgery. The high metabolic needs of the newborn, and in particular the preterm infant, make them prone to hypoglycemia. This may be asymptomatic or produce apnea, lethargy, jitteriness, or seizures. There is a potential for serious cerebral insult as a result.[14–16] There are a number of situations in which to anticipate hypoglycemia, which are listed in Table 13-4.

Blood sugar levels should be monitored with Dextrostix and treated if low (<40 mg%), while awaiting the blood glucose level. Normal requirements of glucose are 4–6 mg/kg/min. However, the sick infant often requires 6–12 mg/kg/min to maintain normal blood glucose levels.

If the infant shows signs of hypoglycemia, in addition to a constant infusion of 6–12 mg/kg/min one should administer a small bolus of 200 mg/kg, i.e., 2 ml/kg of a 10 percent glucose solution. This is preferable to the higher concentrations (25–50%) formerly advocated which leads to rebound hypoglycemia from a large insulin stimulus. In addition, a bolus of a hyperosmolar solution, such as 50 percent glucose, may be associated with intraventricular hemorrhage in the low-birth-weight infant.

Hyperglycemia may lead to a serious osmotic diuresis from glycosuria. Severe hyperglycemia occasionally results in hypertonic non-ketotic coma, and may be seen in very-low-birth-weight infants who are unable to handle increased glucose loads. Should the reduction of glucose administered not lead to a satisfactory fall in the blood sugar level, then soluble insulin (0.1 units/kg) may be necessary with careful monitoring to avoid hypoglycemia. Glucose containing solutions should be administered at constant maintenance rates; a fluid bolus to replace volume deficit should be in the form of a non-glucose containing solution (e.g., lactated Ringer's solution), this is best delivered via a separate "piggy-backed" IV system.

RENAL FUNCTION

In addition to urine output, urine analysis, and specific gravity, the measurement of blood urea nitrogen (BUN) and creatinine levels provide valuable information about renal function. The creatinine value is more significant than the BUN. Renal function may be depressed following severe hypoxemia and ischemia to the kidneys, and this must be considered when titrating the fluids to be infused. Other causes for renal failure include congenital abnormalities of the kidneys and urogenital tract, or renal vein thrombosis. Temporary evidence of renal failure may be seen in infants given indomethacin for promoting closure of the patent ductus arteriosus.[17] The presence of renal failure must always be considered, since many anesthetic drugs are excreted by the kidneys. This may lead to prolonged actions of these drugs with an increased potential for toxic effects (see Chapter 6 and 7). Antibiotics may attain toxic levels in the newborn with renal failure if the dose is not appropriately readjusted.

LIVER FUNCTION AND JAUNDICE

Of importance to the anesthesiologist is the fact that liver function is immature in the neonate, and particularly in the preterm infant. This necessitates careful titration of drugs metabolized by the liver (e.g., narcotics, barbiturates). Jaundice is frequently present for a number of reasons, and may be particularly marked in the preterm infant. Elevated levels of bilirubin carry the risk of kernicterus, particularly in low birth weight infants who are severely ill with hypoxemia, acidosis, and hypoproteinemia.[18] Agents which displace bilirubin from albumin binding sites should be avoided (e.g., furosemide, sulfonamides, and medications containing benzoate preservative such as diazepam).[19] In addition to displacing bilirubin, benzoates are responsible for a toxic syndrome in newborns, presenting as floppiness, seizures, acidosis, and hypotension.[20] Chloramphenicol should be avoided in the newborn because of a history of deaths due to cardiovascular collapse ("grey baby syndrome") associated with its use. This is due to conjugation of the drug in the liver, and delayed excretion which leads to toxic levels.

COAGULATION

At birth all neonates should have received an injection of vitamin K_1 (1 mg) to prevent hemorrhagic disease. A history of maternal anticonvulsant therapy may have significant effects on the newborn's clotting factors, which are similar to the effect of the lack of vitamin K.[21] Neonatal sepsis may present with thrombocytopenia and disseminated intravascular coagulopathy (DIC).

SUSCEPTIBILITY TO INFECTION

One should always have a high index of suspicion in the neonate for the presence of sepsis. The clinical picture is often subtle, presenting as lethargy, apnea, abdominal distension, poor feeding, or cyanosis. Appropriate cultures (blood, urine, trachea, and cerebrospinal fluid) are necessary before antibiotic therapy is commenced. The immature immune system makes the neonate particularly susceptible to infection, especially with gram-negative bacteria. The morbidity and mortality from neonatal infection is significant. All individuals handling the neonate must therefore be careful to take appropriate precautions, i.e. scrupulous hand washing and aseptic techniques at all times.

ASSOCIATED MEDICAL CONDITIONS

Not infrequently the infant scheduled for surgery may be suffering from an associated medical condition (e.g., respiratory distress syndrome, bronchopulmonary dysplasia, congenital heart disease, or disseminated intravascular coagulopathy). It is a good rule to remember that the infant with a congenital anomaly requiring surgery may well have other anomalies. The association of specific anomalies with those that require surgical intervention is discussed under the respective conditions.

NUTRITION

While calories for growth are not of prime consideration during a surgical procedure, this factor must be considered in the overall management, especially in the preterm infant. When it is anticipated that the gastrointestinal tract will require a prolonged period of recovery (e.g., gastroschisis) central line placement for hyperalimentation should be considered.

THE FAMILY

With all anesthetic and surgical procedures in the infant, the anesthesiologist should endeavor to establish a rapport with the parents; their hopes and expectations for a normal, healthy infant have not been realized, and this is a unique and very stressful situation. Compassion and understanding are an important and necessary part of the anesthesiologist's role as a total physician. At times the parents, especially the mother, may be absent as a result of the transfer of the infant to a regional tertiary care center. A phone call may help to alleviate some of the anxieties and concerns.

MONITORING AND EQUIPMENT

Conditions that require emergency surgery in the neonate are often accompanied by a multitude of medical problems, and as a consequence management and monitoring considerations can become quite complex. Aside from the minimum standard monitoring equipment (i.e., ECG, chest or esophageal stethoscope, blood pressure cuff with a Doppler flow detector, and temperature probe), it is extremely helpful to include some method to assess the patient's oxygenation and expired carbon dioxide. Rapid decreases in arterial oxygen content in neonates after brief periods of ventilatory compromise, coupled with the risk of retrolental fibroplasia (RLF) when safe levels of arterial oxygen saturation are exceeded, dictate the need for specific monitoring. The transcutaneous oxygen analyzer has several drawbacks for intraoperative use, including incompatibility with inhalational agents unless a special membrane is utilized.[22] A more recent noninvasive device, pulse oximetry, may prove to be particularly useful for infants in whom the risk of intra-arterial monitoring cannot be justified.[23,24] This device will diagnose hypoxemia but not hyperoxia.

In the neonate, changes in blood pressure, heart rate, and the tonal quality of heart sounds are excellent indicators of intravascular volume status and depth of anesthesia. Under most circumstances, the addition of a urinary catheter to quantify urine output is sufficient to monitor fluid balance in prolonged cases. In cases in which major blood or fluid losses are expected, or the physiology is complicated by the presence of cardiac disease, central venous catheters, or occasionally pulmonary artery catheters, are warranted. Any neonate with significant underlying respiratory or cardiac impairment, including hemodynamic instability secondary to intravascular volume depletion, should have an intra-arterial catheter placed for measuring blood pressure, arterial blood gases, and serum chemistries (Figure 13-1). Many neonates will arrive in the operating room from the ICU with an umbilical arterial line. Unless immediate operation is imperative, the time should be taken to replace this line with a radial arterial catheter, preferably on the right side to measure preductal oxygen tension. The possibility of an unobserved disconnection occurring beneath the surgical drapes, resulting in significant blood loss and disruption of monitoring, makes umbilical arterial or venous lines less reliable under operative conditions. In addition, umbilical venous lines can become wedged in the liver because of an inability to traverse the ductus venosus. In this position, infusion of hypertonic solutions may lead to parenchymal necrosis and ultimately fibrosis.[25,26]

Nonrebreathing (open) circuits are simple and effective for delivering anesthetic agents to infants weighing less than 10 kilograms (Chapter 23). The system must have provisions for a humidifier to warm and hydrate the anesthetic gases. The anesthesia machine should also provide compressed air in addition to oxygen and nitrous oxide. The use of air provides the ability to regulate inspired oxygen in cases where nitrous oxide is contraindicated and hyperoxic levels must be avoided.

Efforts must be taken to reduce the infant's heat loss which occurs by convection and radiation to the environment. Basic measures should include adjusting the ambient temperature in the operating room to 28–30°C (83–86°F) and fitting the operating room table with a warming blanket.[27] A radiant warmer positioned over the infant until completion of the surgical "prep" will also significantly decrease heat loss. Covering the infant's head with a stocking cap will prevent a major source of heat loss.[28] Preventative measures must extend into the period after surgery, since hypothermia is a common complication during transport of the patient to the ICU. The infant's body should be enclosed in plastic wrap and/or warm blankets before being placed in a prewarmed isolette (see Chapter 3). Hemodynamic monitoring appropriate for the infant's condition should continue until safe transfer to the ICU is completed.

ANESTHETIC MANAGEMENT

With the exception of those infants who require emergency endotracheal intubation, the initial decision in planning the anesthetic is whether aspiration precautions are indicated. Clearly, disorders that involve an actual or functional ileus or bowel obstruction make protection from aspiration a priority. The choice then remains between an awake intubation and a rapid-sequence induction and intubation. Awake intubation is recommended in the presence of upper airway abnormalities, or in any moribund neonate. However, for a vigorous infant with a normal airway, a controlled rapid-sequence induction with cricoid pressure is a justifiable alternative. Of special concern is the ease with which endobronchial intubation

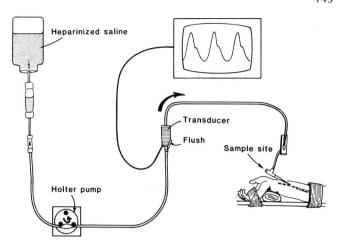

Figure 13-1. Equipment utilized for radial artery cannulation in neonates. Note the Holter pump, which controls the volume of heparinized saline administered to the infant.

occurs with a change in head position (Figure 13-2). Care must be taken to ensure equality of breath sounds after the head is positioned for surgery.

In contrast to the previously described patients, there is a group of respiratory disorders, including tracheoesophageal fistula, congenital lobar emphysema, and bronchogenic cysts, where anesthesia by inhalation induction with spontaneous respiration is recommended. This can be accomplished after an awake intubation or via a face mask, until the infant is at an appropriate depth of anesthesia for intubation. Spontaneous respiration avoids the possible untoward effects of excessive positive pressure ventilation.

Neonatal responses to the potent volatile agents differ from those of older infants and children in several important ways. It has been established that the minimum alveolar concentration (MAC) of an anesthetic is higher in children than adults.[29,30] However, early studies of MAC did not identify neonates as a separate group from infants. This has recently been reassessed, and data have shown that MAC in the first month of life is significantly below previously published values.[31] For example, MAC for halothane was determined to be 1.2 percent in infants, but only 0.87 percent for neonates. Neonates have previously been reported to have an increased sensitivity to cardiovascular depression from volatile agents. However, in view of the new data on MAC, it is evident that most investigators were not administering equipotent anesthetic doses, i.e., one MAC, to all patients.[32,33] When newborns were studied at corrected MAC levels, the incidence of hypotension and bradycardia was comparable to that found in older infants and children.[31]

The effects of potent inhalation anesthetic agents on neonatal respiratory physiology also differ quantitatively from their effects on children and adults. There is evidence that neonates, and premature infants in particular, are more sensitive to anesthetic-induced decreases in respiratory drive and attenuation of the ventilatory response to hypoxia.[34] It is significant that these alterations in neurogenic control of respiration occur at subanesthetic concentrations encountered

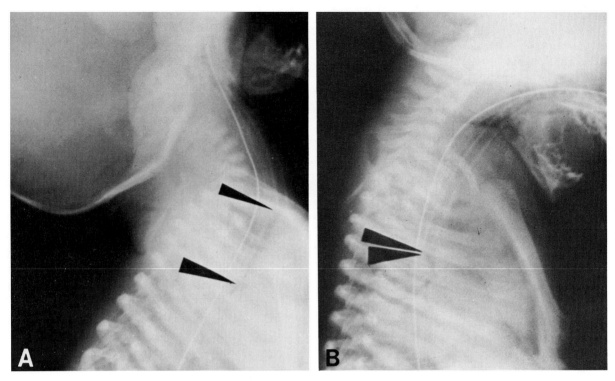

Figure 13-2. Radiographs illustrate the effect of head position on endotracheal tube placement. The upper arrow indicates the tip of the endotracheal tube; the lower arrow the tip of the carina. Note the marked excursion of the tip of the tube with head flexion. (B). (Reproduced with permission from Todres ID, et al: *J Pediatr* 89:126–127, 1976.)

in the recovery period. This is an important concern for preterm infants with a history of apnea and bradycardia, because these effects may induce life-threatening postoperative apnea.[35,36] As a consequence this special group of neonates deserves prolonged (12–24 hours) postanesthetic monitoring of their respiratory status, even after elective procedures that might otherwise be accomplished on an outpatient basis.

The narcotic analgesics also produce significant degrees of ventilatory depression, although full evaluation of their effects in neonates is lacking. Recently fentanyl has become among the most commonly used narcotics in neonatal anesthesia. It is felt that the respiratory drawbacks are more than compensated for by the fact that, in conjunction with muscle relaxants and nitrous oxide, fentanyl produces a minimum of detrimental hemodynamic alterations.[37] The potential for significant bradycardia induced by high doses of fentanyl can be counterbalanced by the choice of a muscle relaxant which produces tachycardia, e.g., pancuronium. Whenever narcotics are used on neonates, particular attention must be paid to the adequacy of respiration postoperatively.

Sustained hypertension (systolic pressure above 80–90 mmHg) has been implicated in episodes of cerebral hemorrhage in asphyxiated premature infants, probably as a result of loss of autoregulation, so that the cerebral circulation varies directly with the blood pressure.[38] For this reason low concentrations of halothane or isoflurane (0.25–0.5 MAC) can be used to supplement the anesthetic if hypertension becomes a persistent problem.

Care in protecting the newborn at risk for retrolental fibroplasia (RLF) must also be factored into the anesthetic management. The high risk group is preterm infants born less than 34 weeks after conception. These infants remain at risk

until they are beyond the age of 42–44 weeks postconception.[39] Recommended safe levels of arterial oxygen tension are between 60–90 torr, and oxygenation should be monitored at a preductal location, such as the right radial artery. Appropriate inspired oxygen concentrations may be achieved by mixing oxygen with air and/or nitrous oxide. However, oxygen should *not* be restricted if the infant is hypoxemic. Other poorly understood factors apart from hyperoxia have been incriminated as being associated with RLF.[40,41] Recent evidence suggests increases in $PaCO_2$ may also be a provoking factor.[42]

RESPIRATORY DISORDERS IN THE NEONATE

GENERAL PRINCIPLES

Assessment of neonates with respiratory distress requires knowledge of their baseline respiratory parameters. The normal breathing rate in a full-term newborn is approximately 40 breaths per minute, and in the preterm infant it is approximately 60 breaths per minute.[42] A unique feature of the premature infant's respiration is the variations in rhythm known as "periodic" breathing, in which evenly spaced breaths are interrupted by short periods of apnea (Fig 2-3). This is considered a normal pattern in newborns unless the apneic periods extend for more than 10 seconds.[44] There are also notable differences in the arterial blood gases of neonates; the pH (7.30–7.35), PaO_2 (60–80 torr), $PaCO_2$ (30–35 torr), and bicarbonate (19–20 mEq/l), are lower than older infants (see Table 13-2).[45] In contrast to adults, a PaO_2 of 60–80 torr is more than adequate for their metabolic needs, because the hematocrit in the neonate is usually 55–60 percent resulting in a high total oxygen content.

Signs of respiratory distress are varied and include apnea, tachypnea and grunting respirations, tachycardia, cyanosis, suprasternal, intercostal and subcostal retractions, and stridor. Accentuation of periodic breathing, including prolonged apnea (longer than 15–20 seconds) may be a late sign of respiratory compromise, which results from the effects of hypoxia or hypercarbia on the central nervous system. In comparison to the full-term infant, premature infants have a blunted respiratory response to hypercarbia.[45,46] In addition, they do not sustain an increase in ventilation in the face of hypoxia, and therefore develop respiratory failure rapidly.[47–49]

The presence of specific clinical signs may help clarify the possible diagnosis and indicate the direction of further investigative studies. For example, rapid respiration without severe chest retractions often reflects congenital heart disease, whereas rapid respirations with grunting and marked chest retractions will often indicate pulmonary pathology. In addition, crying will often improve the infant's color with respiratory disease, and increase cyanosis with cardiac disease. Choking and cyanosis that accompany feeding are characteristic of choanal atresia and tracheoesophageal fistula. Stridor that begins at birth is a prominent feature of obstructive lesions such as laryngeal webs and subglottic stenosis. In contrast, a later progressive onset of stridor and wheezing is associated with subglottic tumors, bronchogenic and pulmonary cysts, and congenital lobar emphysema.

SPECIFIC CONDITIONS

Choanal Atresia

Choanal atresia results when either the bony or membranous portions of the nasopharynx fail to undergo perforation during development; the incidence is one in 8000 births.[50] Few problems occur when the obstruction is unilateral, but bilateral choanal atresia can produce acute respiratory distress at birth. At this time the newborn is an obligate nasal breather and remains so for the first 6–8 weeks of life.[51,52] Although choanal atresia may present immediately after birth, the first indication for many that the nasopharynx is not patent is cyanosis and choking from aspiration during feeding. The diagnosis is established by physical examination (i.e., if a suction catheter cannot be advanced into the nasopharynx), or by x-ray, using contrast media to demonstrate the obstruction. Surgical correction in the neonatal period is necessary in order to prevent repeated aspiration and subsequent pulmonary infection.[53]

Choanal atresia is not generally associated with other major craniofacial anomalies, and therefore the infants airway is usually normal in all other respects.[53] Anesthetic management must take into account the obligatory oral route for air entry; therefore awake intubation or the early placement of an oral airway is necessary to maintain adequate air exchange. The early introduction of an oral airway may be better tolerated if the palate and tongue are anesthetized with small amounts of topical viscous lidocaine.

Laryngeal or Tracheal Web

Tracheal obstruction presenting in the neonatal period may be due to an incomplete fibrous membrane (web) that occludes the laryngeal opening or, more commonly, the

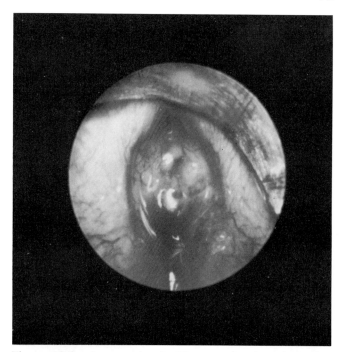

Figure 13-3. Laryngeal web. Photograph taken through a bronchoscope showing a membranous web with near complete occlusion of the larynx (courtesy of Dr. S. Kim).

subglottic tracheal lumen (Figure 13-3).[54] Signs of acute respiratory distress are present at birth, with stridor most prominent. On occasion it is possible to bypass this life-threatening obstruction by inserting an endotracheal tube stented with a stylette which breaks through the web, thus establishing a safe airway. If intubation is unsuccessful, cricothyroid puncture with an IV catheter may be effective. Usually the obstruction can be resected through a bronchoscope, and the patient will recover with few sequelae.

Congenital Subglottic Stenosis

This condition causes neonatal respiratory distress, but the presentation is usually less acute than for a web. When narrowing of the tracheal lumen is severe, or involves a substantial segment, management with a tracheostomy is necessary. Long-term treatment includes repeated bronchoscopic dilatations or stenting of the stenotic segment, and steroid injection to limit formation of granulation tissue.[55,56]

Anesthetic management of the initial bronchoscopic evaluation is most safely accomplished with general anesthesia given through a face mask with assisted ventilation until the nature and extent of the subglottic stenosis is defined. An endotracheal tube should then be placed if tracheostomy is to follow. Future anesthetic procedures are thus simplified following tracheostomy, since direct connection to the tracheostomy tube with an appropriately sized straight connector provides an immediate route for administration of anesthetic gases and positive pressure ventilation. Decannulation is often accomplished by the age of 2–5 years, but in some situations, the clinical course may be complicated by the therapy itself, which can cause excessive mucosal damage of the trachea.

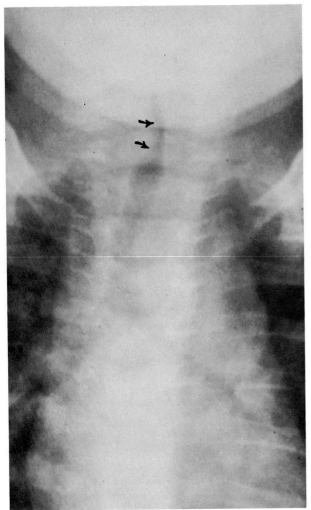

Figure 13-4. AP chest film in a patient with a subglottic hemangioma shows marked tracheal narrowing (arrows). Note the asymmetrical narrowing; in infectious croup the subglottic narrowing is concentric. (Courtesy Dr. P. Donahoe)

Post-traumatic Subglottic Stenosis

Subglottic stenosis may follow trauma from tracheal intubation, especially when the endotracheal tube has been a "tight fit." This complication should be seen infrequently if special attention is paid to selecting an endotracheal tube which will permit an air leak at a peak inspiratory pressure of 20–30 cm H_2O.

Subglottic Hemangioma

Airway obstruction from a subglottic hemangioma rarely presents with immediate respiratory distress, but develops over a period of weeks as the hemangioma, which is present from birth, enlarges. Hemangiomas are seen more commonly than other obstructing masses, such as cystic hygroma or teratoma.[57] The presence of other hemangiomas on the body surface of an infant with stridor should suggest the possibility of subglottic hemangioma as a cause for the infant's airway obstruction.[58]

Although some infants with subglottic hemangioma have a history of respiratory symptoms, particularly intermittent stridor or noisy breathing, acute respiratory arrest may be the first presentation (Figure 13-4). The trauma of coughing from an upper respiratory tract infection is often an instigating factor in the infant's respiratory decompensation.[59] Intubation at this time, although frequently necessary, is not without the danger of causing hemorrhage. In cases of airway obstruction from an unknown cause, the initial intubation should be accomplished with an endotracheal tube that is smaller than usual.

Esophageal Atresia and Tracheoesophageal Fistula

Esophageal atresia may occur as an isolated lesion, as may tracheoesophageal fistula (TEF). In 90 percent of cases, however there is the coexistence of esophageal atresia and TEF.[60,61] In these cases the upper esophagus ends in a blind pouch, and the fistulous connection occurs in the distal trachea; as a result, gastric juice can reflux into the trachea and be aspirated into the lungs, producing a severe chemical pneumonitis. Effective swallowing is impossible and thus saliva accumulates in the esophageal pouch, acting as another source for aspiration. Attempted feedings cause choking, cyanosis, and regurgitation.

The diagnosis is established by the inability to pass a nasogastric tube into the stomach. X-ray will confirm the diagnosis, showing the catheter coiled in the blind upper esophageal pouch. X-ray of the abdomen showing bowel gas indicates the presence of a tracheoesophageal fistula. On occasion the bowel may become markedly distended and impede respirations. In the less common condition of TEF without esophageal atresia (H-type), x-ray studies may be inconclusive and direct examination through bronchoscopy may be necessary to locate the fistula.

TEF occurs in association with a number of other congenital anomalies.[62] It is part of the VATER, syndrome which is a constellation of malformations consisting of vertebral defects, anal atresia, TEF with esophageal atresia, and radial and renal dysplasia.[63] Chromosomal abnormalities, cardiac anomalies, imperforate anus, and duodenal atresia are also commonly associated with TEF. Recent advances in management have reduced the mortality to less than 10 percent. The most important factors influencing mortality are the severity of the associated anomalies and extreme prematurity.[60,61,64,65]

Immediate management consists of placing the infant prone and in a head-up position to prevent gastric juice reflux and aspiration. A catheter placed in the upper esophageal pouch is connected to constant suction to prevent aspiration of saliva. Continuous subclinical aspiration results in chronic pulmonary injury and airway hyperreactivity in the majority of these patients; therefore the anesthesiologist should anticipate potential pulmonary complications.[66] The infant may require supplemental oxygen for aspiration pneumonitis, and in severe cases may require tracheal intubation and ventilation.

Anesthetic management includes securing venous access, hydrating the infant, and placing an arterial line to monitor blood gases. Special considerations for the anesthetic include:

1. Awake intubation.
2. Avoidance of vigorous positive pressure ventilation to prevent gastric inflation; this has led to rupture of the stomach.
3. Strict attention to changes in ventilation throughout the surgical procedure, as obstruction of the trachea often

occurs when the surgeon retracts the lung during the repair.

4. Adequate re-expansion of the compressed lung at the conclusion of the surgical procedure.

5. Postoperative care in the intensive care unit, including constant assessment of pulmonary and hemodynamic status. Effort is made to extubate these infants as soon as possible to minimize the stress on tracheal suture lines.

In most cases the fistula enters the trachea posteriorly a short distance above the carina. Therefore correct positioning of the endotracheal tube is a matter of a few millimeters; this is critical because one needs to have the tube *distal* to the fistula to avoid inflation of the stomach. Some surgeons prefer to place a gastrostomy prior to the repair to avoid abdominal inflation. One method of achieving proper endotracheal tube placement is to intubate a main stem bronchus (usually right), and slowly withdraw the tube until breath sounds and chest expansion first become equal. This should place the distal end of the tube just above the carina. Monitoring should include a stethoscope placed on the left chest in the axilla to detect any accidental displacement of the endotracheal tube into the right main stem bronchus.

A rare form of this anomaly is laryngotracheoesophageal cleft. The cleft usually begins at the larynx. It may be small or extend the entire tracheal length to the carina. The symptoms are similar to those with TEF, i.e., choking during feeding, cyanosis, and distress from aspiration pneumonitis. In severe cases the condition has a high mortality. Repair is often difficult and complicated by breakdown of the tracheal suture line necessitating frequent corrective surgical procedures.

Congenital Bronchogenic and Pulmonary Cysts

The formation of bronchogenic or pulmonary cysts is caused by the isolation of primordial respiratory tissue from the body of the developing respiratory system.[67] The location and size of a cyst will determine whether the lesion causes sufficient respiratory difficulty in the neonatal period to prompt medical intervention. Early diagnosis is of importance, since both varieties of cysts have the potential to cause acute respiratory failure or arrest. Many patients with congenital cysts are only diagnosed after the rupture of the cyst, which results in hemorrhage and bronchopleural fistula formation; this sequence of events often presents as "sudden death."[67,68]

Most bronchogenic cysts are centrally located within the mediastinum, and account for 5–10 percent of all posterior mediastinal masses.[69] Cysts formed at the carina are most likely to cause respiratory compromise, the severity of which parallels the size of the lesion.[70] The natural history of carinal cysts is usually marked by nonspecific respiratory symptoms in the neonatal period, which may dramatically progress to respiratory arrest at several weeks of age. The clinical syndrome is similar to that of lobar emphysema, since the enlarging carinal cyst partially obstructs one or both main stem bronchi, causing air trapping.[71] In contrast, cysts in the paratracheal region, hilum, or within the pulmonary parenchyma, produce a more chronic course in which infection and abscess formation are prominent. These patients are usually brought to medical attention in late infancy and early childhood.[68,72]

The management of an infant with respiratory distress from a congenital cyst is aimed at minimizing the expansion of the lesion during the preoperative period. If respiratory failure requires emergency intubation, ventilation should be accomplished at the lowest possible peak inspiratory pressure. Patients with continued respiratory or cardiovascular compromise may require acute decompression of the cyst, by needle aspiration, or thoracostomy. This should be reserved for extreme cases, as it may result in spillage of infected cyst contents into healthy lung tissue.

In stable patients, spontaneous ventilation should be maintained during induction of anesthesia, and after intubation, until the chest is open. This is mandatory in patients who have a large cyst under tension, or air trapping during expiration. To avoid increasing the volume of the lesion, nitrous oxide should *not* be used. Unless the clinical condition or blood gases justify using 100 percent oxygen, it should be mixed with compressed air to attain the appropriate FiO_2.

Once the thorax is open, muscle relaxants may be administered and controlled ventilation instituted. Cysts that are air-filled pose little problem. However, fluid-filled or abscessed cysts that connect with the tracheobronchial tree can spill into the healthy (downside) lung. Double lumen tubes are not an option in infants, but the endotracheal tube may be advanced into the main stem bronchus of the unaffected lung, and/or the surgeon can temporarily occlude the bronchus and pulmonary artery of the affected lung until the lesion is resected. Selective bronchial blocking can also be accomplished by using a balloon-tipped embolectomy catheter (Fogarty) placed under direct bronchoscopic control.[73,74]

There are no other major congenital anomalies associated with either bronchogenic or pulmonary cysts, and therefore the prognosis for full recovery of these infants after surgical resection is excellent.

Congenital Lobar Emphysema

In the majority of cases of congenital lobar emphysema (CLE) only one lobe is affected, most commonly the left upper lobe. Occasionally an entire lung is involved.[75,76] In approximately ten percent of patients there is coexistent congenital heart disease.[77]

The clinical presentation is one of progressive respiratory distress with unilateral thoracic hyperexpansion, atelectasis of the contralateral lung, and mediastinal shift (Figure 13-5). As the emphysematous segment increases in size, the intrathoracic pressure rises. Cardiovascular compromise, due to the high intrathoracic pressure impeding both the venous return and ventricular outflow, may become a significant feature. Emergency thoracostomy may be required in extreme cases to stabilize the patient until transfer to the operating room is accomplished.[76]

Intraoperative management is similar to that discussed in the section on cystic lesions, with primary emphasis on minimizing positive pressure ventilation and maintaining spontaneous respiration until thoracotomy decompresses the lungs.[78] The patient may require assisted ventilation to assure adequate oxygenation, in which case it is crucial to allow adequate time for expiration. Nitrous oxide is absolutely contraindicated, since it can precipitate an increase in the volume of the lobe, resulting in acute decompensation. The surgeon should be present in the operating room during induction of anesthesia.

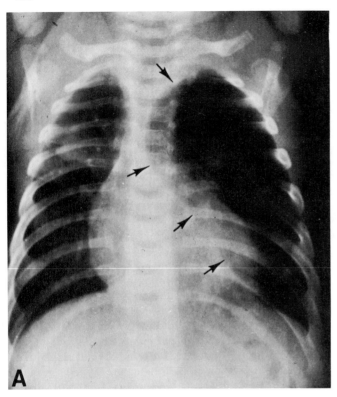

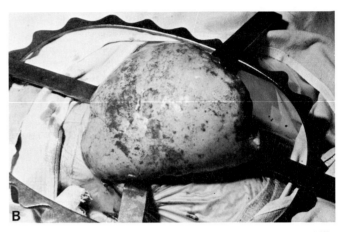

Figure 13-5. X-ray from a patient with CLE (A) demonstrates hyperinflation of the left lung with herniation across the midline (arrows) and mediastinal shift. Intraoperative photograph (B) shows the emphysematous lobe bulging through the thoractomy incision. (Reproduced with permission from Coté CJ: Anesthesiology 49:296, 1978.)

Diaphragmatic Hernia

The incidence of congenital diaphragmatic hernia (CDH) is one in 2,500 live births. Approximately one in four newborns with CDH have associated congenital anomalies. Embryologically this condition develops when, in its normal process of migration, the midgut returns to the abdominal cavity prematurely before the diaphragm has completely formed.[79] Congenital diaphragmatic hernia is therefore characterized by the presence of abdominal viscera in the chest (Figure 13-6). This usually includes the stomach, small or large intestine, and occasionally the liver and spleen. Frequently there is an accompanying malrotation of the gut. The herniation occurs most often through the pleuroperitoneal sinus (foramen of Bochdalek) on the left; much less commonly the herniation occurs through the substernal sinus (foramen of Morgagni). Pulmonary hypoplasia occurs on the affected side, and in some cases in the opposite lung as well. The degree of pulmonary hypoplasia is usually the determining factor in the outcome. If the herniation occurs later in the development of the lungs, there is more functional lung tissue, and the prognosis is better.[80]

Congenital diaphragmatic hernia remains one of the most challenging problems for the surgeon and anesthesiologist. The persistent high mortality (greater than 50%) when presenting with severe symptoms in the first six hours of life has led to a multitude of approaches to the management.[81] Immediately after birth the infant is usually cyanotic, and has tachypnea and chest retractions. In rare cases, the initial signs will be of intestinal obstruction from strangulation of the bowel. In the classic presentation there is decreased chest movement on the affected side, a shift of the cardiac impulse to the opposite side, and a scaphoid abdomen. Breath sounds are absent on the affected side, while bowel sounds may be heard in the chest. Roentgenographic studies are diagnostic, showing gas-filled loops of bowel in the chest with marked shift of the mediastinum to the opposite side (Figure 13-6). This may be confused with congenital cystic lung disease. Blood gas analysis may reflect severe hypoxemia, hypercarbia, and acidemia. Hypercarbia (occurring both immediately before and within two hours of surgery) that is unresponsive to vigorous hyperventilation is associated with a mortality rate of 90 percent.[82] These patients have bilateral pulmonary hypoplasia and severe preductal shunting. Those who respond well to hyperventilation with a reduction in $PaCO_2$ have a more favorable outcome. Acute respiratory decompensation is often a result of pneumothorax of the contralateral lung which may occur before, during, or after surgery.[83]

The urgency of an operation is generally related to the degree of cardiorespiratory distress. In the severely distressed infant the priority in management consists of establishing an airway by means of awake oral intubation and instituting rapid, low volume, controlled respirations to avoid high peak inflation pressures. A nasogastric tube is inserted to decompress the stomach. Once attention has been given to treatment of hypoxemia and hypercarbia, an intravenous line is secured, and depending on the severity of acidemia, sodium bicarbonate (2 mEq/kg) may be administered. Surgical decompression is then carried out as expeditiously as possible. Monitoring of these patients consists of the electrocardiogram, esophageal stethoscope, and blood pressure with Doppler flow probe. Some form of monitoring peripheral oxygen tension, such as pulse oximetry or a transcutaneous electrode, and end-tidal carbon dioxide measurements are extremely helpful. The surgical procedure should *not* be delayed to place an arterial line, but after decompression is accomplished a *right* radial arterial line will aid in postoperative management. The preferred anesthetic agents are narcotics (fentanyl) and muscle relaxants. Nitrous oxide is avoided because of its potential for increasing bowel distension. Prior to decompression, 100 percent oxygen should be administered to treat the underlying hypoxemia. Potent inhalational agents are to be avoided, since their myocardial depressant effects may potentiate any existing cardiovascular compromise. Once the chest is decompressed, inhalational agents may be used to supplement the anesthesia.

A major determinant in the outcome of these infants is the degree and reversibility of the pulmonary artery hypertension in the postoperative period. Recent efforts have focused on methods of reducing pulmonary artery hypertension caused by a hyperactive pulmonary vasculature. During periods of increased pulmonary artery pressure, blood flow is reestablished through the ductus arteriosus and foramen ovale, thus bypassing the lungs. This leads to progressive hypoxemia, acidemia, and death, unless the sequence is rapidly reversed. Factors which provoke pulmonary artery vasoconstriction (i.e., hypoxemia, hypercarbia, acidemia, and hypothermia) must be avoided.[84] Noxious stimuli, such as pain and endotracheal tube suction, may contribute to the development of pulmonary artery hypertension. In an attempt to minimize these effects, a prolonged "anesthetic state" is maintained with the use of infusions of narcotics (e.g., fentanyl) and muscle relaxants.[85] Hyperventilation to a pH of 7.5–7.60 is used to augment pulmonary vasodilation. The benefit of pharmacologic vasodilator therapy remains controversial. Anecdotal reports of early successes with vasodilators, such as tolazoline, isoproterenol, prostaglandin E_1 and nitroglycerin, have not always been followed with consistently good results.[86] Dopamine is frequently used for its inotropic effects and maintenance of systemic vascular resistance. Extracorporeal membrane oxygenation (ECMO) has been used recently with some success following repair of the diaphragmatic hernia in infants with severe ductal shunting. The wide variety of treatment regimens for postoperative management of CDH is a testament to their ineffectiveness, and the mortality from this lesion remains unacceptably high.

GASTROINTESTINAL DISORDERS

PRINCIPLES OF MANAGEMENT

Newborns with gastrointestinal pathology are among the sickest infants cared for in the operating room. Advanced cases of bowel obstruction, frequently coupled with sepsis, cause severe abdominal distension with respiratory compromise, intravascular volume depletion, acidosis and cardiovascular depression. These combine to produce a neonate in extremis. Such moribund infants usually need urgent tracheal intubation, gastric decompression, and fluid resuscitation before surgery can proceed. Awake intubation to prevent pulmonary aspiration of gastric contents is indicated.

Anesthetic techniques that minimize cardiovascular depression and peripheral vasodilatation are utilized. A combination of muscle relaxants and narcotics that support the heart rate is well tolerated. Potent inhalation agents are best used in

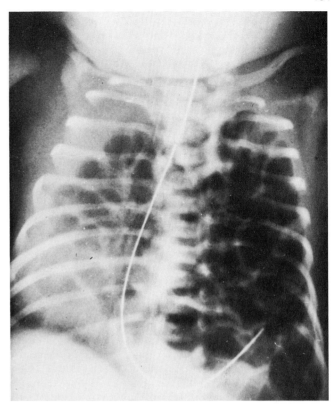

Figure 13-6. Chest radiograph of a neonate with a left diaphragmatic hernia. Note the nasogastric tube placed to decompress the stomach, which resides in the chest; the heart is markedly deviated to the right.

low concentrations as an adjunt to narcotic/relaxant anesthesia. Nitrous oxide should be avoided as it can acutely increase the bowel distension. Analgesia and muscle relaxation is usually continued into the postoperative period, since these patients frequently benefit from mechanical ventilation until abdominal distension diminishes.

Very large fluid volumes, sometimes several times the infant's blood volume, may be needed to maintain adequate blood pressure; assessment of peripheral perfusion, urinary output, and central venous pressure are guidelines for the degree of fluid resuscitation. Increased fluid requirements extend into the first few postoperative days and often must be administered at the cost of generalized edema. The need for a route for parenteral nutrition justifies maintaining central venous access, in spite of the risks of infection and central vein thrombosis. The recent advances in total parenteral nutrition (TPN) has made a significant contribution to reducing the mortality associated with gastrointestinal diseases in the neonatal period.[87,88]

SPECIFIC CONDITIONS

Omphalocele and Gastroschisis

These conditions represent congenital defects of the newborn's abdominal wall associated with herniation of the abdominal viscera. The incidence is one in 5,800 births for omphalocele, and one in 15,000 for gastroschisis.[89] Omphalocele is caused by the failure of the gut, which normally develops within the yolk-sac membranes, to migrate back into the abdominal cavity.[90,91] As a consequence, a membranous sac overlies the herniated viscera so the bowel is morphologically and functionally normal. The pathogenesis of gastroschisis is thought to be due to an intrauterine occlusion of the omphalomesentric artery, which results in a full-thickness defect in the abdominal wall, lateral to the umbilicus (usually to the right).[92] The bowel then herniates through this defect, and is exposed to amniotic fluid in utero and to the atmosphere following birth. This leads to edema and inflammation of the exposed bowel, which becomes dilated, forshortened, and functionally abnormal. A large percentage of these patients are of low birth weight (40%) and premature (30%).[93] Omphalocele is also a feature of the Beckwith-Wiedemann syndrome, which is associated with severe hypoglycemia.[94]

Exstrophy of the bladder and congenital heart disease comprise the majority of the important anomalies associated with omphalocele.[95] The coexistence of other malformations, low birth weight, and prematurity, has a significant effect on the mortality of these patients; those with major anomalies have a mortality rate as high as 65 percent, while the mortality drops to 12 percent in infants with isolated omphaloceles.[93] In contrast, the only significant anomalies (10%) associated with gastroschisis are of the intestines, such as small bowel atresia and malrotation, which are now considered part of the gastroschisis anomaly.[96,97] The overall mortality for gastroschisis is low (less than 10%) since the introduction of TPN. There is often need for prolonged nutritional support until the initially abnormal bowel begins to function.[98] The excellent surgical outcome with gastroschisis is encouraging, since the incidence of this anomaly has increased markedly over the last 20–30 years.[96,99–101]

In gastroschisis and ruptured omphalocele the large exposed surface of the inflamed intestine gives rise to severe fluid and heat loss, leading to hypovolemic shock and hypothermia. This requires urgent treatment with a combination of lactated Ringer's solution and 5 percent albumin, commencing with 20 ml/kg as a bolus, and continuing with additional amounts as needed to achieve a stable hemodynamic status.[102] Loss of heat is also a significant problem, and hypothermia is a frequent complication of transport and surgery.[93] To minimize these losses the extra-abdominal bowel should be covered with saline-soaked gauze and a layer of plastic wrap. Abdominal distension should be treated with a nasogastric tube to avoid regurgitation and aspiration of the stomach contents.

The infant's nasogastric tube is suctioned prior to awake intubation, to ensure airway protection. Muscle relaxants are an essential part of the management, since they facilitate reduction of the eviscerated bowel. For small defects primary closure is satisfactory, and there are usually minimal difficulties postoperatively. Large defects frequently cannot be closed without seriously jeopardizing the infant's respiratory status by critically impeding diaphragmatic excursions.[103] This leads to progressive atelectasis of the lower lobes of the lungs and respiratory failure. Greatly increased abdominal pressure places undue stress on the closure, which can result in dehiscence, a complication with high mortality. With large defects, therefore, a prosthetic Silon pouch is created to enclose the bowel and cover the defect.[104,105] This is then treated with staged reductions over a period of days or weeks, the length of time being guided by close assessment of the infant's ventilatory adequacy (Figure 13-7). During this entire period the neonate will remain intubated and will require ventilatory support. TPN is an important part of the management, since the bowel may take some weeks before enteral feedings are tolerated.

Hypertrophic Pyloric Stenosis

Hypertrophy of the muscularis layer of the pylorus causes a varying degree of gastric outlet obstruction, a common surgical problem in the neonate. The incidence is approximately one in 500 live births, and the majority of patients are male (4:1).[106]

The disorder is usually recognized by 4–6 weeks of age with the onset of classic projectile vomiting following feedings. In many infants the diagnosis is confirmed on abdominal examination by the presence of a firm "olive-sized" mass in the pyloric region. If the abdominal examination is equivocal, a radiologic study with barium should provide the correct diagnosis. A history of a barium swallow should always be specifically elicited during the preanesthetic interview, since the presence of barium in the stomach must be considered in the anesthetic management.

The primary physiologic derangement is fluid and electrolyte depletion from persistent vomiting, which ultimately produces a hypochloremic, hypokalemic metabolic alkalosis.[107] Dehydration is a more consistent finding than metabolic alkalosis; as many as 40 percent of infants with pyloric stenosis have normal electrolyte values. Surgical correction of the defect must be preceded by correction of the fluid deficit and electrolyte imbalance with appropriate intravenous solutions.

All neonates with pyloric stenosis need gastric suctioning with a *large-bore* catheter prior to induction of anesthesia, irrespective of the duration of fasting. This is of particular importance if the infant was given a barium swallow, since pulmonary aspiration of barium produces a severe chemical pneumonitis. Intravenous cimetidine may have a role in the premedication of these infants, but this approach requires further study.

All infants with pyloric stenosis should have intravenous lines placed prior to surgery. Rapid-sequence induction, and intubation with application of cricoid pressure, is therefore readily accomplished. In less vigorous infants awake oral intubation may be expeditiously and relatively atraumatically performed, with preservation of laryngeal reflexes to guard against aspiration. The choice between narcotics and inhalation agents is an individual preference. The use of muscle relaxants allows one to optimize the surgical conditions and minimize the dose of inhalational agents, thus providing for a rapid recovery from anesthesia. Nitrous oxide may be used in these cases, since the bowel obstruction is not complete, nor is there accompanying ileus. Extubation is carried out with the infant fully awake and vigorous.

If the patient is well stabilized preoperatively, the postanesthetic recovery is rapid, and feeding can begin within hours. Most infants may be discharged in 24–48 hours following surgery.

Duodenal Atresia

Duodenal atresia is associated with a high incidence (20%) of other congenital anomalies, the most significant ones, in terms of their medical implications, are trisomy 21 and cardiac defects. Other gastrointestinal malformations, such as esophageal atresia and imperforate anus, frequently occur in the same infant. Failure of the developing gut to recanalize is proposed as the developmental defect in duodenal atresia,

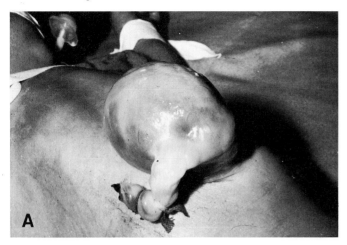

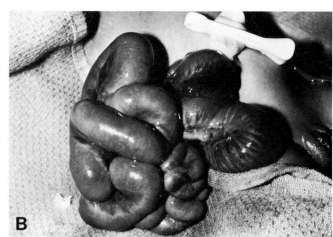

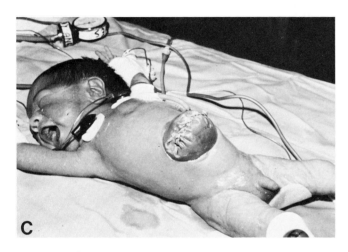

Figure 13-7. Large omphalocele (A) covered with membranous sac. Defect arises at the umbilicus. Large gastroschisis is shown in (B). Note absence of membranous sac. Silon pouch (C) is used to cover large gastroschisis. (Courtesy Dr. S. Kim)

although some cases of duodenal obstruction are caused by extrinsic compression from an annular pancreas.[108] A maternal history of polyhydramnios is a suggestive finding, which is also true for the other intestinal obstructive lesions.[109]

The diagnosis is usually straightforward; bilious vomiting beginning soon after birth is the classic clinical presentation. X-ray confirmation is made by the presence of the "double-bubble" sign formed by air contrast of the dilated stomach and proximal duodenum. The remaining bowel is devoid of air, and therefore abdominal distension is minimal.

The risk of bile and gastric fluid aspiration is significant, even after decompression by a nasogastric tube, so precautions must be taken to prevent regurgitation and aspiration during induction through awake intubation, or rapid-sequence induction with cricoid pressure. Intraoperative fluid resuscitation is required, but is less than in lower intestinal obstruction. The mortality from duodenal atresia repair is low and dependent on the severity of the associated anomalies rather than the intestinal obstruction.

Atresia of the Small Intestine

Compared to duodenal atresia, the majority of small bowel atresias are due to intrauterine mesenteric vascular occlusion and not defective embryogenesis.[110] The clinical syndrome is similar to duodenal atresia, except that abdominal distension and intravascular volume depletion are more prom-

inent features. In neonates with isolated jejunal or ileal atresia the outlook for recovery is good. In a proportion of these infants, however, intestinal atresia occurs in association with malrotation of the gut, volvulus, abdominal wall defects, and prematurity, which increase the overall mortality.[111]

Malrotation and Midgut Volvulus

During development, as the bowel migrates from the yolk sac back into the abdomen, interruption or incomplete rotation of the intestines around the fixed mesentery results in the condition known as malrotation. In addition to producing abnormal anatomic positioning (i.e., the ileocecal valve positioned in the right upper quadrant), malrotation predisposes the bowel to formation of atretic segments and the dire complication of midgut volvulus. These both result from kinking or compression of the vascular supply within the twisted mesentery.

Early recognition of this developmental anomaly is vital to the outcome, since in cases of midgut volvulus any delay may result in necrosis of the entire small intestine.[111] Rapidly increasing abdominal girth and passage of blood in the stool are ominous signs, in which case immediate surgical intervention is imperative. Fluid and electrolyte resuscitation may therefore have to be undertaken intraoperatively, with the aid of central venous and intra-arterial pressure monitoring. Prolonged ICU admission with long-term parenteral nutritional support can be expected, and even with the best of care the mortality in these neonates is quite high.

Necrotizing Enterocolitis (NEC)

This is a serious and potentially life-threatening condition occurring in the newborn. Its onset is usually within the first two weeks of life, and it may occur as early as the first day of life (16% of cases). It is a condition of low birth weight infants in particular, characterized by partial or generalized necrosis of the mucosa and sometimes the submucosa of the small and/or large bowel. It is often associated with high risk factors such as premature rupture of the membranes with chorioamnionitis, birth asphyxia, shock (inadequate perfusion), respiratory distress syndrome, patent ductus arteriosus, and recurrent apnea.[112,113] Added risk factors include umbilical vessel catheterization and infusion of hypertonic solutions. Infectious agents may be responsible, as the condition has occurred in outbreaks and has been associated with specific bacterial and viral organisms. In addition, overzealous feeding and hyperosmolar formulas have been incriminated; most cases have followed feeding.[114,115]

Signs may be subtle, such as abdominal distension and gastric residuals, or more overt, with blood in the stools. Spells of apnea and bradycardia, as well as temperature instability, may occur. Thrombocytopenia is often present. X-rays of the abdomen may reveal a fixed loop of bowel and edema of the bowel wall. A definitive diagnosis on x-ray is characterized by pneumatosis intestinalis or intramural air. In severe cases air is sometimes seen in the portal venous system.[116]

In the early phase of the disease, before progression to necrosis and perforation, infants respond well to medical therapy. This includes nasogastric suctioning, resuscitation with fluids and electrolytes, and systemic antibiotic therapy. All enteral feeds are stopped and the bowel is placed at complete rest.[117–119] The indication for surgical intervention in the course of the disease is evidence of bowel perforation or peritonitis. Toward this end, the infant is monitored closely with repeated abdominal x-rays to screen for perforation. The stools are monitored for the presence of occult blood. Other signs, such as abdominal wall edema, hyperemia, and tenderness of the abdomen, suggest possible peritonitis and the need for surgical exploration.

Anesthetic management includes fluid and electrolyte resuscitation, platelets, and fresh frozen plasma (FFP) for thrombocytopenia and disseminated intravascular coagulation (DIC), correction of acid–base abnormalities, hypocalcemia, and the placement of arterial and central venous catheters. It should be noted that these infants are critically ill and require large volumes for resuscitation, thus necessitating several large-bore intravenous lines. This disease often results in generalized peritonitis, analogous to a peritoneal burn, so it is not unusual to require one or more blood volumes of 5 percent albumin or FFP to maintain intravascular volume. The need for pharmacologic cardiovascular support, usually dopamine, is common. A central venous line will help in the postoperative monitoring and provide a route for total parenteral nutrition, which will be required for some weeks. Postoperative respiratory support may be necessary. Prognosis with medical therapy is usually very good. A number of these infants, however, develop late strictures of the colon, which require resection.[120] There is a high mortality when perforation has occurred.

Meconium Ileus

This condition occurs in 10–15 percent of newborns with cystic fibrosis, and symptoms of intestinal obstruction begin soon after birth. It presents either as terminal ileal obstruction caused by viscid meconium, or as bowel atresia. All infants with distal small bowel atresia should therefore be screened for cystic fibrosis. Perforation with peritonitis may complicate the course. In the past, surgical intervention was required to clear the obstructing viscid meconium. However, most cases now can effectively be treated by hyperosmolar enemas with, for example, meglumine diatrizoate (Gastrografin).[121,122] It is important to appreciate that the hyperosmolar agent will draw water into the gut and can produce severe hypovolemia and electrolyte imbalance. In these instances intravenous fluid replacement is necessary and hydration should be closely monitored following the procedure. When enema treatment is ineffective operative treatment is carried out; meconium is removed, and the gut is irrigated with acetylcysteine.

Hirschsprung's Disease

Hirschsprung's disease is the result of an absence of parasympathetic ganglion cells (Auerbach's and Meissner's plexus) in the large intestine, producing a non-peristaltic segment of variable length, and a tonically contracted anorectal sphincter.[123] The defect is usually confined to the rectosigmoid but can involve the entire colon. Neonates who develop a functional obstruction at the level of the affected segment are diagnosed early, but some patients are not recognized until months of increasing constipation prompts investigation.[124] Progression of this disease causes the normal bowel to become dilated, and ultimately either a perforation occurs or the condition known as "toxic megacolon" (enterocolitis) intervenes. Enterocolitis is caused by invasion of the bowel wall, and then the blood stream, by enterobacteria and their toxins.[125] Either of these conditions can be lethal but the infant with toxic megacolon is most at risk because actual or incipient septic shock is the presenting condition. Corrective measures to restore hemodynamic stability and treatment for sepsis must be instituted before surgery. Once one of these complications has occurred the mortality increases dramatically (to 30–35%).[125]

Imperforate Anus

As an isolated anomaly imperforate anus presents no specific anesthetic problems beyond those of anesthetizing a neonate. In 25–75 percent of cases, however, other congenital malformations are present, and their seriousness is the primary determinant of morbidity and mortality.[126,127] Ten percent of infants with imperforate anus also have esophageal atresia with and without a tracheoesophageal fistula. The presence of this anomaly must therefore be specifically excluded. Some of these neonates demonstrate all the malformations which comprise the VATER syndrome. Other intestinal atresias which complicate the management also occur in patients with anorectal malformations. Genitourinary anomalies comprise the largest group associated with imperforate anus, but only the more serious defects, such as bilateral renal dysgenesis/agensis have a major impact on mortality.[128–130]

Provided the infant has no other congenital malformations and the imperforate anus is noted shortly after birth, before signs of obstruction and ileus develop, the anesthetic risk is reduced to little more than that of elective surgery. Except for defects that involve only the superficial layers, which can be corrected at the first procedure, most newborns undergo a colostomy, and complete reconstruction is undertaken at a later time. In complex malformations with genitourinary involvement, a series of staged operations can be expected.

REFERENCES

1. Goudsouzian NG, Morris RH, Ryan JF: The effects of a warming blanket on the maintenance of body temperatures in anesthetized infants and children. *Anesthesiology* 39:351–353, 1973

2. Wilkinson A, Yu VY: Immediate effects of feeding on blood-gases and some cardiorespiratory functions in ill newborn infants. *Lancet* 1:1083–1085, 1974

3. Keens TG, Bryan AC, Levison H, et al: Developmental pattern of muscle fiber types in human ventilatory muscles. *J Appl Physiol* 44:909–913, 1978

4. Usher R, Lind J: Blood volume of the newborn premature infant. *Acta Paediatr Scand* 54:419–431, 1965

5. Usher R, Shephard M, Lind J: The blood volume of the newborn infant and placental transfusion. *Acta Paediatr Scand* 52:497–512, 1963

6. Gross GP, Hathaway WE, McGaughey HR: Hyperviscosity in the neonate. *J Pediatr* 82:1004–1013, 1973

7. Brinkman CR, Johnson GH, Assali NS: Hemodynamic effects of bradycardia in the fetal lamb. *Am J Physiol* 223:1465–1469, 1972

8. Engelke S, Shah BL, Vasan U. et al: Sodium balance in very low-birth-weight infants. *J Pediatr* 93:837–841, 1978.

9. Fanaroff AA, Wald M, Gruber HS, et al: Insensible water loss in low birth weight infants. *Pediatrics* 50:236–245, 1972

10. Oh W, Karecki H: Phototherapy and insensible water loss in the newborn infant. *Am J Dis Child* 124:230–232, 1972

11. Scanlon JW, Krakaur R: Hyperkalemia following exchange transfusion. *J Pediatr* 96:108–110, 1980

12. Maisels MJ, Li TK, Piechocki JT, et al: Effect of exchange transfusion on serum ionized calcium. *Pediatrics* 53:683–686, 1974

13. Simmons MA, Adcock EW, III, Bard H, et al: Hypernatremia and intracranial hemorrhage in neonates. *N Engl J Med* 291:6–10, 1974

14. Baens GS, Lundeen E, Cornblath M, et al: Studies of carbohydrate metabolism in the newborn infant. VI. Levels of glucose in blood in premature infants. *Pediatrics* 31:580–589, 1963

15. Fluge G: Clinical aspects of neonatal hypoglycemia. *Acta Paediatr Scand* 63(6):826–832, 1974

16. Milner RD: Neonatal hypoglycemia. *J Perinat Med* 7(4):185–194, 1979

17. Yeh TF, Luken JA, Thalji A, et al: Intravenous indomethacin therapy in premature infants with persistent ductus arteriosus—a double-blind controlled study. *J Pediatr* 98(1):137–145, 1981

18. Gartner LM, Snyder RN, Chabon RS, et al: Kernicterus: High incidence in premature infants with low serum bilirubin concentrations. *Pediatrics* 45:906–917, 1970

19. Brodersen R: Prevention of kernicterus, based on recent progress in bilirubin chemistry. *Acta Paediatr Scand* 66:625–634, 1977

20. Lovejoy FH, Jr: Fatal benzyl alcohol poisoning in neonatal intensive care units. A new concern for pediatricians. *Am J Dis Child* 136:974–975, 1982

21. Mountain KR, Hirsh J, Gallus AS: Neonatal coagulation defect due to anticonvulsant drug treatment in pregnancy. *Lancet* 1:265–268, 1970

22. Sugioka K, Woodley C: The use of transcutaneous oxygen electrodes in the presence of anaesthetic agents. *Can Anaesth Soc J* 28:498–505, 1981

23. Yelderman M, New W, Jr: Evaluation of pulse oximetry. *Anesthesiology* 59:349–352, 1983

24. Mihm FG, Halperin BD: Noninvasive detection of profound arterial desaturations using a pulse oximetry device. *Anesthesiology* 62:85–87, 1985

25. Erkan V, Blankenship W, Stahlman MT: The complications of chronic umbilical vessel catheterization. *Pediatr Res* 2:317, 1968

26. Brans YW, Ceballos R, Cassady G: Umbilical catheters and hepatic abscesses. *Pediatrics* 53:264–266, 1974

27. Hey E: Thermal neutrality. *Br Med Bull* 31(1):69–74, 1975

28. Stothers JK: Head insulation and heat loss in the newborn. *Arch Dis Child* 56:530–534, 1981

29. Nicodemus HF, Nassiri-Rahimi C, Bachman L, et al: Median effective doses (ED_{50}) of halothane in adults and children. *Anesthesiology* 31:344–348, 1969

30. Gregory GA, Eger EI, II, Mynson ES: The relationship between age and halothane requirement in man. *Anesthesiology* 30:488–491, 1969

31. Lerman J, Robinson S, Willis MM, et al: Anesthetic requirements for halothane in young children 0–1 month and 1–6 months of age. *Anesthesiology* 59:421–424, 1983

32. Gregory GA: The baroresponses of preterm infants during halothane anesthesia. *Can Anesth Soc J* 29:105–107, 1982

33. Diaz JH, Lockhart CH: Is halothane really safe in infancy? *Anesthesiology* 51:S313, 1979

34. Knill RL, Manninen PH, Clement JL: Ventilation and chemoreflexes during enflurane sedation and anesthesia in man. *Can Anaesth Soc J* 26:353–360, 1979

35. Steward DJ: Preterm infants are more prone to complications following minor surgery than are term infants. *Anesthesiology* 56:304–306, 1982

36. Liu LMP, Coté CJ, Goudsouzian NG, et al: Life threatening apnea in infants recovering from anesthesia. *Anesthesiology* 59:506–510, 1983

37. Robinson S, Gregory GA: Fentanyl-air-oxygen anesthesia for ligation of patent ductus arteriosus in preterm infants. *Anesth Analg* 60:331–334, 1981

38. Lou HC, Lassen NA, Friis-Hansen B: Impaired autoregulation of cerebral blood flow in the distressed newborn infant. *J Pediatr* 94:118–121, 1979

39. Quinn GE, Betts EK, Diamond GR, et al: Neonatal age (human) at retinal maturation. *Anesthesiology* 55:S326, 1980

40. Lucey JF, Dangman B: A reexamination of the role of oxygen in retrolental fibroplasia. *Pediatrics* 73:82–96, 1984

41. Merritt JC, Sprague DH, Merritt WE, et al: Retrolental fibroplasia: A multifactorial disease. *Anesth Analg* 60:109–111, 1981

42. Wolbarsht ML, Georse GS, Kylstra J, et al: Does carbon dioxide play a role in retrolental fibroplasia? *Pediatrics* 70:500–501, 1982

43. Nelson NM: Respiration and circulation after birth, in CA Smith, NH Nelson (eds): *The Physiology of the Newborn Infant.* Springfield, Charles C. Thomas, 1976, pp 117–262

44. Kelly DH, Shannon DC: Treatment of apnea and excessive periodic breathing in the full-term infant. *Pediatrics* 68:183–186, 1981

45. Koch G, Wendel H: Adjustment of arterial blood gases and acid base balance in the normal newborn infant during the first week of life. *Biol Neonat* 12:136–161, 1968

46. Frantz ID, Adler SM, Thach BT, et al: Maturational effects on respiratory responses to carbon dioxide in premature infants. *J Appl Physiol* 41:41–45, 1976

47. Rigatto H, Brady JP, Torre Verduzio R: Chemoreceptor reflexes in preterm infants. I. The effect of gestational and

postnatal age on the ventilatory response to inhalation of 100% and 15% oxygen. *Pediatrics* 55:604–613, 1975

48. Rigatto H, Torre Verduzio R, Cates DB: Effects of O_2 on the ventilatory response to CO_2 in preterm infants. *J Appl Physiol* 39:896–899, 1975

49. Ceruiti E: Chemoreceptor reflexes in the newborn infant: Effect of cooling on the response to hypoxia. *Pediatrics* 37:556–563, 1966

50. Nasal Obstructions, in Avery ME, and HW Taeusch (Eds): Schaffer's Diseases of the Newborn, 5th Edition. Saunders, Philadelphia 1984, pp 120–121

51. Jazbi B: Choanal Atresia, in Jazbi (ed): *Pediatric Otorhinolaryngology.* New York, Appleton-Century-Crofts, 1980, pp 159–164

52. Winther LK: Congenital choanal atresia. *Arch Dis Child* 53:338–340, 1978

53. Devgan BK, Harkins WB: Congenital choanal atresia—20 years experience. *Int Surg* 62(8):397–399, 1977

54. Holinger PH, Brown WT: Congenital webs, cysts, laryngoceles and other anomalies of the larynx. *Ann Oto Rhin Laryn* 76:744–752, 1967

55. Otherson HB: Tracheal stenosis. *J Pediatr Surg* 9:683–690, 1974

56. Stridors in the Newborn, in Avery ME and HW Taeusch (Eds): 5th Edition, Schaffer's Diseases of the Newborn. Saunders, Philadelphia, 1984, pp 122–127

57. Seid AB, Colton R: Tumors of the larynx, trachea and bronchi, in CD Bluestone, SE Stool (eds): Pediatric Otolaryngology, vol II. Philadelphia W.B. Saunders, 1983, pp 1312–1320

58. Lampe I, LaTourette HB: Management of hemangiomas in infants. *Pediatr Clin North Am* 6:511–528, 1959

59. Leiken-Sohn JR, Benton C, Cotton R: Subglottic hemangioma. *J Otolaryngol* 5:487–491, 1976

60. Louhimo I, Lindahl H: Esophageal atresia: Primary results of 500 consecutively treated patients. *J Pediatr Surg* 18:217–229, 1983

61. Woolley MM: Esophageal atresia and tracheoesophageal fistula 1939 to 1979. *Am J Surg* 139(6):771–774, 1980

62. Greenwood RD, Rosenthal A: Cardiovascular malformations associated with tracheoesophageal fistula and esophageal atresia. *Pediatrics* 57:87–91, 1976

63. Barry JE, Auldist AW: The Vater association: One end of a spectrum of anomalies. *Am J Dis Child* 128:769–771, 1974

64. Holder TM, Ashcraft KW: Developments in the care of patients with esophageal atresia and tracheoesophageal fistula. *Surg Clin North Am* 61(5):1051–1061, 1981

65. Rickham PP: Infants with esophageal atresia weighing under 3 pounds. *J Pediatr Surg* 16:595–598, 1981

66. Milligan DW, Levison H: Lung function in children following repair of tracheoesophageal fistula. *J Pediatr* 95:24–27, 1979

67. Kirwan WO, Walbaum PR, McCormack RJM: Cystic intrathoracic derivatives of the forgut and their complications. *Thorac Cardiovasc Surg* 28:424–428, 1973

68. Crawford TJ, Cahill JL: Surgical treatments of pulmonary cystic disorders in infancy and childhood. *J Pediatr Surg* 6:251–255, 1971

69. Intrathoracic Tumors and Cysts, in ME Avery and HW Taeusch (Eds): Schaffer's Diseases of the Newborn. 5th Edition Saunders, Philadelphia 1984, pp 204–213

70. Eraklis AJ, Griscom NT, McGovern JB: Bronchogenic cysts. *New Engl J Med* 281:1150–1155, 1969

71. Weichert RF, Lindsay EJ, Pearce CW, et al: Bronchogenic cyst with unilateral obstructive emphysema. *J Thorac Cardiovasc Surg* 59:287–289, 1970

72. Buntain WL, Isaacs H, Jr., Payne VC, Jr., et al: Lobar emphysema, cystic adenomatoid malformation, pulmonary sequestration and bronchogenic cysts in infancy and childhood. *J Pediatr Surg* 9:85–92, 1974

73. Rao CC, Krishna G, Grosfeld JL, et al: One-lung pediatric anesthesia. *Anesth Analg* 60:450–452, 1981

74. Hogg CE, Lorhan PH: Pediatric bronchial blocking. *Anesthesiology* 33:560–562, 1970

75. Murray GF: Congenital lobar emphysema. *Surg Gyn Obstet* 124:611–625, 1967

76. Hendren WH, McKee DM: Lobar emphysema in infancy. *J Pediatr Surg* 1:24–39, 1966

77. Pierce W, deParedes C, Friedman S, et al: Concomittant congenital heart disease and lobar emphysema in infants. *Ann Surg* 172(5):951–956, 1970

78. Coté CJ: The anesthetic management of congenital lobar emphysema. *Anesthesiology* 49:296–298, 1978

79. Schaffer AJ, Avery ME: Disorders of the diaphragm, in ME Avery and HW Taeusch (eds): Schaffer's *Diseases of the Newborn,* Philadelphia, W.B. Saunders, 1984, pp 189–192 5th Edition

80. Nguyen L, Guttman FM, et al: The mortality of congenital diaphragmatic hernia. Is total pulmonary mass inadequate, no matter what? *Ann Surg* 198:766–770, 1983

81. Reynolds M, Luck S, Lappen R: The "critical" neonate with diaphragmatic hernia: A 21-year perspective. *J Pediatr Surg* 19:364–369, 1984

82. Bohn DJ, James I, Filler RM, et al: The relationship between $PaCO_2$ and ventilation parameters in predicting survival in congenital diaphragmatic hernia. *J Pediatr Surg* 19:666–671, 1984

83. Hansen F, James S, Burrington J, et al: The decreasing incidence of pneumothorax and improving survival of infants with congenital diaphragmatic hernia. *J Pediatr Surg* 19:383–388, 1984

84. Rudolph AM, Yuan S: Response of the pulmonary vasculature to hypoxia and H^+ ion concentration changes. *J Clin Invest* 45:399–411, 1966

85. Vacanti JP, Crone RK, Murphy JD, et al: The pulmonary hemodynamic response to perioperative anesthesia in the treatment of high-risk infants with congenital diaphragmatic hernia. *J Pediatr Surg* 19:672–679, 1984

86. Drummond WH, Gregory GA, Heymann MA, et al: The independent effects of hyperventilation, tolazoline, and dopamine on infants with persistent pulmonary hypertension. *J Pediatr* 98(4):603–611, 1981

87. Filler RM, Erakilis AJ, Rubin VG, et al: Long term parenteral nutrition in infants. *New Engl J Med* 281:589–594, 1969

88. Fox HA, Krasna IH: Total intravenous nutrition by peripheral vein in neonatal surgical patients. Pediatrics 52:14–17, 1973

89. Kim SH: Omphalocele. Surg Clin NA: Pediatric Surgery. WW Hendren (Ed), 56(2):361–372, 1976

90. deVries PA: Pathogenesis of gastroschisis and omphalocele. *J Pediatr Surg* 15:245–251, 1980

91. Thomas DF, Atwell JD: The embryology and surgical management of gastroschisis. *Br J Surg* 63:893–897, 1976

92. Hoyme HE, Higginbottom MC, Jones KL: The vascular pathogenesis of gastroschisis: Intrauterine interruption of the omphalomesenteric artery. *J Pediatr* 98:228–231, 1981

93. Stringel G, Filler RM: Prognostic factors in omphalocele and gastroschisis. *J Pediatr Surg* 14:515–519, 1979

94. Combs JT, Grunt JA, Brandt IK: New syndrome of neonatal hypoglycemia associated with visceromegaly, macroglossia, microcephaly and abnormal umbilicus. *New Engl J Med* 275:236–243, 1966

95. Greenwood RD, Rosenthal AM, Nadas AS: Cardiovascular malformations associated with omphalocele. *J Pediatr* 85;818–821, 1974

96. King DR, Saurin R, Boles T: Gastroschisis update. *J Pediatr Surg* 15:553–557, 1980

97. Moore TC: Gastroschisis and omphalocele clinical differences. *Surg* 82:561–568, 1977

98. Filler RM, Eraklis AJ, Das JB, et al: Total intravenous nutrition:

An adjunct to the management of infants with ruptured omphalocele. *Am J Surg* 121:454–459, 1971

99. Mabogunje OA, Mahour GH: Omphalocele and Gastroschisis. Trends in survival across two decades. *Am J Surg* 148:679–686, 1984

100. Wayne ER, Burrington JD: Gastroschisis. *Am J Dis Child* 125:218–227, 1973

101. Mayer T, Black R, Matlak ME, et al: Gastroschisis and omphalocele: An eight year review. *Ann Surg* 192:783–787, 1980

102. Philippart AI, Canty TG, Filler RM: Acute fluid volume requirements in infants with abdominal wall defects. *J Pediatr Surg* 7:553–558, 1972

103. Ein SH, Rubin SZ: Gastroschisis-primary closure or silon pouch. *J Pediatr Surg* 15:549–552, 1980

104. Schuster SR: A new method for the staged repair of large omphaloceles. *Surg Gynecol Obstet* 125:837–850, 1967

105. Schwartz MZ, Tyson KRT, Milliorn K, Lobe TE: Staged reduction using a silastic sac is the treatment of choice for large congenital abdominal wall defects. *J Pediatr Surg* 18:713–719, 1983

106. Disorders of the Stomach. In ME Avery and HW Taeusch (eds): Schaffer's *Diseases of the Newborn*. Philadelphia, W.B. Saunders, 1984, pp 340–346

107. Touloukian RJ, Higgins E: The spectrum of serum electrolytes in hypertrophic pyloric stenosis. *J Pediatr Surg* 18:394–397, 1983

108. Boyden EA, Cope JA, Bill AH, Jr: Anatomy and embryology of congenital intrinsic obstruction of the duodenum. *Am J Surg* 114:190–202, 1967

109. Lloyd JR, Clatworthy HW, Jr.: Hydramnios as an aid to the early diagnosis of congenital obstruction of the alimentary tract. *Pediatrics* 21:1065–1073, 1958

110. Louw JH: Jejunoileal atresia and stenosis. *J Pediatr Surg* 1:8–23, 1966

111. Bishop HC: Small bowel obstructions from pediatric surgery. *Surg Clin North Am* 56(2):329–348, 1976

112. Kosloske AM: Pathogenesis and prevention of necrotizing enterocolitis: A hypothesis based on personal observation and a review of the literature. *Pediatrics* 74(6):1086–1092, 1984

113. Kliegman RM, Fanaroff AA: Necrotizing enterocolitis. *N Engl J Med* 310(17):1093–1103, 1984

114. Barlow B, Santulli TV: Importance of multiple episodes of hypoxia or cold stress on the development of enterocolitis in an animal model. *Surgery* 77:687–690, 1975

115. Franz ID III, L'Heureux P, Engel RR, et al: Necrotizing enterocolitis. *J Pediatr* 86:259–263, 1975

116. Leonidas JC, Hall RT, Amoury RA: Critical evaluation of the roentgen signs of neonatal necrotising enterocolitis. *Ann Radiol* 19:123–132, 1976

117. Brown EG, Sweet AY: Preventing necrotizing enterocolitis in neonates. *JAMA* 240:2452–2454, 1978

118. Kliegman RM, Fanaroff AA: Neonatal necrotizing enterocolitis: A nine-year experience. *Am J Dis Child* 135:603–607, 1981

119. Santulli TV, Schullinger JN, Heird WC, et al: Acute necrotising enterocolitis in infancy: A review of 64 cases. *Pediatrics* 55:376–387, 1975

120. Krasna IH, Becker JM, Schneider KM, et al: Colonic stenosis following necrotizing enterocolitis of the newborn. *J Pediatr Surg* 5:200–206, 1970

121. Rowe MI, Seagram G, Weinberger M: Gastrografin-induced hypertonicity. The pathogenesis of a neonatal hazard. *Am J Surg* 125:185–188, 1973

122. Noblett HR: Treatment of uncomplicated meconium ileus by Gastrografin enema: A preliminary report. *J Pediatr Surg* 4:190–197, 1969

123. Tiffan ME, Chandler LR, Faber HK: Localized absence of the ganglion cells of myenteric plexus in congenital megacolon. *Am J Dis Child* 59:1071–1078, 1940

124. Swenson I, Shuman JO, Fisher JH: Diagnosis of congenital megacolon: An analyses of 501 patients. *J Pediatr Surg* 8:587–594, 1973

125. Schnaufer L: Hirschsprung's Disease. *Surg Clin North Am* 56(2):349–359, 1976

126. Santulli TV, Schullinger JN, Kiesewetter WB, et al: Imperforate anus: A survey from the members of the Surgical Section of the AAP. *J Pediatr Surg* 6:484–492, 1971

127. Atkins JC, Kiesewetter WB: Imperforate anus. *Surg Clin North Am* 56(2):379–394, 1976

128. Singh MP, Haddadin A, Zachary RB, et al: Renal tract disease in imperforate anus. *J Pediatr Surg* 9:197–202, 1974

129. Smith ED: Urinary anomalies and complications in imperforate anus and rectum. *J Pediatr Surg* 3:337–342, 1968

130. Wiener ES, Kiesewetter WD: Urologic abnormalities associated with imperforate anus. *J Pediatr Surg* 8:151–159, 1973

14

Pediatric Emergencies

I. David Todres
Charles B. Berde

Anesthesiologists may become involved in pediatric emergencies both in the administration of anesthetics for emergency surgery and in their roles as consultants for airway management, resuscitation, and intensive care. This chapter will outline basic principles of resuscitation, describe the approach to anesthetic management for emergency pediatric surgery, and outline selected common clinical problems, including basic pathophysiology, management in the emergency room or intensive care unit, and anesthetic considerations for the operating room.

RESUSCITATION

ORGANIZATION

As with adults, the approach to the pediatric emergency patient begins with assessment of the adequacy of the Airway, Breathing, and Circulation, and restoration of these "ABCs" if any are deficient. Several basic points in pediatric cardiopulmonary resuscitation (CPR) deserve mention. A resuscitation effort should be organized and methodical. There should be a single, highly trained individual who directs the effort and to whom all questions are referred. If too few people are present, a call for assistance should be made; conversely if too many bystanders are present, they should be sent away. The use of "code" teams should be encouraged. Unlike adult arrests, the majority of which are primarily cardiac in origin, a great number of pediatric arrests begin with loss of airway patency (e.g., epiglottitis, foreign bodies, or croup), loss of respiratory drive (e.g., apnea, coma secondary to head injury, or metabolic derangement), or respiratory failure and fatigue (e.g., asthma, bronchiolitis, or pneumonia). It is therefore worth emphasizing that restoration of airway patency and ventilation of the lungs with 100 percent oxygen should be considered primary in every arrest *before* preoccupation with the ECG, vascular access, and medications. Airway management should be delegated to experienced individuals when available. A systematic teaching effort in pediatric CPR should be in effect, with regular "mock codes" conducted by residents, nurses, and attending physicians from the anesthesia department, emergency ward, and the intensive care unit.

AIRWAY MANAGEMENT

Clearing the airway first involves opening the mouth and anterior displacement of the mandible with extension at the atlanto-occipital joint. Extreme neck extension in small children may obstruct the airway. Oral airways may be required when head extension and mandibular displacement are inadequate. Following airway opening and application of 100 percent oxygen, ventilation should be assessed. If inadequate, a bag and mask should be used. If the appropriate size bag and mask are unavailable, use mouth-to-mouth breathing. Face mask and bag ventilation, or mouth-to-mouth breathing, should precede efforts to intubate the trachea, and intubation efforts should not result in prolonged periods without ventilation. For patients in cardiorespiratory arrest, oral intubation under direct vision is preferred because it is the quickest and most direct method. For patients in respiratory failure with effective circulation, the intubation technique chosen depends on a number of factors including age, size, underlying disease (neck fracture, jaw wired, coagulopathy), state of consciousness, and ability to resist attempts at intubation. "Blind" nasal intubation is rarely performed in the child. In small children, a nasal tube can cause considerable bleeding from the adenoids, and the cephalad or anterior position of the larynx may make the blind approach more difficult. Blind nasal intubation may increase

Table 14-1

Guidelines for Chest Compression and
Ventilatory Rates During Cardiopulmonary
Resuscitation (CPR)

Age	Chest Compressions	Ventilatory Rates
Neonate	120	40
Infant	100	20
Child	80	16
Adolescent	60	12

Note the consistent ratio of 5:1 for all ages; except the
neonate which is 3:1.

edema or bleeding in a burned or otherwise inflamed airway, which would make subsequent attempts to visualize the larynx more difficult. However, nasotracheal intubation under direct vision, with the aid of a Magill forceps, is often the preferred route for stabilization.

The use of muscle relaxants for intubation is predicated on confidence in one's ability to intubate rapidly, or to ventilate adequately by mask if attempts at intubation fail. If the suction fails, or the resuscitation bag valve becomes stuck with secretions, or the laryngoscope does not work, etc., there is a risk associated with the use of relaxants; it is imperative that the benefits of their use outweigh the risk. Conversely, if the equipment is readily available and functional, if there are experienced individuals present, and if a patient cannot be intubated by a nasal or oral approach with the aid of topical anesthesia, sedation, or force (for example, a patient in severe status epilepticus with clenched teeth), then muscle relaxants may be invaluable. For situations in which a patient cannot be ventilated by mask or intubated, physicians should be prepared to perform cricothyroidotomy with a 12-, 14-, or 16-gauge intravenous catheter-over-the-needle set. (Fig. 5-15) The catheter can be attached to the adapter from a 3 millimeter endotracheal tube, which can then be connected to a breathing circuit or oxygen-insufflation system. A recent study confirms that in animals with weights up to 30 kilograms, such a system can support oxygenation for up to 30 minutes, allowing for more definitive airway management.[1]

CHEST COMPRESSION

Ensuring adequate perfusion while effectively ventilating the patient is essential when circulation has failed. Chest compression/ventilation rates are described in Table 14-1. The optimal method for chest compression in the neonate is encircling the chest with both hands (Figure 14-1).[2] In the young child the heel of one hand should suffice, while in the child over approximately eight years of age the traditional two-handed adult method is employed.[3]

Synchronization of compressions and ventilation is a subject of debate. However, present recommendations consist of a sequence of compressions alternating with ventilation for most effective oxygenation. An alternative technique (i.e., simultaneous compressions and ventilation) appears on preliminary study to provide better perfusion than standard CPR techniques. However, at this stage it is still considered experimental.[4,5]

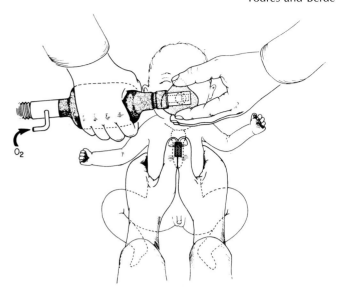

Figure 14-1. Chest encircling method for cardiac compression of the neonate; recent guidelines recommend thumb pressure just below the nipple line.[63] (Reproduced with permission from Todres ID, Rogers MC: Methods of external cardiac massage in the newborn infant. *J Pediatr* 86:781–782, 1975.)

VASCULAR ACCESS

Venous access in pediatric resuscitation may be difficult because children have small veins, the veins may be hidden within adipose tissue, and many acute situations follow intravascular volume depletion with associated venoconstriction. Efforts to cannulate jugular or subclavian veins should not impede airway and ventilatory efforts. If peripheral access is not readily available, it is often more reasonable to insert a femoral venous line or a saphenous vein cutdown. It should be emphasized that sources of bleeding and fluid loss may be subtle, and that constant reassessment of the adequacy of fluid and blood replacement is necessary.

In pediatric resuscitations the patient may be intubated before venous access is obtained. In these cases, many drugs, including epinephrine, atropine, and lidocaine (*not* calcium, dextrose, or bicarbonate), may be readily absorbed through the tracheal-bronchial mucosa via the endotracheal tube.[6]

DRUGS

Drug dosage in pediatric resuscitations may often be a problem. In following "milligram/kilogram" rules, decimal point errors are made, leading to serious errors in drug dosage. We recommend that physicians who deal with pediatric resuscitation infrequently, but handle adult "codes" often, should keep in mind the following simple algorithm in Table 14-2. The guidelines are based on age because physicians are generally more accurate in estimating age than weight. As with all medication regimens, doses should be scaled upwards or downwards according to individual situations. These guidelines give an estimate in emergency situations, and provide a check for the correct order of magnitude of doses derived from milligram/kilogram estimates. Precise dosage recommendations can be found in the table on the inside cover.

ANESTHESIA FOR EMERGENCY PEDIATRIC SURGERY

Emergency anesthetic care begins with assessment of the urgency of the child's problems and an ordering of priorities. For example, in the child with an epidural hematoma and a closed femoral fracture, treatment of the former condition by emergency craniotomy takes precedence over setting of the fracture. Some general principles are outlined in the following sections.

HISTORY AND PHYSICAL EXAMINATION

Unless the condition is so urgent that immediate resuscitation and intervention are needed, one should begin with a preoperative history and physical examination to assess the problem, with special attention being paid to medications, allergies, and any existing medical conditions.

RESUSCITATION

For critically ill and profoundly hypotensive patients who need an immediate operation, one should begin by establishing a clear airway and providing oxygenation and ventilation, and hemodynamic support with fluids, blood, and vasopressors. Under these circumstances, only scopolamine or diazepam for amnesia, and neuromuscular blocking agents for immobility, should be used; when conditions stabilize, other agents (narcotics, inhalation anesthetics) can be added as tolerated.

AIRWAY CONTROL

Some urgent situations are characterized by a compromised airway, such as epiglottitis, croup, and laryngeal trauma. In these situations, the urgency of securing the airway takes priority despite the risks associated with a "full stomach" (see section on full stomach below). In adults, such situations are often managed by awake intubation, either under direct laryngoscopy, "blind" nasal intubation, or by using a fiberoptic laryngoscope. Such an approach is favored in many situations because it "doesn't burn bridges," i.e., the patient maintains spontaneous ventilatory efforts. While such an approach is useful in many types of respiratory failure in infants and children, it may often seriously impair an already compromised airway in children who struggle during intubation attempts. An alternative approach is to anesthetize the child with halothane in oxygen, maintain and assist spontaneous ventilatory efforts, and perform laryngoscopy under deep inhalation anesthesia.

"FULL STOMACH"

Children approaching emergency surgery must be considered to have a "full stomach." Even those who have not recently eaten may have considerable gastric contents because of the increased acid secretion and delayed gastric emptying caused by acute pain and fear. When the child's problem is not urgent, it may be appropriate to delay surgery for a period of six to eight hours (using intravenous fluids to prevent deficits) to increase the likelihood of an empty stomach. If a delay of at least two hours is possible, there may be an indication for the use of cimetidine (7.5 mg/kg) and metoclopramide (0.2–0.4 mg/kg)

Table 14-2

Guidelines for Approximate Estimation of Drug Dosages in Children

Age	Fraction of adult dose
7 yr	1/2 (0.5)
1 yr	1/4 (0.25)
1 mo	1/8 (0.125)
Newborn	1/10 (0.10)

by an intravenous or intramuscular route in order to decrease gastric acidity and increase gastric emptying.[7,8] Whenever there is a possibility of a full stomach, and careful physical examination of the airway reveals no specific likelihood of a difficult intubation, it is generally best to proceed with a rapid sequence induction. This consists of preoxygenation, cricoid pressure, rapid administration of an induction agent such as thiopental and a muscle relaxant such as succinylcholine, followed by laryngoscopy and intubation.[9,10] Although this sequence is ideal for protection against aspiration pneumonitis, it carries a number of associated risks (e.g., an inability to intubate the trachea), which must be weighed against the benefit of diminished risk of aspiration. As noted earlier, such an approach presumes that intubation will be straightforward, or at least that ventilation with a mask while maintaining cricoid pressure will be possible. It should be noted that in such a sequence the ability to intubate is presumed, not tested. The smaller the child, the more rapidly the patient will become hypoxemic during apnea due to the smaller ratio of functional residual capacity to oxygen consumption.[11] Whereas most adults can maintain oxygenation for up to eight minutes of apnea following denitrogenation, newborns can become hypoxemic in less than one minute. Rapid-sequence induction can also be a considerable source of risk for patients with cardiovascular disease. It is difficult to titrate the anesthetic dose to the patient's needs in a controlled fashion, and a given dose of thiopental may lead to either profound hypotension due to myocardial depression and vasodilatation (especially in patients who are hypovolemic or who have high levels of sympathetic tone), or to severe hypertension due to inadequate anesthesia. If there is a contraindication to the use of succinylcholine (e.g., crush injury, acute burns, myopathy, or malignant hyperthermia), a rapid induction may be accomplished by use of a non-depolarizing relaxant without significant histamine release, such as pancuronium or vecuronium usually in a dose of 1.5–2.0 times the ED_{95}.

HYPOVOLEMIA AND INTRAVASCULAR VOLUME EXPANSION

When it is not urgent to operate immediately, it is advisable to replace fluid and electrolyte deficits and severe blood loss prior to induction. Mild to moderate deficits can be replaced with crystalloid solutions. In severe hypovolemia, with ongoing blood loss, 5 percent albumin is a useful intravascular volume expander while awaiting blood. The rational use of blood component therapy is discussed in Chapter 11.

HYPOVOLEMIA AND KETAMINE

Ketamine is often favored as an induction agent in hypovolemic patients. Ketamine is a very good analgesic and supports blood pressure by its action in releasing endogenous catecholamines.[12] In large doses, however, it may be a direct myocardial depressant.[13] Small induction doses (1–2 mg/kg IV) in moderately hypovolemic patients carry less risk. The concommitant use of diazepam has been reported to diminish the incidence of bad dreams and other unpleasant emergence phenomena, but diazepam has also been reported to attenuate the catecholamine release by ketamine, and this may diminish its margin of safety in the setting of uncorrected hypovolemia.[14]

PREMEDICATION

Premedication for emergency procedures is generally administered by the intravenous route. For children who are hemodynamically stable, who have no airway compromise, and especially for those who are in pain, narcotics are recommended. Anesthetics currently in use rarely cause profuse secretions, and therefore the use of antisialogogues prior to induction should be reserved for specific indications. In infants and small children, intravenous administration of anticholinergics immediately prior to induction has three potential benefits; (1) maintenance of cardiac output by increasing heart rate, (2) prevention of reflex bradycardia secondary to airway manipulations, and (3) prevention of bradycardia secondary to either succinylcholine or halothane.

ANXIETY AND FEAR IN PATIENTS AND PARENTS

Emergency surgery is generally a great source of fear and anxiety to both children and their parents. A calm and reassuring presence on the part of the anesthesiologist can be of great benefit to both parties, and can make induction of anesthesia smoother. The importance of clear and straightforward explanation of all procedures to children and their parents cannot be overemphasized.

SPECIAL PROBLEMS

AIRWAY PROBLEMS

General Principles of Airway Management

The general principles of managing acute upper airway obstruction must be appreciated. Once the basic principles of airway management have been followed then the specific therapy for the underlying cause may be undertaken.

The child presenting in the emergency room with acute upper airway obstruction may exhibit inspiratory stridor, tachypnea, sternal and intercostal retractions, agitation (which may be due to hypoxemia), cyanosis, and tachycardia. It is important to appreciate that the child may show few of these symptoms and signs, yet progress rapidly to a life-threatening state.

The initial response to this critically ill child should be to administer oxygen to correct hypoxemia and to keep the child as calm as possible to prevent dynamic collapse of the airway

(Fig. 5-8).[15] Evaluation should then proceed according to the degree of respiratory distress. If the child is not cyanotic and has stable vital signs, then roentgenographic evaluation of the airway may be helpful in clarifying the cause of the obstruction.[16] When this is undertaken it is essential that the child be accompanied to the x-ray facility by personnel skilled and equipped to manage any airway compromise. In addition, the x-rays should be performed with the child in the upright position to avoid further airway obstruction associated with the supine position.

Blood gas analysis is not vital; whether a PaO_2 is 80 torr or 60 torr will not alter clinical events or the therapeutic response of the anesthesiologist. It is also difficult to interpret the PaO_2 when the precise amount of inspired oxygen is uncertain. While the $PaCO_2$ may provide a useful index of ventilatory efforts, obtaining an arterial sample may be attended by severe distress, and may dangerously compromise oxygenation. The procedure to obtain the blood sample may be so disturbing to the child that severe dynamic airway collapse may accentuate respiratory failure. It is thus a risk versus benefit issue, and the balance appears in most situations to swing toward the risks outweighing the benefits.

The need for insertion of an intravenous line also is usually not immediate. Placement of an intravenous line may also upset the child and also produce severe dynamic collapse of the airway. The primary focus of attention should be on the major problem, which is the airway. Placement of the intravenous line is deferred to the operating room, following induction of anesthesia.

Should the degree of upper airway obstruction be potentially life-threatening, the child is transported to the operating room where, under controlled anesthesia and monitoring, a clear airway is established. In the operating room the parents may be invaluable in pacifying the child in the anesthetic induction phase preventing further hypoxemia from dynamic airway collapse that occurs with crying and agitation. The parents' presence in an operating room is certainly an extraordinary procedure, but we have found it to be a humane and extremely helpful one for the child with severe airway compromise. Parents need be present only for the induction phase. In the operating room, our practice is to induce the child with halothane in oxygen, in either the sitting or supine position, depending on the child's degree of respiratory distress. Anesthesia is induced with a face-mask technique utilizing cricoid pressure to avoid aspiration from a full stomach. The cricoid pressure is established at a level of light anesthesia, when the child is able to tolerate it. If the anesthesiologist lays his or her fingers gently over the neck and gradually increases the pressure, then effective cricoid pressure may be obtained without distress to the child.

With the child lightly anesthetized and having adequate air exchange, an intravenous line is inserted and appropriate fluids and drugs administered. These children may be significantly dehydrated, especially if febrile with a prolonged period of inadequate oral intake. We therefore recommend rapid rehydration with 10–30 ml/kg of lactated Ringer's solution. In addition, the early administration of a vagolytic agent (e.g., atropine at a dosage of 0.02 mg/kg), is helpful in (1) diminishing secretions, (2) increasing heart rate and thus maintaining cardiac output in the face of myocardial depressant effects of the potent inhalational agents, and (3) blocking vagal reflexes associated with laryngoscopy and bronchoscopy.

The use of muscle relaxants to secure a clear airway is

fraught with potential dangers. This is because once the child is paralyzed, efforts at ventilation may be ineffective. Therefore it is vital that the anesthetic induction proceed with spontaneous respiratory efforts; this is a principle that applies to all children with compromised or potentially compromised airways.

As induction proceeds and the pupils begin to center, the child with chest-wall retractions may be helped by introducing continuous positive airway pressure (4–8 cm H_2O); this is effected by adjusting the "pop-off" valve, while allowing spontaneous respirations. This will aid in stabilizing the airway opposing the forces of dynamic airway collapse. As anesthesia is deepened, hypoventilation may occur, in which case the child's respirations must be assisted to prevent hypoxemia and hypercarbia. The child anesthetized with halothane is particularly prone to cardiac arrthythmias should hypercarbia develop. The use of an end-tidal CO_2 monitor may be helpful in guiding the degree of necessary assisted ventilation. With airway obstruction and potential hypoventilation, the induction process is slow. The anesthesiologist must be aware of this, as laryngoscopy performed at a "light level" may induce dangerous laryngospasm. We therefore wait until the child's eyes are centered and the rectus abdominus muscles are flaccid. Laryngoscopy is then performed and the larynx examined; the cause of the obstruction may then be evident (e.g., the swollen red epiglottis and aryepiglottic folds). If the supraglottic structures are normal and the cause of obstruction remains unclear, then bronchoscopy may be indicated to establish the cause of airway obstruction beyond the glottis (e.g., foreign body in the trachea or bronchus). Throughout the procedure close attention to the heart rate by means of a precordial stethoscope and electrocardiogram is important. *Slowing of the heart rate is indicative of hypoxemia and requires urgent attention.* Pulmonary edema may occasionally complicate airway obstruction from any cause and aggravate existing hypoxemia.[17]

When bronchoscopy is required, initial orotracheal intubation may be helpful in providing a clear airway and a route for aspiration of secretions. Once stabilized in this manner, the surgeon can then unhurriedly and in a well controlled situation perform the bronchoscopy. The procedure continues with the ventilating bronchoscope. It is important for the surgeon and anesthesiologist to have good rapport, since they are "sharing" the airway. There must be adequate ventilation and adequate visualization. This means that at regular intervals each of these must be alternated so that the child does not suffer from either inadequate bronchoscopic examination or from hypoxemia and hypercarbia. If at any time the child suddenly becomes cyanotic or bradycardic, the bronchoscope should immediately be withdrawn into the trachea, and the child ventilated effectively. To prevent hypoxemia, the anesthetic gas is carried in oxygen only. With the diagnostic evaluation completed, an endotracheal tube may need to be placed for therapeutic reasons. At this stage one may elect to change an orotracheal intubation to the nasotracheal route for better stability.

UPPER AIRWAY PROBLEMS

Epiglottitis

This is a life-threatening infection due to *Haemophilus influenzae*. The rapid onset and progression necessitates urgent diagnosis and treatment. In addition to the presenting symptoms of upper airway obstruction, the child with epiglottitis classically will demonstrate *drooling* and difficulty with swallowing. Usually the child is one to seven years of age, but the condition may occur in older children and adults.[18–20]

Our approach to this problem when it is diagnosed is to establish an artificial airway in all cases through endotracheal intubation. Tracheostomy is an alternative procedure preferred by some where there is less experience with stabilizing an endotracheal tube.[21]

Inspection of the epiglottis in the emergency room may increase airway obstruction by mechanisms previously discussed (viz, dynamic airway collapse), and therefore should be avoided. In the more stable child, x-ray confirmation of the diagnosis may be useful but is only undertaken when the clinical presentation is atypical. X-ray examination should be undertaken only if skilled personnel and adequate equipment can accompany the child to the x-ray facility.

In evaluating the x-ray for epiglottitis special attention should be given to the aryepiglottic folds, which may be inflamed and edematous prior to involvement of the epiglottis itself (Figure 14-2). Hence the condition should more appropriately be considered as a supraglottitis. The child in severe distress is immediately moved from the emergency room to the operating room in a well coordinated manner, under the supervision of the anesthesiologist, surgeon, and pediatrician. As described in the section on principles of management, the presence of the parents during transport and induction of anesthesia is particularly valuable in this condition.

After anesthetizing the child with halothane and oxygen (muscle relaxants are avoided because of the potential danger of loss of airway control), securing an intravenous line, rehydration and administration of atropine, an endotracheal tube is passed orally. A stylette is invaluable as it will give stability to the tube and allow its introduction through a partially obstructed orifice. If the epiglottis appears normal during laryngoscopy, inspection of the aryepiglottic folds is carried out, noting edema and inflammatory change. The tube chosen should be one size smaller than that ordinarily selected, to allow passage through the obstructed glottic opening and to avoid pressure necrosis.

If the anesthesiologist is unable to intubate the child, the surgeon who is standing by with bronchoscopy equipment should attempt to establish an airway either via the bronchoscope or, failing this, perform an urgent tracheostomy or cricothyrotomy.

Changing the oral endotracheal tube to a nasotracheal tube must only be performed if there is complete confidence in this procedure. If oral intubation was especially difficult, the tube should be left in place and well secured. At this time cultures are taken of the epiglottis and blood, and the patient is started on ampicillin and chloramphenicol intravenously, because of ampicillin-resistant strains of *H. influenzae*. The child is returned to the intensive care unit, making certain that his or her arms are in restraints to avoid accidental extubation.

Morphine (0.1 mg/kg) or diazepam (0.1–0.3 mg/kg) is administered intravenously to sedate the child. When sedation is administered, the child must be closely observed for potential respiratory depression. The tube is left in place for 36–48 hours. At this time an air leak usually appears around the tube, signalling the possibility of safe extubation. The child should also be improved clinically, i.e., less toxic, with a decreased fever and no respiratory distress. To confirm the time of safe extubation the child is given atropine (0.02 mg/kg), metho-

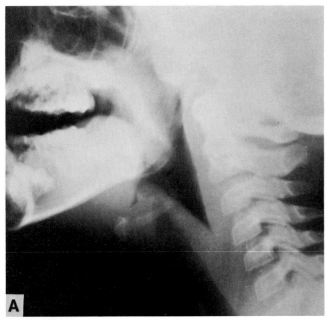

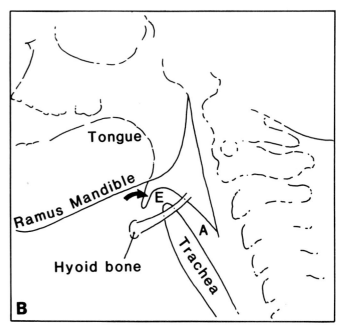

Figure 14-2. (A) Lateral neck roentgenogram of epiglottitis. (B) Line drawing of laryngeal structures. Note the marked thickening of the aryepiglottic folds (A), loss of the vallecula (arrow), and swelling of the epiglottis (E).

hexital (1–2 mg/kg), and succinylcholine (1 mg/kg) intravenously. The child is ventilated through the endotracheal tube and laryngoscopy is performed. If the supraglottic structures are considerably less edematous, with good visualization of the larynx, the child is then allowed to awaken. Once adequate respirations have returned, the child is extubated. Antibiotic therapy, which is modified according to the blood culture results, continues for 10 days.

The anesthesiologist should be aware that metastatic sites of infection may occur, leading to pleural, pericardial, or joint effusions, as well as pneumonia and meningitis (although the latter association is extremely rare).[22] The use of steroids to decrease swelling remains a controversial issue; studies are inconclusive at present.[23]

Laryngotracheobronchitis

This is a common condition in children from six months to six years of age. Occasionally it presents with life-threatening airway obstruction.[24,25] The etiology is usually viral; bacterial tracheitis due to *Staphylococcus* may present as a severe croup-like syndrome.[26] The differential diagnosis includes epiglottitis or foreign body (tracheal or esophageal). Usually the history and presentation are straightforward; however, roentgenographic evaluation may be helpful. This should be performed only when the child is stable and under the supervision of skilled personnel (Figure 14-3).

The onset of the disease is insidious. The child demonstrates a low-grade fever and a "croupy" cough with inspiratory stridor and chest retractions. When the condition is severe, the respiratory distress manifests as cyanosis in room air, severe sternal and costal retractions, and marked tachypnea and tachycardia. In this situation, in addition to giving oxygen for the associated hypoxemia, more aggressive therapy is indicated to relieve the obstruction. At this stage inhalation of nebulized racemic epinephrine (0.5 ml in 3 ml saline) with oxygen through a face mask may dramatically relieve the obstruction.[27,28] In a child who responds to racemic

epinephrine inhalation, repeated treatments one to four hours apart are often necessary. The child may experience a rebound effect, with increasing obstruction following an initial clearing of the airway. For this reason, children receiving racemic epinephrine therapy should be observed closely in the hospital setting.

If treatment with racemic epinephrine inhalation is unsuccessful, the underlying problem, in addition to edema, may be obstruction due to thick inspissated secretions. In this situation relief of the obstruction must be obtained through endotracheal intubation (our preference), or tracheostomy, both followed by vigorous suctioning. This procedure should be performed in the operating room under controlled anesthetic conditions as for the child with epiglottitis.

In the operating room the endotracheal tube selected should be at least one size smaller than would normally fit to avoid aggravating the subglottic edema and possibly causing subglottic stenosis. In children under two years of age a three millimeter internal diameter (ID) tube is used. After orotracheal intubation the tube may be changed to the nasotracheal position for improved stability. Our practice has been to intubate the trachea with an endotracheal tube for the child with life-threatening airway obstruction. However, some institutions have preferred to perform a tracheostomy under these circumstances because of the concerns for the development of subglottic stenosis.[29] This complication is now less commonly seen, since the introduction of implant-tested endotracheal tubes, and more importantly, insertion of smaller diameter tubes.[30] Should a tracheostomy be performed it should be noted that sudden cardiovascular collapse during the performance of the tracheostomy may indicate the presence of a tension pneumothorax. This occurs as a result of the very high negative pressure generated, which leads to dissection of air along paratracheal fascial planes and into the pleural cavity.

Steroid therapy has been advocated by some investigators, but their beneficial effects are still equivocal.[31,32] The child is

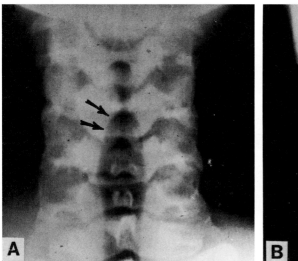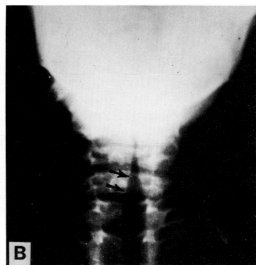

Figure 14-3. (A) Roentgenogram of the normal upper airway (A–P). Note the region below the vocal cords is rounded (arrows). (B). "Croup": markedly edematous tissue (arrows) fills in the normally rounded area forming a "sharpened pencil".

closely monitored in the intensive care unit, and special care is given to endotracheal suctioning of inspissated secretions. The tube is usually left in place for three to five days.

The time for extubation will depend on when the air leak develops around the tube indicating resolution of the subglottic pathology. With an adequate air leak (appearing at 10–20 cm H_2O peak inflation pressure) awake extubation may be undertaken in the pediatric ICU. Morphine given intravenously may be helpful if the child is especially anxious. Where there is minimal air leak (at pressures above 30 cm H_2O), then extubation is more safely carried out in the operating room under general anesthesia. Following extubation, the child is closely observed for retractions and tachycardia. When stabilized, the child is returned to the pediatric ICU. The degree of respiratory difficulty following extubation occasionally necessitates re-insertion of the endotracheal tube. In the pediatric ICU, stridor due to glottic edema after extubation may necessitate treatment with racemic epinephrine inhalation. A single dose of steroids prior to extubation is thought by some investigators to protect against post-extubation edema.

Foreign Body Aspiration

Any child who arrives at the emergency room with a presumptive diagnosis of foreign body aspiration requires emergency therapy. The child who is cyanotic, agitated, tachypneic, and tachycardic is in a life-threatening state. A history of choking and cyanosis while eating (particularly peanuts and popcorn), must arouse the strongest suspicion of foreign body aspiration. *The wheezing child may not necessarily be asthmatic but may be a child who has aspirated a foreign body.*[33,34] Agitation may be interpreted as a state of emotional upset when it is due to serious underlying hypoxemia.

If the child is severely distressed, immediate plans should be made to remove the foreign body in the operating room. If the child is stable, then roentgenographic examination of the airway may be helpful in identifying and localizing the foreign body. However, it should be appreciated that most foreign bodies are not radiopaque. Atelectasis or hyperinflation are often clues to the presence of a foreign body (Figure 14-4).

The removal of the foreign body requires skilled anesthesia and surgery. Anesthetic problems include hypoxemia and possible hypercarbia. The potential full stomach of the child will test the skill of the anesthesiologist. In addition, prolonged anesthetic induction must be anticipated due to the ventilation/perfusion ($\dot{V}/\dot{Q}$) abnormality associated with airway obstruction. The principles of anesthetic management are similar to those used with epiglottitis.

There has been much concern about forcing the foreign body distally in the airway, with assisted ventilation during anesthetic induction. For this reason spontaneous ventilation is advocated. However, our primary concern must be to provide optimal oxygenation and ventilation, especially when anesthetic induction includes inhalational agents (e.g., halothane), which are potent respiratory depressant and arrhythmia producing agents. Therefore gentle assisted ventilation may be necessary.

If a peanut has been aspirated, bronchoscopy should be undertaken without delay; there is an intense reaction in the bronchus to the peanut oil that may lead to complete obstruction and atelectasis. The swelling of the bronchial wall makes removal much more difficult. Once the foreign body has been removed, further management should include support for the family; there is often much guilt accompanying this incident. The parents should be counseled to prevent future mishaps of this nature.

In a child with a suspected foreign body aspiration causing airway obstruction, one must consider the possibility that the foreign body has impacted in the esophagus and has produced airway compression (Figure 14-5).

LOWER AIRWAY OBSTRUCTION

The anesthesiologist should be familiar with the conditions of bronchiolitis and status asthmaticus. In terms of pathology, lower airways (terminal bronchioles) are obstructed

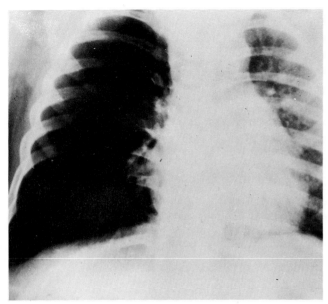

Figure 14-4. Roentgenogram of the chest demonstrating marked right sided hyperinflation due to airtrapping from ball-valve effect of the foreign body.

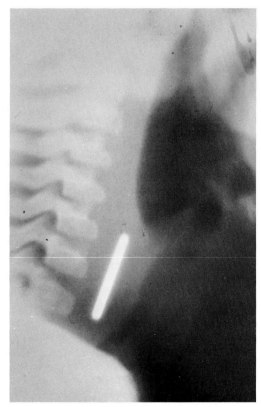

Figure 14-5. Roentgenogram of the lateral neck. Note tracheal compression from foreign body (coin) in the esophagus.

by edema, bronchiolar cellular infiltrate, mucous plugs, and varying degrees of bronchospasm. In the young infant with bronchiolitis, bronchospasm is thought to be less significant due to the relative lack of smooth muscle in the terminal bronchioles.[35] Bronchospasm becomes a critical factor in the child with asthma.

The obstruction of the terminal airways leads to trapping of air, with hyperinflation of the chest and an increase in the physiological dead space. This leads to an increase in the work of breathing in order to maintain a satisfactory $PaCO_2$. Ventilation/perfusion inequality develops, leading to hypoxemia. With increased distress, respiratory failure supervenes.

Early in the course of the illness, compensation may lead to a lower than normal $PaCO_2$. Increasing severity of the disease is reflected in increasing hypoxemia, hypercarbia, and acidosis. If this trend is not checked, progression to respiratory failure, myocardial depression, pulmonary hypertension, and death may follow.

Bronchiolitis

Viruses, especially respiratory syncytial virus (RSV) are the major etiologic agents of bronchiolitis; *M. pneumoniae* and *H. influenzae* are less frequent causes. The disease usually affects infants one to six months of age, although it may occur up to 12 months of age. It occurs especially in epidemic form during the winter months.[36,37]

The disease begins with an upper respiratory infection and fever. Tachypnea and retractions occur, and are usually associated with wheezing. The chest is hyperinflated, and diffuse crepitations are heard over both lung fields. The liver is displaced downwards as a result of the hyperinflation. Cardiac failure is likely to occur if the infant has underlying heart disease. Progressive exhaustion results in hypercarbia and respiratory failure. The diagnosis is usually established by the typical clinical picture. Detection of immunofluorescent antibodies for the respiratory syncyctial virus is easily accom-

plished through nasopharyngeal washings. The disease should not be confused with bronchopneumonia and cardiac failure.

The primary focus of treatment is administration of oxygen for the hypoxemia. Nebulized mist is traditionally used, but has not been shown to have any scientific merit.[38] Fluids are given through a nasogastric tube or intravenously.

Assisted ventilation is required for the small number of children who develop respiratory failure. Indications for ventilation will depend on the clinical picture and blood gas levels. There is no absolute $PaCO_2$ number which will dictate this course of action. The outcome is usually favorable. A significant number of the children will have episodes of asthma later in their lives.

Asthma and Status Asthmaticus

Asthma is characterized by recurrent episodes of wheezing or dyspnea associated with widespread narrowing of the intrapulmonary airways. A cardinal feature of the disease is its reversibility, either spontaneously or with therapy.[39–41] The wheezing in asthma is predominately expiratory. The anesthesiologist must appreciate that wheezing is not synonymous with bronchospasm. Although asthma is the commonest cause of wheezing in childhood, other causes must be considered (Table 14-3).

The asthmatic attack presents with increasing severity of airway obstruction. Wheezing with increasing cough and sputum production is seen. It is important to appreciate the fact that with increasing fatigue expiratory efforts may no longer generate a wheeze.

When there is an unsatisfactory response to three consecutive injections of epinephrine at 15-minute intervals, the term status asthmaticus is applied. At this point increasing dyspnea, fatigue with hypoxemia, and hypercarbia become life-threatening, and therapy is urgent. Aminophylline is administered as a continuous infusion or slow bolus with monitoring of the theophylline levels (therapeutic level should be 10–20 μg/ml). Corticosteroids and inhaled beta-adrenergic agents (e.g., metaproterenol) may be helpful in checking the progress of the disease (Table 14-4).[42–44] Should the disease progress in spite of this therapy, admission to the intensive care unit is required, where intravenous isoproterenol, under strict monitoring control, may be beneficial. If this therapy is ineffective or the child presents in extremis, however, then tracheal intubation and mechanical ventilation are necessary. Control of ventilation with the aid of muscle relaxants is often helpful. Atelectasis, pneumothorax, and pneumomediastinum are complications associated with this therapy.

Table 14-3

Causes of Wheezing in Children

Acute
  Foreign body in trachea, bronchus or esophagus
  Viral bronchiolitis
Recurrent or Persistent
  Asthma
  Foreign body
  Bronchiolitis, inhalation injury
  Cystic fibrosis
  Vascular ring
  Tracheal web or stenosis, bronchial stenosis
  Tracheomalacia
  Mediastinal glands (tuberculosis), cysts, tumors
  Obliterative bronchiolitis
  α_1-antitrypsin deficiency

Table 14-4

Drugs for the Treatment of Status Asthmaticus

Drug	Route of Administration	Dosage	Side Effects
β-adrenergic agents*			All β-adrenergic agents
Epinephrine			
Aqueous 1:1000	Subcutaneous	0.01 ml/kg (maximum 0.3 ml) q 15 min × 3	CNS stimulation Anxiety, restlessness Tremor Cardiac Tachycardia
Terbutaline	Subcutaneous	0.01 ml/kg (maximum 0.25 ml) q 30 min × 2	
Isoproterenol	IV	Start at 0.1 μg/kg/min; increase as tolerated	
Xanthine agent			
Aminophylline	IV	5 mg/kg loading dose over 15 min; then 0.9 to 1.1 mg/kg/hr; measure serum theophylline concentrations	CNS stimulation Anxiety, restlessness Seizures Cardiac Tachycardia Arrhythmias Renal Diuresis Gastrointestinal Nausea, vomiting
Corticosteroids			
Hydrocortisone	IV	7mg/kg stat and 7 mg/kg 24 hr by continuous infusion or 2 mg/kg/6 hr	Electrolyte imbalance, hypokalemia, hyperglycemia, fluid retention
Methylprednisolone		2 mg/kg stat and 2 mg/kg/24 hr by infusion or 0.5 mg/kg/6 hr	

* Parenteral forms.

Table 14-5

Effects of Low Perfusion on Organ Systems of the Body

- Respiratory failure due to development of adult respiratory distress syndrome (ARDS)
- Renal failure. The occurrence of renal failure significantly increases morbidity
- Cerebral edema with confusion and coma
- Decreased liver function with depressed drug metabolism and diminished clotting factors
- Gastrointestinal tract necrosis and bleeding
- Adrenal failure (uncommon)—more likely to occur in septic shock

In the child with an acute asthmatic attack who requires emergency surgery, one should first attempt to control bronchospasm and optimize oxygenation. However, the urgency of the surgical problem must be taken into account.

Induction of anesthesia may be carried out with traditionally used agents, i.e., thiopental or ketamine. Histamine releasing agents (e.g., morphine, curare) should be avoided, since equally efficacious alternative agents are available. Anesthesia is best maintained with potent inhalational agents, such as halothane, which at times appear to have effective bronchodilator properties.[45] Atropine has some bronchodilating effects but has the disadvantage of drying secretions, which may lead to mucous plugging.[46] However, atropine is indicated in this situation primarily for its cardiac vagolytic actions.

In the operating room, the occurrence of wheezing during anesthesia will necessitate an investigation of the underlying cause. It should be appreciated that wheezing under these circumstances may be due to mechanical problems related to the endotracheal tube (e.g., endobronchial intubation, plugging or kinking of the endotracheal tube, or herniation of the cuff).

For elective surgery, extubation is preferably carried out with the patient at a "deeper level" to prevent endotracheal, tube-induced bronchospasm.[47] For emergency surgery with a full stomach, however, extubation should be carried out with the patient awake with intact upper airway reflexes.

CIRCULATION (SHOCK)

The child presenting with a surgical emergency may be in a state of shock. Shock is defined as a condition where perfusion of blood to vital organs, with oxygen and substrate, is inadequate to meet metabolic demands. This inadequacy of blood flow may be due to:

- Hypovolemia (hypovolemic shock)—from loss of blood, plasma, electrolytes.
- Cardiac pump failure (cardiogenic shock)—sepsis, hypoxemia, tamponade.
- Loss of peripheral vascular resistance (toxic shock)—from sepsis, drug overdose, anaphylaxis.

In children, *hypovolemic shock is by far the most important cause*. Metabolic effects of hypovolemic and cardiogenic shock include lactic acidosis produced from anaerobic glycolysis due to diminshed oxygen transport to the tissues. In septic shock (high output shock), oxygen transport is not initially compro-

mised. Other factors that are not well understood account for the significant morbidity and mortality in this form of shock. The effects of low perfusion on organ systems of the body are presented in Table 14-5.

Hypovolemic Shock

Blood loss from trauma is the most common cause of shock in the child. Remember that the bleeding may be "hidden," as in an intra-abdominal rupture of liver or spleen. It should be appreciated that in the child compensatory mechanisms (e.g., vasoconstriction) to maintain perfusion are very active. The child may lose up to one quarter of his or her blood volume without changes in the heart rate or blood pressure. In addition, the child may focus attention on a minor injury, overlooking a more catastrophic one. It is therefore very easy for the anesthesiologist or surgeon to overlook the extent and gravity of the situation. Plasma loss is especially associated with burns and peritonitis. Electrolyte loss is commonly seen with diarrhea and vomiting, and also with ileus and intestinal obstruction. In sepsis, plasma proteins and electrolytes are lost via "leaking capillaries" (third space loss), and hypovolemia may be a significant component of septic shock.

Management of shock requires an evaluation of the degree of hemodynamic compromise and a search for its underlying cause. A secure intravenous line through which blood and fluids may be rapidly pumped is necessary. Blood and fluid resuscitation is carried out while attempts are being made to stop ongoing bleeding. A useful approach to fluid resuscitation is shown in the algorithm (Figure 14-6). In addition to fluid resuscitation, attention must be paid to adequacy of oxygenation and ventilation. Adequacy of perfusion and response to treatment includes monitoring the parameters outlined in Table 14-6. The type of fluid infused remains a matter of debate, with some proponents of crystalloid resuscitation and others of colloid infusions.[48,49] Blood should be transfused if indicated as soon as appropriate crossmatching has been carried out. However, at times the urgency of the situation demands the use of either O-negative blood or type specific non-crossmatched blood.

Cardiogenic Shock

Cardiogenic shock is much less common in children; causes include myocarditis, sepsis, hypoxemia, pericardial tamponade (blood or air), primary heart disease, arrhythmias, or pneumothorax with mediastinal shift and decreased venous return. Cardiac output is the product of stroke volume and heart rate. Stroke volume is a function of preload, afterload, and myocardial contractility. The treatment of cardiogenic shock will depend upon identification of and treatment of the underlying cause. In addition, monitoring of preload, afterload, and contractility will facilitate the choice of appropriate therapy (vasodilator, vasoconstrictor, or inotrope). The use of a flow-directed pulmonary artery catheter (Swan-Ganz catheter) provides measurement of left-sided filling pressure, and through thermodilution, measurement of cardiac output and peripheral vascular resistance.[50]

Septic Shock

The pathophysiology of septic shock may involve several mechanisms. Sepsis will cause a profound vasodilatation, and a loss of peripheral vascular resistance leading to profound hypovolemia. Circulation is shunted away from capillary beds.

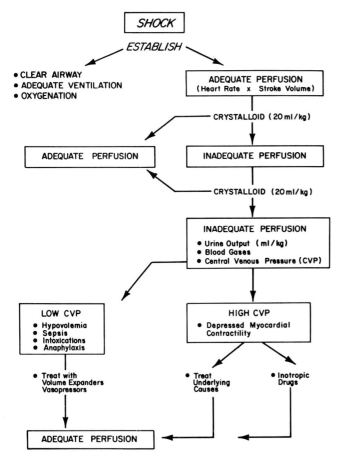

Figure 14-6. Algorithm for the management of the child in shock.

Table 14-6

Parameters of Adequacy of Perfusion

- Level of consciousness (head injury may confuse this evaluation)
- Perfusion of extremities—capillary refill and warmth
- Heart rate
- Blood pressure
- Urine output—greater than 1 ml/kg/hr
- pH—metabolic acidosis may indicate inadequate perfusion

vasodilatation, and hypotension. Treatment consists of ensuring adequate air exchange and oxygenation, administration of alpha-adrenergic agents to reestablish peripheral vascular resistance, beta-agonists to relieve bronchoconstriction, corticosteroids to diminish mediator formation and release, antihistamines to prevent ongoing release of histamine and fluids to support intravascular volume.[53]

STATUS EPILEPTICUS

A child is considered to be in status epilepticus when he or she has tonic–clonic movements for more than twenty minutes, or recurrent convulsions without recovery of consciousness between seizures. Seizures increase metabolic demands through their indirect effects on muscle metabolism and their direct effects on increasing the brain's metabolic requirements.[54,55] Thus, prevention of morbidity and mortality is related both to termination of the increased metabolic demands (stopping the seizures) and to maintenance of substrate supply by ensuring adequate oxygenation, ventilation, systemic and cerebral perfusion, and glucose stores. Status epilepticus is common in children with preexisting seizure disorders who have intercurrent infections, inadequate anticonvulsant drug levels, or noncompliance with medications. Deaths from status epilepticus may occur from compromise of ventilation and circulation by overzealous administration of anticonvulsants without adequate attention to respiratory and circulatory support.

Airway and Ventilation

The initial approach to the child with prolonged seizures is to establish a *patent airway,* administer supplemental oxygen, and assess ventilation. For many patients, an oral airway is very helpful for establishing and maintaining airway patency. Oral airways may also serve as bite blocks to help prevent injuries to the tongue and teeth. If the patient has an adequate natural airway, use the oral airway as the bite block only, since advancement of the airway posteriorly may provoke gagging and vomiting. For many patients, oral secretions and vomitus may occlude the airway. Increased muscle tone may make it difficult to ventilate these patients adequately with a bag and mask. In these cases tracheal intubation serves both to establish a patent airway and to help protect against aspiration pneumonitis. Assessment of the adequacy of ventilatory efforts can be difficult. Tonic–clonic movements can confuse the observer's interpretations of chest wall and diaphragmatic movements, and make auscultation of the chest difficult. Furthermore, these patients have a waxing and waning of their respiratory efforts. Oxygen demand and carbon dioxide production are also increased during seizures. For these rea-

Despite high cardiac output, tissue delivery of oxygen and substrate is compromised. In addition, sepsis may depress myocardial contractility. Sepsis may also lead to severe pulmonary artery hypertension and ventilation/perfusion abnormalities. Many children will initially have a hyperdynamic circulation, i.e., cardiac output will be greater than normal. This contrasts with hypovolemic shock and cardiogenic shock, where cardiac output is reduced. As septic shock progresses, however, the condition changes to a low output state with a very significant increase in morbidity and mortality. Management includes eliminating the underlying cause (e.g., appropriate antibiotics for meningococcemia), and the use of volume expanders and cardiac and vasoactive drugs (see Chapter 15, Tables 15-3 and 15-4). Corticosteroids have traditionally been recommended in overwhelming shock, but their effect on survival remains undetermined.[51,52]

Anaphylactic Shock

Anaphylaxis is the result of a hypersensitivity reaction to foreign substances, such as insect bites, drugs (IV, IM, PO), radiographic contrast media, or food. This response is mediated through immunoglobulin E (IgE), slow reacting substance of anaphylaxis (SRS-A, now identified as leukotrienes), and other compounds. *Anaphylactoid* reactions have a similar clinical manifestation, but are not mediated through IgE. In either situation the patient may present with laryngeal or bronchiolar edema, urticaria, generalized swelling and profound

sons, we recommend early intubation and assisted or controlled ventilation when there is uncertainty about the patient's respiratory efforts. The stomach should be routinely emptied with a nasogastric tube.

Circulation

The adequacy of blood pressure and systemic perfusion should be ensured. Patients are commonly hypertensive during seizures; hypotension should suggest causes such as drug effects (e.g., rapid administration of diphenylhydantoin), septicemia, or hypovolemia.

Intravenous Access and Laboratory Studies

Intravenous access must be secured, a blood sample taken for Dextrostix (Ames Division, Miles Laboratories, Inc., Elkhurst, IN) and blood glucose, electrolytes, and calcium Depending on the circumstances, it may be appropriate to include a toxic screen, anticonvulsant levels, and a blood culture. A bolus of glucose (0.5 gm/kg), or 2 ml/kg of 25 percent dextrose in water should be administered.

Anticonvulsants

Phenobarbital is traditionally the initial drug used to control seizures. If this is inadequate, then additional drug therapy is instituted—diphenylhydantoin, diazepam.

Phenobarbital. Phenobarbital (10 mg/kg initially, followed by an additional 10 mg/kg if seizures persist) is intermediate in onset (approximately 15 minutes) between diazepam and diphenylhydantoin. It has a prolonged anticonvulsive effect and causes some sedation and respiratory depression, particularly when administered in combination with diazepam. Although we strongly recommend the intravenous route for acute situations, it should be noted that phenobarbital can be given intramuscularly, resulting in a somewhat slower onset of action. In a situation in which there is difficult venous access, questionable ventilation, and only one physician or other trained individual present, it may be prudent to give phenobarbital intramuscularly while securing the airway; this approach would be preferred over ignoring the airway during prolonged attempts to start an intravenous line. If a patient has received a loading dose of phenobarbital (i.e., 20 mg/kg) and still has seizures, it is prudent to begin loading with diphenylhydantoin. Drug levels should be monitored, and drug dosages titrated to higher therapeutic levels.

Diphenylhydantoin. Diphenylhydantoin (10 mg/kg initially, followed by an additional 10 mg/kg if seizures persist) is extremely effective. Unlike diazepam and phenobarbital, it does not significantly depress respiration or sedate the child; these features make it especially useful in an acute setting, where ongoing neurologic assessment is required. Depending on the dose and the rate of administration, it is usually effective in about 30 minutes. Diphenylhydantoin must be infused in saline; dextrose causes immediate precipitation in the tubing. It should be administered at rates not greater than 1 mg/kg/min; more rapid administration can cause cardiac conduction disturbances and hypotension.

Diazepam. Diazepam (0.2–0.5 mg/kg) is the most rapidly acting agent in common use for terminating tonic–clonic movements; onset of effect occurs in one to two minutes. The duration of the anticonvulsant effect is very brief; it is there-

fore necessary to follow diazepam with other agents. Respiratory depression is common, especially when diazepam is administered in combination with phenobarbital. Administration of diazepam therefore requires that the physician be fully prepared to provide respiratory support. Diazepam is usually administered as a slow intravenous bolus; it is prone to precipitate in intravenous fluids if given as an infusion or mixed with other medications.

Anesthetics and Muscle Relaxants

A great majority of patients will stop tonic–clonic movements with the drug therapy described above; if they do not, use of anesthetics (such as thiopental) and neuromuscular blockers (such as curare or pancuronium) may be required. In this situation electroencephalographic monitoring to detect continuing seizure activity is essential.

Prevention of Injuries

Attention must be directed toward the prevention of injuries to the tongue, teeth, head, neck, back, and extremities due to tonic–clonic movements.

Establishing the Cause

Early in the course of treatment of status epilepticus, attention should be directed towards a differential diagnosis of the underlying causes of the seizure. A history of preexisting seizure disorder, infection, trauma, metabolic derangement, tumor, or systemic disease will often, but not always, clarify the cause. The head should be examined for evidence of trauma. The neck should be stabilized in all cases of suspected cervical trauma. Neurologic examination may be confusing; for example, focal deficits immediately following a seizure may reflect a structural lesion in the central nervous system, or a postictal (Todd's) paralysis with temporary and essentially reversible loss of function. Neurologic consultation and judiciously chosen diagnostic studies (CT scan, lumbar puncture, and EEG) should be obtained whenever the diagnosis is unclear. Treatable causes of seizures should always be sought first. The child with seizures occasionally presents with high fever, impending or active shock, and an appearance suggestive of overwhelming septicemia. This may occur in previously healthy infants and children, or it may occur in susceptible groups, including children with immunodeficiencies or malignancies. In these latter circumstances, it may be appropriate to obtain only a blood culture before administration of broad-spectrum antibiotics, such as ampicillin and chloramphenicol, and defer lumbar puncture. The reason for this approach is to avoid delaying urgent treatment of a life-threatening condition and the associated risks of performing the procedure with a patient in severe shock.

POISONING

Ingestions of toxic material in childhood are a phenomenon of two age groups; children under age five, and adolescents. The former frequently ingest medications and toxic substances found around the house; 90 percent of such ingestions occur in the home. Adolescents ingest alcohol and abuse drugs, for recreation, in response to peer pressure, and as a suicide attempt or gesture.

In many situations when the ingestion is recent, if the ingested substance is not caustic to the esophagus or the airway, it is possible to prevent absorption of considerable portions of the ingested material by use of emetics (Ipecac), adsorbents (activated charcoal), and cathartics (magnesium citrate).[56]

The anesthesiologist is consulted when there is apnea or hypoventilation with the need for assisted ventilation, when there is depression of protective airway reflexes, and when there is a need for protection of the airway from aspiration of gastric contents by use of an endotracheal tube. Depressed airway reflexes contraindicate the use of emetics; in this situation, passage of a nasogastric tube with an unprotected airway can also lead to vomiting and aspiration. In securing the airway, the anesthesiologist should be aware that assessment of the depth of a patient's sensorial depression may be subtle. Vomiting and aspiration may be triggered by laryngoscopy and intubation attempts, even in patients who appear deeply comatose.

Prior to laryngoscopy, the means for delivering positive pressure ventilation with oxygen, as well as suction, atropine, succinylcholine, laryngoscopes, and endotracheal tubes should be at hand. These patients should be preoxygenated, and cricoid pressure should be applied prior to intubation. Rapid changes in level of central nervous system depression may occur. Thus, if an oral tube is inserted, it is essential that a bite block or an oral airway be placed. Our general dictum is that *whenever a patient's ability to ventilate and protect his or her airway is questionable, the trachea should be intubated and ventilation assisted.*

In addition to airway protection, the anesthesiologist may be of help in the assessment and management of the hemodynamic effect of ingested medications (e.g., arrhythmias secondary to tricyclics, myocardial depression secondary to barbiturates). Familiarity with the pharmacology of many of the agents ingested (barbiturates, narcotics, anticholinergics), and facility with the clinical assessment of drug-induced depression of consciousness and cardiorespiratory reflexes make the anesthesiologist particularly helpful in the management of these problems.

TRAUMA

Trauma is a major cause of morbidity and mortality for infants and children. Automobile accidents, homicide, suicide, drowning, burns, and home accidents (falls, electrical injuries), are all common, frequently fatal, and, tragically, often preventable.[57]

EMERGENCY ROOM MANAGEMENT

Anesthesiologists should familiarize themselves with the equipment and protocols of the emergency room in their hospital before they attend to emergencies.

In the emergency room management of the trauma patient, rapid establishment of provisional diagnoses, and ordering of priorities are essential. The approach to the patient begins with support of respiration and circulation and control of external hemorrhage as outlined earlier. In establishing an airway, the possibility of laryngeal, tracheal, or bronchial injury must be considered. Trauma patients frequently have variations in their level of consciousness, and are at risk for hypoventilation and aspiration of gastric contents; they must be observed constantly as other diagnostic and therapeutic measures proceed.

Table 14-7

Priorities in Emergency Trauma Management

- Cardiorespiratory function
- External hemorrhage
- Injuries to great vessels
- Retroperitoneal injury
- Intraperitoneal injury
- Intracranial injury
- Burns and extensive soft-tissue injuries

In the emergency room, tracheal intubation of most patients with major trauma will proceed either with the patient awake, or as a rapid sequence with succinylcholine and judiciously chosen amounts of ketamine, thiopental, or methohexital. An exception is the child with severe head trauma and increased intracranial pressure. In these circumstances, adequate doses of thiopental, lidocaine, and/or fentanyl, with a relaxant such as pancuronium, may prevent further rises in intracranial pressure during intubation (see Chapter 17).

The anesthesiologist will commonly attend to respiratory and circulatory function for patients with major trauma, while surgical colleagues attend to diagnostic measures. It is important for the anesthesiologist to assess, with the surgeons, the probable nature of the injuries, so that they can evaluate the magnitude of bleeding, the anticipated physiologic effects of the injury and the nature of the surgical procedures planned. The order of priorities is presented in Table 14-7.[58] The approach to diagnosis and treatment is dictated by the degree of urgency. For example, a child with blunt abdominal trauma and profound shock would undergo urgent exploration in an attempt to stem the bleeding; a child with blunt abdominal trauma who is alert, has a blood pressure of 100/60, and has left shoulder pain and abdominal tenderness might undergo radiographic studies or abdominal paracentesis to establish a diagnosis. It is generally the task of the surgeon and radiologist to decide which studies are appropriate in a given situation. The responsibility of the anesthesiologist in these situations is to ensure that if the child is transported for these diagnostic studies there will be adequate attention to respiratory and circulatory function en route to and during these procedures.

The basic principles in the management of trauma proceed along similar lines in children and adults, with some minor differences. In young children, the clinical signs of major injury may be less apparent than in older patients. Since children cannot always verbalize their complaints, clinicians must look beyond the sites of visible injury or the sites of chief complaint. For example, a child with hip pathology may complain that his knee hurts, and a child with major abdominal injury and a femoral fracture may only complain about the fracture. Moreover, a child can often sustain major blood loss (up to 25% of their circulating blood volume) with a minimal change in vital signs. The clinician may therefore have little warning before severe hypovolemic shock ensues.

The spectrum of thoracoabdominal trauma is also somewhat different for children. Abdominal trauma is much more common than thoracic trauma,[59] and blunt trauma is much more common than penetrating trauma. Accidents involving automobiles are the single most common cause of abdominal trauma in children. In thoracic trauma, hemothorax and pneumothorax are common, and chest tube placement may be life-saving. The greater mobility of the mediastinum in children makes it more likely that tension pneumothorax will lead to hemodynamic compromise. Pneumothorax in children is frequently not heralded by rib fractures because of the child's compliant chest wall.

Head injury is common in childhood. Considerations related to airway and ventilatory management and intracranial pressure control are discussed in Chapter 17. The principles are similar to those in adults, with some differences. In newborns, traumatic delivery can lead to skull fractures and intracranial hematomas. Unlike adults, intracranial bleeding in newborns and infants can lead to hypovolemic shock, since the head is a larger fraction of the newborn's body, and the open fontanelles provide greater compliance and space for proportionately more blood loss.

Spinal cord injuries in children are relatively uncommon; they are most frequently seen in newborns after vaginal breech deliveries and in adolescents following falls, diving, or automobile injuries.

Child abuse should be considered when the history of the trauma appears improbable. Fundoscopic examination may disclose retinal hemorrhages, which will suggest occult head injury including subdural hematomas. Examination of the skin may show bruises of various ages, and a skeletal survey may reveal multiple fractures of various ages, occurring most typically at the metaphyses of long bones. It is the responsibility of every physician involved, including the anesthesiologist, to be aware of the possibility of abuse and to report their observations accurately to the appropriate authorities in their hospital. On occasion, a child who has previously been silent in the company of his or her parents will tell operating room or recovery room personnel about the events surrounding their injuries; such reports should be recorded and appropriate referrals should be made. Often abused children, particularly sexually abused children, are terrified of painful procedures and anesthesia; the need for sensitivity and reassurance in these settings cannot be overemphasized.

OPERATING ROOM MANAGEMENT

The general considerations of anesthetic management of the pediatric emergency, as outlined previously in the section on anesthesia for emergency surgery, are applicable for operating room management of the trauma patient as well. Establishment of the type of monitoring will depend on the particular circumstance. For a child who is critically ill, surgery should proceed without delay, and initially the monitoring may include only a stethoscope, blood pressure cuff, ECG, and a urinary catheter. As conditions permit, hemodynamic monitoring with arterial and central venous catheters may be established.[50,60,61] Arterial catheters are helpful in situations in which there is (1) a concern regarding the adequacy of ventilation and a need to sample arterial blood gases, (2) a need for frequent and repeated blood sampling (severe hemorrhage or metabolic derangement), (3) hemodynamic instability, and (4) a need to know and alter the blood pressure rapidly, such as with intracranial aneurysms. *In a setting with acute blood loss, establishment of secure large bore venous access is of higher priority than arterial access.* Following initial attention to ventilation and restoration of perfusion with infused fluids, blood, and vasopressors as needed, the anesthesiologist then begins to address the less acute but important concerns. If it

has not been possible to administer anesthetics or amnesics initially, they are administered in graded doses as soon as some stability is achieved. There is evidence in adult victims of major trauma that recall is very common; it is likely that this is at least as common in children.[62]

Hypothermia can exacerbate acidosis, cause arrythmias, potentiate neuromuscular blockade, and exacerbate coagulopathy. It occurs very commonly in victims of major trauma. As early as possible, measures to warm the patient should be instituted; these include warming the inspired gases, warming of blood and intravenous fluids, use of warming blankets, wrapping the head and extremities (cellophane, towels, plastic bags), and increasing the room temperature.

REFERENCES

1. Coté CJ, Jones D, Eavey RD, et al: Percutaneous cricothyrotomy with simple intravenous equipment. Section on Anesthesiology, American Academy of Pediatrics, Atlanta, April, 1985
2. Todres ID, Rogers MC: Methods of external cardiac massage in the newborn infant. *J Pediatr* 86:781–782, 1975
3. Standards and guidelines for cardiopulmonary resuscitation (CPR) and Emergency Cardic Care (ECC). *JAMA* 244:453–509, 1980
4. Donegan JH: New concepts in cardiopulmonary resuscitation. *Anesth Analg* 60:100–107, 1981
5. Chandra N, Rudikoff M, Weisfeldt ML: Simultaneous chest compression and ventilation at high airway pressure during cardiopulmonary resuscitation. *Lancet* 1:175–178, 1980
6. Roberts JR, Greenberg MI, Knaub MA, et al: Blood levels following intravenous and endotracheal epinephrine administration. J. Am. Coll. Emerg. Phys. *JACEP* 8:53–56, 1979
7. Goudsouzian NG, Coté CJ, Liu LMP, et al: The dose–response effects of oral cimetidine on gastric pH and volume in children. *Anesthesiology* 55:533–536, 1981
8. Albibi R, McCallum RW: Metoclopramide: Pharmacology and clinical application. *Ann Intern Med* 98:86–95, 1983
9. Sellick BA: Cricoid pressure to control regurgitation of stomach contents during induction of anesthesia. *Lancet* 2:404–406, 1961
10. Salem MR, Wong AY, Fizzotti GF: Efficacy of cricoid pressure in preventing aspiration of gastric contents in paediatric patients. *Br J Anaesth* 44:401–404, 1972
11. Cross KW, Tizard JPM, Trythall DAH: The gaseous metabolism of the newborn infant. *Acta Paediatr Scand* 46:265–285, 1957
12. White PF, Way WL, Trevor AJ: Ketamine—its pharmacology and therapeutic uses. *Anesthesiology* 56:119–136, 1982
13. Schwartz DA, Horwitz LD: Effects of ketamine on left ventricular performance. *J Pharmacol Exp Ther* 194:410–414, 1975
14. Jackson APF, Dhadphale PR, Callaghan ML, et al: Haemodynamic studies during induction of anaesthesia for open-heart surgery using diazepam and ketamine. *Br J Anaesth* 50:375–378, 1978
15. Wittenborg MH, Gyepes MT, Crocker D: Tracheal dynamics in infants with respiratory distress, stridor, and collapsing trachea. *Radiology* 88:653–662, 1967
16. Kushner DC, Harris GB: Obstructing lesions of the larynx and trachea in infants and children. Radiol Clin *North Am* 16: 181–194, 1978
17. Travis KW, Todres ID, Shannon DC: Pulmonary edema associated with croup and epiglottitis. *Pediatrics* 59:695–698, 1977
18. Blanc VF, Weber ML, Leduc C, et al: Acute epiglottitis in children: Management of 27 consecutive cases with nasotracheal intubation, with special emphasis on anaesthetic considerations. *Can Anaesth Soc J* 24:1–11, 1977
19. Lazoritz S, Saunders BS, Bason WM: Management of acute epiglottitis. *Crit Care Med* 7:285–290, 1979

20. Maze A, Bloch E: Stridor in pediatric patients. *Anesthesiology* 50:132–145, 1979

21. Oh TH, Motoyama EK: Comparison of nasotracheal intubation and tracheostomy in management of acute epiglottits. *Anesthesiology* 46:214–216, 1977

22. Molteni RA: Epiglottitis: Incidence of extra epiglottic infection. *Pediatrics* 58:526–531, 1976

23. Adair JC, Ring WH: Management of epiglottis in children. *Anesth Analg* 54:622–625, 1975

24. Davis HW, Gartner JC, Galvis AG, et al: Acute upper airway obstruction: Croup and epiglottitis. *Pediatr Clin North Am* 28:859–880, 1981

25. Baker SR: Laryngotracheobronchitis—a continuing challenge in child health care. *J Otolaryngol* 8:494–500, 1979

26. Jones R, Santos JI, Overall JC: Bacterial tracheitis. *JAMA* 242:721–726, 1979

27. Taussig LM, Castro O, Beaudry PH, et al: Treatment of laryngotracheobronchitis (croup). *Am J Dis Child* 129:790–793, 1975

28. Adair JC, Ring WH, Jordan WS, et al: Ten year experience with IPPB in the treatment of acute laryngotracheobronchitis. *Anesth Analg* 50:649–655, 1971

29. Downes JJ, Striker TW, Stool S: Complications of nasotracheal intubation in children with croup. *N Engl J Med* 274:226–227, 1966

30. Allen TH, Steven IM: Prolonged nasotracheal intubation in infants and children. *Br J Anaesth* 44:835–840, 1972

31. Leipzig B, Oski FA, Cummings CW, et al: A prospective randomized study to determine the efficacy of steroids in treatment of croup. *J Pediatr* 94:194–196, 1979

32. Tunnessen WW, Feinstein AR: The steroid–croup controversy: An analytic review of methodologic problems. *J Pediatr* 96:751–756, 1980

33. Blazer S, Naveh Y, Friedman A, et al: Foreign body in the airway. *Am J Dis Child* 134:68–72, 1980

34. Cohen SR, Herbert WI, Lewish GB, Jr, et al: Foreign bodies in the airway: Five year retrospective study with special reference to management. *Ann Otol Rhinol Laryngol* 89:437–442, 1980

35. Milner AD, Henry RL: Acute airway obstruction in children under five. *Thorax* 37:641–645, 1982

36. Wohl ME, Chernick V: State of the art: Bronchiolitis. *Am Rev Resp Dis* 118:759–781, 1978

37. McConnochie KM, Roghmann KJ: Bronchiolitis as a possible cause of wheezing in childhood: New evidence. *Pediatrics* 74:1–10, 1984

38. Bau S, Aspin N, Wood DE, et al: The measurement of fluid deposition in humans following mist tent therapy. *Pediatrics* 48:605–612, 1971

39. Commey JOO, Levison H: Physical signs in childhood asthma. *Pediatrics* 58:537–541, 1976

40. Blair H: Natural history of childhood asthma. *Arch Dis Child* 52:613–619, 1977

41. Todres ID: Asthma and status asthmaticus. *Semin Anesth* 3:98–105, 1984

42. Hendeles L, Weinberger M, Johnson G: Monitoring serum theophylline levels. *Clin Pharmacokinet* 3:294–312, 1978

43. Garra B, Shapiro GG, Dorsett CS, et al: A double-blind evaluation of the use of nebulized metaproterenol and isoproterenol in hospitalized asthmatic children and adolescents. *J Allergy Clin Immunol* 60:636–638, 1977

44. Downes JJ, Wood DW, Harwood I, et al: Intravenous isoproterenol infusion in children with severe hypercapnia due to status asthmaticus. Effects on ventilation, circulation, and clinical score. *Crit Care Med* 1:63–68, 1973

45. Hirshman CA, Berman NA: Halothane and enflurane protect against bronchospasm in an asthma dog model. *Anesth Analg* 57:629–633, 1978

46. Chick TW, Jenne JW: Comparative bronchodilator responses to atropine and terbutaline in asthma and chronic bronchitis. *Chest* 72:719–723, 1977

47. Schnider SM, Papper EM: Anesthesia for the asthmatic patient. *Anesthesiology* 22:886–892, 1961

48. Virgilio RW, Rice CL, Smith DE, et al: Crystalloid versus colloid resuscitation: Is one better? A randomized clinical study. *Surgery* 85:129–139, 1979

49. Tranbaugh RF, Lewis FR: Crystalloid versus colloid for fluid resuscitation of hypovolemic patients. *Adv Shock Res* 9:203–216, 1983

50. Todres ID, Crone RK, Rogers MC, et al: Swan-Ganz catheterization in the critically ill newborn. *Crit Care Med* 7:330–334, 1979

51. Crone RK: Acute circulatory failure in children. *Pediatr Clin North Am* 27:525–538, 1980

52. Perkin RM, Levin D: Shock in the pediatric patient. Part I. *J Pediatr* 101:163–169, 1982
Perkin RM, Levin D: Shock in the pediatric patient. Part II. *J Pediatr* 101:319–331 1982

53. Lucke WC, Thomas H, Jr: Anaphylaxis: Pathophysiology, clinical presentation and treatment. *J Emerg Med* 1:83–95, 1983

54. Volpe JJ: Neonatal seizures. *Clin Perinatol* 4:43–63, 1977

55. Delgado-Escueta AV, Wasterlain C, Treiman DM, et al: Management of status epilepticus. *N Engl J Med* 306:1337–1340, 1982

56. Holazo AA, Colburn WA: Pharmacokinetics of drugs during various detoxification procedures for overdose and environmental exposure. *Drug Metab Rev* 13:715–743, 1982

57. Rivera FP: Traumatic deaths of children in the United States: Currently available prevention strategies. *Pediatrics* 75:456–462, 1985

58. Streichen F. Emergency Management of the severely injured child, in Ravitch MM, Welch KJ, Benson CD, et al. (eds): *Pediatric Surgery.* Chicago, Yearbook Medical Publishers, 1979, pp 101–110

59. Welch KJ. Abdominal Injuries, in ed. Ravitch MM, Welch KJ, Benson CD, et al. (eds): *Pediatric Surgery.* Chicago, Yearbook Medical Publishers, 1979

60. Coté CJ, Jobes DR, Schwartz AJ, et al: Two approaches to cannulation of a child's internal jugular vein. *Anesthesiology* 50:371–373, 1979

61. Todres ID, Rogers MC, Shannon DC, et al: Percutaneous catheterization of the radial artery in the critically ill neonate. *J Pediatr* 87:273–275, 1975

62. Bogetz MS, Katz JA: Recall of surgery for major trauma. *Anesthesiology* 61:6–9, 1984

63. Standards and guidelines for cardiopulmonary resuscitation and emergency cardiac care. JAMA 255:2843–2989, 1986.

15

Cardiovascular Physiology and Pharmacology in Children: Normal and Diseased Pediatric Cardiovascular Systems

Paul R. Hickey
Robert K. Crone

The cardiovascular system of the infant differs from the adult in its physiologic and pharmacologic responses. Maturation of the cardiovascular system is rapid and dramatic in the perinatal period. The infant's cardiovascular physiology is therefore quite unlike the adult, especially during the first year. By age four or five, the cardiovascular system is essentially that of a small, very fit adult.

A host of congenital and environmental factors, such as toxins, infectious agents, radiation, and chemotherapy, interact with and alter the normal sequence of cardiovascular growth and development. Some factors affect primarily the cardiovascular system, while others cause secondary change in normal cardiovascular development through alterations in the pulmonary or other body systems. Congenital heart defects, however, are the primary factors altering postnatal cardiovascular development.

In healthy children, administration of anesthesia must be based on knowledge of cardiovascular development and the functional limitations present at any particular age; anesthesia in children with congenital and acquired heart disease should be based on this knowledge as well as the physiologic deviations resulting from the cardiac disease process.

Although the incidence of congenital heart defects has not changed, in the past several decades dramatic advances have been made in operative repair. As a result, more children with congenital heart disease are surviving after correction, and are subsequently presenting for other operative procedures. "Repair" of congenital heart defects does not necessarily result in normal cardiopulmonary physiology. Various kinds of cardiovascular dysfunction are irreversible and therefore remain after repair. In addition, the repair itself may cause some cardiovascular dysfunction. Knowledge of the cardiac dys-

function remaining after correction is important in order to deliver appropriate anesthetic management.

The normal developmental physiology of the infant cardiovascular system will be reviewed as a basis for understanding alterations in normal cardiovascular development. Departures from adult cardiovascular physiology and pharmacology which are particularly relevant to anesthetic management will be noted.

CARDIOVASCULAR PHYSIOLOGY IN CHILDREN

Our knowledge of cardiovascular physiology in infants and children stems primarily from animal studies of fetal, newborn, and young animals, as well as clinical studies. Extrapolation of these data is limited by species differences. Because of changes in the cardiovascular system with birth and growth, studies done at one point in this developmental continuum have limited applicability to other points. Thus, many of the data available must be extrapolated across both developmental and species differences in an attempt to understand pediatric cardiovascular physiology and pharmacology.

TRANSITIONAL CIRCULATION

The transition from fetal to adult circulation is a complex and incompletely understood process. The fetal circulation is a parallel circulation; both left and right ventricles supply systemic cardiac output (Figure 15-1). Oxygenated blood comes from the placenta via the ductus venosus and inferior vena cava. This oxygenated blood is shunted primarily across the

FETAL CIRCULATION (PARALLEL)

TRANSITIONAL CIRCULATION (SERIES OR PARALLEL)

NORMAL CIRCULATION (SERIES)

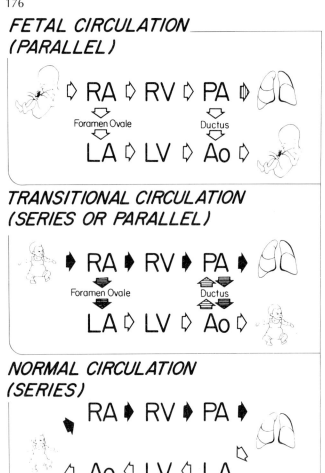

Figure 15-1. Schematic representation of course of circulation during transition from fetal type circulatory pattern to adult type circulatory pattern. Dark arrows represent totally desaturated blood, shaded arrows, partially desaturated blood, and light arrows represent saturated blood.

foramen ovale and ejected by the left heart into the ascending aorta. Return from the superior vena cava is directed primarily into the right ventricle and is ejected into the pulmonary artery, where most of the flow is shunted across the ductus arteriosus into the descending aorta so that pulmonary blood flow is minimal (seven percent of combined ventricular output).

The normal adult circulation is a series circulation, where each ventricle pumps the entire cardiac output into either the pulmonary or systemic circulation. At birth the abrupt transition to the adult circulatory pattern therefore imposes new demands upon the neonatal cardiovascular system, necessitating an intermediate stage, the transitional circulation.

The hemodynamic changes occurring at birth are outlined in Table 15-1. Before birth the fetal heart is well adapted to its parallel circulation, but it is poorly adapted to the loads placed on it by the abrupt change to the series, extrauterine adult type circulation that now incorporates the pulmonary circuit for oxygenation. During the time required to adapt to the altered demands of neonatal and infant life, cardiovascular reserve is much less than that found in late childhood and adulthood.

While the transition to an extrauterine type circulation is commonly thought to occur in minutes, the actual process may take hours, days, or even weeks as the fetal cardiovascular and pulmonary vascular systems adapt to the new demands. While removal of the placenta from the circulation, and expansion of the lungs, are abrupt events, the other changes in the circulatory pattern shown in Table 15-1 occur over a protracted period of time and require normal development. During these changes the infant's circulation is best thought of as an intermediate, transitional system that is initially quite unstable. The transitional circulation then becomes progressively more stable as developmental changes progress (Figure 15-1).

The primary factors in the instability of the transitional circulation are the ductus arteriosus, foramen ovale, pulmonary vascular resistance (PVR), and the immature heart. The instability of the newborn circulatory system is reasonably well tolerated and self-correcting as normal developmental mechanisms eliminate the causes of the instability. However, a number of conditions listed in Table 15-2 cause prolongation and exacerbation of the period of neonatal circulatory instability. The transitional circulation of the neonate immediately after birth is shown schematically in Figure 15-2. Pulmonary vascular resistance is high, and right-to-left shunting can take place across the patent ductus arteriosus (PDA) and foramen ovale, resulting in desaturation of the descending and ascending aorta respectively. This configuration has been inaccurately termed "persistent fetal circulation," although the placenta is no longer involved in the circulation.

As PVR decreases in the first few days of life, pulmonary artery pressures fall, the foramen ovale closes functionally, and shunting across the ductus arteriosus becomes left-to-right

Table 15-1

Hemodynamic Changes at Birth

Right Ventricle	Left Ventricle
Decreased afterload	Increased afterload
Decreased pulmonary vascular resistance	Low resistance placenta removed
Ductal closure	Ductal closure
Small increase in volume load	Large increase in volume load
66% of C.O. to 100% C.O.	34% cardiac output to 100+% cardiac output
Foramen oval closes	Increased pulmonary venous return
	Transient left-to-right ductal shunt

Table 15-2

Conditions Prolonging
Transitional Circulation

Prematurity
Pulmonary disease
    Hypoxemia
    Hypercarbia
Congenital heart disease
Sepsis
Acidosis
Hypothermia
High altitude
Prolonged stress

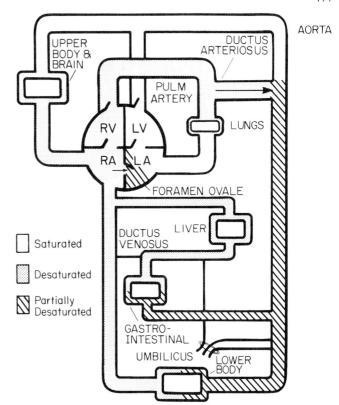

TRANSITIONAL CIRCULATION
HIGH PULMONARY VASCULAR RESISTANCE

Figure 15-2. Schematic diagram of transitional circulation of the neonate when pulmonary vascular resistance is high. Desaturated blood is shunted from the right atrium (RA) across the foramen ovale to partially desaturate the left atrial (LA) blood. Although not shown for purposes of clarity, this partially desaturated blood will flow into the left ventricle (LV) where it will be ejected into the ascending aorta and thence the upper half of the body. Fully desaturated blood from the pulmonary artery is shunted right-to-left across the patent ductus arteriosus into the descending aorta, desaturating the blood there.

(Figure 15-3). As the ductus arteriosus closes, usually by the second or third day of life, the circulation assumes the normal, adult pattern.

It has become increasingly clear that in the first weeks of postnatal life many of the normally occurring changes in the circulation may be prolonged, delayed, or reversed by the conditions listed in Table 15-2.

Most of the congenital problems requiring surgical intervention in the neonatal period, such as congenital diaphragmatic hernia, tracheoesophageal fistula, and intestinal obstruction, are associated with the conditions outlined in Table 15-2. Surgical and anesthetic manipulations further destabilize the transitional circulation, prolonging and increasing the shunting normally seen in this period. While persistence of the transitional circulation usually is potentially hazardous, in certain types of severe congenital heart disease the transitional circulation persists and is beneficial in maintaining life until operative intervention can be undertaken. In any case, an understanding of the factors governing the transitional circulation is thus vital for anesthetic care of all neonates.

Ductus Arteriosus

Closure of the ductus arteriosus occurs in two stages in normal infants, functional and anatomic.[1] Functional closure usually takes 24–48 hours; anatomic closure may take several weeks.[2,3] Until anatomic closure takes place many stimuli can cause the ductus to reopen (Table 15-2).

Functional Closure. Functional closure of the ductus arteriosis is due to contraction of its spirally arranged medial muscular layer; the mechanisms behind this contraction are not entirely understood.[1] A rise in the PaO_2 passing through the ductus is probably the most important factor.[4] This may only be true in the mature infant, however, since data from the fetal lamb demonstrate that the immature ductus does not contract even in extremely high concentrations of oxygen. The amount of contraction in response to increasing PaO_2 becomes greater, and the level of PaO_2 required to initiate a response falls, as full gestational age approaches.[5]

Prostaglandins E_1 and E_2 (PGE_1 and PGE_2) have been shown to markedly relax the ductus arteriosus, at both low and high arterial oxygen tensions.[6] It is now thought that high levels of circulating or locally produced prostaglandins help keep the ductus open during fetal life. In contrast to the low levels found in adults, these high levels are probably due in part to low fetal blood flow in the lungs, where prostaglandins

are metabolized, and in part to a substantial production of prostaglandins by the placenta. By using an inhibitor of prostaglandin synthesis, indomethacin, ductal closure can be induced in the neonatal period.[7]

While the ductus is only functionally closed, it is still responsive to changes in PaO_2 and PGE_1 infusion; reopening has been documented in a functionally closed ductus in infants older than seven days of age.[8–10] Presence of any of the factors listed in Table 15-2 can prolong patency, and thus prolong shunting in either direction through the persistent or reopened ductus, depending on relative pulmonary and systemic pressures.

Shunting through the patent ductus has been reported to be right-to-left, even in normal infants, for the first several hours of life.[11] Shunting then becomes predominantly left-to-right during the remainder of its patency, which may last up to two or three days in healthy full-term infants. Using pulsed Doppler echocardiography, patency has been documented in 20 percent of healthy infants at 48 hours of age.[12]

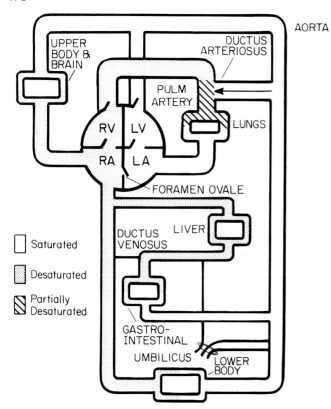

TRANSITIONAL CIRCULATION
LOW PULMONARY VASCULAR RESISTANCE

Figure 15-3. Schematic diagram of the transitional circulation of the neonate when the pulmonary vascular resistance has fallen. Foramen ovale is closed and no intracardiac shunting can occur at that point. Left-to-right shunting of fully saturated blood from the aorta is shunted across the patent ductus arteriosus into the pulmonary artery so that pulmonary arterial blood becomes only partially desaturated.

Anatomic Closure. After muscle contraction causes functional obliteration of the lumen by an infolding of the intima, permanent sealing of the lumen is produced by disruption and proliferation of subintimal layers, and hemorrhagic necrosis. This results in connective tissue formation and fibrosis, which is usually complete by two to three weeks of age. When ductal tissue is abnormal, the ductus can continue to be patent through infancy into adulthood.[1]

Pulmonary Vascular Resistance (PVR)

Pulmonary vascular resistance declines rapidly at birth, due in part to the expansion of the lungs with gas, and in part to direct exposure of pulmonary resistance vessels to alveolar oxygen. The fall in PVR and pulmonary arterial pressure continues at a rapid pace for the first day or two of life; by 24 hours of age pulmonary artery pressure usually falls below systemic pressure in normal infants. Both pulmonary vascular resistance and pressure continue to fall at a moderate rate throughout the first five or six weeks of life, and then at a more gradual rate for two to three years.[13,14]

The initial rapid fall of PVR in the first day of life is largely independent of growth and developmental changes. However, for pulmonary artery pressure and vascular resistance to fall to adult levels, there must be extensive remodeling of the

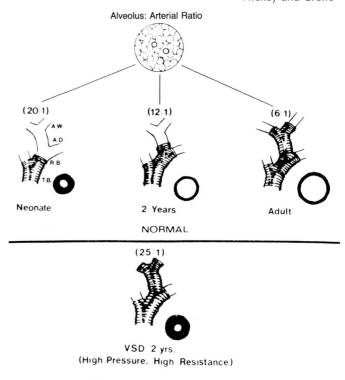

Figure 15-4. Developmental changes in peripheral pulmonary arterial tree in normal children and children with large left-to-right shunt (VSD). (Page 1117, Rabinovitch M, et al. Lung Biopsy in Congenital Heart Disease: A Morphometric Approach to Pulmonary Vascular Disease, Circulation 58:1107–1122, 1978. Reproduced with permission.)

pulmonary arterial tree. The thick muscular walls of the newborn pulmonary arteries thin dramatically as the muscle coat extends peripherally; the number of arterioles for each alveolus increases, and the arteriole lumen diameter also increases (Figure 15-4).[15,16] When any of the factors listed in Table 15-2 intervene during the neonatal period, this developmental fall in PVR may slow or even reverse, as in the case of some forms of congenital heart disease. This is exemplified by the pulmonary arterial vessels from a child with a ventricular septal defect (VSD) shown in Figure 15-4.

In the early neonatal period, PVR remains elevated and the muscular pulmonary bed is highly reactive. Noxious stimulation during this period can cause marked increases in PVR. The degree of hypoxic pulmonary vasoconstriction seen in normal newborns is much greater than in adults.[17] This vasoconstriction, when added to the already high PVR, can raise pulmonary arterial pressure in excess of systemic arterial pressure in the neonate, resulting in intermittent or continuous right-to-left shunting through the ductus arteriosus, foramen ovale, or other intracardiac defects.

Foramen Ovale

The foramen ovale closes functionally when mean left atrial pressures exceed mean right atrial pressures; this probably happens in the first few hours after birth. Atrial pressures measured in normal newborns in the first 14 hours of life showed an average mean left atrial pressure of 9 mm Hg, and an average mean right atrial pressure of 4.5 mm Hg.[18] Left-to-right shunting through the normal foramen ovale is prevented by the septum primum acting as a one-way flap valve. This functional closure does not become anatomically fixed until well into the first year of life. Probe patency of the foramen ovale exists in 50 percent of individuals up to five years of age, and in more than 25 percent over 20 years of age.[19] Any of the conditions in Table 15-2 which raise pulmonary arterial pressures can result in right-to-left shunting through the foramen ovale for at least the first month or two of life, and probably for much longer in many individuals.

This shunting across the foramen ovale has been demonstrated in both newborns with congenital heart disease and those with normal hearts having "persistent fetal circulation" with pulmonary hypertension.[20] It occurs because the increased right ventricular afterload raises right ventricular filling pressure, and therefore right atrial pressure, to levels in excess of those in the left atrium. In infants without pulmonary hypertension, coughing or the Valsalva maneuver have been shown to transiently increase right atrial pressures, resulting in right-to-left atrial shunting through the foramen ovale. This is probably the mechanism of "paradoxical" embolization of air or particulate matter into the left side of the circulation; this can also occur in adults.

DEVELOPMENTAL CHANGES IN THE CARDIOVASCULAR SYSTEM

The Heart

Gross Structural Changes. The changing demands on the heart during the postnatal period and later infancy are reflected in gross structural changes in the heart. At birth, right and left ventricular size and wall thickness are virtually equal, with the right ventricle being slightly heavier.[21] During the neonatal period, volume load and afterload on the left ventricle both increase appreciably, whereas there are only minimal increases in volume load, and substantial decreases in afterload, on the right ventricle. In response, the left ventricle becomes larger and more thickly walled than the right ventricle; by four weeks of age the left ventricle weighs more than the right.[22]

This process continues throughout infancy and early childhood, until the left ventricle becomes approximately twice as heavy as the right, which is the normal relationship in the adult.[21] This relative growth of the left ventricle and regression of the right ventricle are reflected in the right-to-left shift of QRS forces in the precordial leads of the electrocardiogram during infancy, and have also been demonstrated by echocardiography.[23,24]

Ultrastructural and Enzymatic Development. Concurrently with the physiologic and gross structural changes described above, changes also take place in the ultrastructure of the myocardial cells. At birth myofiber cells are small and round, with chaotically arranged myofibrils. This is in distinct contrast to the long cells with orderly rows of sarcomeres in adult myocardial tissue. Intercalated disks and the transverse tubular system are either absent or poorly developed in neonatal hearts, and appear only gradually. Nuclei, surface membranes, and other noncontractile mass needed for the synthesis of proteins during the active phase of myofiber hyperplasia and hypertrophy during infancy take up a relatively large proportion of the myofiber.[25] The result is that the fraction of cellular mass dedicated to contractile protein in the neonatal and infant myofiber is considerably less than that in the adult myofiber (30% versus 60%).[26] These differences in the organization, structure, and contractile mass of the young myofiber are partly responsible for the decreased functional capacities of the young heart.

Significant increases in enzymatic activity and aerobic capacity have been demonstrated in ventricular muscle mitochondria in the postnatal period.[27,28] During this same period mitochondria have been shown to change from relatively rudimentary structures with random intracellular distribution to structures with complex cristal development, which are carefully aligned and distributed among the myofibrils. The hearts of fetal animals are known to have a large anaerobic capacity, and fetal atrial and ventricular muscle tissue have been shown to be dependent on anaerobic metabolism.[29] This explains the high tolerance for hypoxia documented in newborn lambs and seen clinically in human newborns.[31] As changes in enzymatic activity and mitochondrial development progress during the neonatal and infant periods, this tolerance to hypoxemia is lost.

Electrophysiologic Changes. The electrophysiology of the myocardium changes as the cells mature; these postnatal changes coincide with alterations in the structure of the myofiber outlined above. These maturational changes in cellular morphology are accompanied by an increase in the ability of the cellular membrane and other subcellular organelles to sequester calcium.

Repolarization in neonatal Purkinje fibers of animals is consistently faster than adult fibers.[32,33] Action potential configurations differ between adult and neonatal Purkinje fibers in that neonatal action potentials are significantly shorter. Notable differences have been found between responses of adult and neonatal Purkinje fibers to ionized calcium and potassium.[32] Ionic events in the immature heart may thus differ significantly from the adult heart, until maturation of membranes and development of the sarcoplasmic reticulum and the transverse tubule system is complete. These differences in electrophysiology and, inferentially, membrane structure, may partially explain the different responses of the immature heart to various drugs, including anesthetics. This may also account for neonatal tolerance for heart rates of 200 or more, which would result in cardiovascular collapse in the adult.

Humoral and Autonomic Nervous Development in the Heart

The development of the autonomic innervation of the cardiovascular system is incomplete at birth. Significant changes take place during infancy, but the exact timing of these changes in the human is unknown, since large interspecies differences occur in autonomic development. Sympathetic innervation of the heart is known to be incomplete at birth, as evidenced by decreased cardiac catecholamine stores.[34] In addition, histochemical studies have demonstrated progressive ingrowth of sympathetic nerve endings in fetal and newborn hearts, and denervation-type hypersensitivity (lack of innervation) to norepinephrine has been found in neonatal sheep and dogs.[35,36] Recent studies in neonatal dogs have confirmed that adrenal integrity and circulating catecholamines are important in enabling the newborn ventricle to respond appropriately to sympathetic stimulation.[35,37]

Parasympathetic innervation of the heart has been shown

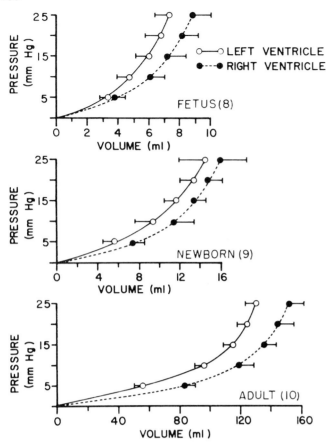

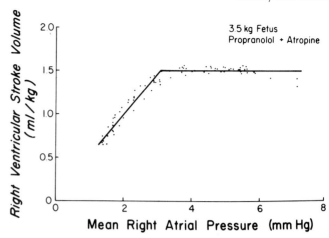

Figure 15-6. Right ventricular stroke volume and right atrial pressure relationships in a sheep fetus. Solid lines are linear regression lines. (Page H658, Thornburg KL, et al: Filling and arterial pressures as determinants of RV stroke volume in the sheep fetus. Am J Physiol 244:H656–H663, 1983. Reproduced with permission.)

Figure 15-5. Comparison of ventricular pressure–volume curves for fetal, newborn, and adult sheep. Differences between ventricles are significant only in adult. (Page 1288, Romero T, et al: A comparison of pressure-volume relations of the fetal, newborn, and adult heart. Am J Physiol 222:1285–1290, 1972. Reproduced with permission.)

to be complete at birth in newborn puppies when sympathetic responses were not present.[38] This is confirmed in human neonates and infants by the increased vagal tone that is often seen clinically.

Peripheral Circulation

Sympathetic innervation of peripheral tissues also appears to continue postnatally; vascular tone in the newborn also seems to be under more humoral than nervous control. Animal studies in postnatal puppies have shown that sympathetic nerve stimulation did not result in peripheral vasoconstriction until four weeks of age.[39] Harlequin color changes in the human newborn are thought to reflect immaturity of the peripheral circulation, as vasodilation of half of the body and blanching of the other half occur, with sharp midline demarcation.[40]

Functional Capacities of the Immature Heart

The maturational changes in the cardiovascular system outlined above result in alteration of the functional characteristics of the cardiovascular system. These functional limitations of neonatal and infant hearts must be understood in order to administer anesthetics safely.

The shift of the circulation to a series arrangement in the early neonatal period increases flows through relatively small

ventricles which had previously been handling only part of the systemic cardiac output in a parallel, fetal-type circulation. Immature hearts are significantly less compliant than adult hearts. This is due partly to their ultrastructure, since the immature myocardial cells have half as much elastic contractile mass and twice as much stiff membrane mass by weight, and partly to the increased flows in relatively small chambers. After birth, 100 percent of the total cardiac output passes through *each* ventricle in the series circulation, whereas prior to birth only a fraction of total cardiac output flowed through each ventricle. The results of these two factors are apparent in the pressure–volume relationships in the newborn ventricle shown in Figure 15-5.

Both ventricles are relatively noncompliant compared to the adult. This has two functional implications. First, the reduced compliance, together with the similarity in size and wall thickness during the first month of life, makes the interrelationship of ventricular function much more intimate.[21] Failure of either ventricle, resulting in increased filling pressures, quickly causes septal shift and encroachment on stroke volume of the opposite ventricle. Thus, in contrast to adults, congestive heart failure quickly becomes biventricular in infants.

The second functional implication is that the reduced compliance of these small hearts makes them very sensitive to volume overload and relatively restricted in their ability to change stroke volume. Figure 15-6 shows the Starling curve for the right ventricle of a full-term sheep fetus just before birth. Although stroke volume does change with filling pressure, the range over which increasing filling pressure results in increases in stroke volume is very restricted. The plateau of the Starling curve is reached at the very low filling pressures of 4 mm Hg, and stroke volume actually falls off at a filling pressure of about 7 mm Hg.[42] This function curve is clearly shifted to the left compared to older children and adults.

While cardiac output is not completely rate-dependent at low filling pressures, small amounts of fluid rapidly bring filling pressures to the plateau of the function curve where stroke volume is fixed; at this point output is strictly rate-dependent. Additional small amounts of fluids will push filling pressures to the descending part of the curve, where the ventricle begins to fail; because of the interdependence of ventricular function mentioned above, failure of the other ventricle will immediately ensue. Function curves for the left ventricle are similar to that shown for the right.[43–45] *Thus the normal immature heart is very sensitive to volume loading.* As growth and development of the heart occurs, the ascending limb of the Starling curve becomes longer and shifts to the right toward higher pressure levels, and the flat portion of the curve is reached at higher levels of filling pressure.

The immature structure of the young heart also results in poor tolerance for increased afterload on either side of the circulatory system. The rate and magnitude of active tension development by isolated immature ventricular muscle is decreased compared to mature muscle.[41] When afterload is increased to mean adult levels, both left and right ventricles in the intact immature heart are unable to sustain stroke volumes and filling pressures rise quickly. As afterload increases, the Starling function curve flattens and its peak is reached at even lower filling pressures, effectively shifting the ventricular function curve in a way similar to a negative inotrope.

The net result of these considerations is that the functional capacity of the neonatal and infant heart is generally reduced in proportion to age, and as age increases functional capacity increases. Increments of either preload or afterload result in failure of the young heart to adjust its cardiac output in the way that adult hearts do. *The stress of either volume or pressure loading is therefore handled poorly by the normal young heart.* The time over which growth and development overcome these limitations is uncertain and variable. When adult levels of systemic arterial pressure and PVR are achieved (by ages three or four), the above functional limitations probably no longer apply.

ALTERATIONS OF DEVELOPMENT AND FUNCTION BY PEDIATRIC HEART DISEASE

CONGENITAL HEART DISEASE

Normal cardiac and vascular development appears to the dependent on normal blood flow and pressure. Generally speaking, children with congenital heart disease have significant abnormalities of systemic and pulmonary flow and resistance, and therefore reduced functional cardiac reserve relative to their age.

The Pulmonary Circuit

Increased Flow. Increases in pulmonary blood flow and pressure resulting from left-to-right shunting can retard the normal decline in PVR and eventually cause pulmonary vascular disease similar to that shown in Figure 15-4.[46–48] Elevations in PVR become permanent (pulmonary artery hypertension) because of interference with normal growth and development of the pulmonary arterial tree.[49] This is true especially in lesions with high pulmonary blood flow, such as large ventricular septal defects, atrioventricular canal, transposition of the great arteries, and large patent ductus arteriosus. In lesions with high pulmonary flows, even where pulmonary pressures are intially normal (such as atrial septal defect and anomalous pulmonary venous return) pulmonary

vascular disease may result.[49,50] Although pulmonary vascular disease does not usually occur until after the first year of life, in complete atrioventricular canal, it may occur earlier.[51]

Decreased Flow. Decreased flow in the pulmonary circulation also results in abnormal development. In children with pulmonary atresia and hypoplastic left heart syndrome, there are significant abnormalities in size, number, and muscularity of small pulmonary arteries at birth.[49]

The Ventricles

Volume Overload. Volume overload of cardiac chambers results in dilatation, hypertrophy, and hyperplasia (in early postnatal life).[52] Exactly when these cardiac responses to increased volume loads become detrimental to normal cardiac function is unclear. However, volume overload results in symptoms of congestive heart failure in many infants with severe congenital heart disease. The extent to which these changes are reversible, resulting in return to normal cardiac function, also is unclear. The premature infant with a large left-to-right shunt through a PDA usually shows a remarkably rapid decrease in left ventricular dilatation following ductal closure.[53,54] In older children, however, with volume overload secondary to a large left to right shunt through a VSD, the left ventricular enlargement, hypertrophy, and decreased ejection fraction associated with volume overload may all remain to some degree postoperatively despite surgical closure of the defect by the age of five.[55] Another study has shown depressed velocity indices of left ventricular contraction in adolescents and young adults whose VSD was closed at seven years of age.[56] On the other hand, normal values of left ventricular (LV) volume, wall mass, and ejection fraction were found in infants whose VSDs were closed at one year of age.[57] Conversely, even in adults after closure of a small VSD in late childhood, resting and exercise left ventricular ejection fractions are abnormal.[58] It appears that earlier repair of these and other lesions results in less permanent injury to the heart and more nearly normal function in later life.

In children with VSDs and left-to-right shunts, hypertrophy of anomalous right ventricular muscle bundles has resulted in the development of right ventricular outflow tract obstruction, increasing pressure loads on the right side.[59]

Increased pressure and volume loads seen in lesions such as tetralogy of Fallot result in both left and right ventricular dysfunction, some of which can persist after repair.[60–62] When repaired in infancy, however, left ventricular function in patients with tetralogy of Fallot has been shown subsequently to be normal.[63] Full recovery of normal right ventricular function seems to be related to absence of respiratory failure.[64]

Pressure Overload. Pure pressure loads caused by congenital defects also result in significant dysfunction. When the right ventricle functions from birth under systemic pressure loads in congenitally corrected transposition of the great arteries where the aorta is connected to the right ventricle and receives fully saturated blood, systemic (right) ventricular dysfunction occurs by the time of adolescence.[65] Similarly, after atrial repair of transposition of the great arteries (Mustard or Senning) during early childhood, significant abnormalities of right ventricular function may also exist, since it functions as the systemic ventricle under high systemic afterload.[65,66] In patients with other lesions, significant ventricular dysfunction persists after repair of a variety of lesions, including atrial septal defects, aortic and pulmonic stenosis, and tricuspid atresia.[67]

Even in relatively simple congenital defects, such as coarctation of the aorta, there are significant abnormalities in cardiovascular development resulting from the disturbed physiology due to the primary defect in the aortic isthmus. In some cases these abnormalities remain even after correction. In patients whose coarctation was repaired, residual hypertension, often with accompanying left ventricular hypertrophy, has been reported in 20–25 percent of patients, even in those whose coarctation was repaired during infancy.[68,69] There is some evidence that this hypertension may be partly due to altered baroreceptor function.[70] In these patients cardiac index and exercise tolerance are often quite normal. On the other hand, after "repair" of more complex defects such as tricuspid atresia, cardiac index and cardiovascular responses to exercise are abnormal, despite lack of overt symptoms.[71] Therefore patients presenting for anesthesia who have congenital heart disease should be considered to have some degree of cardiac dysfunction even after repair of their congenital heart disease, both as a consequence of the congenital defect as well as the surgical procedure itself.

Myocardial and Valvular Dysfunction Following Repair

Scarring and fibrosis in ventricular muscle resulting from ventriculotomy and ischemic injuries during operation can result in dysfunction in the postoperative period which is additive to that produced by the lesion itself.[67] Transannular outflow patches, unvalved conduits, valvotomies, and valvuloplasties can all result in valvular insufficiency, and thus in increased ventricular volume loads.[72,73] Similarly, these procedures, as well as construction of intra-atrial or intraventricular baffles, can also result in obstruction to blood flow from valvular stenosis or outflow tract obstruction. Increased afterloads can result on either side of the circulation. Although children with these problems are usually identified by their symptomatology, asymptomatic patients may have milder decreases in cardiac reserve that become important during the stress of subsequent anesthesia and operation.

Conduction Disturbances Following Repair

Injury to the conduction systems of the heart during cardiac surgery has been well documented.[74] Atriotomy may disturb the sinoatrial node and the atrial conduction pathways. Ventriculotomy may injure the conduction system, producing right bundle branch or complete heart block. These effects may not appear until years after surgery. Ventricular arrhythmias and conduction disturbances are most commonly seen after correction of tetralogy of Fallot, VSD, and complete atrioventricular canal.[74] Supraventricular arrhythmias, and sinus node dysfunction such as sick sinus syndrome, are generally seen after surgery for transposition of the great arteries and atrial septal defects.[75] Besides direct injury to conduction systems, injury to nutrient coronary arteries and lymphatics may be responsible for electrophysiologic abnormalities.[76] The contribution of these conduction abnormalities to postoperative cardiac dysfunction may be obvious, as in complete heart block, or more subtle and uncertain, as in right bundle branch block.[77]

These rhythm disturbances may be unmasked for the first time or be exacerbated by the stress of anesthesia or the anesthetic agents. For example halothane, by prolonging A–V nodal conduction time, can induce reentry arrhythmias in the A–V node, and can induce release of catecholamines.[78,79] Many other effects of anesthetic agents on the conduction system of the heart are known that are beyond the scope of this chapter. When coupled with postoperative ventricular dysfunction, however, arrhythmias provoked by anesthesia (which are normally well tolerated) may cause significant introperative hemodynamic problems.

ACQUIRED HEART DISEASE IN CHILDREN

Infectious Disease of the Heart and Pericardium

Group A streptococcal infections can result in acute rheumatic fever. While the incidence of this problem is decreasing, it still occurs. Myocarditis is part of the acute phase; this can be severe, with associated ventricular dysfunction and cardiomegaly. Myocarditis progresses to death in two to three percent of cases.[80] Recurrent and severe rheumatic fever is associated with the development of valvular disease, predominantly mitral and, to a lesser degree, aortic.[81] Although uncommon in developed countries, both early valvular insufficiency and later stenosis can occur in childhood, requiring operation as early as six years of age.[82]

Hypertrophy and dilatation, with diminution of cardiac reserve, are the consequences of volume overload of the left ventricle with valvular insufficiency; these consequences are similar to those seen in volume overload from intracardiac shunts. Abrupt onset of insufficiency is poorly tolerated, however, even in children. Obstruction to the pulmonary return resulting from mitral stenosis can result in pulmonary congestion and hypertension, and eventually right ventricular failure. Anesthetic management in these patients is very similar to that in adults with acquired valvular heart disease, except that similar amounts of valvular disease are better tolerated in children.[83,84]

Myocarditis from many nonspecific causes, including viral infection, can cause significant myocardial dysfunction. Mild cases probably go undetected, but when cardiomegaly is present clinical ventricular dysfunction usually occurs.[85]

Pericardial disease frequently accompanies infectious disease of the myocardium in children and can result in purulent pericarditis, acute cardiac tamponade, and constrictive pericarditis. The effects of pericardial disease on cardiac function are usually limitation both of ventricular filling and of stroke volume, thus reducing cardiac output. Heart rate then becomes a primary determinant of cardiac output, as in the neonate. Because of the already limited stroke volume in infants and neonates, and the relatively large pericardial surface-area-to-volume ratio in small hearts, pericardial disease in infants can rapidly become symptomatic. Small amounts of pericardial effusion may initially be well tolerated, but sudden decompensation as a result of tamponade can occur with less warning than in adults. Cardiac output must be sustained by adequate filling pressures, high heart rates, and avoidance of positive pressure ventilation until decompression. Anesthetics that depress the myocardium are generally avoided.[86]

Cardiac Manifestations of Systemic Diseases

Many systemic diseases have important cardiac manifestations in childhood, such as Marfan's syndrome, Down's syndrome, and systemic and pulmonary hypertension. Less frequently Hurler's and Hunter's syndromes, other mucopolysaccharidoses, mucolipidoses, glycogen storage disease, and several forms of muscular dystrophy, have associated cardiac dysfunction.[87]

Marfan's Syndrome. Cardiac abnormalities seen in Marfan's syndrome generally result from degenerative changes in abnormal tissue rather than structural defects present at birth. Mitral insufficiency is most frequently seen, followed by aortic dilatation with aortic insufficiency in the second decade of life.[88] The clinical symptoms of one of these cardiovascular problems generally are seen in 50 percent of Marfan's patients by the age of 21.[87] The resulting hemodynamic problems are similar to those seen in young patients with mitral or aortic insufficiency resulting from rheumatic disease. However, aortic dissection in older children and adolescents with Marfan's can occur spontaneously, and is certainly a consideration in the anesthetic management.

Down's Syndrome. Frequently Down's syndrome patients present to the anesthesiologist for noncardiac operations with previously undetected or untreated congenital heart disease. Congenital heart defects are frequent in this syndrome, with approximately 12 percent of patients having clinically apparent heart disease, and 60 percent having cardiac defects at autopsy.[89] Complete atrioventricular canal, VSD, PDA, and tetralogy of Fallot, in that order, are the most common cardiac lesions. These patients have an increased tendency to develop pulmonary vascular disease, partly because of the high incidence of pulmonary hypoplasia.[90,91] Other than the pulmonary hypoplasia, their cardiovascular pathophysiology does not differ from patients without Down's syndrome who have identical cardiac lesions. The incidence of respiratory complications with anesthesia is therefore high in these children, and special attention must be paid to the airway and secretions. Mortality rates in cardiac surgery are little higher than those in the non-Down's population.[92,93] Although suggestions that atropine be avoided in these patients have appeared, a recent study reports no problems with atropine premedication in Down's children.[94–96]

Systemic Hypertension. The incidence of systemic hypertension during childhood and adolescence is poorly defined. Usually in young children, causes such as coarctation of the aorta and renal problems become apparent on investigation. There is, however, an increasing number of older children and adolescents identified with primary hypertension. The hemodynamic consequences are primarily left ventricular hypertrophy and the accelerated development of atherosclerotic disease. In rare cases, hypertensive crises with acute left ventricular failure and seizures will occur in young patients. More commonly, the anesthesiologist will encounter young hypertensive patients in the operating room who have been treated with diuretics, beta blockers, vasodilators and other antihypertensive agents.[97,98] Problems occurring with these patients intraoperatively are very similar to adult hypertensive patients, except that the risks of coronary artery disease and perioperative ischemia are much lower.

Pulmonary Hypertension. Pulmonary hypertension in children has a much more ominous prognosis than systemic hypertension, unless associated with increased pulmonary blood flow and a normal PVR, as in young children with left-to-right shunting in various forms of congenital heart disease. The causes of pulmonary hypertension in children are numerous, including congenital heart disease, pulmonary disease of various causes, airway disease, acute or chronic hypoxemia, structural disorders of the chest wall and spine (e.g., scoliosis), and idiopathic pulmonary hypertension. In pediatric anesthesia, persistent pulmonary hypertension of the newborn with a prolonged transitional circulation is a serious problem.

Unless the underlying etiology of the pulmonary hypertension can be identified and corrected before irreversible pulmonary vascular obstructive disease has occurred, pressure overload of the right ventricle will result in hypertrophy and eventual failure that is progressive and inexorable. Sudden death in patients with pulmonary hypertension is well documented and is probably due to ventricular arrhythmias or acute right ventricular failure. Cardiac catherization by itself carries appreciable risk in these patients, and sudden death has been reported during pulmonary angiography.[99,100]

Drug therapy to reduce pulmonary hypertension in children has generally been disappointing, although many drugs have been tried.[101] Little has been written about the management of pulmonary hypertension during anesthesia, but risk of significant morbidity and mortality in the perioperative period is commonly thought to be high, although no studies have been done to support this belief. When the underlying cause of the pulmonary hypertension is identified and corrected by operation, risk is generally thought to be much lower. In the newborn, however, because of high baseline PVR, even repair of a lesion such as congenital diaphragmatic hernia does not result in immediate correction of pulmonary hypertension. Severe instability in the intraoperative and postoperative period can result.[102] In any pediatric patient with pulmonary hypertension, anesthetic management should include close monitoring and use of those techniques minimizing PVR (see Chapter 16).

Developmental Alterations with Cardiomyopathies

Hypertrophic Cardiomyopathy. In idiopathic hypertrophic subaortic stenosis (IHSS), also known as hypertrophic cardiomyopathy, muscle cells are bizarrely arranged in the myocardial tissue; the functional meaning of this observation is unclear. Of more functional import is the gradual development of left ventricular outflow obstruction due to apposition of a hypertrophied ventricular septum with an anteriorly tethered mitral valve leaflet. The resulting obstruction causes dynamic pressure overload of the left ventricle, resulting in further hypertrophy, reduced compliance, and gradual loss of functional capacity. Progressive heart failure in infancy from this cause has been documented.[103]

Infants with symptomatic hypertrophic cardiomyopathy differ from older children with the disease in that they often have associated right ventricular outflow tract gradients accompanied by right ventricular hypertrophy and cyanosis, in addition to their left ventricular outflow tract gradients.[103] Cyanosis is presumably due to right-to-left shunting across the foramen ovale in the presence of right ventricular hypertension. Onset of symptoms in infancy or childhood carries a poor prognosis, since half of these patients die or experience clinical deterioration early in life.[104]

Hypertrophic cardiomyopathy is a frequent cause of

sudden death in well conditioned adolescents, especially during strenuous activity.[105] Death or syncope is thought to result from either dysrhythmias or an acute increase in left ventricular outflow obstruction. Treatment of these patients in childhood with beta blockers (propranolol) and calcium channel blockers (verapamil) has been shown to be effective in decreasing left ventricular outflow tract gradients and increasing cardiac output.[105,106]

No studies of the responses of these children to anesthesia are available. Maintenance of filling pressures and afterload are known to be important in diminishing or abolishing outflow tract gradients. Clinical experience indicates that high filling pressures, and use of phenylephrine to maintain peripheral vascular resistance, will improve cardiac output. Intraoperative use of propranolol and verapamil must be cautious if the patient is in congestive failure, but these drugs should be continued preoperatively if they have been taken on a daily basis. Halothane has been administered with good results in adults, but in infants with congestive failure it should be used with caution.[107]

Endocardial Fibroelastosis. Endocardial fibroelastosis is a poorly defined entity associated with a wide variety of heart diseases in children. It also occurs as a primary disease, without other demonstrable cardiac disease, presenting with symptoms of congestive heart failure. It is difficult to distinguish from viral myocarditis, which some investigators feel is the etiology of endocardial fibroelastosis.[108]

Hemodynamic findings in children include elevation of left ventricular filling pressures and decreases in contractility. Mild pulmonary hypertension occurs in about 25 percent of younger children with this disorder, whereas older children have more marked pulmonary hypertension.[109] Cardiac output is maintained until late in the progress of the disease. Progressive heart failure and death occur in about a third of affected children, another third survive but with persistent symptoms or cardiomegaly, and the other third recover completely.[110]

Treatment of primary endocardial fibroelastosis with digitalis and diuretics is the only known effective therapy; surgical treatments have met with failure. No studies of anesthesia in these children are available, but avoidance of anesthetic agents known to cause myocardial depression, and availability of inotropic support would seem indicated.

Adriamycin (Anthracycline) Cardiomyopathy. The anthracycline antineoplastic agents adriamycin and daunomycin are used with increasing frequency; unfortunately these agents also cause an unpredictable, dose-related cardiomyopathy. Both acute and chronic manifestations of cardiac toxicity can result from treatment; isolated reports of cardiovascular complications during and after administration of anesthesia have occurred.[111,112]

Clinically apparent left ventricular dysfunction appears in less than 2 percent of patients receiving less than a 550 mg/m^2 cumulative dose of either drug, but its appearance is unpredictable. In a study of pediatric patients receiving adriamycin, a history of past or present clinical congestive heart failure was found to be the best predictor of intra-anesthetic cardiovascular complications.[113]

CARDIOVASCULAR PHARMACOLOGY IN CHILDREN

Drugs used to manipulate the cardiovascular system have not been well studied in children; doses and effects are derived from clinical experience and extrapolation of adult data.[114]

VASOPRESSORS AND INOTROPIC AGENTS

The aim of vasopressor therapy is generally to increase perfusion pressure and thus flow to critical organs, preferably without decreasing individual organ flow or total cardiac output. Agents useful in achieving these goals will vary depending on which organ is being hypoperfused, the clinical setting, and the individual response of each patient. Generally speaking, perfusion pressure is not as critical in children because of the low incidence of atherosclerotic arterial disease. Large increases in afterload without inotropic support are poorly tolerated by immature hearts. Increases in afterload may result in decreases in cardiac output, so that pure alpha adrenergic agonists are seldom useful in infants, except as brief, temporizing measures. Effects and doses of vasopressors and inotropic agents are summarized in Table 15-3.

Epinephrine (Adrenaline)

Epinephrine has alpha-, beta$_1$-, and beta$_2$-agonist properties. At lower doses it can result in increased inotropy and decreased systemic vascular resistance (SVR). At higher doses SVR tends to increase.[117] Although very useful for short periods and in emergencies, it is generally replaced with drugs such as dopamine for long-term use in order to preserve renal blood flow.

Norepinephrine (Noradrenaline)

Norepinephrine, the naturally occurring mediator of sympathetic activity, has both alpha and beta effects which are dose-dependent. At birth, norepinephrine accounts for 80–90 percent of the circulating catecholamines, in contrast to the adult where epinephrine is the major circulating catecholamine.[115,116] In lower doses, the positive inotropic and moderate peripheral vasoconstrictive effects are useful, but as doses increase, marked peripheral vasoconstriction is seen, which occurs at the expense of splanchnic and renal blood flow. Higher doses may actually decrease cardiac output.[117] Norepinephrine is infrequently used in children except for very short periods.

Dopamine

Dopamine is a unique sympathomimetic amine which is an alpha-, beta-, and delta-agonist, and thus selectively dilates splanchnic, renal, and cerebral vessels. At lower doses dopaminergic effects predominate and SVR decreases. In intermediate doses positive inotropic effects predominate, with somewhat less chronotropy than other inotropic agents. At high doses alpha effects predominate and SVR tends to increase. In young children, higher doses of dopamine may be needed for similar effects, probably because of decreased releaseable stores of norepinephrine in the myocardium of immature ventricles.[118–121]

At present dopamine is probably the most clinically useful vasopressor in children; this is in part due to its beneficial effects on the renal circulation and its relative lack of associated arrhythmias and tachycardia.[119,122–124] There is some contro-

Table 15-3

Inotropes and Vasopressors in Children

Agent	Doses (IV)	Peripheral Vascular Effect	Cardiac Effect	Conduction System Effect
Digoxin (Total digitalizing dose; see text for rate)	20 μg/kg premature 30 μg/kg neonate (0–1 mo) 40 μg/kg infant (<2 yr) 30 μg/kg child (2–5 yr) 20 μg/kg child (>5 yr)	Increases peripheral vascular resistance 1–2+; acts directly on vascular smooth muscle	Inotropic effect 3–4+ acts directly	Slows sinus node Decreases AV conduction
Calcium: Chloride Gluconate	10–20 mg/kg/dose (slowly) 30–60 mg/kg/dose (slowly)	Variable; probably depends on blood [Ca^{++}] level	Inotropic effect 3+; depends on blood [Ca^{++}] level	Slows sinus node Decreases AV conduction

Agent	Dose Range	Peripheral Vascular Effect			Cardiac Effect		Comment
		Alpha	Beta$_2$	Delta	Beta$_1$	Beta$_2$	
Phenylephrine	0.1–0.5 μg/kg/min	4+	0	0	0	0	Increases systemic resistance, no inotropy; may cause renal ischemia
Isoproterenol	0.1–0.5 μg/kg/min	0	4+	0	4+	4+	Strong inotropic and chronotropic agent; peripheral vasodilator; reduces preload and pulmonary vasodilator
Norepinephrine	0.1–0.5 μg/kg/min	4+	0	0	2+	0	Increases systemic resistance; mildly inotropic; may cause renal ischemia
Epinephrine	0.1 μg/kg/min 0.2–0.5 μg/kg/min	2+ 4+	1–2+ 0	0 0	2–3+ 4+	2+ 3+	B$_2$ effect with lower doses; best for supporting blood pressure in anaphylaxis and drug toxicity
Dopamine	2–4 μg/kg/min 4–8 μg/kg/min >10 μg/kg/min	0 0 2–4+	0 2+ 0	2+ 2+ 0	0 1–2+ 1–2+	0 1+ 2+	Splanchnic and renal vasodilator; may be used with isoproterenol; increasing doses produce increasing alpha effect
Dobutamine	2–10 μg/kg/min	1+	2+	0	3–4+	1–2+	Less chronotropy and arrhythmias at lower doses. Effects vary with dose similar to dopamine

† Magnitude of peripheral vascular effects & cardiac effects is noted on a scale of 0–4+, estimating the strength of the effect.

versy surrounding its effect on pulmonary vascular resistance. Conflicting clinical studies have reported three varying effects: pulmonary vasoconstriction in adults; no effect on pulmonary vascular resistance in infants and adults; and a decrease in pulmonary vascular resistance in children.[119,123–126] Therefore the response of the pulmonary vasculature to dopamine is variable, as has been reported in infants with persistent pulmonary hypertension.[127] The use of dopamine in conjunction with a vasodilator such as nitroprusside has been quite successful in children, and this may potentially obviate problems with pulmonary vascular resistance.[123,124]

Dobutamine

Dobutamine is a direct acting synthetic amine which probably has some alpha$_1$ activity, as well as strong cardiac beta activity; there is little experience with this drug in children.[128] Effects vary with dosage in a manner similar to that seen with dopamine, except that there is no dopaminergic activity with dobutamine, i.e., there is less preservation of renal blood flow. Its main advantage is purported to be a lower incidence of tachycardia and arrhythmias than isoproterenol.[129]

In a study done in children during cardiac catheterization,

cardiac and stroke index improved without increases in systemic pressure until higher doses were reached.[130] Used in children after cardiac surgery, however, dobutamine did result in significant increases in heart rate.[131,132] Dobutamine has been reported to be more useful for children with cardiogenic shock than those with septic shock, but increases in pulmonary capillary wedge pressure were noted in these children.[133]

Dobutamine does not appear to offer significant advantages over dopamine in children, and has the disadvantage of less published clinical experience. In children who require more inotropy than that provided by dopamine, and who do not tolerate isoproterenol, dobutamine is a possible alternative drug.

Isoproterenol

Isoproterenol is a pure beta-agonist that produces cardiac inotropic and chronotropic effects, with dilatation in skeletal muscle beds and a fall in SVR. Falls in filling pressure can result from these latter effects. Myocardial oxygen consumption is considerably increased by the inotropic and chronotropic effects. High heart rates and increased oxygen consumption are generally well tolerated in young, uncompromised hearts. However, excessive increases in heart rate may limit the use of isoproterenol in compromised hearts, and hypotension is a possibility, especially in the presence of hypovolemia.[129]

Isoproterenol has a number of potential advantages. Decreased sensitivity of the immature myocardium to dopamine may be overcome, its chronotropic effects may be desirable, it is sometimes useful in restoring sinus rhythm, and it is a known bronchodilator. Furthermore, it has been shown to be a pulmonary vasodilator; this effect may be very useful in children with heart disease who frequently have pulmonary artery hypertension.[125]

Phenylephrine

Phenylephrine is a pure alpha-agonist which causes strong peripheral vasoconstriction. In children this is generally not well tolerated because of the lack of inotrophy. However, it may increase cardiac perfusion during hypotensive events. In those cardiac patients whose pulmonary perfusion is dependent on adequate systemic arterial pressures (e.g., those with any kind of systemic to pulmonary shunt, such as a Blalock-Taussig shunt) use of an alpha-agonist may significantly improve arterial oxygenation in cases of hypotension, and thus secondarily improve myocardial performance in spite of the increased afterload.

Digitalis

Digitalis is the prototypical inotropic agent, and is also used to control arrhythmias in children. In addition to its inotropic effects, it reduces sinoatrial node automaticity and atrioventricular conduction, and has some peripheral vasoconstricting effects. It is used in congestive heart failure and for control of supraventricular tachycardias, including atrial fibrillation and flutter, and A–V nodal paroxysmal tachycardia.[134]

Over the last decade there has been much controversy concerning digoxin doses in children. It was previously thought that the therapeutic dose of digitalis was appreciably greater in infants.[135] Infants are known to tolerate greater dosages and serum levels without clinical evidence of toxicity.[136] It has become apparent that the larger doses of digoxin recommended previously frequently resulted in serum

digoxin levels that were in the toxic range.[137] Recent work, however, indicates that lower doses of digoxin result in the same cardiac effects in young children without the dangers of toxicity, so there is now a tendency to decrease previous dosage recommendations.[138,139]

The parenteral doses recommended in Table 15-3 are guidelines; in clinical situations in which rapid digitalization is warranted, half the digitalizing dose should be given initially, then a remaining quarter of the dose in four to eight hours, followed by the last quarter dose in 8–15 hours. However, the onset and severity of digitalis toxicity are unpredictable in the acutely unstable pediatric patient with changing levels of serum potassium, ionized calcium, and pH, so we avoid the use of digitalis in this situation. The need for rapid digitalization is rare intraoperatively, since safer, more rapid acting and predictable agents may often be substituted. Furthermore the efficacy of digitalis in infants with left-to-right shunts and circulatory congestion has been questioned.[140,141]

Calcium

Calcium is an inotropic agent frequently utilized in the operating room, although its effects in children have not been well studied. Because of the unstable calcium metabolism of the neonate, it is an especially useful drug in this age group.[142,143] It is a positive inotropic agent when ionized calcium is low, and in low flow states.[144–146] It should be noted that despite a normal total calcium level, the ionized fraction, important for normal cardiac function, may be low.[147] When ionized calcium levels are normal, the effects of calcium on contractility are much less marked.[148]

Calcium also has numerous effects on the conduction systems of the heart, which are similar to digitalis and opposite to those of potassium.[149] It therefore must be given with caution to patients taking digitalis and also to those with hypokalemia. The most prominant effect on rhythm is bradycardia, especially if administered centrally in children with normal ionized calcium levels. Other effects are controversial, as it has been reported to both decrease and increase peripheral vascular resistance, and to increase pulmonary vascular resistance, particularly in the presence of pulmonary hypertension.[144,145,147,150]

Calcium gluconate is favored for use in children because it is less liable to cause sloughing when given through peripheral lines. Calcium chloride is equally appropriate when given centrally and is three times as potent when administered on a weight basis. When equal amounts of elemental calcium are given, both drugs are equally effective in raising ionized calcium levels.[151] In life-threatening situation, calcium chloride may be more appropriate because of its increased potency by weight.

Calcium is a very useful drug in the operating room because of the instability of calcium metabolism in infants, especially when large quantities of citrated blood are being infused. However, the potential for severe bradycardia when given rapidly should restrict its use to appropriate situations. During open heart procedures, calcium can cause myocardial contracture ("stone heart") when given after myocardial ischemia, probably because of the poorly understood phenomenon of "calcium paradox."[152] In children who require calcium during bypass, myocardial contracture is a particular hazard if the calcium is given immediately upon reperfusion of the heart after a period of cardiac ischemia, or deep

Table 15-4

Vasodilators in Children

Agent	Dose (IV)	Effects		Action and Comments
		Arterial Resistance	Venous Capacitance	
Sodium Nitroprusside	0.5–5.0 μg/kg/min	3+	3+	Direct smooth muscle relaxation Pulmonary vasodilator ? effectiveness
Hydralazine	0.1–0.3 mg/kg bolus	3+	1+	Direct smooth muscle relaxation Pulmonary vasodilator ? effectiveness
Nitroglycerin	0.25–1.0 μg/kg/min	1+	3+	Direct smooth muscle relaxation Pulmonary vasodilator Little experience in children
Phentolamine	20 μg/kg/min	3+	1+	Alpha-blocker, some direct action, little used
Prostaglandin E_1	0.1 μg/kg/min	2+	2+	Direct smooth muscle relaxation Relatively specific for ductal tissue

hypothermic circulatory arrest when the myocardium has not been perfused except for periodic cardioplegic infusions.

VASODILATORS

Vasodilators are used in children for four main purposes; (1) to control systemic hypertension, (2) to increase cardiac output by decreasing afterload, (3) to control pulmonary hypertension, and (4) in attempts to control cardiac shunting.

The use of vasodilators for control of systemic hypertension and for increasing cardiac output in children with congestive heart failure has been quite successful. However, use of vasodilators without concommitant use of inotropic agents to increase cardiac output in the low output state should be initiated very carefully to avoid hypotension and decompensation.

Treatment of pulmonary hypertension and cardiac shunting with vasodilators has shown mixed results. Responses of the pulmonary vasculature, and of cardiac shunting to vasodilators, seem to vary from patient to patient. The primary problem with these two uses is that all currently available vasodilators seem to work on the systemic circulation as well as on the pulmonary circulation. Systemic hypotension during treatment of pulmonary hypertension, and increases in left-to-right shunting, have resulted from attempts to treat these problems with vasodilators. Those vasodilators currently used in children are listed, with their doses, in Table 15-4.

Sodium Nitroprusside

Sodium nitroprusside has been successfully used to reduce afterload, especially in conjunction with dopamine, and to increase cardiac output in children with low output syndrome after cardiac surgery.[123,124,153,154] It has also been reported to be effective when used in children with severe left ventricular dysfunction secondary to various cardiomyopathies, and in children with mitral regurgitation.[155] Sodium nitroprusside, used both intraoperatively and postoperatively to control systemic hypertension during operations such as

coarctation repairs, has been of value. Although this drug has been employed to treat pulmonary hypertension, these attempts have not been uniformly successful.[156–159]

Toxicity of nitroprusside in children with the usual doses employed has generally not been a problem clinically, but at least one death has been reported.[160] Children exhibiting tachyphylaxis who require abnormally high doses should be carefully evaluated for signs of cyanide toxicity.

Hydralazine

Hydralazine has been used to control both pulmonary and systemic hypertension in children. Some efficacy has been reported with oral hydralazine therapy for pulmonary hypertension in adults, but effects in children have been disappointing.[101,161] Acute intravenous use in children has shown no change in pulmonary vascular resistance in two studies; one report documented a decrease in left-to-right intracardiac shunting, while the other showed an increase.[162,163] Another study of intracardiac shunting, in infants with atrioventricular canal defects who were given hydralazine, showed variable results. Pulmonary vascular resistance decreased in the majority, but not all, of these infants.[164] The chronic use of hydralazine in the oral form to control systemic hypertension is the most frequently encountered use in children. It has also been therapeutically employed chronically in children with congestive heart failure.[155] Hydralazine has been suggested as an intraoperative alternative to control systemic hypertension during pediatric procedures, such as repair of coarctation of the aorta.

Nitroglycerin

Nitroglycerin given intravenously as a vasodilator has had little use in children; it is included here because it has relatively unique vasodilating properties, such as differential effects on the venous capacitance bed compared to the arterial resistance bed. No studies of its use in children have been published, but two studies of its effects in adults suggest that it has potential as a pulmonary vasodilator.[158,165] Limited use of intravenous

Table 15-5

Antiarrythmia Agents in Children

Agent	IV Dose	Indications	Comments
Lidocaine	1 mg/kg 20–50 μg/kg/min	Ventricular arrythmias (acute)	Bolus dose may be repeated in 10 minutes
Procainamide	3–6 mg/kg	Ventricular arrythmias	Dose given over 10 minutes
Phenytoin	5 mg/kg	Ventricular arrrythmias Supraventricular arrythmias (digitalis induced)	Dose given over 5 minutes Useful in digitalis toxicity
Bretylium	5–10 mg/kg	Life threatening, refractory ventricular arrythmias	Dose given over 10 minutes, little experience in children
Propranolol	0.01–0.02 mg/kg	Supraventricular arrythmias Ventricular arrythmias	Dose given over 10 minutes Beta-blocker, caution when used in children with CHF or taking calcium channel blocker Also used for control of hypertension
Verapamil	0.125–0.25 mg/kg	Supraventricular tachycardias Atrial flutter-fibrillation	Caution in children with CHF or taking beta blockers

nitroglycerin in neonates in our institution has not been associated with particular problems, except for one case of severe intrapulmonary shunting and arterial hypoxemia.

Tolazoline and Phentolamine

Tolazoline has been used primarily to control pulmonary artery hypertension in children, but it is not uniformly successful and is rarely used now.[127,166–169] Phentolamine, an alpha-blocker, has also been reported to be successful for control of pulmonary hypertension when administered orally in adults, but not in children, where it increased a left-to-right shunt.[163,170]

Prostaglandin E₁

While classified as a vasodilator, PGE₁ is a unique drug which has greatly improved the care of neonates with heart disease. PGE₁ acts directly on vascular smooth muscle; infused at a rate of 0.1 μg/kg/min, it will maintain patency of the ductus arteriosus, or even reopen it, in neonates up to seven days of age and older.[171] This response is dependent on factors such as age and the state of contraction of the ductus.[172] Side effects of apnea, hypotension from systemic vasodilatation, or central nervous system excitability are usually immediately apparent and can be readily managed in the operating room.[173]

This drug is indispensable in patients with ductus-dependent cardiac lesions, such as interrupted aortic arch, critical aortic stenosis, or hypoplastic left heart, where systemic flow is supplied by the ductus. PGE₁ is equally indispensable in pulmonary atresia and critical pulmonic stenosis, where pulmonary blood flow is supplied by the ductus. Infusion of PGE₁ to maintain cardiovascular stability of these neonates in the operating room has been without problems thus far in our experience. It has also been used to treat pulmonary hypertension with varying degrees of success.[174,175]

ANTIARRHYTHMICS

The administration of digoxin in supraventricular tachycardias has been reviewed above. The recommended doses and indication for these drugs are summarized in Table 15-5.[176]

Propranolol

Propranolol is a beta-blocking agent used in children for control of supraventricular tachycardias, hypertension, cyanotic spells in tetralogy of Fallot, and hypertrophic cardiomyopathy.[177–179] For acute control of supraventricular tachycardias in the operating room, and as an adjunctive agent for control of hypertension, doses of 0.01–0.02 μg/kg given over ten minutes are recommended, repeated every six to eight minutes as necessary.[180] Its acute use for cyanotic spells in tetralogy of Fallot has also been advocated.

Propranolol must be used with caution in patients with asthma and congestive heart failure. An additional caution in its intraoperative use is the possibility of perioperative hypoglycemia, especially when used in small children.[181]

Verapamil

Calcium channel blockers, exemplified by verapamil, are becoming the drugs of choice in supraventricular tachycardias. In rapid intravenous doses of 0.125–0.25 mg/kg in infants, verapamil has been shown to be rapidly effective in termination over 90 percent of supraventricular tachycardias without obvious side effects.[182,183] One infant who inadvertently received three times the recommended dose had severe bradycardia and hypotension that was reversed with isoproterenol. Verapamil is also useful in the primary therapy of hypertrophic cardiomyopathy.[106] Use of this or other calcium blockers in children with congestive heart failure or who are taking beta-blockers is uncertain, but experience in adults suggests that caution should be used in this situation. Cardiac decompensation following verapamil therapy for supraventricular tachycardia in three infants with congestive heart failure has recently been reported.[184]

Other Antiarrhythmics

Other drugs utilized acutely in controlling ventricular arrhythmias in children include lidocaine in a dose of 1 mg/kg, and procainamide in a dose of 3–6 mg/kg over five minutes intravenously.[176,180] Administration of much larger doses of procainamide has been reported.[185] Phenytoin has been used in an intravenous dose of 5 mg/kg given over 5 minutes, especially for cases of suspected digitialis toxicity. Oral therapy for chronic control of postoperative ventricular arrhythmias in children has also been described.[176,186] For life-threatening, refractory ventricular arrhythmias unresponsive to other drugs, bretylium given in a dose of 5–10 mg/kg intravenously over 10 minutes is recommended, although there is little experience with the use of bretylium in the pediatric patient.[187]

REFERENCES

1. Heymann MA: Patent ductus arteriosus. In Adams FH, Emmanouilides GC (eds): *Heart Disease in Infants, Children, and Adolescents.* (ed 3). Baltimore Williams & Wilkins, 1968, pp 158–170

2. Moss AJ, Emmanouilides GC, Duffie ER: Closure of the ductus arteriosus in the newborn infant. *Pediatrics* 32:25–30, 1963

3. Gessner IH, Klovetz LJ, Henson RW, et al: Hemodynamic adaptations in the newborn infant. *Pediatrics* 36:752–62, 1965

4. Kovalcik V: The response of the isolated ductus arteriosus to oxygen and anoxia. *J Physiol (Lond)* 169:185–197, 1963

5. McMurphy DM, Heyman MA, Rudolph AM, et al: Developmental changes in constriction of the ductus arteriosus: Responses to oxygen and vasoactive substances in the isolated ductus of the fetal lamb. *Pediatr Res* 6:231–238, 1972

6. Clyman RI, Heymann MA, Rudolph AM: Ductus arterious responses to prostaglandin E₁ at high and low oxygen concentrations. *Prostaglandins* 13:219–223, 1977

7. Friedman WF, Hirschklau MJ, Printz MP, et al: Pharmacologic closure of patent ductus arteriosus in the premature infant. *N Eng J Med* 295:526–529, 1976

8. Moss AJ, Emmanouilides GC, Adams FH, et al: Response of the ductus arteriosus and pulmonary and systemic arterial pressure to changes in oxygen environment in newborn infants. *Pediatrics* 33:937–941, 1964

9. Freed MA, Heymann MA, Lewis AB, et al: Prostaglandin E₁ in infants with ductus arteriosus-dependent congenital heart disease. *Circulation* 64:899–905, 1981

10. Clyman RI, Mauray F, Roman C, et al: Factors determining the loss of ductus arteriosus responsiveness to prostaglandin E. *Circulation* 68:433–436, 1983

11. Arcilla J, Oh W, Wallgreen G, et al: Hemodynamic findings in early and late clamping of the umbilical cord. *Acta Paediatr Scand (Suppl)* 179:25–30, 1967

12. Gentile R, Stevenson G, Dooley T, et al: Noninvasive determination of time of ductal closure in normal newborn infants. *Pediatr Cardiol* 1:177–182, 1979

13. Emmanouilides GC, Moss AJ, Duffie ER, et al: Pulmonary arterial pressure changes in human newborn infants from birth to 3 days of age. *J Pediatr* 65:327–333, 1964

14. Rudolph AM: *Congenital Diseases of the Heart.* Chicago, Yearbook Medical Publishers, 1974, pp 29–48

15. Davies G, Reid L: Growth of the alveoli and pulmonary arteries in childhood. *Thorax* 25:669–681, 1970

16. Hislop A, Reid L: Pulmonary arterial development during childhood: Branching pattern and structure. *Thorax* 28:129–135, 1973

17. James LS, Rowe RD: The pattern of response of pulmonary and systemic arterial pressures in newborn and older infants to short periods of hypoxia. *J Pediatr* 51:5–11, 1957

18. Arcilla J, Oh W, Lind J, Blankenship W: Portal and atrial pressures in the newborn period. A comparative study of infants born with early and late clamping of the cord. *Acta Paediatr Scand* 55:615–625, 1966

19. Scammon RE, Norris EH: On the time of the postnatal obliteration of the fetal blood passages. *Anat Rec* 15:165–180, 1918

20. Kupferschmid C, Lang D: The valve of the foramen ovale in interatrial right-to-left shunt: Echocardiographic, cineangiographic and hemodynamic observations. *Am J Cardiol* 51:1489–1494, 1983

21. Romero T, Covell J, Friedman WF: A comparison of pressure volume relations of the fetal, newborn, and adult heart. *Am J Physiol* 222:1285–1290, 1972

22. Emery JL, Mithal A: Weights of cardiac ventricles at and after birth. *Br Heart J* 23:313–316, 1961

23. Emmanouilides GC, Moss AJ, Adams FH: The electrocardiogram in normal newborn infants: Correlation with hemodynamic observations. *J Pediatr* 67:578–587, 1965

24. Azancot A, Caudell TP, Allen HD, et al: Analysis of ventricular shape by echocardiography in normal fetuses, newborns, and infants. *Circulation* 68:1201–1211, 1983

25. Legato MJ: Ultrastructural changes during normal growth in the dog and rat ventricular myofiber, in Lieberman M, Sano T (eds): *Developmental and Physiological Correlates of Cardiac Muscle.* New York, Raven Press, 1975, pp 249–274

26. Friedman WF: Intrinsic physiological properties of the developing heart. *Prog Cardiovas Dis* 15:87–111, 1972

27. Rolph TP, Jones CT, Parry C: Ultrastructural and enzymatic development of fetal guinea pig heart. *Am J Physiol* 243:H87–H93, 1982

28. Wells RJ, Friedman WF, Sobel BE: Increased oxidative metabolism in the fetal and newborn lamb heart. *Am J Physiol* 222:1488–1493, 1972

29. Jolley RL, Cheddely UH, Newburgh RW: Glucose catabolism in fetal and adult heart. *J Biol Chem* 233:1289–1294, 1958

30. Su JY, Friedman WF: Comparison of the responses of fetal and adult cardiac muscle to hypoxia. *Am J Physiol* 224:1249–1253, 1973

31. Lee JC, Halloran KH, Taylor JFN, et al: Coronary flow and myocardial metabolism in newborn lambs: Effects of hypoxia and acidemia. *Am J Physiol* 224:1381–1387, 1973

32. Ezrin AM, Bassett AL, Gelband H: Cellular electrophysiology in the developing mammalian heart: Modification by antiarrythmic agents, in Roberts WK, Gelband H (eds): *Cardiac Arrythmias in the Neonate, Infant and Child* (ed 2). Norwalk, CT, Appleton-Century-Crofts, 1983, pp 37–58

33. Reder RF, Micros DS, Danilo P, et al: The electrophysiological properties of normal neonatal and adult canine cardiac Purkinje fibers. *Circ Res* 48:658–668, 1981

34. Friedman WF, Pool PE, Jacobowitz D, et al: Sympathetic innervation of the developing rabbit heart: Biochemical and histochemical comparisons of fetal, neonatal, and adult myocardium. *Circ Res* 23:23–32, 1968

35. Geis WP, Tatooles CJ, Priola DV, et al: Factors influencing neurohumoral control of the heart in the newborn dog. *Am J Physiol* 228:1685–1689, 1975

36. Lebowitz EA, Novick JS, Rudolph AM: Development of myocardial sympathetic innervation in the newborn lamb. *Pediatr Res* 6:887–893, 1972

37. Erath HG, Boerth RC, Graham TP: Functional significance of reduced cardiac sympathetic innervation in the newborn dog. *Am J Physiol* 243:H20–26, 1982

38. Sinha SW, Armour JA, Randall WC: Development of autonomic innervation of the heart. *Circulation* 58:Suppl IV:37, 1973

39. Boatman DL, Shaffer RA, Dixon RL, et al: Function of vascular

smooth muscle and its sympathetic innervation in the newborn dog. *J Clin Invest* 44:241–246, 1965

40. Mattensen O, Stovgard Anderson P: Harlequin color changes in the newborn. *Arch Dermatol* 98:41–46, 1968

41. Friedman WF: Intrinsic physiologic properties of the developing heart. *Prog Cardiovas Dis* 15:87–111, 1972

42. Thornburg KL, Morton MJ: Filling and arterial pressure as determinants of RV stroke volume in the sheep fetus. *Am J Physiol* 244:H656–663, 1983

43. Downing SE, Talner NS, Gardner TH: Ventricular function in the newborn lamb. *Am J Physiol* 208:931–937, 1965

44. Kirkpatrick SE, Pitlick PT, Naliboff J, Friedman WF: Frank-Starling as an important determinant of fetal cardiac output. *Am J Physiol* 231:495–500, 1976

45. Brinkman CR, Johnson GH, Assali NS: Hemodynamic effects of bradycardia in the fetal lamb. *Am J Physiol* 223:1465–1469, 1972

46. Heath D, Edwards JE: The pathology of hypertensive pulmonary vascular disease. A description of six grades of structural changes in the pulmonary arteries with special attention to congenital cardiac septal defects. *Circulation* 18:533–547, 1958

47. Haworth SG: Normal pulmonary vascular development and its disturbance in congenital heart disease, in Godman MJ (ed): *Paediatric Cardiology*, vol 4. New York, Churchhill-Livingston, 1981, pp 46–55

48. Rabinovitch M, Haworth SG, Castaneda AR, et al: Lung Biopsy in congenital heart disease: A morphometric approach to pulmonary vascular disease. *Circulation* 58:1107–1122, 1978

49. Hoffman JIE, Rudolph AM, Heyman MA: Pulmonary vascular disease with congenital heart lesions: Pathologic features and causes. *Circulation* 64:873–877, 1981

50. Haworth SG: Pulmonary vascular disease in secundum atrial septal defect in childhood. *Am J Cardiol* 51:265–272, 1983

51. Thgiene G, Maxxucco A, Grisolia EF, et al: Postoperative pathology of complete atrioventricular defects. *J Thorac Cardiovasc Surg* 83:891–900, 1982

52. Graham TP, Jr: Myocardial functional abnormalities in congenital heart disease-effects of cyanosis and abnormal loading conditions, in Godman MJ (ed), *Paediatric Cardiology*, vol 4. New York, Churchhill-Livingston, 1981, pp 103–116

53. Baylen B, Meyer RA, Korfhagen J, et al: Left ventricular performance in the critically ill premature infant with patent ductus arteriosus and pulmonary disease. *Circulation* 55:182–188, 1977

54. Friedman WF, Kirschlaw MJ, Printz MP, et al: Pharmacologic closure of patent ductus arteriosus in the premature infant. *N Engl Med* 295:526–529, 1976

55. Jarmakani JM, Graham TP, Jr, Canent RV, Jr, et al: The effect of corrective surgery on heart volume and mass in children with ventricular septal defect. *Am J Cardiol* 27:254–258, 1971

56. Cordell D, Graham TP, Jr, Atwood GF, et al: Left heart volume characteristics following ventricular septal closure defects in infancy. *Circulation* 54:417–422, 1976

57. Jarmakani JM, Graham TP, Jr, Canent RV, Jr: Left ventricular contractile state in children with successfully corrected ventricular septal defect. *Circulation* 45–47:Suppl I:I102–110, 1972

58. Jablonsky G, Hilton JD, Liu P, et al: Rest and exercise ventricular function in adults with congenital ventricular septal defects. *Am J Cardiol* 51:293–298, 1983

59. Pongiglione G, Freedom RM, Cook D, et al: Mechanism of acquired right ventricular outflow tract obstruction in patients with ventricular septal defect: An angiocardiographic study. *Am J Cardiol* 50:776–780, 1982

60. Lange PE, Onnasch GW, Bernhard A, et al: Left and right ventricular adaptation to right ventricular overload before and after surgical repair of tetralogy of Fallot. *Am J Cardiol* 50:786–794, 1982

61. Borow KM, Green LH, Castaneda AR, et al: Left ventricular function after repair of tetralogy of Fallot and its relationship to age at surgery. *Circulation* 61:1150–1158, 1980

62. James FW, Kaplan S, Schwartz DC, et al: Response to exercise in patients after total surgical correction of tetralogy of Fallot. *Circulation* 54:671–676, 1976

63. Borow KM, Keane JF, Castenada AR: Systemic ventricular function in patients with tetralogy of Fallot, ventricular septal defect and transposition of the great arteries repaired during infancy. *Circulation* 64:878–885, 1981

64. Bove EL, Byrum CJ, Thomas FD, et al: The influence of pulmonary insufficiency on ventricular function following repair of tetralogy of Fallot. *J Thorac Cardiovasc Surg* 85:691–695, 1983

65. Graham TP, Jr, Parrish MD, Boucek RJ, et al: Assessment of ventricular size and function in congenitally corrected transposition of the great arteries. *Am J Cardiol* 51:244–251, 1983

66. Benson LN, Bonet J, McLaughlin P, et al: Assessment of right ventricular function during supine bicycle exercise after Mustard's operation. *Circulation* 65:1052–1059, 1982

67. Graham TP, Jr: Ventricular performance in adults after operation for congenital heart disease. *Am J Cardiol* 50:612–620, 1982

68. Glancy DL, Morrow AG, Simon AL, et al: Juxtaductal aortic coarctation: Analysis of 84 patients studied hemodynamically, angiographically, and morphologically after age 1 year. *Am J Cardiol* 51:537–551, 1983

69. Pollack P, Freed MD, Castaneda AR, et al: Reoperation for isthmic coarctation of the aorta: Follow-up of 26 patients. *Am J Cardiol* 51:1690–1694, 1983

70. Beekman RH, Katz BP, Moorehead-Steffens C, et al: Altered baroreceptor function in children with systolic hypertension after coarctation repair. *Am J Cardiol* 52:112–117, 1983

71. Shachar GB, Fuhrman BP, Wang Y, et al: Rest and exercise hemodynamics after the Fontan procedure. *Circulation* 65:1043–1048, 1982

72. Ebert PA: Second operation for pulmonary stenosis or insufficiency after repair of tetralogy of Fallot. *Am J Cardiol* 50:637–640, 1982

73. Roberts WC: Valvular residua and sequelae after operation for congenital heart disease, in Engle MA, Perloff JK (eds): *Congenital Heart Disease after Surgery*. New York, Yorke Medical Books, 1983, pp 133–147

74. Vetter VL, Horowitz LN: Electrophysiologic residua and sequelae of surgery for congenital heart defects. *Am J Cardiol* 588–604, 1982

75. Martin TC, Smith L, Hernandez A, et al: Dysrythmias following the Senning operation for dextro-transposition of the great arteries. *J Thorac Cardiovasc Surg* 85:928–932, 1983

76. Bharati S, Lev M: Sequelae of atriotomy and ventriculotomy on the endocardium, conduction system and coronary arteries. *Am J Cardiol* 50:580–587, 1982

77. Tamer D, Wolff GS, Ferrer P, et al: Hemodynamics and intracardiac conduction after operative repair of tetralogy of Fallot. *Am J Cardiol* 51:552–556, 1983

78. Atlee JL, Kreul JF, Rusy BF: Halothane depression of A-V conduction studied by electrograms of the bundle of His in dogs. *Anesthesiology* 36:112–118, 1972

79. Morrow DH, Logic JR, Haley JV: Antiarrhythmic anesthetic action. I: The effect of halothane on canine intracardiac impulse conduction during sinus rhythm. *Anesth Analg* 56:187–193, 1977

80. United Kingdom and United States Joint Report: The natural history of rheumatic fever and rheumatic heart disease: Ten-year report of a cooperative trial of ACTH, cortisone and aspirin. *Circulation* 32:457–467, 1965

81. Kaplan S: Chronic rheumatic heart disease, in Adams FH, Emmanouilides GC (eds): *Heart Disease in Infants, Children and Adolescents* (ed 3). Baltimore, Williams & Wilkins, 1983, pp 522–564

82. John S, Bashi VV, Jairaj PS, et al: Closed mitral valvotomy: Early results and long term follow-up of 3724 consecutive patients. *Circulation* 68:891–896, 1983

83. Kaplan JA (ed): *Cardiac Anesthesia.* New York, Grune & Stratton, 1979

84. Tarhan S (ed): *Cardiovascular Anesthesia and Postoperative Care.* Chicago, Year Book Medical Publishers, 1982

85. Noren GR, Kaplan EL, Stanley NA: Nonrheumatic inflammatory diseases, in Adams FH, Emmanouilides GC (eds): *Heart Disease in Infants, Children, and Adolescents* (ed 3). Baltimore, Williams & Wilkins, 1983, pp 576–595

86. Lake CL: Anesthesia and pericardial disease. *Anesth Analg* 62:431–443, 1983

87. Adams FH, Emmanouilides GC, (ed): *Heart Disease in Infants, Children, and Adolescents* (ed 3). Baltimore, Williams & Wilkins, 1983

88. Phornphutkul C, Rosenthal A, Nadas AS: Cardiac manifestations of Marfan syndrome in infancy and childhood. *Circulation* 47:587–596, 1973

89. Greenwood RD, Nadas AS: The clinical course of cardiac disease in Down's syndrome. *Pediatrics* 58:893–897, 1976

90. Yamaki S, Horeiuchi T, Sekino Y: Quantitative analysis of pulmonary vascular disease in simple cardiac anomalies with the Down's syndrome. *Am J Cardiol* 51:1502–1506, 1983

91. Cooney TP, Thurlbeck WM: Pulmonary hypoplasia in Down's syndrome. *N Engl J Med* 307:1170–1173, 1982

92. Kobel M, Creighton RE, Steward DJ: Anesthetic considerations in Down's syndrome: Experience with 100 patients and a review of the literature. *Can Anaesth Soc J* 29:593–598, 1982

93. Katlic M, Clark EB, Neill C, et al: Surgical management of congenital heart disease in Down's syndrome. *J Thorac Cardiovasc Surg* 74:204–209, 1977

94. Smith RM: *Anesthesia for Infants and Children* (ed 4). St Louis, C.V. Mosby, 1980, p 537

95. Harris WS, Goodman RM: Hyper-reactivity to atropine in Down's syndrome. *N Engl J Med* 279:407–410, 1968

96. Wark HJ, Overton JH, Marian P: The safety of atropine premedication in children with Down's syndrome. Anaesthesia 38:871–874, 1983

97. Mirkin BL, Sinaiko A: Clinical pharmacology and theraputic utilization of antihypertensive agents in children, in New MI, Levine LS (eds): *Juvenile Hypertension.* New York, Raven Press, 1977 pp 345–78

98. Sinaiko AR, Mirkin BL: Clinical pharmacology of antihypertensive drugs in children. *Pediatr Clin North Am* 25:137–157, 1978

99. Keane JF, Fyler DC, Nadas AS: Hazards of cardiac catheterization in children with primary pulmonary vascular obstruction. *Am Heart J* 96:556–558, 1978

100. Snider GL, Ferris E, Gaensler EA, et al: Primary pulmonary hypertension: A fatality during pulmonary angiography. *Chest* 64:628–635, 1973

101. Rabinovitch M: Pulmonary hypertension, in Adams FH, Emmanouilides (eds): *Heart Disease in Infants, Children, and Adolescents* (ed 3). Baltimore, Williams & Wilkins, 1983, pp 687–692

102. Vacanti JP, Crone RK, Murphy J, et al: Treatment of congenital diaphragmatic hernia with chronic anesthesia to control pulmonary artery hypertension. *Anesthesiology* 59:A436, 1983

103. Maron BJ, Tajik AJ, Ruttenburg HD, et al: Hypertrophic cardiomyopathy in infants: Clinical features and natural history. *Circulation* 65:7–17, 1982

104. Fiddler GL, Tajik AJ, Weidman WH, et al: Idiopathic hypertrophic subaortic stenosis in the young. *Am J Cardiology* 42:793–799, 1978

105. Maron BJ, Roberts WC, Epstein SE: Sudden death in hypertrophic cardiomyopathy: Profile of 78 patients. *Circulation* 65:1388–1395, 1982

106. Spicer RL, Rocchini AP, Crowley DC, et al: Hemodynamic

effects of verapmil in children and adolescents with hypertrophic cardiomyopathy. *Circulation* 67:413–420, 1983

107. Morrow AG, Reitz BA, Epstein SE, et al: Operative treatment in hypertrophic subaortic stenosis. *Circulation* 52:88–102, 1975

108. Hutchins GM, Vie SA: The progression of interstitial myocarditis to idiopathic endocardial fibroelastosis. *Am J Pathol* 66:483–496, 1972

109. McLoughlin TG, Schiebler GL, Krovetz LJ: Hemodynamic findings in children with endocardial fibroelastosis. Analysis of 22 cases. *Am Heart J* 75:162–166, 1968

110. Hastreiter AR, Miller RA: Management of primary endomyocardial disease. The myocarditis-endocardial fibroelastosis syndrome. *Pediatr Clin North Am* 11:401–430, 1964

111. Smith RM, DasGupta V: Adriamycin cardiotoxicity. *Anesth Rev* 8:14–19, 1981

112. Caviale P, McClellan EL: Adriamycin toxicity: Effects in subsequent anesthesia and surgery. *J Kans Med Soc* 82:553–554, 1981

113. Burrows FA, Hickey PR, Kalin SA: Complications of anesthesia in adriamycin treated pediatric patients. *Can Anaes Soc J* 32:149–157, 1985

114. Gorodischer R: Cardiac drugs, In Jaffe SJ (ed) *Pediatric Pharmacology: Therapeutic Principles in Practice.* New York, Grune & Stratton, 1980, pp 281–304

115. Eliot RJ, Lam R, Leake RD, et al: Plasma catecholamine concentrations in infants at birth and during the first 48 hours of life. *J Pediatr* 96:311–315, 1980

116. Chernow B, Rainey TG, Lake CR: Endogenous and exogenous catecholamines in critical care medicine. *Crit Care Med* 10:409–416, 1982

117. Innes IR, Nickerson M: Norepinephrine, epinephrine and the sympathomimetic amines, In Gillam AG, Goodman LS, Gillman A (eds): *The Pharmacological Basis of Theraputics.* New York, MacMillan, 1980, pp 477–513

118. Driscoll DJ, Gillette PC, Ezrailson EG, et al: Inotropic response of the neonatal canine myocardium to dopamine. *Pediatr Res* 12:42–45, 1978

119. Lang P, Williams RG, Norwood WI, et al: Hemodynamic effect of dopamine in infants after corrective cardiac surgery. *J Pediatr* 96:630–634, 1980

120. Harris WH, Van Petten GR: The effects of dopamine on blood pressure and heart rate of the unanesthetized fetal lamb. *Am J Obstet Gynecol* 130:211–215, 1978

121. Privitera PJ, Loggie JMH, Gaffney TE: A comparison of the cardiovascular effects of biogenic amines and their precursors in newborn and adult dogs. *J Pharmacol Exp Ther* 166:293–298, 1969

122. Driscoll DJ, Gillette PC, McNamara DC: The use of dopamine in children. *J Pediatr* 92:309–314, 1978

123. Stephenson LW, Edmunds LH, Raphaely R, et al: Effects of nitroprusside and dopamine on pulmonary arterial vasculature in children after cardiac surgery. *Circulation* 60:I104–110, 1979

124. Williams DB, Kiernan PD, Schaff HV, et al: The hemodynamic response to dopamine and nitroprusside following right atrium-pulmonary artery bypass (Fontan procedure). Ann Thorac Surg 34:51–57, 1982

125. Mentzer RM, Alegre CA, Nolan SP: The effects of dopamine and isoproternol on the pulmonary circulation. *J Thorac Cardiovasc Surg* 71:807–814, 1976

126. Holloway EL, Polumbo RA, Harrison DC: Acute circulatory effects of dopamine in patients with pulmonary hypertension. *Br Heart J* 37:482–485, 1975

127. Drummond WH, Gregory GA, Heyman MA: The independent effects of hyperventilation, tolazoline, and dopamine on infants with persistent pulmonary hypertension. *J Pediatr* 98:603–611, 1981

128. Kenakin TP: An in-vitro quantitative analysis of the alpha-adrenoreceptor partial agonist activity of dobutamine and its relevance to inotropic selectivity. *J Pharmacol Exp Ther* 216:210–219, 1981

129. Driscoll DJ, Gillette PC, Lewis RM, et al: The comparative hemodynamic effects of isoproterenol, dopamine and dobutamine in the newborn dog. *Pediatr Res* 13:1006–1009, 1979

130. Driscoll DJ, Gillette PC, Duff DF, et al: Hemodynamic effects of dobutamine in children. *Am J Cardiol* 43:581–585, 1979

131. Bohn DJ, Poirier CS, Edmonds JF, et al: The hemodynamic effects of dobutamine after cardiopulmonary bypass in children. *Crit Care Med* 8:367–371, 1980

132. Jose AB, Niguidula F, Botros S, et al: Hemodynamic effects of dobutamine in children. *Anesthesiology* 55:A61, 1981

133. Perkin RM, Levin DL, Webb R, et al: Dobutamine: A hemodynamic evaluation in children with shock. *J Pediatr* 100:977–983, 1982

134. Linde LM, Turner SW, Awa S: Present status and treatment of paroxysmal supraventricular tachycardia. *Pediatrics* 50:127–130, 1972

135. Berman W, Jr, Ravenscroft PJ, Sheiner LB, et al: Differential effects of digoxin at comparable concentrations in tissues of fetal and adult sheep. *Circ Res* 41:635–642, 1977

136. Hayes CJ, Butler VP, Gersony WM: Serum digoxin studies in infants and children. *Pediatrics* 52:561–568, 1973

137. Wettrell G, Andersson KE: Clinical Pharmacokinetics of digoxin in infants. *Clin Pharmacokinet* 2:17–31, 1977

138. Berman W, Jr, Whitman V, Marks KH: Inadvertent over-administration of digoxin to low-birth-weight infants. *J Pediatr* 92:1024–1025, 1978

139. Pinsky WW, Jacobsen JR, Gillette PC, et al: Dosage of digoxin in premature infants. *J Pediatr* 96:639–642, 1977

140. White RD, Leitman PS: A reappraisal of digitalis for infants with left to right shunts and "heart failure." *J Pediatr* 92:867–870, 1978

141. Berman W, Jr, Yabek SM, Dillon T, et al: Effects of digoxin in infants with a congested circulatory state due to a ventricular septal defect. *N Engl J Med* 308:363–366, 1983

142. Tsang RC, Donovan EF, Steichen JJ: Calcium physiology and pathology in the neonate. *Pediatr Clin North Am* 23:611–626, 1976

143. Mizrahi A, London RD, Gribetz: Neonatal hypocalcemia: Its cause and treatment. *N Engl J Med* 278:1163–1165, 1968

144. Stanley TH, Amaral JI, Liu WS, et al: Peripheral vascular versus direct cardiac effects of calcium. *Anesthesiology* 45:46–58, 1976

145. Denlinger JK, Kaplan JA, Lecky JH, et al: Cardiovascular responses to calcium administered intravenously to man during halothane anesthesia. *Anesthesiology* 42:390–397, 1975

146. Drop LJ, Laver MB: Low plasma ionized calcium and response to calcium in critically ill man. *Anesthesiology* 43:300–306, 1975

147. Scheidegger D, Drop LJ, Schellenberg JC: Role of the systemic vasculature in the hemodynamic response to changes in plasma ionized calcium. *Arch Surg* 115:206–211, 1980

148. Drop LJ, Geffin GA, O'Keefe DD, et al: Relation between ionized calcium concentration and ventricular pump performance in the dog under hemodynamically controlled condition. *Med J Cardiol* 47:1041–1051, 1981

149. Waller JL: Inotropes and vasopressors, in Kaplan JA (ed): *Cardiac Anesthesia*, vol 2, *Cardiovascular Pharmacology*. New York, Grune & Stratton, 1983, p 288

150. Lappas DG, Drop LJ, Buckley MJ, et al: Hemodynamic response to calcium chloride during coronary surgery. *Surg Forum* 26:234–235, 1975

151. Cote CJ, Daniels AL, Drop LJ: Comparative hemodynamic and ionized calcium effects of calcium gluconate and calcium chloride. *Anesthesiology* in press

152. Zimmerman ANE, Daems W, Lulsmann WC, et al: Morphological changes of heart muscle caused by successive perfusion with Ca-free and Ca-containing solutions (Ca-paradox). *Cardiovasc Res* 1:201–209, 1967

153. Benzing G, Helmsworth JA, Schrieber JT, et al: Nitroprusside after open-heart surgery. *Circulation* 54:467–471, 1976

154. Faraci PA, Rheinlander HF, Cleveland RJ: Use of nitroprusside for control of pulmonary hypertension in repair of ventricular septal defects. *Ann Thorac Surg* 29:70–73, 1980

155. Beekman RH, Rocchini AP, Dick M, et al: Vasodilator therapy in children: Acute and chronic effects in children with left ventricular dysfunction or mitral regurgitation. *Pediatrics* 73:43–51, 1984

156. Knapp E, Gmeiner R: Reduction of pulmonary hypertension by nitroprusside. *Int J Clin Pharmacol Biopharm* 15:75–80, 1977

157. Beekman RH, Rocchini AP, Rosenthal A: Hemodynamic effects of nitroprusside in infants with a large ventricular septal defect. *Circulation* 64:553–558, 1981

158. Rosenthal MH, Pearl RG, Schroeder JS, et al: Nitroglycerine versus nitroprusside in pulmonary hypertension. *Anesthesiology* 55:A79, 1981

159. Appelbaum A, Blackstone EH, Kouchoukos NT, et al: Afterload reduction and cardiac output in infants early after intracardiac surgery. *Am J Cardiol* 39:445–451, 1977

160. Davies DW, Greiss L, Steward DJ: Sodium nitroprusside in children: Observations on metabolism during normal and abnormal responses. *Can Anaesth Soc J* 22:553–560, 1975

161. Rubin LJ, Peter RH: Oral hydralazine therapy for primary pulmonary hypertension. *N Engl J Med* 302:69–73, 1980

162. Beekman RH, Rocchini AP, Rosenthal A: Hemodynamic effects of hydralazine in infants with a large ventricular septal defect. *Circulation* 65:523–528, 1982

163. Linday LA, Levin AR, Klein AA, et al: Acute effects of vasodilators on left-to-right shunts in infants and children. *Pediatr Pharmacol* 1:267–278, 1981

164. Artman M, Parrish RC, Boerth RJ, et al: Hemodynamic effects of acute hydralazine in infants with atrioventricular canal defects. *Circulation* 66:Suppl II:112, 1982

165. Rao TK, El-Etr AA: Right ventricular function in pulmonary hypertension-role of nitroglycerine. *Anesth Analg* 63:263 (abst), 1984

166. Goetzman BW, Sunshine P, Johnson JD, et al: Neonatal hypoxia and pulmonary vasospasm: Response to tolazoline. *J Pediatr* 89:617–621, 1976

167. Levin DL, Gregory GA: The effect of tolazoline on right-to-left-shunting via a patent ductus arteriosus in meconium aspiration syndrome. *Crit Care Med* 4:304–307, 1976

168. Rudolph AM, Paul MH, Sommer LS, et al: Effects of tolazoline hydrochloride on circulatory dynamics of patients with pulmonary hypertension. *Am Heart J* 55:424–432, 1958

169. Vogel JHK, Cameron D, Jamieson G: Chronic pharmacologic treatment of experimental hypoxic pulmonary hypertension. *Am Heart J* 72:50–59, 1966

170. Ruskin LJ, Hutter AM: Primary pulmonary hypertension treated with oral phentolamine. *Ann Intern Med* 90:772–774, 1979

171. Freed MD, Heyman MA, Lewis AB, et al: Prostaglandin E$_1$ in infants with ductus arteriosus-dependent congenital heart disease. *Circulation* 64:899–905, 1981

172. Clyman RI, Mauray F, Roman C, et al: Factors determining the loss of ductus arteriosus responsiveness to prostaglandin E. *Circulation* 68:433–436, 1983

173. Lewis AB, Freed MD, Heyman MA, et al: Side effects of therapy with prostaglandin E$_1$ in infants with critical congenital heart disease. *Circulation* 64:893–898, 1981

174. Szczerlik J, Dubiel JS, Mysik M, et al: Effects of prostaglandin E$_1$ on the pulmonary circulation in patients with pulmonary hypertension. *Br Heart J* 40:1397–1401, 1978

175. Watkins WD, Peterson MD, Crone RK: Prostacycline and prostaglandin E$_1$ for severe idiopathic pulmonary artery hypertension. *Lancet* 1:1083(letter), 1980

176. Pickoff AS, Singh S, Gelband H: The medical management of cardiac arrythmias, in Roberts NK, Gelband (eds): *Cardiac*

Arrythmias in the Neonate, Infant, and Child (ed 2). Norwalk, NJ, Appleton-Century-Crofts, 1983, pp 297–339

177. Mirkin BL, Siniako A: Clinical pharmacology and theraputic utilization of antihypertensive agents in children, in New MI, Levine LS (eds): *Juvenile Hypertension.* New York, Raven Press, 1977, pp 195–217

178. Ponce FE, Williams LC, Webb HM, et al: Propranolol palliation of tetralogy of Fallot: Experience with long term drug treatment in pediatric patients. *Pediatrics* 52:100–108, 1973

179. Shand DG, Sell CG, Oates JA: Hypertrophic obstructive cardiomyopathy in an infant-propranol therapy for three years. *N Engl J Med* 285:843–844, 1971

180. Gelband H, Rosen MR: Pharmacologic basis for the treatment of cardiac arrythmias. *Pediatrics* 55:59–66, 1975

181. Zeligs MA, Lockhart CH: Perioperative hypoglycemia in a child treated with propranolol. *Anesth Analg* 62:1035–1037, 1983

182. Soler-Soler J, Sagrista-Sauleda J, Cabrera A, et al: Effect of verapamil in infants with paroxysmal supraventricular tachycardia. *Circulation* 59:876–879, 1979

183. Greco R, Musto B, Arienzo V, et al: Treatment of paroxysmal supraventricular tachycardia in infancy with digitalis, Adenosine-5'-Triphosphate, and verapamil: A comparative study. *Circulation* 66:504–508, 1982

184. Epstein BL, Kiel EA, Victorica BE : Cardiac decompensation following verapamil therapy in infants with supraventricular tachycardia. *Pediatrics* 75:737–740, 1985

185. Gelband H, Steeg CN, Bigger JT: Use of massive doses of procainamide in the treatment of ventricular tachycardia in infancy. *Pediatrics* 48:110–115, 1971

186. Garson A, Kugler JD, Gillette PC, et al: Control of late postoperative ventricular arrythmias with phenytoin in young patients. *Am J Cardiology* 46:290–294, 1980

187. Koch-Weser J: Bretylium. *N Engl J Med* 300:473–477, 1979

16

Anesthesia for Children with Heart Disease

Paul R. Hickey

The most important consideration in anesthesia for children with heart disease is the necessity for individualizing care. Each lesion in congenital heart disease is polymorphic; tetralogy of Fallot, for example, can result in severe cyanosis and congestive failure in the first months of life, or can in its milder forms be consistent with virtually normal growth and result in few symptoms during childhood. Uncorrected congenital heart disease presents one set of problems for management during anesthesia, but the growing number of patients who have had "correction" of their congenital heart disease often present a quite different set of problems resulting from their corrective procedures. "Cookbook" approaches in children with heart disease are thus fraught with difficulties.

Anesthetic management of these patients therefore is based on the principles of pediatric anesthetic care outlined in other chapters of this text, as well as on the physiologic and pharmacologic considerations in the pediatric cardiovascular system described in the preceding chapter.

PREANESTHETIC EVALUATION

HISTORY

Evaluation prior to surgery is based on the classic triad of history, physical examination, and laboratory examination. Specific areas in the history must be explored in detail. Cyanosis, whether intermittent or continuous, as well as related stress, squatting, sweating, syncope, and upper extremity hypertension, all are important cardiac symptoms and signs useful in estimating clinical status. Exercise intolerance, feeding intolerance, tachypnea, and failure to thrive early in life are major manifestations of congestive heart failure in young children.

Cardiac medications, past and current, are important aspects of the history, since more children are treated with drugs, such as beta-blockers and calcium channel blockers in addition to digoxin and diuretics. Past episodes of congestive heart failure requiring hospitalization must be carefully reviewed, as must any major systemic disease. Previous surgical procedures, especially cardiac, must be reviewed in detail, along with the anesthetic records. *If previous cardiac surgical procedures have been performed, evidence for residual cardiac dysfunction and rhythm problems must be carefully sought out, and one should never assume that the cardiac lesion is now "cured."* Associated anomalies and their status must be precisely defined.

PHYSICAL EXAMINATION

While specific anatomic diagnoses of congenital heart disease may be difficult to make by physical examination alone, much useful information is gained by a physical examination. Evaluation of respiratory rate and pattern, including associated signs of respiratory distress such as nasal flaring, retractions, grunting, and respiratory alternans, will be helpful in assessing cardiac function, as well as providing a baseline for the judgment of adequacy of ventilation prior to postoperative extubation.

Pulses and their quality in all extremities provide clinical evidence for coarctation, previous sacrifice of a subclavian artery for a Blalock-Taussig shunt, a coarctation repair, or, when coupled with pulse pressure, aortic incompetence. Respiratory variations in pulse pressure may indicate hypovolemia or cardiac tamponade.

The general activity level, cyanosis at rest or during crying, general state of nutrition, height and weight percentile, pedal temperature, presence of enlarged liver and spleen and fullness of the anterior fontanelle, and examination of the chest for scars from previous procedures, all give the clinician much useful information about the child's circulatory status and cardiovascular reserve. These points are noted in addition to the usual preanesthetic examination, which concentrates on the airway, venous access, behavior, relation to parents, and other routine matters of concern to the pediatric anesthesiologist.

LABORATORY EVALUATION

Laboratory data, including echocardiographic examination and cardiac catheterization, are important for an understanding of the pathophysiology. The hematocrit level on admission to the hospital is often the best indicator of the magnitude of right-to-left shunting. Polycythemia with hematocrits above 60 percent complicates management. Consideration of therapy to lower the hematocrit level prior to operation may be indicated if the operative procedure will not correct the problem.

Cardiac catheterization data must be carefully evaluated for right-sided pressures, the site and magnitude of shunting, pressure gradients indicating obstructive lesions, and evidence of regurgitant lesions, as well as systemic saturation and myocardial function.

Response of the pulmonary vasculature to 100 percent inspired oxygen during catheterization is important, especially in patients with pulmonary hypertension. Decreases in pulmonary arterial pressure with 100 percent oxygen indicate a significant reactive component to the pulmonary hypertension. This implies that irreversible pulmonary vascular obstructive disease is not present, so that postoperative pulmonary hypertension is less likely to be a problem.

Pressure, and pressure gradients, must be evaluated in terms of flow. In cases where pulmonary flow is several times the systemic flow, despite pulmonary hypertension of more than half the systemic pressure level, pulmonary hypertension is unlikely to persist after repair of a defect through which a significant left-to-right shunt is occurring. When normal levels of pulmonary flow are restored, pulmonary pressures will generally return to normal. In the case of coarctation of the aorta, small pressure gradients are misleading if cardiac output was low at the time of measurement, since the apparent degree of coarctation and obstruction will be understated.

While catheterization data are important, they may be misleading in a patient who is heavily sedated or anesthetized during the catheterization study. Furthermore these data may be months old, thus bearing little relation to the present clinical status in the rapidly changing cardiovascular system of a child. Raw data obtained during a catheterization are subject to different interpretations; wide variations in calculated shunts, pulmonary-to-systemic flow ratios, and vascular resistance are possible, depending on how the raw data are manipulated. For these reasons, catheterization data require critical interpretation and integration with the clinical picture. Catheterization data that do not fit the present clinical status of the child should be viewed critically.

Two-dimensional echocardiography can provide current, noninvasive information quickly and accurately, supplementing and even replacing catheterization data in some instances. It is an excellent screening tool in sick newborns with suspected congenital heart defects.[1] A screening echocardiogram should be seriously considered before anesthesia in all neonates with multiple congenital abnormalities. Consultations with the child's cardiologist will help in interpretation of echocardiographic and catheterization data and in assessing cardiac reserve.

ANESTHETIC MANAGEMENT

CLASSIFICATION

The conventional classification of children with heart disease into those with cyanotic and those with acyanotic lesions is inadequate for anesthetic management. This conventional classification ignores the dynamic nature of congenital heart disease, the impact of palliative and corrective procedures, and the many variations of each specific lesion. For those who are not widely experienced in caring for children with heart disease, the functional grouping presented in Table 16-1 is useful in the preanesthetic assessment of circulatory status. This classification emphasizes the expected functional defects in the more common forms of pediatric heart disease. In addition to a general functional classification, the most critical areas of each child's pathophysiology usually can be determined from preoperative evaluation and from consultation with pediatric cardiologists. Identification of critical pathophysiology will guide appropriate anesthetic management.

Children with shunting as their primary problem are divided into those with right-to-left and those with left-to-right shunts. In disease which is primarily obstructive (e.g., congenital valvular obstruction, obstruction in the great vessels, or acquired valvular obstruction) the concerns of filling pressure, perfusion pressure, and heart rate become paramount. The same holds true in congenital or acquired regurgitant lesions. When primary myocardial disease is the critical problem, avoidance of myocardial depression and implementation of inotropic support is essential. If pulmonary hypertension is present, then anesthetic management is directed towards minimizing fluctuations in pulmonary artery pressure.

In more complex lesions where the problems of shunting, obstruction, regurgitation, and myocardial disease coexist, the management of multiple areas of pathophysiology will require close attention and planning. An estimate of general functional status, such as that outlined in Table 16-1, together with analysis of the critical elements of the pathophysiology, are much more useful in guiding anesthetic management than a conventional classification system.

PREMEDICATION

Recommendations for specific premedications in pediatric patients with heart disease are legion. We generally omit premedications for infants under six months of age, and often prescribe little or no premedication for older, healthier children with low anxiety levels and with whom good preoperative rapport can be established. In children with severe congestive heart failure or with cyanosis, heavy premedication is generally avoided. Morphine (0.1 mg/kg), with atropine or scopolamine as indicated, is generally well tolerated by the sickest of patients. Glycopyrrolate may be a useful alternative as a long-term antisialogogue. Supplemental premedication with intramuscular ketamine (1–2 mg/kg) in the preoperative facility under the direct supervision of the anesthesiologist, is an excellent compromise. This provides for a quiet child and calm separation from the parents, and minimizes the dangers of unsupervised heavy premedication in sick children with heart disease who may experience an exacerbation of the blunted ventilatory response to hypoxia often seen in congenital heart disease.[2] When ketamine is used in these patients we feel that premedication with an antisialogogue is important.

Table 16-1

Functional Grouping

Group A. Normal functional cardiac status	
PDA	Postoperative (PO) with no residual defect
ASD	PO no residual defect, normal sinus rhythm (NSR)
VSD	PO no residual defect, NSR
VSD	Spontaneous closure
TOF	Corrected, no residual defect, NSR
Other	Anomalous subclavian artery, right aortic arch, dextrocardia and situs inversus, other defects of embryologic and possibly genetic significance, but not affecting cardiac function
Group B. Mild cardiac defect	
VSD	Qp:Qs < 2:1 with normal PA pressure, NSR unoperated, or PO with residual shunt
PS	RV-PA pressure difference 50 mm or less; unoperated or PO
CA	PO normal blood pressure, arm to leg BP difference < 20 mm Hg
ECD	PO with mild residual MI
MI	Congenital MI due to prolapse or other causes; mild, no severe dysrhythmia
TOF	PO mild residual PS ± PI ± small VSD, ± RBBB
Other	Bicuspid aortic valve (BAV) with AI ± LV-aorta pressure difference of 20 mm or less: small atrial or other shunts PO or unoperated with Qp:Qs 1.5:1 or less; peripheral PS mild
Group C. Moderate cardiac defect	
VSD	Qp:Qs > 2:1 and/or with AI, PS, or anomalous RV muscle bundle
PS	RV-PA pressure difference > 50 mm Hg unoperated or PO
CA	Unoperated or PO with BP differences arms and legs > 30 mm Hg and/or arm BP greater than 150/95
TOF	PO with RV-PA pressure difference > 50 mm Hg, grossly dilated or calcified outflow patch, AI or TI or dysrhythmias

Table 16-1 (continued)

AS	Unoperated or PO with LV-aortic pressure difference 20 mm Hg ± AI
TGA	Post-Mustard ± residual shunts or dysrhythmias
Other	Unoperated or PO PDA, ASD, AV canal etc. requiring surgery or reoperation: AI, moderate. Dysrhythmias: sick sinus syndrome, other. Cardiomegaly with C/T ratio 60% ± with any congenital lesion
Group D. Severe cardiac defect	
Cyanotic	
TOF	Unoperated or with palliative shunt, PO open repair with homograft, prosthetic valve, or with severe dysrhythmia
TGA	All not in Group C
SV	All types with or without prior shunts
TA	All types with or without prior shunts
PVOD	Eisenmenger reaction or primary pulmonary hypertension
Other	Truncus variants, pulmonary atresia with VSD, rare cyanotic lesions

Acyanotic

Cardiomyopathy including hypertrophic subaortic stenosis (IHSS) or following fibroelastosis or ligation anomalous left coronary artery, other

LV outflow obstruction, e.g., subaortic tunnel or other unrelieved AS with LV-aortic pressure differences of 80 mm Hg or greater

Dysrhythmias—associated syncope, or requiring pacemaker: prolonged or incapacitating + any cardiac defect

Prosthetic valves: severe AI or MI, other

PDA = Patent Ductus Arteriosus; ASD = Atrial Septal Defect; VSD = Ventricular Septal Defect; TOF = Tetralogy of Fallot; PS = Pulmonic Stenosis; CA = Coarctation of Aorta; MI = Mitral Insufficiency; AS = Aortic Stenosis; TGA = Transposition of Great Arteries; TA = Tricuspid Atresia; PVOD = Pulmonary Vascular Obstructive Disease; ECD = endocardial cushion defect; SV = single ventricle; Qp:QS = pulmonary systemic flow (Reprinted from Moss' Heart Disease in Infants, Children, and Adolescents, 3rd Ed., Adams FH, Emmanouilides G.C. (Eds) Baltimore. William & Wilkins, 528, 1983. With permission.)

Older children with less critical circulatory status often respond well to oral diazepam as a supplement to their intramuscular medication when more premedication is required.

PLANNING

Monitoring, induction, maintenance, emergence, and postoperative care, all are based on the preoperative evaluation and planned procedure, and then modified as required by intraoperative events. In pediatric cardiac patients with diminished cardiac reserve, major surgical procedures have greater potential for adverse effects on the circulation. In minor procedures, the anesthetic itself is the major physiologic stress on the child.

Table 16-2 outlines physiological stresses imposed on cardiac patients by various types of procedures, exclusive of the anesthetic. The magnitude of the management problems, along with suggested minimal monitoring required to deal with these stresses, are included. Obviously, for more critically ill patients, monitoring for any given procedure may need to be more extensive.

MONITORING

Basic monitoring during a minor surgical procedure for the child with mild heart disease (such as a small, asymptomatic patent ductus arteriosus) includes EKG, a precordial or esophageal stethoscope, a temperature probe, and a blood pressure cuff. The addition of a Doppler flow detector facilitates measurement of blood pressure and provides a continuous monitor of blood flow when breath sounds and heart sounds are obscured by "rain out" from the humidification system.

As sicker patients are anesthetized, or more extensive procedures are undertaken, monitoring becomes more extensive. It is debatable at what point an arterial line is indicated, but in any patient with existing arterial desaturation, or the potential for desaturation from right-to-left shunting, even minor procedures might best be carried out with an arterial line. Ability to quickly sample arterial blood gases and continuous display of blood pressure and arterial wave form will enable a more rapid response to circulatory problems, since the tolerance for disturbance of the circulatory status quo in these patients is limited. Radial artery lines are standard, but

Table 16-2

Physiological Stresses and Monitoring During Various Procedures

Procedure	Stresses	Effects	Magnitude	Monitoring
Cardiac Catheterization	Atrial and ventricular ectopy	Cardiac output	Mild & transient	EKG Precordial stethoscope
	Obstruction of stenotic valves and vessels	Cardiac output	Mild & transient	Arterial line
CAT Scan Radiation Therapy	None	—	—	EKG Blood pressure TcO₂ or oximeter (if cyanotic)
Dental & Minor Surgery	Blood loss and fluid shifts Positioning	Preload and electrolytes	Minimal to mild	Same as above, Esophageal stethoscope; larger procedures may need arterial line
Major thoracic, abdominal & orthopedic surgery	Same as above and direct manipulation of lungs, diaphragm, heart and great vessels	Same as above plus PVR & SVR	Moderate to severe	Same as above and arterial line, CVP, and possibly oximeter TcO₂ monitor
Cardiac surgery	All of above	All of above and primary myocardial function	Severe	All of above and intracardiac lines

several other sites can be used, each with its own potential problems.

Monitors of Gas Exchange

Transcutaneous oxygen and carbon dioxide monitors in well perfused patients can be useful supplements, or even occasionally substitutes, for arterial lines when arterial access is a problem or when continuous monitoring of oxygenation is desired. Pulse oximeters can provide the same information with a somewhat faster response time and have the same limitations. A special use of these monitors in neonatal anesthesia is for the detection of right-to-left transductal shunting using preductal and postductal monitors as alternatives to using radial *and* umbilical artery lines. End-tidal carbon dioxide monitors and fiberoptic indwelling oximeters are other means of monitoring both ventilation and pulmonary blood flow in patients whose arterial blood gases are readily affected by alterations in either ventilation or pulmonary blood flow.

Central Venous and Pulmonary Arterial Catheters

Percutaneous central venous lines can be very useful in children with cardiac disease, although their placement in infants can be difficult. For cardiac surgical procedures, cooperative cardiac surgeons will usually have the heart quickly exposed and available for inspection and estimation of filling pressures. Central lines can then be established readily from the field and handed off to the anesthesia team. For long, complex non-cardiac procedures, especially when access to the infant is limited and the heart is not exposed, central venous lines may be very helpful. In small infants, percutaneous insertion of central venous lines through the internal jugular or subclavian route may fail, or be associated with pneumothorax, hemorrhage, and hematoma formation after puncture of major arteries.[3–6] The external jugular vein is probably the

safest route when a line can be successfully threaded (59% in one study of children).[7] In children with unrestrictive intracardiac ventricular or atrial septal defects, including hearts with a single ventricle or single atrium, *the central venous pressure is equivalent to left ventricular filling pressure.*

Pulmonary arterial lines in children *with intracardiac defects* usually provide little more information than a simple central line, are difficult to insert without fluoroscopy, and cannot provide meaningful measurements of cardiac output. In babies with persistent fetal circulation or respiratory failure, and children who have primary myocardial disease or valvular disease and otherwise normal hearts, conventional thermodilution pulmonary arterial lines can be of great value.

Temperature

Temperature monitoring at one site is generally sufficient for non-cardiac procedures, whereas multiple sites, including rectal, core temperature (e.g., esophageal), and a measurement of brain temperature (e.g., nasopharyngeal or tympanic), are used in cardiac procedures employing cardiopulmonary bypass or circulatory arrest. Temperature monitoring at multiple sites allows estimation of tissue perfusion during periods of cooling and warming. Use of multiple temperature monitoring sites during periods of circulatory arrest also assures adequate levels of hypothermia for organ protection, especially protection of the brain, since sizable temperature gradients can develop in the body if insufficient time is allowed during cooling and warming on bypass.

Calcium

Monitoring of *ionized* calcium [Ca⁺⁺] levels in arterial blood is essential during cardiac surgical cases or other cases where significant quantities of citrated blood are infused rapidly or where entire blood volumes are replaced when on cardiopulmonary bypass. Smaller children are especially prone to disturbance of their ionized calcium level when citrated blood is infused, and those with limited cardiac reserve tolerate hypocalcemia poorly. Total serum calcium by itself can be misleading in this regard.

Urine Output

Urine output is often the most readily available index of circulating volume status, and obviously requires monitoring in any prolonged case where cardiac dysfunction or large intravascular and extravascular volume shifts are a possibility. In small children, the small quantity of normal urine flow may be difficult to measure unless small gauge tubing is used to attach an appropriate size urimeter to the urinary catheter. While the patient is on bypass, the amount of hemolysis seen in the urine is a good index of the trauma to blood components from the pump and suctioning.

Airway Pressure

Airway pressure monitoring is essential in the neonate, especially in the premature, and also in infants with a history of bronchopulmonary dysplasia, pneumopericardium, or pneumothorax. In children who are prone to development of pneumopericardium or pneumothorax continuous monitoring of airway pressure will help prevent sudden intraoperative development of these potentially fatal complications. Furthermore, in children with abnormally low pulmonary compliance who are covered with surgical drapes so that chest movement is obscured, airway pressure may be the only good index of the adequacy of ventilation, unless end-tidal $PaCO_2$ or arterial gases are being monitored.

SPECIFIC PROBLEMS DURING ANESTHESIA IN CHILDREN WITH HEART DISEASE

CYANOSIS

Compensatory mechanisms activated when children become cyanotic include polycythemia, increases in circulating blood volume, vasodilation, and metabolic adjustments of factors such as circulating 2,3-diphosphoglycerate (DPG). These adjustments allow better utilization of available oxygen. The increase in blood viscosity with polycythemia leads to increased vascular resistance and sludging, which have resulted in renal, pulmonary, and cerebral thromboses, especially in dehydrated children.[8] Long periods without oral intake both preoperatively and postoperatively should therefore be avoided in children with hematocrits over 60 percent, unless adequate intravenous hydration is supplied.

Coagulopathies are well known in children with cyanotic congenital heart disease, and pulmonary vascular resistance is known to increase more than systemic vascular resistance as the hematocrit increases, further decreasing pulmonary blood flow in patients who already have a compromised pulmonary circulation.[9–12] When the hematocrit reaches 65 percent, polycythemia is no longer advantageous, since the disadvantages of the hydraulic stresses of high blood viscosity outweigh the advantages of increased oxygen-carrying capacity. Reduction of red cell volume has been shown to correct the coagulopathy and also to improve hemodynamics when hematocrit elevations are extreme.[13]

BACTERIAL ENDOCARDITIS PROPHYLAXIS

Children with valvular disease, prosthetic valves, most forms of congenital heart disease, hypertrophic cardiomyopathy (IHSS), mitral valve prolapse, and also postoperative cardiac patients, should have antibiotic prophylaxis for operations.[14] All patients with repaired or corrected cardiovascular lesions continue to receive preoperative and postoperative antibiotic prophylaxis; only uncorrected secundum atrial septal defects, secundum atrial septal defects closed without a patch, and closed patent ductus arteriosus are generally excluded from prophylaxis. The children at highest risk for bacterial endocarditis are those with prosthetic valves, congenital aortic stenosis after valvotomy, and those with systemic-to-pulmonary anastomoses (Blalock-Taussig, etc.).[15] The recommendations for prophylaxis in children are shown in Table 16-3.[16] These should be implemented by the anesthesiologist if not ordered by the surgical team. Those at highest risk should probably have parenteral prophylaxis.

CARDIAC SHUNTING

In congenital heart disease much of the pathophysiology involves communications between chambers or vessels that are normally separate, resulting in shunting of blood flow between ventricles, atria, the great arteries, or a combination of these structures, depending on the nature of the lesion. Management of this shunting is a major consideration during anesthesia and requires an understanding of the factors which control shunting.

Dependent and Obligatory Shunts

Rudolph's distinction between dependent shunting and obligatory shunting is very useful for understanding control of intracardiac shunting.[17] *Dependent shunts* are those in which size and direction of shunting through abnormal cardiac communications depends on the relationship between pulmonary and systemic vascular resistance (SVR), and are thus variable. Dependent shunting occurs between two structures having pressures which are nearly equal, or at least having the same order of magnitude. Dependent shunts include patent ductus arteriosus, simple atrial and ventricular septal defects, and aortopulmonary windows and most other systemic-artery-to-pulmonary-artery shunts, such as Blalock-Taussig, Waterston, and Glenn shunts.

In contrast, *obligatory shunts* are those in which shunting is relatively independent of the relationship between PVR and SVR. Resistances tend to be fixed and blood flow occurs between structures having pressures differing by an order of magnitude. Obligatory shunting occurs between the left ventricle and the right atrium in common atrioventricular canal defects, and between systemic arteries and veins in peripheral arterial venous fistulae.

Special forms of obligatory shunts occur in complex heart disease when partial or complete obstruction to blood flow occurs along with communications between chambers. In tricuspid or mitral atresia, obligatory shunting occurs between the atria because there is no atrial outlet on the side of the atresia. In aortic or pulmonary atresia, likewise, obligatory shunting occurs between either the atria or the ventricles because there is no ventricular outlet. While these special types of obligatory shunts are independent of vascular resistances, they only can occur simultaneously with a dependent type of shunt at another level which provides either pulmonary blood

Table 16-3

Prevention of Bacterial Endocarditis[1]

Procedure	Dosage for Children
Dental & upper respiratory procedures[2]	
Oral[3]	
Penicillin V	≥60 lbs: 2 g 1 hr before surgery then 500 mg q6 h × 8 doses
	<60 lbs: half adult dose 1 hr before procedure, 6 hr later 250 mg q6h × 8 doses
Erythromycin (penicillin allergy)	20 mg/kg 1 hr before procedure, 10 mg/kg 6 hr later × 8 doses
Parenteral[3]	
Ampicillin	50 mg/kg IM or IV 30 min to 1 hr before procedure, repeat once 8 hr later
or Aqueous penicillin G	50,000 units/kg IM or IV 30 min to 1 hr before procedure, repeat once 8 hr later
plus Gentamicin	2.0 mg/kg IM or IV 30 min to 1 hr before procedure, repeat once 8 hr later
Vancomycin (penicillin allergy)	20 mg/kg IV infused over 1 hr, beginning 1 hr before procedure, repeat once 8 hr later
Gastrointestinal & genitourinary procedures	
Parenteral	
Ampicillin	50 mg/kg IM or IV 30 min to 1 hr before procedure, repeat once 8 hr later
plus Gentamicin	2.0 mg/kg IM or IV 30 min to 1 hr before procedure, repeat once 8 hr later
Vancomycin (penicillin allergy)	20 mg/kg IV infused over 1 hr, beginning 1 hr before procedure, repeat once 8 hr later
plus Gentamicin	2.0 mg/kg IM or IV 30 min to 1 hr before procedure, repeat once 8 hr later

1. For patients with valvular heart disease, prosthetic heart valves, most forms of congenital heart disease (but not uncomplicated secundum atrial septal defect), idopathic hypertrophic subaortic stenosis, and mitral valve prolapse.

2. Data are limited regarding the risk of endocarditis with a particular procedure. For a review of the risk of bacteremia with various procedures, see ED Everett, JV Hirschman, *Medicine* 56:61, 1977.

3. An oral regimen is safer and is preferred for most patients. Parenteral regimens are more likely to be effective; they are recommended especially for patients with prosthetic valves, those who have had endocarditis previously, or those taking continuous oral penicillin for rheumatic fever prophylaxis.

(Reproduced and modified with permission from Medical Letter 26:652, 1984)

flow in the case of pulmonary atresia, or systemic flow, in the case of aortic atresia.

When partially obstructive lesions occur simultaneously with communications between chambers, as in pulmonary stenosis with patent ductus or tetralogy of Fallot, the distinctions between the two types of shunts blur. Similarly, when the pressure differential on two sides of a dependent shunt becomes very great, it takes on the characteristics of an obligatory shunt. However, except in the most complex forms of congenital heart disease rarely seen by the nonspecialist, these distinctions between various types of shunting are useful in anesthetic care of most children with congenital heart disease because they predict how shunts will be altered by any given stress.

Restrictive Shunts

The above discussion assumes that the intracardiac and great vessel communications are relatively large and nonrestrictive. When communications are small, the size of the defect itself limits shunting and considerations of relative pulmonary and systemic vascular resistance become correspondingly smaller in determining the amount of shunting. Whenever there is a large pressure differential at the same level of the circulation on either side of a communication, the communication is restrictive; flow is limited across the defect, and other factors determining shunt flow become less important. This is usually the situation in children with mild heart disease that is asymptomatic or minimally symptomatic, such as small atrial and ventricular septal defects, or a small patent ductus arteriosus.

DEPENDENT SHUNTING DURING
ANESTHESIA

In children with dependent shunts, the direction and amount of their shunting is determined by their circulatory dynamics. Control of circulatory dynamics to minimize the shunt is one major goal of anesthetic management. Since

Table 16-4

Techniques to Manipulate Relative Vascular Resistances

Vascular Resistance	Increases	Decreases
Pulmonary	PEEP	Avoid PEEP
	Low FiO$_2$	High FiO$_2$
	Acidosis & high PaCO$_2$	Alkalosis (7.6 pH) & low PaCO$_2$
	Direct manipulation	? Vasodilators
Systemic	Vasoconstrictors	Potent inhalational agents
	Direct manipulation	Vasodilators

shunting in these children is dependent on the relationship between systemic and pulmonary vascular resistances, anesthetic management often revolves around control of relative vascular resistances.

In children with dependent *right-to-left* shunts, decreases in SVR or increases in PVR will increase the shunt. In children with dependent *left-to-right* shunts, increases in SVR and decreases in PVR will increase the shunt. In children with bidirectional or balanced shunting, any change in either vascular resistance will increase net shunt away from the side with elevated vascular resistance.

For practical purposes, acute increases in left-to-right shunts during anesthesia are of clinical importance in only a few situations, such as hypoplastic left heart syndrome or pulmonary atresia when the ductus arteriosus is widely patent, and a substantial "steal" of systemic blood flow by the pulmonary circulation can occur. Except for these few extremely large shunts, left-to-right shunting generally is well tolerated, especially during acute episodes. Shunting from right-to-left, since it is accompanied by at least some degree of arterial desaturation, is relatively poorly tolerated, and is much more frequently a problem during anesthesia.

CONTROL OF SYSTEMIC AND PULMONARY VASCULAR RESISTANCE DURING ANESTHESIA

Manipulation of systemic vascular resistance (SVR) during anesthesia is useful during anesthesia for adult cardiac patients. However, in anesthesia for congenital heart disease there is the additional need to manipulate pulmonary vascular resistance (PVR), which may prove very difficult. The reasons for this are that (1) control of pulmonary resistance is poorly understood, (2) vasoactive drugs usually are distributed on both sides of the circulation, and (3) pharmacological attempts to modify shunting have produced unpredictable results.[18-20]

Despite these problems, a number of techniques have proven useful in manipulating relative pulmonary and systemic resistances (Table 16-4). Potent inhalational anesthetics appear to reduce SVR more than PVR. Pulmonary vascular resistance has been shown to be reduced in children by increasing FiO$_2$ to 1.0, and by hyperventilation to a pH of 7.6 or greater.[21,22] Vasoconstrictors such as phenylephrine increase SVR more than PVR, since these vasoconstrictors are acutely effective in reducing right-to-left shunting and increasing left-to-right shunting in the operating room. Positive end expiratory pressure (PEEP) acidosis, hypothermia, and the use of FiO$_2$ of 0.30 or less all can increase PVR.

During cardiac surgical procedures, a more direct method of selectively increasing PVR or SVR is to have the surgeons place partially obstructing tourniquets around pulmonary arteries or the aorta to increase resistances so that flow in the opposite side of the circulation will increase. Systemic vascular resistance can be increased similarly during abdominal surgery with aortic clamps if higher systemic pressures are needed to perfuse the lungs through a systemic to pulmonary artery shunt. Although these are only temporary measures, they may be useful to reestablish a better relative balance of resistances and a more normal physiology in a deteriorating clinical situation.

CHOICE OF ANESTHETIC TECHNIQUE

Evaluation of the patient and the proposed surgical procedure will be the major considerations in the choice of anesthetic technique. Response to premedication, and the parent–child relationship, may have some further influence on the choice of technique.

INHALATIONAL AGENTS

Conventional inhalation induction, when administered cautiously, may be used safely in many children with heart disease, primarily those in functional groups A and B (see Table 16-1). However, in children with more severe heart disease (functional groups C and D), use of the potent inhalational agents considerably narrows the margin of safety and probably should be avoided. While there are theoretical differences in uptake and distribution of inhalational anesthetics in children with intracardiac shunting, these considerations are of little practical importance in clinical anesthesia, as has been shown in children with left-to-right shunts.[23]

Halothane

Studies have shown a greater than 50 percent incidence of hypotension with bradycardia in infants with *normal cardiovascular systems* during induction with halothane.[24,25] A study of ventricular function during halothane induction of normal infants showed decreases in stroke volume and ejection fraction of 38 percent.[26] Uptake of halothane in infants less than three months of age has been demonstrated to be considerably more rapid than in adults; the infant's myocardial concentrations probably increase more rapidly than the adult's.[27] While the effects of halothane on the human neonatal myocardium are unknown, it has been shown that young rats have a reduced cardiovascular tolerance for halothane, while requiring greater amounts for anesthesia.[28] The maximum alveolar concentration (MAC 1.2%) for halothane in infants one to six months of age also has been shown to be the highest of any age group.[29] This increased anesthetic requirement in infants, combined with the immaturity of their cardiovascular system, partly explains the cardiovascular intolerance for halothane in infants.[24–26]

In neonates, the cardiovascular system is even more immature, and though their MAC for halothane is lower (0.87%), it is still higher than in adults.[29] Atropine has been used intramuscularly before induction to partially compensate for the myocardial depression of halothane by reducing bradycardia and hypotension.[24]

Isoflurane

Isoflurane induction in infants might be thought to be less detrimental to the cardiovascular system; however, a 32 percent decrease in heart rate and a 40 percent decrease in blood pressure on induction have been demonstrated in healthy infants under six months of age.[30] In addition, a high incidence of laryngospasm (30%) also occurred in this study.[30] Inadequate ventilation from laryngospasm, or from other causes, will quickly lead to large increases in PVR secondary to hypoxemia and hypercarbia. This is poorly tolerated in small children with heart disease, especially in the presence of actual or potential right-to-left shunts with pulmonary hypertension.

The above studies, along with our clinical experience, suggest that potent inhalational agents may be an unwise choice for induction in young infants with severe cardiac disease. Use of atropine, combined with a slow induction with halothane, may be well tolerated in children with mild to moderate heart disease. In children of any age with marginal cardiovascular reserve, and in those with severe desaturation of systemic arterial blood due to right-to-left shunting, the myocardial depression and systemic hypotension from potent inhalational agents are poorly tolerated. A more appropriate use of these anesthetic agents in children with severe heart disease is the use of small concentrations to control hypertensive reponses after induction.

Nitrous Oxide

The use of nitrous oxide for anesthetic maintenance in congenital heart disease is controversial. In all children with shunts there is potential for micro- and macrobubbles of air from multiple intravenous lines, which can be shunted directly into the systemic circulation. Routine use of air traps in intravenous lines in patients with known intracardiac defects should be combined with careful purging of air bubbles from all intravenous lines. Use of nitrous oxide may cause these bubbles to expand, increasing obstruction to blood flow in arteries and capillaries. The effects of venous air embolism on the circulation have been shown to be exaggerated by the presence of nitrous oxide, even in the absence of paradoxical embolization.[31] In patients with preexisting right-to-left shunts, paradoxical air embolism is clearly a potential problem, but even patients with large left-to-right shunts can transiently reverse their shunts. This is especially true during coughing or a Valsalva maneuver, when the normal transatrial pressure gradient is reversed; several studies have demonstrated right-to-left shunting of microbubbles of air after injection of saline into the right atrium during these maneuvers.[32–34] Since coughing and Valsalva maneuvers often occur during an anesthetic, even the most rigorous attention to air

bubbles in intravenous lines may not prevent some small amounts of air from reaching the systemic circulation. When the left heart is exposed to the atmosphere during cardiac surgery, the same considerations of arterial air embolism apply.

An additional problem is the increase in PVR with nitrous oxide reported in adults.[35,36] On this basis, it has been suggested that in children with limited pulmonary blood flow or with pulmonary hypertension, use of nitrous oxide should be avoided because it may further increase pulmonary hypertension or further decrease pulmonary blood flow. No studies of nitrous oxide effects on PVR in children have been published.

Another problem with nitrous oxide is a decrease in PaO_2 because of the consequent decrease in FIO_2. Our clinical experience suggests PaO_2 is much more dependent on intracardiac mixing than on FIO_2, and use of 40–50 percent oxygen and air usually result in little change in PaO_2 when the cyanosis is due to cardiac problems. The known negative inotropic effect of nitrous oxide is also well documented; this effect can cause marked myocardial depression in abnormal hearts. We use nitrous oxide freely if well tolerated in patients without shunting, avoiding its use in those patients with severely depressed myocardial function. In patients with intracardiac shunts, it occasionally is used to speed induction in more healthy patients, but it is generally avoided after cardiopulmonary bypass.

INTRAMUSCULAR AND INTRAVENOUS ANESTHETICS

Intravenous and intramuscular induction techniques are safe and effective in neonates and infants with severe cardiac disease. They are also effective in older children with a minimum of functional cardiac reserve.

Ketamine

When intravenous access is a problem, intramuscular ketamine (5–10 mg/kg) is well tolerated in sick children with cyanosis and/or congestive heart failure.[37,38] Concommitant intramuscular succinylcholine is used to facilitate control of the airway. Use of atropine or scopolamine to offset the secretions often produced by ketamine is helpful. Although increases in PVR have been reported in adults following ketamine, in well premedicated children ketamine causes no change in PVR when the airway is maintained and ventilation is supported.[39,40] In children with congenital heart disease, the ejection fraction has been shown to be well preserved during ketamine anesthesia.[41] Our clinical experience with IM ketamine has been excellent with most forms of heart disease, including those with limited pulmonary blood flow and cyanosis. Ketamine is also used for short, nonsurgical procedures such as a CAT scan, radiotherapy, and cardiac catheterization.[42]

When intravenous access is readily available in patients with marginal cardiac reserve, several techniques may be used for induction. Ketamine (1–2 mg/kg IV), is an excellent induction agent with most forms of congenital heart disease. Relative contraindications to the use of ketamine may be coronary insufficiency caused by anomalous coronary artery, severe critical aortic stenosis, or hypoplastic left heart syndrome with aortic atresia and hypoplasia of the ascending aorta. These patients are prone to ventricular fibrillation because of relative coronary insufficiency; tachycardia and catecholamine release with ketamine may predispose the patients in this group to ventricular fibrillation.

Fentanyl

As in adults with severe cardiac disease, high-dose intravenous fentanyl, given together with pancuronium and with 100 percent oxygen, or air and oxygen, is an excellent induction technique in very sick children with all forms of congenital heart disease. When fentanyl or other narcotics are used with nitrous oxide, the negative inotropic effects of nitrous oxide may appear, especially in sicker patients.[36,44] The high-dose fentanyl technique has been reported to be effective in premature neonates undergoing ligation of a patent ductus arteriosus.[45] In high risk, full-term neonates, and older infants with severe congenital heart disease, use of the high-dose fentanyl technique in doses of up to 75 μg/kg, given with pancuronium, results in minimal hemodynamic changes on induction and intubation, and only mild hemodynamic responses to surgical incision generally occur.[46] Transcutaneous PO_2 levels are well maintained and actually improve during induction, intubation, and surgical stimulation, even in cyanotic children.[46] Changes in cardiac index, SVR, and PVR in infants given 25 μg/kg of fentanyl have been shown to be insignificant.[47] The use of pancuronium with the high-dose fentanyl technique is recommended; the vagolytic effects of pancuronium offset the vagotonic effects of fentanyl. The hemodynamic stability reported in infants with high-dose fentanyl and pancuronium may not be found when other muscle relaxants are used.[48] The high-dose fentanyl technique is most suitable for sick infants in whom extubation in the operating room is not planned.

Thiopental

Intravenous induction with thiopental generally is not used in patients with severe cardiac defects, although in a reduced dose of 1–2 mg/kg, it may be quite safe for induction in patients with moderate defects (functional group C). In pediatric patients with minimal or mild cardiac defects (functional group A or B), intravenous induction with larger doses of thiopental (3–5 mg/kg) are usually well tolerated, *provided the patient is not hypovolemic.*

MUSCLE RELAXANTS

Pancuronium has been well studied in children with congenital heart disease and produces no heart rate or blood pressure changes when given slowly.[43] An intubating dose of pancuronium, given as a bolus, may produce tachycardia; this is sometimes desirable to support cardiac output in infants in congestive heart failure whose stroke volume is fixed. Metocurine, as well as vecuronium and atracurium, appear to be largely free of cardiovascular side effects in children, but have not been specifically studied in children with heart disease.

MAINTENANCE

Maintenance of anesthesia in the pediatric heart patient depends on the preoperative status and the response to induction, as well as the surgical procedure and intraoperative events. Whether inhalational agents, additional narcotics, or other intravenous agents are used for maintenance depends on the tolerance of the individual patient and postoperative plans for ventilatory management.

In the child with a congenital heart defect, intraoperative changes in cardiac shunting are a unique problem during maintenance of anesthesia. While it is not always clear whether deterioration in clinical condition in these patients is due to changes in shunting or to primary myocardial dysfunction, the intraoperative events and progress of the anesthetic will usually suggest an etiology. Decreases in arterial oxygenation or systemic blood flow may be due to alterations in intracardiac shunting in these children. When circulating blood volume is adequate, either pharmacologic support (see Chapter 15) or techniques of managing intracardiac shunting (Table 16-4) can be employed.

ANESTHESIA FOR NON-CARDIAC SURGERY IN CHILDREN

Most children with heart disease will be quite stable when presenting for elective non-cardiac surgery and will tolerate a well managed anesthetic. However, their tolerance is often limited during events such as loss of airway patency, hypoventilation, inappropriate amounts and choices of anesthetics, and major intraoperative surgical insults. Children on cardiac medications should have their medications continued up to and including the morning of surgery, except perhaps for diuretics. Anesthetic techniques which provide the largest margin of safety are particularly advisable in these children. Control of ventilation, and the use of 50–100 percent oxygen, is recommended in cyanotic children, those with right-to-left shunts, and children with pulmonary hypertension.

Intraoperative problems such as hypotension and hypoxemia should be aggressively treated using the drugs and techniques outlined in this and the previous chapter. By anticipating most problems, significant clinical deterioration will be prevented, since resuscitation may be difficult in these children.

ANESTHESIA FOR CARDIAC SURGERY

Specific discussion of anesthetic considerations for various repairs of each form of congenital heart disease is beyond the scope of this chapter.[49] Space does not permit discussion of the physiology of cardiopulmonary bypass, deep hypothermia with circulatory arrest, and the anesthetic considerations of these techniques.[50,51] However, a short discussion of the problems which may be encountered during repair of the more common congenital heart lesions—including atrial septal defect (ASD), ventricular septal defect (VSD), tetralogy of Fallot (TOF), coarctation of the aorta, and patent ductus arteriosus (PDA)—is presented below, with a brief discussion of the management of cardiopulmonary bypass for repair of congenital heart disease.

CARDIOPULMONARY BYPASS

Management of cardiopulmonary bypass in children with congenital heart disease differs considerably from that in adult patients with acquired heart disease. Perfusion of the child during bypass is controlled primarily by pump flows; arterial pressures are generally of less concern in the pristine arterial tree of the child. Pump flows as high as 150–175 ml/kg/min are utilized in the neonate weighing two or three kilograms. At these flows, mean arterial pressures during bypass are often around 30 mm Hg. As children become older, lower flows are employed until the standard adult flows of 50–70 ml/kg/min are used in children weighing over 50 kilograms. As the child ages, perfusion pressures will generally increase. Since mean arterial pressures are lower than in adults, it is important that no obstruction of venous inflow to the heart exists during bypass, especially in the superior vena cava. If high venous pressures are present in the head during bypass, cerebral perfusion can be markedly decreased in children with low mean arterial pressures. When caval tapes are tightened, it is therefore especially important to check for signs of superior or inferior vena caval obstruction, including pressures in a central venous line positioned distal to the caval tape.

The best available indicator of perfusion during bypass in children is the rate of cooling or warming in various parts of the body, determined by using multiple temperature probes. Core temperature, as measured by esophageal temperature, generally changes most quickly, followed by a lag of several degrees of the nasopharyngeal or tympanic temperature, indicating the degree of perfusion of the brain. A somewhat larger lag is seen in the rectal temperature, or skin temperature of the extremities, since these areas reflect more peripheral perfusion. Temperature gradients between these areas will decrease as a steady state is reached. The same gradients will generally be seen in reverse order during warming. Deviations from the normal temperature gradients seen on warming and cooling require investigation as to their cause, since these abnormal gradients may indicate problems with perfusion of the involved area of the body or incorrect temperature probe placement. When there is no warming or cooling taking place, urine output and systemic acid–base balance are the best available indicators of perfusion.

Although the indicated perfusion rate by the pump head may be high, unless control of all sources of systemic-to-pulmonary shunts is established in patients with congenital heart disease, much of the perfusion from the pump will circle through the lungs and return to the pump as a result of a VSD or an ASD, without perfusing the systemic circulation. While discrete shunts, such as the Blalock-Taussig or the Waterston, may be ligated prior to bypass, many children with cyanotic disease will have extensive aorticopulmonary collaterals that cannot be easily controlled. Under these conditions pump flow rates bear little relation to systemic flow, and other indicators of perfusion outlined above must be employed. An abnormally low perfusion pressure on bypass in the face of high pump flows should bring to mind the possibility of an open systemic-to-pulmonary shunt.

Management of ventilation and the lungs during bypass is controversial, but during partial bypass some ventilation is probably indicated, if only to oxygenate the small amount of blood being ejected from the heart so that the coronaries which receive the bulk of this blood will not be perfused with desaturated blood. At a minimum, flow of 100 percent oxygen into the lungs should continue, even if no mechanical ventilation takes place, so that apneic oxygenation will occur until pulmonary blood flow ceases. Frequent visual checks of arterial and venous lines at the pump will give an estimate of the difference in oxygen saturation, and oxygen consumption. These impressions are periodically confirmed by checks of venous and arterial blood gases, along with the determinations of electrolytes, glucose, hematocrit, and ionized calcium. Addition of blood, sodium bicarbonate, calcium, heparin, potassium, and crystalloid solutions to the pump reservoir, along with gas flow through the oxygenator, will be guided by these values.

Determinations of the need for vasopressor and inotropic support in weaning from bypass are facilitated by close observation of the surgical field during bypass, and especially by the behavior of the heart during the rewarming phase. Arrhythmias, coronary perfusion problems, and the state of myocardial contractility can be estimated from the behavior of the heart during this period. Separation from bypass should be accomplished in concert with the surgical team. While monitoring lines often give an excellent idea of how the heart is functioning, slavish adherence to the numbers thus produced, without visual confirmation of cardiac filling pressures and performance, can lead to numerous errors. In congenital heart operations, problems with oxygenation following bypass are due to deficiencies in pulmonary blood flow as frequently as to deficiencies in ventilation. In patients who are not doing as well as expected in the post-bypass period, there is a high possibility of missed or residual lesions in congenital heart repairs. This should be carefully considered.

ATRIAL SEPTAL DEFECT (ASD)

These defects are relatively benign in childhood and except for rare, large defects, children are usually asymptomatic or mildly symptomatic (see Table 16-1, functional group A or B, rarely C). Even with the larger ostium primum type of defects, symptoms tend to be mild unless associated with appreciable mitral regurgitation; this lesion is properly termed an incomplete atrioventricular canal.

In isolated ASDs repaired during childhood, most anesthetic agents are well tolerated. Pulmonary vascular resistance usually remains normal during childhood, and pulmonary artery pressures are only mildly elevated due to the moderate left-to-right shunting. The shunt is not large because the gradient across the atrial septum is small. Transient reversal of this gradient, and thus shunting itself, is possible with coughing and Valsalva maneuver, or events such as loss of the airway and severe hypoventilation. Systemic air embolization and/or arterial desaturation can result. Eisenmenger physiology, where high pulmonary blood flow results in markedly elevated PVR and permanent reversal of atrial shunting, is rarely seen, since surgical repair is now usually carried out at a younger age.

Repairs are straightforward, except when a sinus venosus type of septal defect is encountered and the septal patch must be placed to baffle pulmonary venous return from the right lung into the left atrium. If not appreciated and corrected this defect will result in a continued left-to-right shunt and volume overload of the right heart as pulmonary venous blood from the right lung returns to the right atrium.

Cardiopulmonary bypass time is short, separation from bypass is uncomplicated, and patients can often be extubated in the operating room or in the intensive care unit shortly after arrival.

VENTRICULAR SEPTAL DEFECT (VSD)

In childhood a VSD may be a serious problem. This is primarily because the pressure gradient between the two communicating chambers tends to be high. Since PVR falls during early infancy, right ventricular pressure falls, and thus the amount of dependent shunting across the ventricular septum becomes large. Severe pulmonary hypertension in childhood is a possibility if large lesions are uncorrected. Congestive heart failure early in life generally results from large VSDs.

Elevated right-sided pressures are present when the defects are large. When the defect is small this lesion behaves more like an ASD. After the initial physiologic fall in PVR during infancy, PVR often remains low early in childhood, although pulmonary artery pressures are somewhat elevated because of the large left-to-right shunts and correspondingly high pulmonary blood flows. If the lesions are not repaired until late in childhood, however, pulmonary vascular disease may have developed from the high flows and pressure. In that event, PVR may remain elevated even after flow has dropped to normal following repair.

When defects are large, with pulmonary/systemic flows (QP/QS) greater than two to one, and congestive failure exists (functional group C), more problems may be encountered on induction of anesthesia. Only low concentrations of potent inhalational agents will be tolerated without appreciable systemic hypotension. If right ventricular pressures are close to systemic pressures, relatively little systemic hypotension will cause the dependent type shunt to reverse; the left-to-right shunt now becomes right-to-left, with systemic desaturation and further myocardial dysfunction leading to progressive hypotension. Intravenous induction techniques, such as ketamine or fentanyl, maintain systemic arterial pressures and are generally safer.

If the defect is small so that the heart is able to support the shunting without congestive failure, and right-sided pressures are mildly elevated (functional group B), a cautious inhalation induction, bearing in mind the limited cardiac reserve, may be well tolerated.

Regardless of induction technique and size of VSD, if the airway becomes obstructed or alveolar hypoventilation supervenes, PVR will increase markedly, increasing right ventricular pressures and possibly reversing the dependent shunt, even when systemic pressures are maintained. The degree of airway obstruction or hypoventilation tolerated will depend on resting levels of right ventricular pressure.

If shunt reversal should occur and the child becomes cyanotic, an alpha-adrenergic agent (such as phenylephrine) to support systemic pressure, establishment of an airway, and hyperventilation with 100 percent oxygen will usually permit a return to baseline pulmonary arterial and right ventricular systolic pressure, with resumption of left-to-right shunting. In clinical practice the tendency should be to err on the side of using techniques that lower PVR and maintain SVR, tending to slightly increase the left-to-right shunt. The higher the probability of right-to-left shunting, the more important this approach becomes.

Once induction is accomplished, maintenance of anesthesia is generally smooth until cardiopulmonary bypass. Although VSD repair is often straightforward, a number of problems can occur. Outflow tract obstruction can sometimes result either in the left or right ventricle when the VSD is high, and the ventricle malaligned so that closure of the defect crowds either the pulmonary or aortic valve orifice. A redundant outflow patch can cause the same problem.

Injury to the bundle of His, with complete heart block, may require pacemaker support to allow weaning from bypass. A more common problem is that of residual muscular type VSDs that are undiagnosed preoperatively. These may be difficult to find among the trabeculated interior of the right ventricle even when specifically sought. The resulting residual left-to-right shunting through these unsuspected defects may make weaning from bypass difficult, and complicate the anesthetic course after bypass and the postoperative course in the intensive care unit, because of low output. If problems are encountered after the repair, drawing a pulmonary artery blood sample and comparing its saturation to a simultaneous mixed venous sample from the right atrium will reveal if there is any significant increase in oxygen saturation in the right ventricle, indicating a residual shunt.

Children having small defects, with short bypass times and benign intraoperative courses, can be extubated in the operating room, but as defects become larger and bypass times lengthen, extubation may be safer if delayed until later on the day of operation. In the more severe forms of VSD, with marked congestive failure, prolonged bypass times, deep hypothermic circulatory arrest, and possible intraoperative ventriculotomy, extubation must be guided by the postoperative clinical course.

TETRALOGY OF FALLOT (TOF)

This lesion varies widely in its severity. Infants may become cyanotic and have frequent "tet spells" in the first six months of life, requiring palliation with a Blalock-Taussig shunt, or repair in infancy. In its more mild forms, no palliation is needed and children may be largely asymptomatic and acyanotic through early childhood.

In the more severe forms, large amounts of valvular and outflow obstruction of the right ventricle rapidly leads to systemic pressures in that chamber, with right-to-left shunting intermittently or continuously through the VSD. Stress may lead to increases in both right ventricular outflow obstruction and PVR, increasing right-to-left shunting and resulting in severe cyanosis, a "tet spell."

Pulmonary vascular resistance is usually normal because the pulmonic stenosis and right-to-left shunting protect the vascular bed of the lungs from both the high pressure in the right ventricle and high flow seen in VSDs with left-to-right shunts.

Maintenance of systemic pressures and a patent airway are critical during induction of anesthesia. If patients are extremely cyanotic and polycythemic, adequate preoperative hydration is necessary. In severe cases, techniques using 100 percent oxygen, with fentanyl and pancuronium as the baseline anesthetic, are satisfactory. Ketamine also is an excellent induction agent *as long as* the airway is maintained and ventilation is controlled. Increases in PVR associated with ketamine in children probably are secondary effects of the respiratory depression with hypoventilation and loss of airway.[40]

If a cyanotic spell develops during induction, or prior to initiation of cardiopulmonary bypass, or especially during manipulation of the great vessels with cannulation, initial treatment should be as outlined for reversal of shunt in VSDs. This includes hyperventilation with 100 percent oxygen, a bolus of phenylephrine, and elevation of the legs to increase central blood volume. As an alternative or addition to the steps above, propranolol (0.005 mg/kg initially, then increasing as needed) has been used intravenously to abort spells. Morphine (0.1-0.2 mg/kg) has also been used to abort spells, although it may not be as useful in a well anesthetized and narcotized patient.

Intraoperative problems include residual right ventricular outflow obstruction, pulmonic insufficiency as the result of resection of the pulmonic stenosis or a transannular outflow patch, partial or complete heart block, and residual VSDs. Some patients have peripheral pulmonic stenosis, which may not be appreciated at catheterization because pulmonary arteriograms usually cannot be done without great risk.

Most TOF patients have at least some degree of right ventricular dysfunction after repair, which is additive to myocardial dysfunction resulting from bypass itself. Pulmonary insufficiency of some degree, and right ventricular dysfunction resulting from right ventriculotomy, are always present, along with a right bundle branch block. If residual pulmonic obstruction, shunting, or peripheral pulmonic stenosis are added, right ventricular function can be severely compromised, requiring significant inotropic support. Pulmonary artery saturations of greater than 80 percent during ventilation with an FIO_2 of 0.5 generally indicate a significant residual left-to-right shunt.[52] Residual shunts of this magnitude may make the intraoperative course following bypass and the postoperative course in the intensive care unit difficult.

Because of these problems, children undergoing surgery for TOF are generally not extubated until the day following the operation, unless the defects are mild and the intraoperative course has been totally benign.

COARCTATION OF THE AORTA

This lesion may have a great range of presentations, from critical coarctations in the sick, acidotic newborn (functional group D), where the ductus arteriosus supplies the great majority of the systemic perfusion to the lower half of the body, to asymptomatic older children (functional group B) whose coarctation is discovered incidentally and who have only minimal upper extremity hypertension.

The neonate with critical coarctation will require prostaglandin E_1 infusion to maintain ductal patency, improve systemic perfusion, and hopefully correct acidosis. Induction must be carefully carried out to maintain cardiovascular stability in the face of a large right-to-left shunt to the lower half of the body. Some stability is provided by the more normal arterial saturations in the upper half of the body perfused by the left ventricle, but myocardial depressant anesthetics are still poorly tolerated. The asymptomatic older child will probably tolerate a smooth induction by any of a number of techniques. The potential for shunting is virtually nil, and cardiac reserve is usually good.

Intraoperative problems related to the procedure will be different in these two types of patients. Retraction of the lung in the lateral position may have profound consequences on arterial oxygenation, especially in the neonate whose transitional circulation is still unstable. Use of the subclavian flap angioplasty technique for repair renders the left arm useless for intraoperative blood pressure measurements.

Cross clamping of the aorta is generally well tolerated in the neonate, since the isthmus of the aorta has little flow through it. In the older child, especially those with preexisting hypertension of the upper extremity, cross clamping of the aorta may result in systolic pressures in the upper half of the body approaching 200 mm Hg. Although aggressive treatment of this may appear indicated, the anesthesiologist should be aware that perfusion of renal, hepatic, and especially spinal cord vascular beds is dependent on high arterial pressures in the upper half of the body when the thoracic aorta is cross clamped. Lowering arterial pressures in the upper half of the body below preanesthetic levels may predispose the kidney and the spinal cord to ischemic damage. Recent animal studies have shown that while use of vasodilators such as nitroprusside may improve the circulation above the occlusion, the mean arterial pressure and organ perfusion below the occlusion decreases. This has been associated with paraplegia in dogs.[53,54]

In children with coarctation, especially after a short cross-clamp time, the decline in arterial pressure with removal of the cross clamp is usually mild to moderate, and quickly rises again if central blood volume is adequate. More severe falls in pressure may be treated with partial reapplication of the clamp and gradual removal. Extubation in the operating room for older patients with coarctation is routine, whereas sick neonates and infants are usually ventilated at least overnight.

PATENT DUCTUS ARTERIOSUS (PDA)

A PDA may vary greatly in its severity. A large PDA in the newborn may cause congestive failure and ventilator dependence, particularly in the premature infant (functional group D); a small PDA may remain undetected during early childhood in asymptomatic children (functional group B).

Considerations on induction are similar to those in coarctation of the aorta in patients of similar age and preoperative condition, except that left-to-right shunting with pulmonary overperfusion and systemic underperfusion must be considered. Low diastolic pressure, and pulmonary "steal" from the systemic circulation, can result in decreased organ perfusion. In neonatal lambs with left-to-right ductal shunting, perfusion of the myocardium, gastrointestinal tract, and even the brain, increases significantly when the ductus is obliterated.[55] Elevated pulmonary artery pressures with the potential for reversal of shunting are rarely encountered in this lesion, except in older patients with end-stage pulmonary vascular obstructive disease and a large PDA. Transient reversal of shunting across the ductus with desaturation of blood going to the lower half of the body can occur, as it does in neonates with "persistent fetal circulation."

PRINCIPLES OF POSTOPERATIVE CARDIAC CARE

The timing of extubation and the intensity of care during recovery will be based on the preoperative assessment of the child's cardiopulmonary status, the procedure performed, and the assessment of intraoperative events, including the course of the anesthetic; this is no different than for the child with a normal cardiovascular system.

In a child with heart disease the determination must be made regarding how much the anesthetic and surgical procedure have further disturbed the preexisting homeostasis of the abnormal cardiopulmonary system. After cardiac procedures, an estimate is made of the degree of correction of cardiovascular physiology, and how much temporary dysfunction will result from factors such as cardiopulmonary bypass and surgical trauma. After procedures such as cardiac catheterization, CAT scans, or minor dental procedures, the child's physiology will be little disturbed by the procedure, and only the effects of the anesthetic need be considered. In these situations, even in children with severe cardiac defects, extubation immediately following the procedure should be possible after a brief, well managed anesthetic. If the procedure is prolonged and the patient is slow to awaken, extubation should be delayed. Even mild hypoventilation secondary to residual anesthetic in the postoperative period may result in hypoxic vasoconstriction and increases in PVR. Children with either significant potential for right-to-left shunting, limited pulmonary blood flow, or pulmonary hypertension, have little tolerance for hypoventilation and should be wide awake with an unobstructed airway before extubation.

In patients with severe polycythemia from chronic arterial desaturation, postoperative hydration is as important as preoperative hydration, especially when the hematocrit is above 60 percent. Postoperative intravenous hydration should be continued until the child has a good oral intake with no nausea and vomiting.

When abdominal or thoracic procedures are performed, the threshold for employing postoperative ventilatory support decreases as the cardiac defect becomes more severe, especially when large amounts of fluid and blood have been given. Just as the effects of intraoperative ventilation on relative PVR are important in altering shunting, they are equally important in the postoperative course (Table 16-4).

Pediatric cardiac patients who required inotropic and pressor support intraoperatively will usually require intensive care postoperatively. Transport of these patients to the intensive care area should be accomplished expeditiously, and with monitoring appropriate to the length of the transport and the patient's condition prior to transport. Continuation of the pressor support is essential during transport, especially since children who require this support are prone to become unstable. The stresses involved in transport, and the often unavoidable changes in the rate of administration of drugs and intravenous fluids during transport, make this a particularly vulnerable period. Portable, battery operated infusion pumps must be utilized for long transports, especially when inotropic agents are required. The utmost vigilance must be maintained during preparations for transfer, as well as during and after transfer into the intensive care unit. Frequent interruptions in monitoring and a high need for therapeutic interventions during transport have been reported in children following cardiothoracic surgery.[56] In our experience hypovolemia is the most frequent problem during and immediately after transport, and immediate availability of blood and blood products is imperative during this period.

After cardiac surgical procedures, the rapidity with which cardiac tamponade may cause cardiovascular collapse must be appreciated. Tamponade may occur even with apparently adequate drainage from chest and mediastinal tubes. In small children, the small volume of the pericardial space leads to rapid onset of tamponade with few preliminary warning signs. The small caliber drainage tubes used in infants are easily clotted or sequestered from the area of tamponade so that they became ineffective.

The use of adequate sedation to prevent movement has been shown to decrease oxygen consumption in the postoperative period.[57] The use of muscle relaxants may not further reduce oxygen consumption significantly in patients who are not actively moving, but will often facilitate control of ventilation to optimize shunting and oxygenation. The use of fentanyl with muscle paralysis, and use of pancuronium as a continuation of anesthesia postoperatively for hours or days, has been reported to help control pulmonary hypertension

and shunting after repair of congenital diaphragmatic hernia.[58] This technique has also been applied to the postoperative care of neonates and infants with highly reactive pulmonary circulations following repair of congenital heart disease. The use of moderately high doses of fentanyl to blunt the stress responses of the pulmonary circulation to noxious stimuli such as endotracheal suctioning has been demonstrated to be effective in infants.[59]

OUTCOME OF ANESTHESIA IN CHILDREN WITH HEART DISEASE

Children with heart disease have an increased incidence of cardiovascular complications during anesthesia and surgery, but the magnitude of this risk has not been well documented. In 1966, a 3 percent anesthetic mortality was reported in infants under one year of age undergoing cardiac surgery.[60] Few data are available which document modern mortality from anesthesia in children with heart disease, but a well managed anesthetic should rarely contribute to mortality even in the sickest children with cardiac disease.[61]

REFERENCES

1. Linday LA, Ehlers KH, O'Loughlin JE, et al: Noninvasive diagnosis of persistent fetal circulation versus congenital cardiovascular defects. Am J Cardiol 52:847–851, 1983
2. Edelman NH, Lahiri S, Braudo L, et al: The blunted ventilatory response to hypoxia in cyanotic congenital heart disease. N Engl J Med 282:406–411, 1970
3. Prince SR, Sullivan RL, Hackel A: Percutaneous catheterization of the internal jugular vein in infants and children. Anesthesiology 46:362–364, 1977
4. Groff DB, Ahmed N: Subclavian vein catheterization in the infant. J Pediatr Surg 9:171–174, 1974
5. Groff DB: Complications of intravenous hyperalimentation in newborns and infants. J Pediatr Surg 4:460–464, 1969
6. Coté CJ, Jobes DR, Schwartz AJ, et al: Two approaches to cannulation of a child's internal jugular vein. Anesthesiology 50:371–373, 1979
7. Humphrey MJ, Blitt CD: Central venous access in children via the external jugular vein. Anesthesiology 57:50–51, 1982
8. Phornphutkul C, Rosenthal A, Nadas AS: Cerebrovascular accidents in infants and children with cyanotic congenital heart disease. Am J Cardiol 32:329–334, 1973
9. Kontras S, Sirak H, Newton W: Hematologic abnormalities in children with congenital heart disease. JAMA 195:611–615, 1976
10. Ekert H, Sheers M: Preoperative and postoperative platelet function in cyanotic congenital heart disease. J Thorac Cardiovasc Surg 67:184–190, 1974
11. Lister G, Hellenbrand WE, Kleinman CS, et al: Physiologic effects of increasing hemoglobin concentration in left-to-right shunting in infants with ventricular septal defects. N Engl J Med 306:502–506, 1982.
12. Fouron JC, Hebert F: The circulatory effects of hematocrit variations in normovolemic newborn lambs. J Pediatr 82: 995–1003, 1973
13. Mauer H, McCue C, Robertson L, et al: Correction of platelet dysfunction and bleeding in cyanotic congenital heart disease by simple red cell volume reduction. Am J Cardial 35:831–835, 1975
14. Committee on Prevention of Rheumatic Fever and Bacterial Endocarditis of the American Heart Association: Prevention of bacterial endocarditis. Circulation 56:139A, 1977
15. Kaplan EL, Rich A, Gersony W, et al: A collaborative study of infective endocarditis in the 1970's. Emphasis on infections in patients who have undergone cardiovascular surgery. Circulation 59:327–335, 1979

16. Prevention of bacterial endocarditis. *Med Lett Drugs Ther* 26:3–4, 1984

17. Rudolph AM: *Congenital Diseases of the Heart.* Chicago, Yearbook Medical Publishers, 1974, pp 29–48

18. Beekman RH, Rocchini AP, Rosenthal A: Hemodynamic effects of nitroprusside in infants with a large ventricular septal defect. *Circulation* 64:553–558, 1981

19. Beekman RH, Rocchini AP, Rosenthal A: Hemodynamic effects of hydralazine in infants with a large ventricular septal defect. *Circulation* 65:523–528, 1982

20. Linday LA, Levin AR, Klein AA, et al: Acute effects of vasodilators on left-to-right shunts in infants and children. *Pediatr Pharmacol* 1:267–278, 1981

21. Drummond WH, Gregory GA, Heyman MA, et al: The independent effects of hyperventilation, tolazoline, and dopamine on infants with persistent pulmonary hypertension. *J Pediatr* 98:603–611, 1981

22. Peckham GJ, Fox WW: Physiologic factors affecting pulmonary artery pressure in infants with persistent pulmonary hypertension. *J Pediatr* 93:105–110, 1978

23. Tanner G, Angers D, Barash PG, et al: Does a left-to-right shunt speed the induction of inhalational anesthesia in congenital heart disease? *Anesthesiology* 57:A427, 1982

24. Friesen RH, Lichtor JL: Cardiovascular depression during halothane induction in infants: A study of three induction techniques. *Anesth Analg* 61:42–45, 1982

25. Diaz JH, Lockhart CH: Is halothane really safe in infancy? *Anesthesiology* 51:S313, 1979

26. Lichtor JL, Beker BE, Ruschhaupt DG: Myocardial depression during induction in infants. *Anesthesiology* 59:A452, 1983

27. Brandom BW, Brandom RB, Cook DR: Uptake and distribution of halothane in infants: In vivo measurements and computer simulations. *Anesth Analg* 62:404–410, 1983

28. Cook DR, Brandom BW, Shiu G, et al: The inspired median effective dose, brain concentration at anesthesia, and cardiovascular index for halothane in young rats. *Anesth Analg* 60:182–185, 1981

29. Lerman J, Robinson S, Willis MM, et al: Anesthetic requirements for halothane in young children 0–1 and 1–6 months of age. *Anesthesiology* 59:421–424, 1983

30. Friesen RH, Lichtor JL: Cardiovascular effects of inhalation induction with isoflurane in infants. *Anesth Analg* 62:411–414, 1983

31. Mehta M, Sokoll MD, Gergis SD: Effects of venous air embolism on the cardiovascular system and acid base balance in the presence and absence of nitrous oxide. *Acta Anaesthesiol Scand* 28:266–274, 1984

32. Banas JS, Meister SG, Gazzaniga AB, et al: A simple technique for detecting small defects of the atrial septum. *Am J Cardiol* 28:467–471, 1971

33. Kronik G, Mosslacher H: Positive contrast echocardiography in patients with patent foramen ovale and normal right heart hemodynamics. *Am J Cardiol* 49:1806–1809, 1984

34. Gross CM, Wann S, Johnson GL: Valsalva maneuver echocardiography: A new technique for improved detection of right-to-left shunting in patients with systemic embolism. *Am J Cardiol (Abst)* 49:955, 1982

35. Schulte-Sasse U, Hess Wolfgang, Tarnow J: Pulmonary vascular responses to nitrous oxide in patients with normal and high pulmonary vascular resistance. *Anesthesiology* 57:9–13, 1982

36. Lappas DG, Buckley MJ, Laver MB, et al: Left ventricular performance and pulmonary circulation addition of nitrous oxide to morphine during coronary-artery surgery. *Anesthesiology* 43:61–67, 1975

37. Levin RM, Seleny FL, Streczyn MV: Ketamine–pancuronium–narcotic technique for cardiovascular surgery in infants—a comparative study. *Anesth Analg* 54:800–805, 1975

38. Vaughan RW, Stephen MD: Ketamine for corrective cardiac surgery in children. *South Med J* 66:1226–1230, 1973

39. Gassner S, Cohen M, Aygen M, et al: The effect of ketamine on pulmonary artery pressure: An experimental and clinical study. *Anaesthesia* 29:141–146, 1974

40. Hickey PR, Hansen DD, Cramolini MD: Pulmonary and systemic responses to ketamine in infants with normal and elevated pulmonary vascular resistance. *Anesthesiology* 62:287–293, 1985

41. Bini M, Reves JG, Berry D, et al: Ejection fraction during ketamine anesthesia in congenital heart diseased patients. *Anesth Analg (Abst)* 60:186, 1984

42. Coppel DL, Dundee JW: Ketamine anesthesia for cardiac catheterization. *Anaesthesia* 27:25–31, 1972

43. Maunuksela EL, Gattiker RI: Use of pancuronium in children with congenital heart disease. *Anesth Analg* 60:798–801, 1981

44. Motomura S, Kissin I, Aultman DF, et al: Effects of fentanyl and nitrous oxide on contractility of blood-perfused papillary muscle of the dog. *Anesth Analg* 63:47–50, 1984

45. Robinson S, Gregory GA: Fentanyl–air–oxygen anesthesia for ligation of patent ductus arteriosus in preterm infants. *Anesth Analg* 60:331–334, 1981

46. Hickey PR, Hansen DD: Fentanyl and sufentanyl–oxygen–pancuronium anesthesia for cardiac surgery in infants. *Anesth Analg* 63:117–124, 1984

47. Hickey PR, Hansen DD, Wessel D, et al: Pulmonary and systemic hemodynamic responses to fentanyl in infants. *Anesth Analg* 64:483–486, 1985

48. Salmenpera M, Peltola K, Takkunen O, et al: Cardiovascular effects of pancuronium and vecuronium during high-dose fentanyl anesthesia. *Anesth Analg* 62:1059–1064, 1983

49. Beynen FM, Tarhan S: Anesthesia for repair of congenital heart defects. In Tarhan S (ed): *Cardiovascular Anesthesia and Postoperative Care.* Chicago, Yearbook Medical Publishers, 1982, pp 73–180

50. Ionescu MI: *Techniques in Extracorporeal Circulation* (ed 2). London, Butterworth, 1981

51. Utley JR (ed): *Pathophysiology and Techniques of Cardiopulmonary Bypass,* vol I & II. Baltimore, Williams & Wilkins, 1982 & 1983

52. Lang P, Chipman CW, Siden H, et al: Early assessment of hemodynamic status after repair of tetralogy of Fallot: A comparison of 24 hour (intensive care unit) and 1 year postoperative data in 98 patients. *Am J Cardiol* 50:795–799, 1982

53. Gelman S, Reves JG, Fowler K, et al: Regional blood flow during cross-clamping of the thoracic aorta and infusion of sodium nitroprusside. *J Thorac Cardiovasc Surg* 85:287–291, 1983

54. Symbas PN, Pfaender LM, Drucker MH, et al: Cross-clamping of the descending aorta: Hemodynamic and humoral effects. *J Thorac Cardiovasc Surg* 85:300–305, 1983

55. Baylen BG, Ogata H, Ikegami M, et al: Left ventricular performance and regional blood flows before and after ductus arteriosus occlusion in premature lambs treated with surfactant. *Circulation* 67:837–843, 1983

56. Sudan N, Kosarussavadi B, Rothstein P, et al: Transport of children following cardiothoracic surgery. *Anesthesiology* 55:A337, 1981

57. Palmisano BW, Fisher DM, Willis MM, et al: Effect of paralysis on oxygen consumption in infants after cardiac surgery. *Anesthesiology* 59:A140, 1983

58. Vacanti JP, Crone RJ, Murphy J, et al: Treatment of congenital diaphragmatic hernia with chronic anesthesia to control pulmonary artery hypertension. *Anesthesiology* 59:A436, 1983

59. Hickey PR, Hansen DD, Wessel D: Responses to high dose fentanyl in infants. II. Blunting of stress responses in the pulmonary circulation. *Anesthesiology* 61:In press

60. Strong MJ, Keats AS, Cooley DA: Anesthesia for cardiovascular surgery in infancy. *Anesthesiology* 27:257–265, 1966

61. Hickey PR, Hansen DD, Norwood WI, et al: Anesthetic complications in surgery for congenital heart disease. *Anesth Analg* 63:657–664, 1984

17

Pediatric Neurosurgical Anesthesia

Mark A. Rockoff

The management of a child with neurosurgical disease places great demands upon the anesthesiologist. In addition to problems common to general pediatric anesthesia practice, special considerations must be given to the effects of anesthesia and surgery on the central nervous system. This chapter emphasizes a clinical approach to the evaluation and management of these patients.

PATHOPHYSIOLOGY

INTRACRANIAL COMPARTMENTS

The skull may be compared to a rigid container with nearly incompressible contents. Under normal conditions, the intracranial space is occupied by the brain and its interstitial fluid (80%), cerebrospinal fluid ([CSF] 10%), and blood (10%). In various pathologic states there may be other space-occupying lesions, such as varying amounts of edema, tumor, hematoma, or abscess. For over a century it has been recognized that an increase in volume of one compartment must be accompanied by an approximately equal decrease in volume of the other compartments in order to maintain a normal intracranial pressure (ICP).[1] The brain itself can provide some compensation to offset these pathologic increases of volume within the cranium. This includes intracellular dehydration and a reduction in interstitial fluid volumes. The compensatory mechanisms provided by the other compartments (CSF and blood), however, are better understood and can be more readily altered.

Under normal conditions, CSF exists in dynamic equilibrium with absorption balancing production. The average adult has between 90 and 150 ml of CSF distributed throughout the brain and subarachnoid space. Children have correspondingly

smaller amounts; in neonates, often only a few drops can be obtained from the spinal canal. Production occurs largely, although not exclusively, in the choroid plexus, and renewal occurs about five times each day.[2] Production of CSF is little affected by alterations of intracranial pressure (ICP), and is usually unchanged in children with hydrocephalus. Some drugs (including acetazolamide, furosemide, and steroids) do, at least temporarily, decrease CSF production.[1,3,4] Choroid plexus papillomas which cause overproduction of CSF are rare, but are more likely to occur in childhood.

Absorption of CSF is not well understood, but it appears that the arachnoid villi are important sites for reabsorption of some CSF into the venous system. One-way valves exist between the subarachnoid space and the sagittal sinus that, in man, open at about five torr. Reabsorption increases with elevation of ICP. There are many conditions which can result in decreased CSF absorption (intracranial hemorrhage, central nervous system infections, and possibly congenital malformations), presumably through obstruction of arachnoid villi and/or pathways of CSF flow.[5] In infancy, if external ventricular drainage is employed, over 100 ml/day of CSF may be obtainable.

CSF translocation initially compensates for any addition to intracranial volume and prevents elevation of ICP. This translocation occurs through the foramen magnum to the distensible spinal subarachnoid space. As pressure increases, and especially if changes are sudden, brain distortion develops that can block the pathways of CSF flow. The loss of this compensatory mechanism can lead to a significant elevation of ICP, and can result in rapid clinical deterioration. Ultimately, herniation of brain tissue results. In the presence of open fontanelles and open cranial sutures, these effects may be attenuated by increasing head circumference. It is important

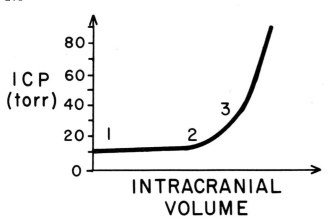

Figure 17-1.   Idealized intracranial compliance curve.

to note, however, that herniation can still occur in patients with open fontanelles if acute, severe increases in ICP develop.

INTRACRANIAL PRESSURE

In children the signs of increased ICP may not be apparent on clinical examination. Pupillary dilatation, increasing blood pressure, and bradycardia may be absent in the presence of intracranial hypertension, or may occur with normal ICP.[6,7] When associated with increased ICP, they are usually late and dangerous signs.[8] Papilledema may not be present even in children dying as a result of intracranial hypertension.[9] A diminished level of consciousness, especially when associated with abnormal motor responses to painful stimuli, is frequently associated with elevated ICP.[6] Computerized tomography (CT) brain scanning is extremely helpful by demonstrating small or obliterated ventricles or basilar cisterns, hydrocephalus, intracranial masses, or midline shifts. It is important to note that increases in ICP occurring soon after head injury in children are not often due to intracranial hematomas (as in adults), but are more likely secondary to diffuse brain swelling caused by excessive cerebral blood volume.[10]

Techniques used to monitor ICP in adults have been useful in children.[11-14] Unfortunately, ventricular catheters may be difficult to insert in conditions where they are most needed, e.g., severe brain swelling associated with small ventricles. Subarachnoid bolts are most commonly used to monitor ICP, but are difficult to stabilize in infants less than one year of age because of the thin calvarium. An epidural transducer secured noninvasively to the anterior fontanelle has been used to assess neonatal ICP and it may be surgically implanted in patients of any age.[14,15]

As with adults, normal values for ICP are generally accepted as less than 15 torr. On occasion children with intracranial pathology and a normal baseline ICP may exhibit pressure waves, which should be considered abnormal.[6] In the presence of open fontanelles, significant increases in head circumference can occur with ICP in the "normal range." Furthermore, ICP abnormalities can exist without bulging fontanelles, especially if changes develop slowly.

INTRACRANIAL COMPLIANCE

Knowledge of the ICP itself does not always indicate how much compensatory ability remains. If the ICP is abnormally elevated, then compensation has failed. If the ICP is within the normal range, however, dangerously increased intracranial volume may or may not be present. Intracranial compliance (the change in pressure that occurs with change in volume) is a concept that may be applied to intracranial dynamics.[16] Figure 17-1 represents a theoretical relationship between the addition of volume to intracranial compartments and intracranial pressure. The actual shape of the curve depends upon the time over which the volume increases and the relative size of the compartments. At normal intracranial volumes (point 1), ICP is low (high compliance), and it remains so with an added volume increment. If volume increases fast enough, compensatory abilities will be exceeded. Further addition of volume will cause increases in pressure. This can occur while the actual level of ICP is still within normal limits (point 2), but the compliance at this stage is low. When the ICP is already elevated, further volume expansion results in rapid ICP elevation (point 3). In an individual patient, compliance can be evaluated by injecting small amounts of saline into a ventriculostomy catheter, or can be more safely estimated by observing the response of ICP to various extraneous stimulating procedures, such as endotracheal suctioning.

CEREBRAL BLOOD FLOW (CBF) AND CEREBRAL BLOOD VOLUME (CBV)

Intracranial blood volume represents another compartment through which compensatory mechanisms influence the ICP. Although CBV occupies only a small proportion (10%) of the intracranial space, dynamic blood-volume-related changes occur that are often initiated by anesthesia or intensive care procedures. As with other vascular beds, most blood is contained in the low-pressure, high-capacitance venous system.[17] Increases in intracranial volume are met initially by decreases in cerebral venous blood volume. This is apparent in hydrocephalic infants, in whom a shift of venous blood from intracranial to extracranial vessels produces distended scalp veins.[18] Ultimately, increased CBV results in elevation of ICP.

CBV is usually proportional to CBF, and is affected by many homeostatic mechanisms. In the normal adult, CBF is approximately 55 ml/100 g of brain tissue/min.[19] This is almost 15 percent of the cardiac output for an organ that represents only two percent of body weight. In small children CBF accounts for an even greater percentage of cardiac output.[2]

CBF is regulated to match the metabolic needs of the brain. The mechanism for this coupling is probably mediated by a local hydrogen ion effect upon cerebral vessels. Factors which result in acidosis (hypoxia, hypercarbia, ischemia) cause cerebrovascular dilatation, which augments CBF and increases CBV. Similarly, a reduction in brain metabolism normally reduces CBF and CBV. If this metabolic autoregulation is impaired (because of brain injury), blood flow then becomes dependent upon factors other than demand. When CBF exceeds that required for metabolic needs, "luxury perfusion" or "hyperemia" is said to exist. Many pharmacologic agents act directly upon the cerebral vasculature and, as will be discussed later, affect CBF and CBV. Neurogenic influences also play a role in the regulation of CBF, but are poorly understood.

CEREBRAL PERFUSION PRESSURE (CPP)

At present, CBF determinations are difficult to perform, require expensive specialized equipment, and are limited to investigational centers. However, as with the use of blood pressure to estimate cardiac function (without the knowledge of cardiac output or systemic vascular resistance), CPP is a helpful guide to the adequacy of the cerebral circulation.[20] Cerebral perfusion pressure is defined as the blood pressure gradient across the brain, and is the difference between mean systemic arterial pressure at the entrance to the brain minus mean exit pressure. When ICP is elevated, it then replaces central venous pressure in the calculation of CPP. In the supine patient, the mean cerebral perfusion pressure (CPP) can for practical purposes be considered equal to the mean systemic arterial blood pressure ($\overline{BP}$) minus the mean intracranial pressure ($\overline{ICP}$). If the brain and the heart are positioned at different levels, all pressures must be referenced to the head level.

AUTOREGULATION

In the absence of brain injury, CBF remains constant over a wide range of perfusion pressures[1,19] (Figure 17-2). Autoregulation enables brain perfusion to remain stable with moderate changes in BP or ICP. Normally, with low ICP and low venous pressure, BP approximates perfusion pressure. Constant CBF occurs in healthy adults with a $\overline{BP}$ between 50 and 150 torr. In chronic hypertensive states, both the upper and lower limits of autoregulation are elevated. Although the limits of autoregulation are not known for children or neonates, autoregulation is probably intact at lower absolute values than in adults.

The mechanism by which autoregulation is maintained is partly mediated through myogenic control of arteriolar resistance. Therefore, with falling perfusion pressure, cerebral vessels dilate to maintain CBF, thereby increasing CBV. With increasing perfusion pressure, cerebral vasoconstriction occurs, and CBF is maintained with a lower CBV. Abrupt pronounced elevations in BP can cause early breakthrough of the upper limits of autoregulation and result in locally increased CBF. Outside the limits of autoregulation, CBF becomes passively dependent upon changes in perfusion pressure. Even small BP decreases may then result in ischemia, while BP elevations increase CBV and, therefore, ICP.

Within a wide range of PaO_2, CBF remains constant (Figure 17-2). Only when PaO_2 decreases below about 50 torr does CBF increase in adults. At about 35 torr, CBF increases approximately 32 percent, and at 15 torr CBF is about four times normal. The resultant increase in CBV causes large elevations in ICP when intracranial compliance is low. This limit for PaO_2 may be even lower in neonates. Hyperoxia produces little decrease in CBF.

In the physiologic range, CBF is most sensitive to $PaCO_2$ (Figure 17-2). Between about 20–80 torr, CBF increases with increasing $PaCO_2$. In the adult, with a normal CBV of approximately 130 ml, an increase in $PaCO_2$ to a level of 60 torr results in an increased volume of about 33 ml. If compliance is high, this volume added as a result of hypercarbia will be buffered by CSF translocation. In poorly compliant states, dangerous elevations in ICP may result. This ability of CBF and, therefore, CBV to change with $PaCO_2$ is the basis for therapeutic hyperventilation to reduce ICP. The effects of hyperventilation in neonates have not been closely examined, and reducing $PaCO_2$ to less than 20 torr may be effective and useful in reducing ICP in certain brain-injured children.[10] It is always important, however, to prevent a significant decrease in blood pressure due to mechanical hyperventilation in order to avoid compromising cerebral perfusion.

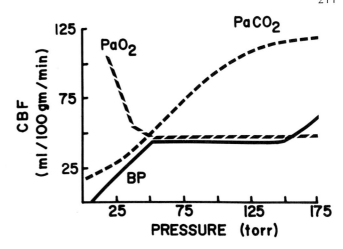

Figure 17-2. The effect of mean blood pressure, PaO_2, and $PaCO_2$ on cerebral blood flow in the normal brain. (From Shapiro HM: *Anesthesiology* 43:447, 1975, with permission.)

Autoregulation of CBF may be disrupted in areas of damaged brain.[21] Blood vessels in an ischemic zone are subjected to hypoxia, hypercarbia, and acidosis, which are all potent stimuli for vasodilatation. These vessels then assume a fixed, maximal reduction in cerebrovascular tone, known as "vasomotor paralysis." Furthermore, through unknown mechanisms, small localized lesions may result in autoregulation difficulties in areas far removed from the site of injury.[22] In addition, the extent of autoregulation impairment is variable in brain-damaged patients, and even techniques which measure CBF may not detect localized changes. CBF determinations have shown that a common response to head injury in pediatric patients is an early hyperemic response characterized by an unexplained increase in CBF.[6] Although ICP may be normal in these patients, because the increased CBV is compensated for, compliance is often reduced (Figure 17-1, point 2).

In summary, the normal brain maintains a system of regulation which matches cerebral blood supply to metabolic demand. The cerebral blood volume varies inversely with cerebrovascular resistance. The injured brain may not be able to compensate for increases in intracranial volume that occur secondary to changes in intracranial blood volume or secondary to the injury itself. Furthermore, autoregulation may be lost entirely, or in specific sites in a random and non-quantifiable manner. The knowledge of normal brain physiology and the secondary changes that occur during pathological states form the basis for safe anesthetic management of these children.

ANESTHETIC MANAGEMENT

PREOPERATIVE EVALUATION

The evaluation of the child before surgery has been discussed (see Chapter 4). Nevertheless, due to special concerns relevant to patients with neurologic disorders, certain aspects of this preoperative visit should be emphasized. A careful history of food or drug allergies, eczema, or asthma may provide a warning of possible adverse reaction to the contrast agents frequently used for neuroradiological studies. Medical problems commonly associated with pediatric patients should be sought, since they may also affect the anesthetic technique. For example, halothane, which increases CBF, may be indicated for children with severe asthma despite the presence of an intracranial lesion. Prior episodes of croup may influence the choice of endotracheal tube size for prolonged procedures. Large adenoids make nasotracheal intubation more difficult. The use of aspirin for headache may cause bleeding abnormalities; high-dose steroids given in the recent past would require continuation (and often augmentation) in the perioperative period. Anticonvulsant drugs may alter metabolism of other medications; they should also be maintained perioperatively.

The physical examination should include a neurological assessment, particularly regarding signs of intracranial hypertension. Examination of pupillary responsiveness and equality will detect benign congenital anisocoria or other preoperative abnormalities. Motor weakness may affect ability to cough and breathe adequately, impaired gag and swallowing mechanisms may interfere with airway protection, and muscle dysfunction may alter the response to muscle relaxants or confuse assessment of their effectiveness. The physical examination should also detect preoperative pulmonary dysfunction (such as aspiration pneumonia) and disorders of hydration (which may be secondary to prolonged vomiting, poor appetite, diabetes insipidus, inappropriate antidiuretic hormone secretion, or iatrogenic dehydration caused by fluid restriction or osmotic agents). Accurate weight of the patient is necessary to guide drug, fluid, and blood replacement. Baseline vital signs, including temperature, blood pressure, heart rate, and respiratory rate, should be recorded.

Laboratory data should include a hematocrit. Additional studies, such as a chest x-ray, urinalysis, EKG, clotting parameters, serum electrolytes and osmolality, blood urea nitrogen and creatinine, pH, and blood gas analysis may be appropriate. Occasionally urine osmolality and electrolytes may also be helpful. A blood sample should be sent to the blood bank for typing and crossmatching.

PREMEDICATION

Premedication is frequently withheld from pediatric neurosurgical patients. The exception is the rare child with an intracranial aneurysm, where premedication is essential to avoid agitation. Narcotics and sedatives are not administered on the wards to patients with intracranial hypertension, central nervous system depression, or hypotonia, since the effects of the drugs are unpredictable in these patients, and respiratory depression or airway obstruction may occur. Atropine is usually avoided, since its vagolytic effect often dissipates by the time of induction, and the drying effect is disturbing to the patient and usually unnecessary. Atropine or its pharmacologic equivalent may be administered during induction if required. Pentobarbital (4–5 mg/kg) or diazepam (0.2–0.5 mg/kg) may be given orally with a small amount of water 1.0–1.5 hours preoperatively to very anxious and alert patients.

As an alternative to oral or intramuscular premedication, methohexital, 20–30 mg/kg, may be given rectally as a ten percent solution in sterile water.[23] This will result in sedation sufficient to permit intravenous catheter placement or smooth inhalation induction. Although not studied, rectal barbiturates probably lower ICP in a similar way to intravenous barbiturates if airway obstruction is prevented. Methohexital should

be avoided in patients with psychomotor, temporal, or mixed seizure disorders, since it may induce convulsions under these conditions;[24] rectal thiopental in the same dosage may be preferable in these circumstances.[25] Chloral hydrate (20–50 mg) has also been useful in infants and can be administered orally as well as rectally.[26]

MONITORING

Minimum monitoring for pediatric anesthesia includes a stethoscope (precordial or esophageal), electrocardiogram, and observance of temperature (core or axillary) and blood pressure (with the appropriate size of cuff by auscultation, palpation, oscillotonometry or Doppler). End-tidal carbon dioxide monitors, neuromuscular blockade monitors, electroencephalograms, evoked potentials, precordial Dopplers, and ICP monitoring devices are used for the same indications as in adults.[27–29]

Urinary output should be closely monitored during prolonged procedures (longer than six hours), during cases with expected large blood loss, or when the use of osmotic diuretics is indicated. An infant "feeding tube" may be substituted for a Foley catheter in smaller infants. Collection into a syringe will facilitate accurate assessment of hourly output. The use of osmotic agents, however, makes urine output a poor guide to intravascular volume status, because the diuresis produced may occur even in the presence of a low intravascular volume.

Small patient size should not preclude the use of invasive monitoring, and may actually be an indication for a more aggressive approach since life-threatening events can occur rapidly in small children. Intra-arterial catheters (22–24 gauge) can be placed percutaneously (or by cutdown) in the radial, dorsalis pedis, or posterior tibial arteries, even in infants weighing less than 1,000 grams. In the first days of life the umbilical artery can be cannulated. It is important to zero the arterial transducer at the level of the head, if head and heart positions differ, so that cerebral perfusion pressure may be calculated. The lateral corner of the eye is at about the level of the foramen of Monro and is a convenient landmark.

Percutaneous central venous cannulation may be indicated for procedures involving major blood loss or possible air embolism. Percutaneous central vein cannulation (external or internal jugular, or femoral vein) using the Seldinger technique has been useful in the smallest children.[30] Anticubital vein cannulation may also provide central venous access; however, this route is technically more difficult in small children. Umbilical vein cannulation in the first few days of life offers an alternative. Children with raised intracranial pressure may not be ideal candidates for internal jugular vein cannulation because of possible impairment of cerebral venous drainage.

SPECIAL PROBLEMS

Positioning

Access to the patient is a common problem in pediatric anesthesia. Disconnection of catheters under drapes can rapidly result in disaster. In small children, slight displacement of an endotracheal tube can result in either extubation or bronchial intubation. It is our practice to have the major intravenous port under direct vision so as to assure accurate administration of all medications, fluids, and blood. In addition, it is

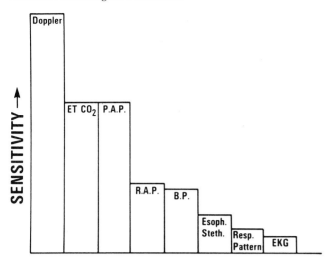

Figure 17-3. Relative sensitivity of air embolism monitoring modalities—end-expired CO_2, (ET CO_2) pulmonary artery pressure (PAP), right atrial pressure (RAP). (Courtesy of Dr. J. Drummond)

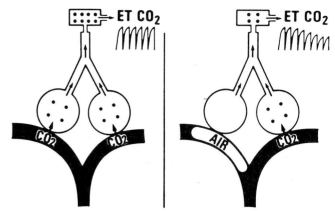

Figure 17-4. Mechanism of decreased end-tidal CO_2 following an air embolus. (Courtesy of Dr. J. Drummond)

vital to have a well lit "tunnel" where possible, to enable access to the airway. We also check the color of the nail beds and capillary perfusion with the aid of a flashlight when the child is obscured by the surgical drapes. The liberal use of tincture of benzoin and adhesive tape is employed in order to prevent accidental displacement of all monitoring devices.

Unusual positioning may also create other dangers for the patient. Care must be taken to assure that movement will not occur that might result in dangerous stretching of nerves (such as an arm falling over the side of the operating table) or compression of vital areas (such as eye or chin compression if the head moves off the headrest). Watertight eye pads and ophthalmic wetting agents should be used to keep the eyes closed and protected from surgical prep solutions and the dangers of corneal drying. Extremes of head position may cause brainstem compression in patients with posterior fossa pathology (mass lesions or Arnold-Chiari malformation).[31]

Fortunately, use of the sitting position appears to be less popular among pediatric neurosurgeons. Some pediatric centers have abandoned the sitting position entirely for posterior fossa craniotomies. In any case, it is rarely used for children under three years of age.[32] In the prone position, care must be taken to assure free abdominal wall motion to avoid impairment of respiration or increased intra-abdominal pressure resulting in increased epidural venous pressure. The child is usually supported by padding under the chest and pelvis. It is unavoidable that some anesthetic equipment must be temporarily disconnected to facilitate positioning of the patient, but constant attention should be directed toward the heart tones audible with the esophageal stethoscope. Periods of monitoring "blackout" should be kept to a minimum.

If the sitting position is used, the danger of air embolization increases as the distance between the head and the heart increases.[33] This is especially true during craniotomy, since large venous channels held open by passage through bone may remain patent. Air emboli can also occur in the supine position, especially in small children undergoing large craniotomy with the head of the bed elevated. As can be seen from Figure 17-3, the characteristic murmur and cardiovascular changes which occur with air embolization are late signs. End-tidal

carbon dioxide monitoring is more helpful than simple auscultation. When a sudden decline in end-expired carbon dioxide concentration occurs in the absence of arterial hypotension, it is diagnostic of air embolism (Figure 17-4).[33] When arterial hypotension accompanies the event, the diagnosis by end-tidal carbon dioxide monitoring is more difficult, because hypotension also produces ventilation and perfusion abnormalities. End-tidal nitrogen monitoring is not affected by blood pressure changes, but is less widely available and too insensitive. A precordial Doppler should always be utilized, since it provides the earliest warning of air embolism.[34–37] It is usually placed over the fourth or fifth intercostal space at the right sternal border, where it best detects right-sided heart tones. Two dimensional echocardiography may be the most sensitive method of detecting small air emboli, but is not easily utilized.

A central venous catheter should be placed just above the right atrium to provide a means of evacuating entrained air. The position of the catheter is confirmed by chest x-ray, by transducing intravascular pressures, or by electrocardiographic monitoring.[27] If reasonable attempts to secure central venous access are unsuccessful, it is possible to proceed safely with operations in the sitting position if great attention is devoted to both Doppler and end-tidal CO_2 monitoring. If a CVP is present, appropriate Doppler position can be confirmed by listening for characteristic sounds after rapid administration of saline into the central venous catheter.[35] The peripheral intravenous injection of up to 0.5 ml of carbon dioxide gas has been used in adults, but may not be entirely benign if unsuspected intracardiac shunting occurs.[27] Potential cardiac shunts exist in many otherwise healthy children, and may be significant if pulmonary hypertension develops acutely after large air emboli.[38]

Management of Air Embolism

If air embolization is detected, treatment must be prompt.[36] The surgeon should immediately be notified so the wound may be packed or covered with saline. Lowering the head of the table and compressing the jugular veins when they are accessible can prevent further air entrainment. The addition of positive end expiratory pressure will increase venous pressure, but may aggravate an already decreasing blood pressure. Nitrous oxide should be discontinued to prevent expansion of air bubbles due to the greater solubility of nitrous oxide compared to nitrogen. Attempts should be made to aspirate air from the central venous catheter, but this is usually

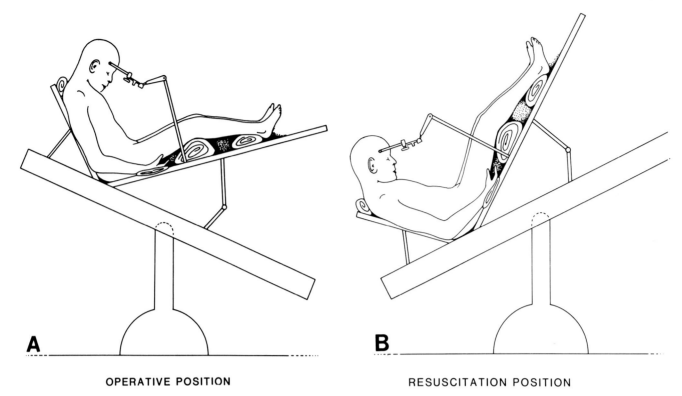

A   **B**

OPERATIVE POSITION   RESUSCITATION POSITION

Figure 17-5. Resuscitation from the modified standard sitting position. Normal operative position (A), and resuscitation position (B). Note that the position can be expiditiously changed by one control of the operating table.

not successful unless substantial and continued amounts of air are entrained. Pressor support and full resuscitative efforts, as well as a change in the position of the table, may be necessary in extreme cases (Figure 17-5).[39] Once the patient is stabilized anesthesia can be readministered. Nitrous oxide can be reinstituted provided the end-tidal carbon dioxide has returned to baseline values and does not decrease again.

Temperature Control

Hypothermia is a common problem in pediatric neurosurgical patients. Children have a greater surface-area-to-weight ratio, and are usually less well insulated with fat. Central nervous system abnormalities themselves, such as hydrocephalus, may predispose the child to autonomic dysfunction and temperature instability.[40,41] Cases are often performed in rooms not designed for pediatric anesthesia.

Although mild hypothermia may be beneficial in paralyzed patients, since it decreases brain energy requirements, the deleterious effects become important during the recovery period. Shivering will not only raise ICP, but will markedly increase oxygen consumption. Metabolic acidosis will depress cardiac output, and arrhythmias commonly occur below 28°C.[42,43] If the patient is to remain under the control of neuromuscular blocking agents, as well as sedated, then mild hypothermia is acceptable. Temperature regulation is considered in greater detail in Chapter 3.

Blood Replacement

Blood loss is difficult to estimate accurately in neurosurgical procedures, since much of the loss is absorbed by the drapes. Irrigation solutions also confuse sponge weights and

suction measurement. Accuracy can be improved if all suctioned blood is collected in calibrated bottles (such as empty 250 ml IV fluid bottles) accessible to the anesthesiologist.

Much blood loss occurs with the initial surgical exposure because of the scalp's marked vascularity. Although bleeding from bone is difficult to control, scalp losses can be decreased by the subcutaneous infiltration of lidocaine with 1:200,000 epinephrine, or diluted concentrations of epinephrine in saline. No more than 3 mg/kg of lidocaine should be used at one time. If the standard solution of 0.5 percent lidocaine with 1:200,000 epinephrine is used, 0.5 ml/kg will deliver less than a toxic dose of either agent. When greater volumes are necessary, this solution can be effectively diluted with an equal volume of saline. The use of lidocaine also provides additional anesthesia for the initial stimulation caused by surgical incision.

Blood replacement principles have been discussed in Chapter 11; however, it is important to consider possible adverse effects that large volumes of crystalloid solutions may have upon cerebral edema formation. In order to minimize exacerbation of cerebral edema all blood losses should be replaced with colloid solutions (five percent albumin, plasma, whole blood, or packed cells) on a milliliter-for-milliliter basis.

Induction

Any patient with an elevated ICP should ideally have an IV line secured in place prior to induction of anesthesia. The use of local anesthetic drugs minimizes the trauma of IV placement and alterations of ICP. If attempts to insert a catheter provoke crying and struggling, making the procedure extraordinarily difficult, the child probably has adequate intracranial compliance to tolerate an inhalation induction.

Spontaneous hyperventilation with oxygen, and the use of mannitol may improve intracranial compliance in the cooperative child.[44]

An important goal during induction is to minimize life-threatening increases in ICP. Therefore ketamine should not be used for induction of anesthesia, since numerous cases of sudden and severe increases in ICP have been reported following ketamine administration, especially in infants and children with hydrocephalus.[45-47] Barbiturates are the induction agents of choice because they cause a decrease in cerebral blood flow and metabolism and, therefore, ICP.[48,49] Thiopental (4-6 mg/kg) and methohexital (1-2 mg/kg) are IV induction agents with ICP-lowering properties. Small doses may also be effective in preventing or treating brief increases in ICP that may accompany painful stimuli. Longer-acting agents, including pentobarbital (3-30 mg/kg) and phenobarbital (50-150 mg/kg), may also be used if prolonged recovery time is not a concern.[50,51] These latter agents are more likely to be used in the ICU in association with ICP monitoring in patients failing conventional therapy for intracranial hypertension. All barbiturates can lower blood pressure and, therefore, should be used with caution in the presence of hypovolemia.

Succinylcholine is frequently used to facilitate intubation because of its rapid action and brief duration. However, it may induce dangerous hyperkalemia in muscular dystrophy, crush injury, burns, spinal cord dysfunction, encephalitis, multiple sclerosis, stroke, or tetanus.[52-57] The dose required for intubation is 1-1.5 mg/kg IV, or 4 mg/kg IM.[58] It is helpful to pretreat children with IV atropine (0.01 mg/kg, with a total dose of at least 0.1 mg) in order to prevent life-threatening bradycardia.

Although succinylcholine may cause a small transient increase in intracranial pressure in some patients, this is not usually of clinical significance.[59,60] The effects upon ICP of a small, defasciculating dose of non-depolarizing muscle relaxant are unknown. Most important, intubation should be rapid and atraumatic to avoid the known ICP-increasing effects of hypoxia, hypercarbia, coughing, bucking, and light anesthesia.[36]

If no airway problems are anticipated, and a lengthy procedure is planned, non-depolarizing agents can be used to facilitate intubation. Pancuronium (0.1 mg/kg) is particularly useful in small children, since its vagolytic properties often increase the heart rate and thus maintain optimal cardiac output. Increasing the dose will affect a more rapid onset, and this is useful when succinylcholine is contraindicated. Curare (0.5 mg/kg) can also been used in children. However, histamine release may have adverse effects in the form of reducing blood pressure and increasing ICP.[61,62] Atracurium may also have a similar effect, especially if large doses (greater than 0.5 mg/kg) are given to facilitate a rapid induction.[63] Muscle relaxants should be avoided or carefully titrated if the neurosurgeon plans direct nerve stimulation.

Controlled hyperventilation, narcotic administration, and supplemental barbiturates prior to intubation will improve cerebral compliance and minimize the increases in ICP caused by laryngoscopy and intubation. Lidocaine (1.5 mg/kg) has been shown to blunt the ICP-increasing effect of laryngoscopy and intubation when given a few minutes prior to these procedures in patients with poor intracranial compliance.[64] Osmotic agents (mannitol, in a dose of 0.25-1.0 g/kg) and diuretics (furosemide, in a dose of 1 mg/kg) may also be used

to improve intracranial compliance.[65] Rapid administration of mannitol may result in sudden systemic vasodilation resulting in decreased CPP.[66] There is danger of causing renal dysfunction when the serum osmolality exceeds 340 milliosmoles/kg.

A technique employing fentanyl (5-15 μg/kg) along with nitrous oxide, barbiturates, and muscle relaxants is commonly utilized in neurosurgical anesthesia.[36] It offers the advantages of maintaining cardiovascular stability (especially in the sitting position), and allows for prompt recovery even after prolonged procedures. It may be used even in very small children.

If surgery is elective and there is no increase in ICP, rectal barbiturates as previously described are particularly useful, especially for children under five years of age who may resist separation from their parents and become frightened by the smell of anesthetic agents. Once consciousness is blunted, an intravenous catheter can be placed, or an inhalation induction performed. Older children will usually cooperate with an inhalation induction when offered as an alternative to an intravenous injection. In the absence of intracranial hypertension, intubation can be performed with deep halothane. If elevated ICP is a concern, then inhalation of halothane to light levels of anesthesia will allow one to secure intravenous access. Early hyperventilation prior to introduction of potent inhalation agents appears to blunt the ICP-increasing effects secondary to cerebral vasodilatation in adults, but the effect of this maneuver in children is unknown.[67] It would certainly appear safer, however, to introduce muscle relaxants with low levels of halothane. The deep level of anesthesia compatible with intubation using inhalation agents alone will lower blood pressure and simultaneously elevate ICP in patients with poor intracranial compliance.

Endotracheal Intubation

Oral intubation is usually preferred because it is expeditious, thus minimizing laryngoscopy and apnea time. A nasotracheal tube may be inserted, however, if ICP has been controlled, since this position offers more stability. If oral tubes are used, they should be placed on the side of the mouth that will be upward, so that saliva which may drain during the case will not loosen the tape. Adhesive drapes can be used to protect the endotracheal tube and its tape from surgical prep solutions. A nasogastric tube is usually inserted after intubation to decrease the amount of air and fluid in the stomach.

Maintenance

Local anesthesia is usually not sufficient for children. It may occasionally be utilized to facilitate CSF drainage prior to induction. Local anesthesia may be supplemented with intravenous sedation in selected older children for brief, radiologic procedures involving little stimulation.

General anesthesia is usually required for most neurosurgical procedures. Ventilation is controlled whenever intracranial hypertension is a factor, and in all infants. Although respiratory function does provide another monitor of brainstem function during spontaneous ventilation, this appears to be outweighed by the safety of controlled hyperventilation during craniotomy.[68]

The effects of commonly used agents on cerebral blood flow are shown in Figure 17-6. All halogenated agents are cerebral vasodilators, and high concentrations of these agents are avoided when ICP is elevated, at least until the dura is opened.[36,69] Halothane is often chosen·since it provides a smooth inhalation induction. Enflurane, especially when com-

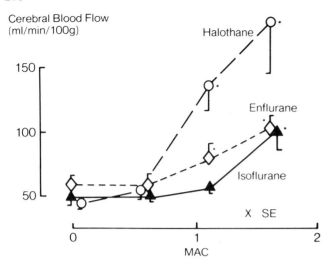

Cerebral Blood Flow
(ml/min/100g)

Figure 17-6. Effects of anesthetic agents on cerebral blood flow (CBF). (From Eger EI, II: *Isoflurane (Forane): A Compendium and Reference.* Madison, WI, Ohio Medical Products, 1981, with permission.)

bined with hyperventilation, may be epileptogenic.[70] Isoflurane seems to produce the smallest increase in CBF at similar depth of anesthesia when compared with halothane or enflurane. It may be the volatile agent of choice once induction has been performed.[71–75] Nitrous oxide may increase ICP in patients with poor cerebral compliance, but this effect appears to be prevented by combining its use with barbiturates or diazepam.[66] The halogenated inhalation agents also cause a dose-dependent decrease in blood pressure due to myocardial depression plus peripheral vasodilation. This makes their use for procedures in the sitting position more hazardous.

Controlled Hypotension

Elective, controlled hypotension may be useful in otherwise healthy patients for certain neurosurgical procedures. This is considered in greater detail in Chapter 12. In the case of extensive reconstructive surgery it appears to reduce blood loss when combined with elevation of the operative site. For surgery of intracranial aneurysms or arteriovenous malformation, it may reduce the tension in the abnormal blood vessels and increase the safety of surgical manipulation. Controlled hypotension should not be used in the presence of increased ICP, since all hypotensive agents cause cerebral vasodilatation, thus increasing ICP and decreasing CPP.

Controlled hypotension is generally induced with potent inhalational agents, e.g., halothane used in combination with ganglionic blockers (trimethaphan, pentolinium) or vasodilators (nitroprusside, nitroglycerine). Although the absolute limits of acceptable hypotension are unknown, a mean blood pressure greater than 40 torr (for small infants) or 50 torr (for older children) appears safe. At the completion of the procedure, the operative site should always be inspected after blood pressure is returned to normal, and systemic hypertension should be avoided to decrease the likelihood of postoperative bleeding.

Awakening from Anesthesia and Postoperative Care

Awakening and extubation should be smooth in order to prevent fluctuations in ICP and venous pressure. Intravenous lidocaine (1–1.5 mg/kg) just prior to extubation may diminish coughing on the endotracheal tube and provide a smooth extubation. A small dose of fentanyl may have the same effect. Neuromuscular blockade should be pharmacologically reversed with atropine (0.02–0.03 mg/kg) and neostigmine (0.06–0.08 mg/kg), since even slight residual paralysis is poorly tolerated. The conditions of adequate air exchange and alert mental status must be met prior to extubation. If there is danger of postoperative increases in ICP the patient should remain intubated.

Repeated neurologic examinations are most important in following postoperative progress.[20] Deterioration in neurologic function is often a complication of intracranial bleeding. For this reason it is usually desirable to have the child as fully alert as possible immediately after the operation. Intracranial pressure can only be carefully followed in unconscious patients by the continuous monitoring of ICP. CT scans are extremely helpful in evaluating either rising ICP or deteriorating neurologic status. Cranial ultrasound diagnosis may be useful if the fontanelles are still open. Careful assessment of fluid and electrolyte status is necessary to avoid difficulties produced by diabetes insipidus or inappropriate antidiuretic hormone release. Portable evoked potential monitoring (auditory, visual, somatosensory) can be performed and, is invaluable in detecting brainstem abnormalities in patients who are paralyzed and heavily sedated. Close observation in an intensive care unit familiar with the care of children is vital to the prevention and early detection of all postoperative problems.

SPECIAL PROCEDURES

This section will consider some of the common neurosurgical and neuroradiologic procedures requiring anesthesia.

CRANIOTOMY

Brain tumors are second only to leukemia as a cause of cancer in childhood, and are the most common solid tumors. Therefore, most elective craniotomies in childhood are for tumor excision. Contrary to the situation in adults, the majority of pediatric brain tumors are infratentorial. Patients with tumors in the pituitary/hypothalamic region may have preoperative or postoperative hormonal dysfunction, especially diabetes insipidus. Aneurysms presenting in childhood are rare and frequently fatal. Large arteriovenous malformations may present in neonates as congestive heart failure.[77] Repair of either may be associated with massive blood losses.[78,79]

An important consideration in every case is the possibility of raised ICP (see previous sections). Monitoring and venous access should be appropriate for the intended procedure and possible blood losses anticipated. Brainstem manipulation may cause vasomotor instability during the operation or result in postoperative complications including neurological deficits.[80–82]

HEAD INJURY

Accidents are the leading cause of death among children, and head injuries are the major cause of these fatalities. Small children may suffer coincidental cervical spine injuries without radiologic evidence of fracture; great care must be taken during intubation and positioning.[83] The cribriform plate is easily fractured, and nasal tubes of any sort should be avoided or used cautiously if midfacial injury or nasal discharge (CSF, blood) is present.[84] The outlook following severe head injury in childhood is better than after a similar injury in adult life. Contrary to the situation in adults, severe head injuries are usually not associated with intracranial hematomas.[10] In those head-injured patients with severe neurologic dysfunction and abnormal motor responses to painful stimulation, management includes continuous monitoring of ICP; control of raised ICP may be life saving.

CRANIOFACIAL DEFORMITIES

Craniosynostoses, alone or in combination with facial anomalies (Apert's and Crouzon's Syndromes), often entail extensive surgery with massive blood losses.[85–87] Preparations for adequate replacement must be made. Intracranial hypertension may be present if multiple suture fusions occur. Spinal fluid drainage through a lumbar subarachnoid catheter may improve surgical exposure, but should not be utilized if increased ICP is present.

Postoperative intensive care is essential after some of these procedures, especially those involving maxillofacial reconstruction or orbital advancement. Life-threatening postoperative complications have resulted following extensive surgical manipulation. In addition, a completely alert patient with intact airway reflexes is also mandatory in cases of maxillary fixation with the jaws wired shut. In such cases it is common to leave the patient intubated for 24 to 48 hours postoperatively in order to avoid airway complications. Wire cutters, as well as drugs and equipment for emergency airway management should be at the bedside.

HYDROCEPHALUS

To allow for growth, the distal end of a pediatric CSF shunt is usually placed intraperitoneally. In these patients raised ICP usually is present preoperatively. In the case of shunt revision, where only the peritoneal end of the catheter is obstructed, ICP may be reduced prior to induction by tapping the shunt reservoir. The sudden removal of large amounts of CSF from the ventricles, however, may result in upward motion of the brainstem, with resulting signs similar to downward brain herniation. Should this complication occur, replacement of fluid (CSF or saline) can be an effective temporizing measure. Upward herniation as a result of hemorrhage into a posterior fossa tumor may also occur following shunt placement for hydrocephalus prior to a posterior fossa exploration.[88,89] Intravenous catheters should not be placed in the head near a ventriculostomy insertion site because of the dangers of shunt infection. The problems commonly associated with CSF shunting in children have recently been reviewed.[90]

DYSRAPHISM

Dysraphism in the spine (meningomyelocele) or in the head (encephalocele) is often associated with neurologic deficits and hydrocephalus.[91,92] Hydrocephalus usually coexists in those children with neurologic impairment. This is most often due to an associated Arnold-Chiari malformation (a downward displacement of the brainstem structures into a deformity of the upper cervical spine). Extremes of head flexion can cause brainstem compression similar to that produced with posterior fossa tumors. Vocal cord paralysis, leading to stridor and respiratory difficulty, may be associated with the Arnold-Chiari malformation; endotracheal intubation may be required.[31] Neuromuscular blockade should be avoided (or carefully monitored) if the surgeon plans to use a nerve stimulator. Other congenital anomalies must also be considered in these children, but are unusual.

NEURORADIOLOGICAL PROCEDURES

Neuroradiologic procedures may entail special risks. They are usually performed in environments not designed for pediatric anesthesia and far from additional personnel and technical support. Contrast agents may be used, and the danger of allergic reactions to them is always present. The osmotic load of these agents will induce a diuresis, necessitating close monitoring of fluid status. The anesthesiologist must be certain all necessary equipment for the safe conduct of anesthesia is available and functioning.

Computerized Tomography (CT) Scan

The development of CT scanning has been a revolutionary advance in the care of neurosurgical patients. This procedure requires immobilization, but is painless.[93] Intravenous sedation may be used, but young children are well controlled with rectal barbiturates alone.[94] Ketamine may also be used if intracranial hypertension is not a problem. Very small babies and neonates can usually be scanned when they sleep immediately after feeding, but may, after fasting, be sedated with oral or rectal chloral hydrate (20–50 mg/kg). General anesthesia will rarely be necessary. If contrast agents are to be used to enhance CT scanning, an intravenous catheter may be inserted once the child is sedated.

Magnetic resonance imaging can provide even greater anatomic and functional details, but is not widely available. It produces many technical challenges, since any feromagnetic material can be attracted to the strong magnet of the equipment and interfere with the procedure.

Arteriography

The intra-arterial injection of contrast agents produces pain that may cause children to move; general anesthesia usually is required. The rapid injection of contrast material may produce systemic hypotension from vasodilatation. If intracranial hypertension exists, controlled hyperventilation, with the avoidance of halogenated agents is preferred. There is evidence that hyperventilation may even improve the quality of cerebral angiograms by diverting cerebral blood flow from normal areas of brain to areas with impaired autoregulation.[95] The intra-arterial injection of contrast agents may also increase ICP in poorly compliant states, but this may be blunted by small doses of intravenous thiopental immediately prior to the injection.

Pneumoencephalography (PEG)

This procedure is rarely utilized since the advent of CT scanners. If intracranial hypertension is suspected, the study is performed through a ventriculostomy, and not through the lumbar subarachnoid space. The extreme position changes which are used require firm anchoring of all tubes and catheters, as well as the ability to promptly detect patient distress in order to return the patient to the supine position and initiate treatment.

If air is used as the contrast medium, the administration of nitrous oxide will cause uncontrolled expansion of the gas bubble.[96,97] In such circumstances, halothane or isoflurane in oxygen is preferable. On the other hand, this problem may be eliminated if nitrous oxide is injected as the contrast agent. The more rapid absorption from the ventricles appears to reduce post-contrast headache. Unfortunately, larger volumes must be used and the study done quickly before absorption occurs. The rapid or excessive injection of any contrast agent can precipitate an acute increase in ICP. In the presence of a ventriculoatrial shunt, any injected gas may embolize intravascularly.[98]

Myelography, Polytomography

Like pneumoencephalography, these procedures often involve a great deal of patient motion. All lines should be secure, and attention must be devoted to immediate recognition of patient distress in order to initiate therapy. A new water-soluble contrast agent (metrizamide) is being used more frequently in conjunction with CT scanning. It has been recommended that drugs which lower seizure threshold (such as phenothiazines and perhaps butyrophenones) be avoided when this agent is given. The use of intravenous contrast agents and CT scanning of the spine may decrease the need for myelography.

Radiation Therapy

These procedures require that the anesthesiologist observe the patient from outside the room usually via a television screen. EKG and a monitor of respirations should be readily visible. Pulse oximetry is also very useful. Like CT scans, rectal barbiturates or intramuscular ketamine may be all that is required, though absolute immobilization for prolonged periods usually entails general anesthesia.

REFERENCES

1. Shapiro HM: Intracranial hypertension: Therapeutic and anesthetic considerations. *Anesthesiology* 43:445–471, 1975
2. Rosman NP: Increased intracranial pressure in childhood. *Pediatr Clin North Am* 21:483–499, 1974
3. Rubin RC, Henderson ES, Ommaya AK, et al: The production of cerebrospinal fluid in man and its modification by acetazolamide. *J Neurosurg* 25:430–436, 1966
4. Clasen RA, Pandolfi S, Casey D: Furosemide and pentobarbital in cryogenic cerebral injury and edema. *Neurology* 24:642–648, 1974
5. Bell WE, McCormick WF: *Increased Intracranial Pressure in Children* (ed 2). Philadelphia, W.B. Saunders, 1978
6. Bruce DA, Berman WA, Schut L: Cerebrospinal fluid pressure monitoring in children: Physiology, pathology, and clinical usefulness. *Adv Pediatr* 24:233–290, 1977
7. Marshall LF, Smith RW, Shapiro HM: The influence of diurnal rhythms in patients with intracranial hypertension: Implications for management. *Neurosurgery* 2:100–101, 1978
8. McDowall DG: Monitoring the brain. *Anesthesiology* 45:117–134, 1976
9. Chaves-Carballo E, Gomez MR, Sharbrough FW: Encephalopathy and fatty infiltration of the viscera (Reye-Johnson Syndrome): A 17-year experience. *Mayo Clin Proc* 50:209–215, 1975
10. Bruce DA, Gennarelli TA, Langfitt TW: Resuscitation from coma due to head injury. *Crit Care Med* 6:254–269, 1978
11. Hanlon K: Description and uses of intracranial pressure monitoring. *Heart Lung* 5:277–282, 1976
12. Lundberg N: Continuous recording and control of ventricular fluid pressure in neurosurgical practice. *Acta Psychol Neurol Scand* [suppl] 149:1–193, 1960
13. James HE, Bruno L, Shapiro HM, et al: Methodology for intraventricular and subarachnoid continuous recording of intracranial pressure in clinical practice. *Acta Neurochir* 33:45–51, 1976
14. Coroneos NJ, McDowell DG, Pickerodt VWA, et al: A comparison of intra-cranial extradural pressure with subarachnoid pressure. *Br J Anaesth* 43:1198, 1971
15. Vidyasagar D, Raju TNK: A simple noninvasive technique of measuring intracranial pressure in the newborn. *Pediatrics* 59:957–961, 1977
16. Leech P, Miller JD: Intracranial volume-pressure relationships during experimental brain compression in primates. *J Neurol Neurosurg Psychiatry* 37:1099–1104, 1974
17. Shenkin HA, Bouzarth WF: Clinical methods of reducing intracranial pressure. *N Engl J Med* 282:1465–1471, 1970
18. DiRocco C, McLone DG, Shimoji T, et al: Continuous intraventricular cerebrospinal fluid pressure recording in hydrocephalic children during wakefulness and sleep. *J Neurosurg* 42:683–689, 1975
19. Lassen NA, Christensen MS: Physiology of cerebral blood flow. *Br J Anaesth* 48:719–734, 1976
20. Marsh ML, Marshall LF, Shapiro HM: Neurosurgical intensive care. *Anesthesiology* 47:149–163, 1977
21. Lassen NA: Control of cerebral circulation in health and disease. *Circ Res* 34:749–760, 1974
22. Lassen NA, Ingvar DH, Skinhoj E: Brain function and blood flow. *Sci Am* 239:62–71, 1978
23. Goresky GV, Steward DJ: Rectal methohexital for induction of anaesthesia in children. *Can Anaesth Soc J* 26:213–215, 1979
24. Rockoff MA, Goudsouzian NG: Seizures induced by methohexital. *Anesthesiology* 54:333–335, 1981
25. Smith RM: Techniques for the induction of anesthesia, in Smith, RM (ed): *Anesthesia for Infants and Children* (ed 4). St. Louis, C.V. Mosby, 1980, p 153
26. Lees MH, Olsen GD, McGilliard KL, et al: Chloral hydrate and the carbon dioxide chemoceptor response: A study of puppies and infants. *Pediatrics* 70:447–450, 1982
27. Shapiro HM: Monitoring in neurosurgical anesthesia, in Saidman LJ, Smith NT (ed): *Monitoring in Anesthesia*. New York, John Wiley & Sons, 1978, pp 171–204
28. Grundy BL: Intraoperative monitoring of sensory-evoked potentials. *Anesthesiology* 58:72–87, 1983
29. Steinhart CM, Weiss IP: Improved early prognostication using evoked potentials in comatose children. *Crit Care Med* 12:279, 1984
30. Coté CJ, Jobes DR, Schwartz AJ, et al: Two approaches to cannulation of a child's internal jugular vein. *Anesthesiology* 50:371–373, 1979
31. Mullan S, Raimondi AJ: Respiratory hazards of the Arnold-Chiari malformation. *J Neurosurg* 19:675–678, 1962
32. Meridy HW, Creighton RE, Humphries RP: Complications

during neurosurgery in the prone position in children. *Can Anaesth Soc J* 21:445–453, 1974

33. Albin MS, Babinski M, Maroon JC, et al: Anesthetic management of posterior fossa surgery in the sitting position. *Acta Anaesth Scand* 20:117–128, 1976

34. Gildenberg PL, O'Brien RP, Britt WJ, et al: The efficacy of Doppler monitoring for the detection of venous air embolism. *J Neurosurg* 54:75–78, 1981

35. Maroon JC, Albin MS: Air embolism diagnosed by Doppler ultrasound. *Anesth Analg* 53:399–402, 1974

36. Shapiro HM, Aidinis SJ: Neurosurgical anesthesia. *Surg Clin North Am* 55:913–928, 1975

37. Tinker JH, Gronert GA, Messick JM, et al: Detection of air embolism, a test for positioning of right atrial catheter and Doppler probe. *Anesthesiology* 43:104–106, 1975

38. Fischler M, Vourc'h G, Dubourg O, et al: Patent foramen ovale and sitting position. *Anesthesiology* 60:83, 1984

39. Shapiro HM: Neurosurgical anesthesia and intracranial hypertension, in Miller RD (ed): *Anesthesia*. New York, Churchill-Livingstone, 1981, pp 1079–1132

40. Gubbary SS: Derangement of temperature control in hydrocephalus. *Dev Med Child Neurol (suppl)* 13:125–132, 1967

41. Cross KW, Hey EN, Kennaird DL, et al: Lack of temperature control in infants with abnormalities of central nervous system. *Arch Dis Child* 46:437–443, 1971

42. Vandam LD, Burnap TK: Hypothermia. *N Engl J Med* 261:546–553, 595–603, 1959

43. Rosomoff HL: Adjuncts to neurosurgical anaesthesia. *Br J Anaesth* 37:246–261, 1965

44. Shapiro HM: The physiological basis of neurosurgical anesthesia. Lecture 202, Annual Refresher Course Lecture, American Society of Anesthesiology, 1977

45. Lockhart CH, Jenkins JJ: Ketamine-induced apnea in patients with increased intracranial pressure. *Anesthesiology* 37:92–93, 1972

46. Crumrine RS, Nulsen FE, Weiss MH: Alterations in ventricular fluid pressure during ketamine anesthesia in hydrocephalic children. *Anesthesiology* 42:758–761, 1975

47. List WF, Crumrine RS, Cascorbi HR, et al: Increased cerebrospinal fluid pressure after ketamine. *Anesthesiology* 36:98–99, 1972

48. Shapiro HM, Galindo A, Wyte SR, et al: Rapid intraoperative reduction of ICP with thiopentone. *Br J Anaesth* 45:1057–1061, 1973

49. Shapiro HM, Wyte SR, Loeser J: Barbiturate-augmented hypothermia for reduction of persistent intracranial hypertension. *J Neurosurg* 40:90–100, 1974

50. Marshall LF, Smith RW, Shapiro HM: Acute and chronic barbiturate administration in the management of head injury. *J Neurosurg* 50:26–30, 1979

51. Conn AW, Edmonds JF, Barker GA: Cerebral resuscitation in near-drowning. *Pediatr Clin North Am* 26:691–701, 1979

52. Cooperman LH: Succinylcholine-induced hyperkalemia in neuromuscular disease. *JAMA* 213:1867–1871, 1970

53. Cowgill DB, Mostello LA, Shapiro HM: Encephalitis and a hyperkalemic response to succinylcholine. *Anesthesiology* 40:409–411, 1974

54. Roth F, Wuthrich H: The clinical importance of hyperkalemia following suxamethonium administration. *Br J Anaesth* 41:311–316, 1969

55. Smith RB, Grenvix A: Cardiac arrest following succinylcholine in patients with central nervous system injuries. *Anesthesiology* 30:558–560, 1970

56. Tolmie JD, Joyce TH, Mitchell GD: Succinylcholine danger in the burned patients. *Anesthesiology* 28:467–470, 1967

57. Mazze RI, Escue HM, Houston JB: Hyperkalemia and cardiovascular collapse following administration of succinylcholine to the traumatized patient. *Anesthesiology* 31:540–547, 1969

58. Liu LMP, DeCook T, Goudsouzian NG, et al: Dose response to intramuscular succinylcholine in children. *Anesthesiology* 55:599–602, 1981

59. Borman BE, Smith RB, Bunegin L, et al: Does succinylcholine raise intracranial pressure? *Anesthesiology* 53:S–262, 1980

60. March ML, Dunlap BJ, Shapiro HM, et al: Succinylcholine—intracranial pressure effects in neurosurgical patients. *Anesth Analg* 59:550–551, 1980

61. Tarkhanen L, Laitinen L, Johansson G: Effects of d-tubocurarine on intracranial pressure and thalamic electrical impedance. *Anesthesiology* 40:247–251, 1974

62. Savarese JJ: Histamine, d-tubocurarine, and CSF pressure. *Anesthesiology* 42:369, 1975

63. Ali HH, Savarese JJ, Basta SJ, et al: Clinical pharmacology of atracurium: A new intermediate acting nondepolarizing relaxant. *Semin Anesth* 1:57–62, 1982

64. Bedford RF, Winn HR, Tyson G, et al: Lidocaine prevents increased ICP after endotracheal intubation, in Shulman K, Mamarou A, Miller JD, et al (eds): *Intracranial Pressure IV*. Berlin, Springer-Verlag, 1980, pp 595–598

65. Marshall LF, Smith RW, Shapiro HM, et al: Mannitol dose requirements in brain injured patients. *J Neurosurg* 48:169–171, 1978

66. Coté CJ, Greenhow DE, Marshall BE: The hypotensive response to rapid intravenous administration of hypertonic solutions in man and in the rabbit. *Anesthesiology* 50:30–35, 1979

67. Adams RW, Gronert G, Sundt TM, et al: Halothane, hypocapnia and cerebrospinal fluid pressure in neurosurgery. *Anesthesiology* 37:510–517, 1972

68. Michenfelder JD, Gronert FA, Kehder K: Neuroanesthesia. *Anesthesiology* 30:65–100, 1969

69. Smith AL: The mechanism of cerebral vasodilation by halothane. *Anesthesiology* 39:581–587, 1973

70. Neigh JL, Garman JK, Harp JR: The electrencephalographic pattern during anesthesia with ethrane: Effects of depth of anesthesia, $PaCO_2$, and nitrous oxide. *Anesthesiology* 35:482–487, 1971

71. Eger EI, II: Isoflurane: A review. *Anesthesiology* 55:559–576, 1981

72. Todd MM, Drummond JC: A comparison of the cerebrovascular and metabolic effects of halothane and isoflurane in the cat. *Anesthesiology* 60:276–282, 1984

73. Artru AA: Isoflurane does not increase the rate of CSF production in the dog. *Anesthesiology* 60:193–197, 1984

74. Wade JG, Stevens WC: Isoflurane: An anesthetic for the Eighties? *Anesth Analg* 60:666–682, 1981

75. Eger EI, II: *Isoflurane (Forane): A Compendium and Reference.* Madison, WI, Ohio Medical Products, 1981

76. Phirman JR, Shapiro HM: Modification of nitrous oxide-induced intracranial hypertension by prior induction of anesthesia. *Anesthesiology* 46:150–151, 1977

77. Holden AM, Fyler DC, Shilleto J, et al: Congestive heart failure from intracranial arteriovenous fistula in infancy—clinical and physiologic considerations in eight patients. *Pediatrics* 49:30–39, 1972

78. Ishak B, Gutierrez F, Seleny F: Anesthetic management of arteriovenous malformations of the brain in infants and children. *Anesthesiol Rev* 5(2):23–27, 1978

79. Hood JB, Wallace CT, Mahaffey JL: Anesthetic management of an intracranial arteriovenous malformation in infancy. *Anesth Analg* 56:236–241, 1977

80. Allan D, Kim HS, Cox JM: The anesthetic management of posterior fossa explorations in infants. *Can Anaesth Soc J* 17:227–232, 1970

81. Artru AA, Cucchiara RF, Messick JM: Cardiorespiratory and cranial-nerve sequellae of surgical procedures involving the posterior fossa. *Anesthesiology* 52:83–86, 1980

82. Gorski DW, Rao TLK, Scarff TB: Airway obstruction following surgical manipulation of the posterior fossa, an unusual complication. *Anesthesiology* 54:80–81, 1981

83. Babcock JL: Spinal injuries in children. *Pediatr Clin North Am* 22:487–500, 1975

84. Seebacker J, Nozik D, Mathieu A: Inadvertent intracranial introduction of a nasogastric tube, a complication of severe maxillofacial trauma. *Anesthesiology* 42:100–102, 1975

85. Shillito J, Matson DD: Craniosynostosis: A review of 519 surgical patients. *Pediatrics* 41:829–853, 1968

86. Davies DW, Monro IR: The anesthetic management and intraoperative care of patients undergoing major facial osteotomies. *Plast Reconstr Surg* 55:51–55, 1975

87. Finucane BT, Brown RG, O'Brien MS: Anesthesia for craniofacial reconstructive surgery. *Anesthesiol Rev* 7(3):39–43, 1980

88. Epstein F, Murali R: Pediatric posterior fossa tumors—hazards of the preoperative shunt. *Neurosurgery* 3:348–350, 1978

89. Vaquero J, Cabezudo JM, DeSola RG, et al: Intratumoral hemorrhage in posterior fossa tumors after ventricular drainage. *J Neurosurg* 54:406–408, 1981

90. Rockoff MA: Anesthesia for children with hydrocephalus. *Anesthesiol Rev* 6(5):28–34, 1979

91. Schroeder HG, Williams NE: Anaesthesia for meningomyelocoele surgery. *Anaesthesia* 21:57–65, 1966

92. Creighton RE, Relton JES, Meridy HW: Anaesthesia for occipital encephalocoele. *Can Anaesth Soc J* 21:402–406, 1974

93. Aidinis SJ, Zimmerman RA, Shapiro HM, et al: Anesthesia for brain computer tomography. *Anesthesiology* 44:420–425, 1976

94. Kallar SK, Vasinanukorn M, Rah KH, et al: The use of rectal thiopental in children for computerized axial tomography. *Anesthesiol Rev* 7(3):30–33, 1980

95. Dallas SH, Moxon CP: Controlled ventilation for cerebral angiography. *Br J Anaesth* 4:597–602, 1969

96. Saidman LJ, Eger EI, II: Change in cerebrospinal fluid pressure during pneumoencephalography under nitrous oxide anesthesia. *Anesthesioloyy* 26:67–72, 1965

97. Elwyn RA, Ring WH, Loeser E, et al: Nitrous oxide encephalography: 5-year experience with 475 patients. *Anesth Analg* 55:402–408, 1976

98. Paul WL, Munson ES: Gas embolism during encephalography. *Anesth Analg* 55:141–145, 1976

18

Radiologic Procedures

Susan Firestone

The proliferation of computer-assisted radiographic procedures is revolutionizing the diagnosis of disease and rapidly supplanting less sophisticated technology. Techniques such as computerized axial tomography (CAT), digital subtraction angiography, and nuclear magnetic resonance spectroscopy (NMR), are superior to conventional x-ray studies in their accuracy, speed, and reduced radiation exposure. Perhaps the most welcome advantage is their noninvasive nature, which has lowered the threshold of pediatricians to order these examinations. However, one absolute requirement for producing the stunning detail which is characteristic of these imaging techniques is a cooperative patient who will remain motionless for several minutes at a time. Such a goal is clearly unrealistic for the pediatric patient, and therefore requests from the radiologist for general anesthesia for these studies are a growing part of the practice of pediatric anesthesia.

What follows is a discussion of the issues involved in providing clinical anesthesia in the radiology suite, including both environmental and technical considerations.

PHYSICAL LIMITATIONS OF THE RADIOLOGY SUITE

Most anesthesiologists are justifiably uncomfortable providing anesthesia coverage outside of their usual environment, the operating room, where equipment, supplies, and technical assistance are always available.

In the past, design of radiology suites did not account for the need to anesthetize patients, so the basic facilities for anesthesia are absent. By necessity anesthesiologists have had to develop suitable adaptations in their equipment to overcome these physical limitations. For example, nitrous oxide must be supplied by tank, although there is usually wall-supplied oxygen and suction. Forethought about the anesthetic plan is particularly important, since any specialized supplies and drugs that could be needed should be brought to the radiology suite prior to the induction of anesthesia.

Another disadvantage that must be accommodated is that the radiology table usually does not have the capacity for the Trendelenburg position. Furthermore, once positioned for the study, access to the patient is limited by the x-ray source and camera, and this is especially true in the cases of CAT and NMR scans. Radiology rooms tend to be darker than operating rooms, and are generally kept colder (68-70°F) to protect the computer equipment. This is a particularly important disadvantage for pediatric patients, and some method of supplying heat, such as a heated humidifier or radiant warmer, must be utilized during anesthesia. Unfortunately, most heating blankets contain radiopaque coils so they cannot be an option.

Finally, it cannot be overemphasized that even if radiology rooms are short on space, it is mandatory to have a source of positive pressure ventilation ideally an anesthesia machine, for the patient's protection.

GOALS OF ANESTHESIA

The first task in organizing any sensible and safe management is to define the goals, which are different for radiology than for surgical procedures. Just as the type of surgical procedure is one term in the equation for planning an appropriate anesthetic, familiarity with the many radiologic procedures is an equally integral consideration.

The main goal for all procedures is that the patient be immobile to optimize image resolution. This is the primary motivation for the radiologist to consult the anesthesiologist; since the superior resolution of computer-reconstructed im-

Table 18-1

Sedation Regimens

Drug	Dose	Route	Disadvantages, Problems
Chloral Hydrate	30–50 mg/kg	Oral/Rectal	Long onset and duration
"Pedimix"*	0.1 ml/kg	IM	Prolonged duration Respiratory compromise
Ketamine	5–10 mg/kg	IM	Need antisialogogue High study failure rate due to movement Contraindicated with increased ICP
Methohexital	25–30 mg/kg 1–2 mg/kg	Rectal IV	Seizures, rare

*Meperidine, chlorpromazine, promethazine

ages is dependent on the subject remaining motionless. Likewise, movement during radiation therapy (RT) may reduce the success and increase the side effects of the treatment. In the event of movement during this therapy, the target tissue may be underexposed, while adjacent healthy tissues are unnecessarily irradiated by the therapeutic beam.

Another important goal for pediatric patients is amnesia. Considerable effort should be directed towards minimizing the apprehension and unpleasant memories of the child, as well as the parents. In practical terms, many patients undergo a radiologic study in preparation for surgery, so an unsympathetic handling of this anesthetic procedure will influence future successful rapport.

There are other unique characteristics of radiologic procedures that influence the choice of anesthetic. Studies that do not use contrast media usually do not cause pain. For this reason sedation rather than general anesthesia may be preferable for CAT scans and RT. There are, however, periods of discomfort during angiograms that are not limited to the insertion of the guide needle, wire, and catheter. Injection of contrast media during the angiogram causes an uncomfortable burning sensation which can provoke movement at the very moment when the radiographs are being taken. In these instances general anesthesia is preferable to sedation.

General anesthesia is also the safest choice when extensive patient maneuvering is needed during an x-ray study. For example, during a myelogram, the patient may be rotated into extreme positions which mandates general anesthesia with intubation, for airway protection, as well as mechanical ventilation to insure adequate gas exchange.

Prevention of movement is not the only way the anesthesiologist's skill may affect the quality of a radiologic study. Many of the agents used for general anesthesia have profound hemodynamic effects and could be expected to influence the images of procedures that rely on contrast-enhanced regional blood flow. Unfortunately, effects of general anesthesia on the quality of an angiographic study are largely undefined, despite a wealth of knowledge about regional blood flow under anesthesia. There are some data available on the effect of potent inhalation agents and hyperventilation on the quality of cerebral arteriograms.[1–3] Halothane, which causes cerebral vasodilatation, tends to blur fine detail in these studies. Vasoconstriction secondary to hypocarbia, however, has been shown to enhance the definition of the vessels by slowing the

transit time of the injected dye, thereby increasing the relative concentration within the vascular system.[2,3] This effect is particularly helpful in detecting tumor vessels, so a good case can be made for general anesthesia with mechanical ventilation to a PaCO2 of 30–35 torr for cerebral arteriograms.[3,4]

Perhaps the most dramatic instance in which the cardiovascular effects of anesthetic agents can quantitatively alter the results is in cardiac catheterization. This is another area where the essential questions have yet to be systematically investigated. Since decisions about the nature and timing for the surgical intervention are based on absolute hemodynamic values obtained during catheterization, most cardiologists prefer to sedate and restrain their pediatric patients rather than employ general anesthesia. As the hemodynamic effects of anesthetic agents are elucidated it can be anticipated that this practice will change.

ANESTHETIC TECHNIQUES

The most common radiologic procedures performed on pediatric patients that require anesthesia are cranial and body CAT scans, angiograms, and less frequently, myelography, and radiation therapy. Many of these cases can be safely performed on an outpatient basis, even when anesthesia is required. The principles of safe outpatient anesthesia are discussed elsewhere in this text (see Chapter 4) and will not be elaborated here. It does bear repeating that *all radiology outpatients should receive the same high standard of monitoring and recovery room care applied to any anesthetized inpatient.*

The advent of cranial CAT scans has decreased the number of invasive neuroradiologic procedures performed on children. Since the scans are so brief, the majority are suitably done with sedation rather than general anesthesia. The exceptions to this are extremely young patients (under two months of age), any child with preexisting or potential airway compromise, and those undergoing studies of the posterior fossa, which require cervical flexion. These cases are most safely performed under general anesthesia, with an endotracheal tube to provide airway protection.

There are many drug combinations that have successfully been employed to sedate children for CAT scans (Table 18-1) and radiation therapy.[5–9] Chloral hydrate is commonly used by pediatricians for this purpose. The oral dosage is 30–50 mg/kg, and must be administered at least one hour prior to the scheduled procedure to insure maximum effect.[5] Disadvantages of chloral hydrate include its unpleasant taste and odor, the long onset to sedation, and a duration of action several hours longer than is necessary for the study. Further, chloral hydrate sedation may be inadequate (defined as movement during a scan) up to 15 percent of the time.[5]

Another commonly used sedative is the mixture known as "pedimix" or "cardiac cocktail," which consists of 25 mg/ml of meperidine, 8 mg/ml of promethazine, and 5 mg/ml of chlorpromazine. The recommended dosage is 0.1 ml/kg in an intramuscular injection given at least one hour prior to the study, with a maximum dose of two milliliters.[10] This drug mixture has the disadvantage of being a fixed-dose combination, and the suggested dose contains 2.5 mg/kg of meperidine. This amount exceeds the meperidine dose that would normally be given to a patient during a painful surgical procedure, so for CT scans this is an excessively heavy narcotic load which thus incurs a significant risk of respiratory depression. It is notable that this potent mixture, augmented with intramuscular secobarbital, does not significantly improve the study failure rate (12 percent) over chloral hydrate, a much safer drug.[5]

Ketamine was prominent in early studies of anesthesia for CAT scans, but has recently lost favor.[11,12] At a dose of 5–10 mg/kg intramuscularly, it has a suitably short onset and duration of action.[13] However, an antisialogogue must be used as a premedication to prevent the copious secretions that accompany ketamine use. A more serious disadvantage is the frequent nonpurposeful movements that patients may exhibit while anesthetized with ketamine.[7] In addition, because there is a marked increase in intracranial pressure in patients given ketamine, it is contraindicated for any patient with a significant mass lesion or evidence of preexisting intracranial hypertension.[13]

The technique preferred by many anesthesiologists is sedation with a short-acting barbiturate. This is most simply accomplished with a 10 percent solution of methohexital given rectally in a dose of 25–30 mg/kg.[14] The onset of sedation is usually within five or ten minutes, lasts for 30–60 minutes, and can be reinforced with intravenous doses of 1–2 mg/kg.[15] Although the patient will move upon painful stimuli, the sedation is deep enough to easily obtain intravenous access in a restrained limb. Premedication with an antisialogogue is not necessary, and after 60 minutes there is so little residual sedation that it is very satisfactory for outpatients.[15] A theoretical problem with methohexital is that it may induce seizures in patients who have a seizure disorder, (in particular temporal lobe epilepsy), but in practice this is an extremely rare occurrence.[16]

General anesthesia for CAT scans and radiation therapy should be reserved for patients with obvious potential airway problems, infants under two months of age, and those patients in whom sedation has failed. General anesthesia is also the method of choice for children undergoing angiograms and myelograms. These children are always inpatients, so early discharge is not a consideration. Any of the many methods of general anesthesia are acceptable within the confines of the patient's medical condition. As mentioned earlier, hemodynamic considerations often confer an advantage upon a nitrous oxide/narcotic/relaxant technique, since radical position changes are less likely to cause orthostatic blood pressure changes with this method.

The primary complication from any general anesthetic in pediatric patients is airway compromise after extubation, principally laryngospasm and obstruction.[17] Since the recovery room is often remote from the radiology department, the patient should either be fully awake prior to departure or transported to the recovery room before extubation.

CONTRAST MEDIA

Although anesthesiologists are conversant with the pharmacology of many drugs, few are familiar with the contrast media that are routinely used in radiology. The pharmacology and adverse reactions to these compounds have been the topic of comprehensive reviews, so only the pertinent aspects of their clinical pharmacology will be discussed.[18–20]

The most commonly used compounds contain an iodinated anion, which is the radiopaque component, and a cation to prepare the salt. They are all extremely hyperosmolar. For example, Renografin* (meglucamine diatrizoate), one of the most widely used contrast media, is manufactured in several concentrations, the least of which (60 percent solution) has an osmolarity of 1200 mOsm/l. The cardiovascular consequences of systemic injection of hyperosmolar compounds are to increase blood pressure, then decrease both blood pressure and systemic vascular resistance.[21] These changes are usually transient, but in patients with marked hypovolemia, hypotension may be profound. The high osmolarity of these compounds may also pose a serious threat to the red blood cells of patients with sickle cell anemia, so extra care in hydrating them is warranted.[18]

Another result of administering hyperosmolar compounds that are exclusively excreted by the kidney is an obligate diuresis. Maintenance intravenous fluids need to be adjusted to compensate for this extra loss; neglecting it in a small child who is already hypovolemic can precipitate serious hypotension. Diuresis may also reduce the half-life of drugs primarily excreted by the kidney, such as metacurine and pancuronium, and decrease the interval between doses.

Even after brief procedures such diuresis in small children may necessitate catheterization to avoid severe distension of the urinary bladder. In-dwelling bladder catheters, however, should be reserved for prolonged cases.

Dosage and Adverse Reactions

The guideline for maximum dosage of 60 percent Renografin used by pediatric radiologists is 2–3 ml/kg/day for a child of 10 kilograms or less, and 1–2 ml/kg for larger children. Dosages of more concentrated solutions should be adjusted proportionately. The larger dose is required in small children because of their relatively larger blood volume and higher cardiac output, both of which tend to dilute contrast media. Minor overdoses are not usually harmful if the patient receives adequate compensatory fluid volumes, but large overdoses may have grave consequences. These substances are known to have direct glomerular toxicity and can cause permanent renal impairment.[22,23] In animal studies these compounds cross the blood–brain barrier in a dose-dependent fashion at clinically relevant concentrations.[23,24] In principle

_____
* E.R. Squibb & Sons, Princeton, NJ.

Table 18-2

Radiation Exposure

Procedure	Patient's Skin Dose (mrem)
CX Ray (PA view)	30–50[33]
CT scan (single slice)	400–6500[32]
CT scan (full scan)	8,000–10,000[32]
Cardiac angiography	75,000 (not including fluoroscopy)[33]
Fluoroscopy (with image intensifier)	500–2000/min[33]

this leakage into the central nervous system would be enhanced by any process that increases the blood–brain barrier permeability, such as infection, neoplasm, trauma, and intrinsic diseases of the central nervous system, such as multiple sclerosis.[25] Even low concentrations in the central nervous system will cause intractable seizures, which are masked by general anesthesia and only become apparent on emergence.[26,27] The treatment for such seizures is the same as for status epilepticus, which is discussed in Chapter 14. In a large overdose it may take several days for the patient to excrete the dye, and the seizures may continue throughout this time. These serious complications may be avoided by staying within the recommended dose range.

The older iodinated contrast media had much higher incidences of allergic phenomena, but even with current compounds five to eight percent of cases still manifest reactions.[19] These vary in severity from flushing and urticaria to bronchospasm and anaphylaxis. One of the more common symptoms, urticaria, rarely progresses to a more serious reaction.[28] However, significant and prolonged decreases in blood pressure may herald a more severe response. Subjective respiratory distress was the earliest symptom in 20 percent of those patients who ultimately progressed to a fatal outcome; so the anesthetized patient is at a disadvantage.[28] Changes in pulmonary compliance, and signs of periorbital, glossal, or laryngeal edema, may be the first warning in an anesthetized patient. It is therefore imperative that treatment for anaphylaxis be instituted as soon after the diagnosis as possible to decrease the morbidity and mortality. Treatment for anaphylaxis is covered in Chapter 14.

RADIATION PROTECTION

The risk from x-ray exposure engenders a great deal of concern, but continues to be an area of uncertain knowledge for most anesthesiologists. Attention to this problem is often deferred until after the anesthetic has begun, although it is more effective to implement precautions right from the start.

Modern x-ray equipment has many safety features and technological advances that minimize a patient's exposure to radiation, but the anesthesia personnel are still at risk. In one study of various occupational hazards for the anesthesiologist it was found that the mean dosage level of radiation for the study group as a whole was within current federal regulations. Notably, however, there were individuals with excessive exposure to radiation.[29] Fortunately, the study also demonstrated that the heightened awareness of the anesthesiologists participating in the study brought about a decrease in their future

dose levels. It is clear that education about this hazard is an effective preventative measure.

The National Council of Radiation Protection has established safe exposure levels at 100 milliroentgens in a week, or an absorbed dose of 5000 millirems in a year.[29,30] Table 18-2 contains the radiation dose delivered during CAT scans, angiograms and fluoroscopy.[30,31] Even though the anesthesiologist is not in direct line with the x-ray beam, the exposure rate is still influenced by the duration of exposure, distance from the x-ray source, and the protective shielding being used. To reduce duration of exposure, an anesthetic plan can be chosen that allows the anesthesiologist to leave the room during periods of maximum risk, provided that patient and monitor visibility can be maintained. Since exposure received from a source is inversely proportional to the square of the distance from that source, increasing the distance from the x-ray tube substantially reduces exposure. In the case of CAT scans it is advisable to position oneself opposite the direction of rotation of the x-ray source, since the maximum x-ray scatter is in the direction of rotation of the x-ray tubes (Figure 18-1). The usual procedure is for the rotation to alternate directions for each slice, so the anesthesiologist's position will need to change for each film taken, but this maneuver will decrease the dose delivered to one or two millirems each hour.[7] Most angiography machines have lead screening suspended around the x-ray tube that can be lowered into place prior to use. Rolling lead screens equipped with lead glass windows are also available to shield the anesthesiologist from exposure.

Fluoroscopy presents a more serious hazard because the radiation scatter is extremely high (Table 18-2).[31] Unfortunately, it is difficult to avoid exposure from fluoroscopy, since radiologists will use it episodically, often without warning, during initial placement of wires and catheters. It is therefore necessary to wear a lead apron with circumferential body coverage. There are also lead thyroid protectors.

All anesthesia personnel who regularly (i.e., weekly) provide coverage for radiology should wear radiation detection badges. They should be worn on the shirt collar to reflect the maximum exposure to tissues not protected by a lead apron. The badge generally contains a piece of film which is exposed in proportion to the x-ray dose, and is returned each month for calculation of the exposure.

FUTURE PERSPECTIVES

One technologic trend that is germane to anesthesia for radiologic procedures is nuclear magnetic resonance spectroscopy (NMR). NMR imaging is currently at the same stage of development that CAT scanning was five to eight years ago.[34] Many similar issues, such as cost/benefit ratios and its clinical efficacy, have been raised about the use of NMR. However the controversy is resolved, many hospitals already have NMR equipment in place, and more plan to purchase these instruments in the next few years. The speed with which this technology is adopted will depend on the timing of FDA approval, and the willingness of third-party payers to reimburse for these studies.

Although NMR imaging is more tolerant of movement during scanning than CAT, the length of an NMR study, at this time, is 0.5–1.5 hours, which would stress the endurance of most adult patients. Under these conditions, some form of anesthesia would be mandatory for all pediatric patients.

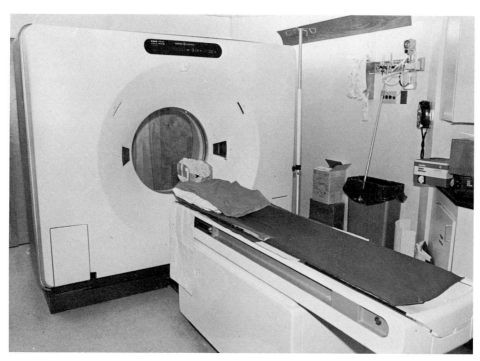

Figure 18-1. CAT scan suite. Note the centrally supplied oxygen, nitrous oxide, suction, and OR plug adaptors on wall. X-ray tube array rotates within the "doughnut" of the gantry, usually alternating directions for each film.

The physical principles of NMR spectroscopy depend upon the simultaneous application of electromagnetic and pulsed radiofrequency fields to a subject. The radiofrequency used is specific for each element with an odd atomic number that can be induced to exhibit nuclear resonance, and the resultant computerized reconstruction can either be an anatomic image, similar to CAT scans or, if phosphorus or potassium are chosen, a functional map of the tissues. "Physiological imaging" is expected to be NMR's primary contribution to noninvasive diagnostic radiology.

In addition to all the standard difficulties of providing anesthesia in the radiology department, the presence of both the electromagnetic field and radiofrequency pulsations in the NMR facility creates unique problems for the anesthesiologist (Figure 18-2). In particular, patients with cardiac pacemakers and ferromagnetic surgical implants (e.g., vascular clips, joint prostheses) are not suitable candidates for exposure to a powerful magnetic field. Many monitoring devices, such as sphygmomanometers and electronic thermometers, contain ferromagnetic parts and are disabled in the NMR room. In fact, the magnet is so powerful that small metallic articles like laryngoscopes and circuit connectors can becomes dangerous projectiles.

The skeleton of the anesthesia machine and gas tanks are also ferromagnetic, and will be attracted to the magnet. Replacing the tanks with ones manufactured of aluminum decreases the ferromagnetic mass. Any large metallic object disrupts the homogeniety of the magnetic field, so placement of the anesthesia machine must take this into account. Such field distortions compromise the equipment's ability to produce a clear image. Since magnetic fields have specific patterns, there are predictable regions of diminished field strength where equipment will be less obstrusive.[35] Perhaps

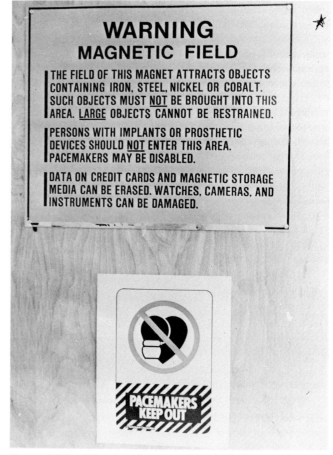

Figure 18-2. Warning sign posted in the hallway and on the door of the NMR suite.

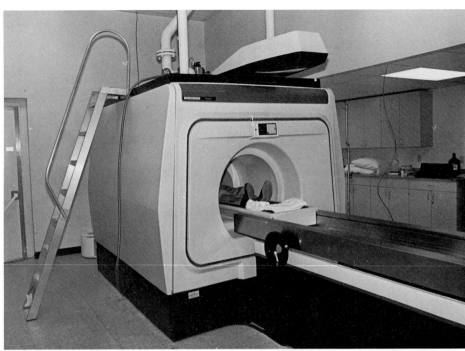

Figure 18-3. NMR scanner with supercooled magnet. Tank and pipes on top of magnet contain liquid nitrogen to cool the magnet. Note small bore and length of tunnel. The child completely disappears into the tunnel during scanning.

the only advantage of the magnetic coils is the by-product, heat, which is beneficial for the pediatric patient.

Electrocardiographic monitoring can still be employed by using heavily insulated cables and placing the monitor in a magnetically null corner of the room. The radiofrequency pulses produce a periodic artifact on the screen, but this pattern can be distinguished from the EKG. An alternate method of blood pressure measurement can be devised by constructing a glass-tube mercury manometer that is mounted in a non-ferromagnetic material. Intermittent temperature monitoring can be accomplished with a conventional thermometer or heat-sensitive adhesive thermometers. Even intravenous catheters must be composed only of plastic, since brands with metallic hubs move upwards towards the magnet, thus dislodging or kinking the line. In summary, all standard equipment must be examined for ferromagnetic components, and suitable replacements must be found.

Recommendations for anesthetic technique for NMR are necessarily based on limited experience, but some constraints are immediately apparent. The tunnel, which is long enough to accomodate the body of an adult (Figure 18-3), severely restricts access to the head, so light general anesthesia with endotracheal intubation, rather than sedation, seems the safest choice.

Additional issues that need to be addressed in the future are the safety for anesthesia personnel of prolonged and repeated exposure to strong magnetic fields, and possible effects of anesthetics on NMR image resolution, especially in physiologic imaging.

As the technology progresses there will continue to be new challenges to our ingenuity in order to provide safe anesthetic care for patients undergoing radiologic procedures.

REFERENCES

1. Campkin TV: General anesthesia for neuroradiology. *Br J Anaesth* 48:789, 1976
2. Edmonds-Seal J, Boulay GH du, Bostock T: The effect of intermittent positive pressure ventilation on cerebral angiography. *Br J Radiol* 40:457–464, 1967
3. Dallas SH, Moxon CP: Controlled ventilation for cerebral angiography. *Br J Anaesth* 41:597–601, 1969
4. Samuel JR, Grange RA, Hawkins TD: Anesthetic techniques for carotid angiography. *Anaesthesia* 23:543–554, 1968
5. Thompson JR, Schneider S, Ashwal S, et al: The choice of sedation for computerized tomography in children: A prospective evaluation. *Radiology* 143:475–479, 1982
6. Aidinis S, Zimmerman R, Shapiro H, et al: Anesthesia for brain computer tomography. *Anesthesiology* 44:420–425, 1976
7. Ferrar-Bechner T, Winter J: Anesthetic considerations for cerebral computer tomography. *Anesth Analg* 56:344–347, 1977
8. Shapiro HM, Aidinis S: Neurosurgical anesthesia. *Surg Clin North Am* 55:913–928, 1975
9. Anderson RE, Osborn AG: Efficacy of simple sedation for pediatric computed tomography. *Radiology* 124:739–740, 1977
10. Committee on Pharmacy and Therapeutics: Clinical Recommendations. Boston, Massachusetts General Hospital, 1985
11. Wilson GH, Fotias NA, Dillon JB: Ketamine: A new anesthetic for use in pediatric neuroroentgenologic procedures. *Am J Roentgenol* 106:434–439, 1969
12. Welborn S: Anesthesia for EMI scanning in infants and small children. *South Med J* 69:1294–1295, 1976
13. Goodman L, Gilman A: *The Pharmacological Basis of Therapeutics* (ed 6) New York, Macmillan, 1980, pp 296–297
14. Goresky GV, Steward DJ: Rectal methohexital for induction of anaesthesia in children. *Can Anaesth Soc J* 26:213–215, 1979
15. Liu LMP, Goudsouzian NG, Liu P: Rectal methohexital premedication in children. *Anesthesiology* 53:343–345, 1980

16. Rockoff M, Goudsouzian N: Seizures induced by methohexital. *Anesthesiology* 54:333–335, 1981

17. Gregory G: *Pediatric Anesthesia*. New York, Churchill-Livingstone, 1983, pp 1–8

18. Goldberg M: Systemic reactions to intravascular contrast media. *Anesthesiology* 60:46–56, 1984

19. Shehadi WH, Toniolo G: Adverse reactions to contrast media. *Radiology* 136:299–302, 1980

20. Shehadi WH: Adverse reactions to intravascularly administered contrast media. *Am J Roentgenol* 124:145–152, 1975

21. Coté CJ, Greenhow DE, Marshall BE: The hypotensive response to rapid administration of hypertonic solutions in man and rabbit. *Anesthesiology* 50:30–35, 1979

22. Ansell G: *Complications in Diagnostic Radiology*. Oxford, Blackwell Scientific Publications, 1976, pp 111–115, 396

23. Port FK, Wagone RD, Fulton RK: Acute renal failure following angiography. *Am J Roentgenol* 121:544–550, 1974

24. Bromen T, Ollon O: The tolerance of cerebral blood vessels to a contrast medium of the diodrast group. *Acta Radiol* 30:326–342, 1948

25. Lampke KF, James G, Erbesfeld M: Cerebrovascular permeability of a water soluable contrast material (sodium diatrizoate). *Invest Radiol* 5:79–85, 1970

26. Hoppe JO, Archer S: X-ray contrast media for cardiovascular angiography. *Angiology* 11:244–254, 1960

27. Ansell G: *Complications in Diagnostic Radiology*. Oxford, Blackwell Scientific Publications, 1976, p 400

28. Lalli AF: Contrast media reactions: Data, analysis, and hypothesis. *Radiology* 134:1–12, 1980

29. Linde HW, Bruce DL: Occupational exposure of anesthetists to halothane, nitrous oxide and radiation. *Anesthesiology* 30:363–368, 1969

30. Code of Federal Regulations, Title 10, 1972

31. National Council of Radiation Protection Reports 17, 33, 34. Washington, DC, 1985

32. Lee S: *Computerized Body Tomography*. New York, Raven Press, 1983, pp 7–8

33. Ansell G: *Complications in Diagnostic Radiology*. Oxford, Blackwell Scientific Publications, 1976, pp 404, 436–437

34. Evens R: Computed tomography—A controversy revisited. *N Engl J Med* 310:1183–1185, 1984

35. Nuclear Magnetic Resonance. American Hospital Association, Hospital Technology Series, vol 2(8), 1983

19

Burns

S.K. Szyfelbein
J.A. Jeevendra Martyn
Charles J. Coté

Every year in the United States over two million people are burned; more than 5,000 are children.[1] Eleven thousand hospital beds are occupied daily by burned patients, at a cost estimated in 1979 to be 1.5 billion dollars.

Burned patients need a high degree of coordinated care, which must be delivered by many specialists. These patients are managed well only through an understanding of the abnormalities associated with burn injury. These abnormalities include metabolic derangements, neurohumoral responses, massive fluid shifts, sepsis, and the systemic effects of massive tissue destruction. This chapter will discuss the pathophysiology, the initial evaluation and resuscitation, and the anesthetic management of the burned pediatric patient. Some of the principles presented are derived from experiences with adult patients and applied to children, whereas others are the result of over 17 years experience in caring for burned children at the Shriners Burns Institute.

PATHOPHYSIOLOGY

A burn is unique among traumatic injuries. It destroys skin, the largest organ of the body, upon which we depend for thermal regulation, fluid and electrolyte homeostasis, and protection against bacterial infection. It is important to appreciate that systemic responses are associated with even minor, localized burn injuries.[2]

In pediatric patients, because of their greater body surface area-to-weight ratios, the clinical symptoms and pathologic changes are relatively more severe and, unfortunately, the gravity of the injury is often underestimated (Figure 19-1).

Soon after injury, massive fluid shifts occur from the vascular compartment into the burned tissue, resulting in sequestration of fluid, even in nonburned areas; this results in significant hemoconcentration.[2–4] Despite the massive fluid loss, systemic blood pressure may be maintained as a result of the outpouring of catecholamines and antidiuretic hormone.[5,6] In the first four days after a burn of moderate size or larger, an amount of albumin equal to twice the total plasma albumin content is lost through the wound. Half this albumin remains sequestered in the extravascular space for three weeks or more.[2] In addition to direct effects of the burn (thrombosis, increased capillary permeability), changes in vascular integrity occur in areas remote from the injury.[4,7] In the pulmonary capillary network these changes can be life-threatening; severe pulmonary edema and vascular congestion may result.

CARDIAC EFFECTS

Immediately after injury, cardiac output is strikingly reduced.[8–12] This decrease is often related to the rapid reduction in circulating blood volume, or to the severe compressive effects of circumferential abdominal burns upon venous return.[11] Despite adequate cardiac filling pressures, however, some patients continue to have reduced cardiac output. This suggests other contributing factors, such as a direct myocardial effect from the burn injury. Some investigators have shown a circulating myocardial-depressant factor (MDF) to exist in both man and laboratory animals, particularly in subjects with extensive third-degree burns.[13,14]

Three to five days following the burn injury the patient develops a hypermetabolic state. This may result in a two- to three-fold *increase* in cardiac output, which persists for weeks

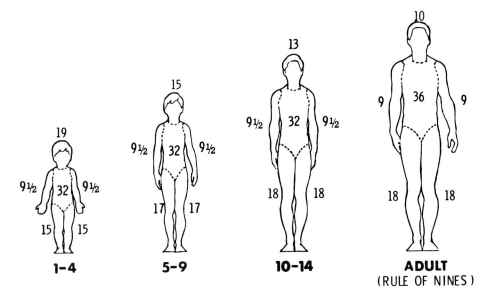

Figure 19-1. This figure represents the different proportions of body surface area for calculation of percent burn according to patient age. Note the large proportion of body surface area the head and face account for in an infant. (Reproduced with permission from Carvajal, et al: *Textbook of Pediatrics*, W.B. Saunders.)

to months. Gram-negative sepsis, however, may cause a depressed cardiac output in some patients.

PULMONARY EFFECTS

Pulmonary function may be adversely affected at several levels. The upper airway is a good heat exchanger; just as cold air is warmed, hot air is cooled. This may, however, cause heat destruction of laryngeal tissues. Thus inspiration of hot air can damage the upper airway and result in airway obstruction secondary to massive edema formation. The upper bronchi may show heat destruction of the ciliated epithelium and mucosa. The lower bronchi and alveoli may be damaged by inhalation of toxic fumes, such as nitrogen dioxide and sulfur dioxide, which combine with water in the tracheobronchial tree to form nitric acid and sulfuric acid. Inhalation of products of wool and cotton combustion results in acid aldehyde formation, which may cause pulmonary edema in concentrations as low as ten parts per million. Combustion of polyurethane containing products (insulation, wall paneling) releases hydrogen cyanide, which can lead to histotoxic hypoxia and death.[15-17] The overall effect of a pulmonary inhalation injury is necrotizing bronchitis, bronchial swelling, alveolar destruction, exudation of protein, loss of surfactant, loss of the protective bronchial lining, and bronchospasm, all of which contribute to the development of bronchopneumonia (Figure 19-2).[18-25] Inhalation of particulate matter (smoke, soot) also results in mechanical obstruction. Edema of the bronchi, combined with loss of integrity of the pulmonary capillary endothelium, results in decreased pulmonary compliance. Chest wall compliance may also be diminished by circumferential chest burns.[26] All of these effects lead to major ventilation–perfusion abnormalities, with resultant hypoxemia and hypercarbia. In addition to direct damage to the respiratory system, extrapulmonary factors such as changes in cardiac output can also contribute to poor oxygenation.[27] Measurement of blood gases alone will not indicate these factors. Rational therapy of reduced arterial oxygen saturation re-

quires measurement of both extra- and intrapulmonary factors contributing to arterial desaturation.[27]

RENAL EFFECTS

Renal function may be adversely affected soon after injury as a result of myoglobinuria and hemoglobinuria. The former is most common in electrical injury, while the latter is seen following severe cutaneous burns. Hypovolemia and hypotension may further aggravate the renal dysfunction, resulting in acute tubular necrosis. Three to seven days after the burn, glomerular filtration rate increases pari passu with cardiac output and metabolic rate increases.[28,29] Patients with greater than 40 percent body surface burn demonstrate renal tubular dysfunction, mainly an inability to concentrate the urine.[5,30] Even during hyperosmolar states antidiuresis is not seen, suggesting an inadequate renal response to antidiuretic hormone (ADH) and aldosterone. Thus it is possible to observe good urine output even in the presence of hypovolemia. Episodic or persistent hypertension is frequent in children; this may in part be mediated by increased renin and catecholamine production.[6,31]

HEPATIC EFFECTS

The liver may be damaged by hypoperfusion during the early post burn phase as a result of hypovolemia, hypotension, hypoxemia, and inhaled or absorbed chemical toxins.[32] Later hepatic dysfunction may result from drug toxicity, sepsis, or blood transfusions. Studies in adults have found increased hepatic blood flow, protein synthesis and breakdown, and increased hepatic gluconeogenesis during the hypermetabolic phase of burn injury. With the onset of sepsis, hepatic glucose output, and alanine uptake may decrease sharply, but hepatic blood flow and oxygen utilization can remain elevated.[33] Although there is a marked reduction in the activity of the hepatic microsomal drug metabolizing system, data on the metabolism of drugs by the liver in acute burn states are

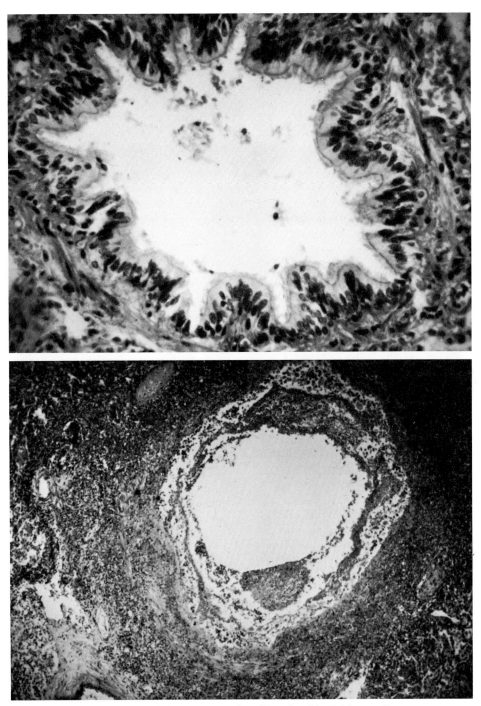

Figure 19-2. Cross section of a normal bronchiole (A). Note the ciliated epithelial layer. Compare to a cross section of a distal bronchiole from a patient who died from an inhalational injury (B). Note the marked thickening of the bronchial wall, the massive inflammatory cell infiltrate, the sloughing of the mucosa, and total destruction of the ciliated collumnar epithelium.

scanty.[32,34,35] Fatty infiltration of the liver has also been reported.[36]

CENTRAL NERVOUS SYSTEM EFFECTS

The central nervous system (CNS) may be adversely affected by inhalation of neurotoxic chemicals, or by hypoxic encephalopathy; other contributing factors include sepsis, hyponatremia, and hypovolemia.[37] The CNS dysfunction includes hallucinations, personality changes, delirium, seizures, and coma.[38] Such effects usually clear after several weeks. The possibility of cerebral edema and increased intracranial pressure (ICP) must be considered during the initial phases of burn injury. Under such circumstances the usual measures for treating ICP would be instituted (osmotic diuretics, moderate hyperventilation, nursing in the head-up position).

HEMATOLOGIC EFFECTS

Blood viscosity may increase, not only as a result of hemoconcentration secondary to fluid shifts, but also as a result of alterations in plasma protein content.[2] The

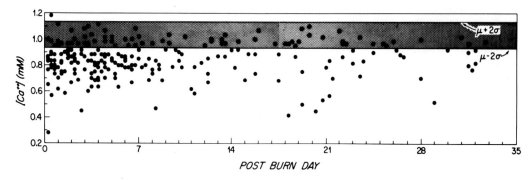

Figure 19-3. This figure represents ionized calcium values from burned children and adults for the first 35 days after burn injury. Note that the majority of values are abnormally low. (Reproduced with permission from Szyfelbein SK, et al: Persistent ionized hypocalcemia during resuscitation and recovery phases of body burns. *Crit Care Med* 9:454–458, 1981)

hematopoietic system is also adversely affected; an ongoing hemolytic anemia secondary to the burn injury is common.[39] In the early stage, thrombocytopenia, secondary to increased platelet aggregation and trapping of platelets in the lungs, is followed by an increase in platelet count 10–14 days after burn injury. This elevation will persist for several months.[40] Often there is an increase in fibrin split products (disseminated intravascular coagulopathy) lasting for three to five days.[41] Factors V and VIII are also increased four to eight times for the first three months after injury.[41]

GASTROINTESTINAL EFFECTS

Gastrointestinal function is diminished immediately following burn injury secondary to the development of gastric and intestinal ileus.[42] Because of the danger of aspiration into the lungs of gastric contents during this time, the stomach should be adequately vented, particularly in patients unable to protect their airway. In patients unable to tolerate enteral feeding, parenteral nutrition must be supplied to prevent tissue protein breakdown.[49,43] Stress ulcers (Curling's ulcer) are associated with any burn injury, and may be life-threatening.[44] Retrospective studies in pediatric burn patients, and prospective studies in adult burn and intensive care patients, indicate that cimetidine in the usual doses may not adequately protect seriously ill patients from increases in gastric acidity.[29,45,46] This may in part be related to pharmacokinetic or pharmacodynamic alterations. Therefore frequent feedings when tolerated and the use of antacids, together with larger or more frequent doses of histamine$_2$ receptor antagonists may help prevent stress ulcers.[29,44,47]

SKIN EFFECTS

Extensive skin destruction results in the inability to regulate body heat, to conserve fluids and electrolytes, or to protect against bacterial invasion. Children have a much greater body surface area-to-weight ratio compared to adults (Figure 19-1), and therefore are even more prone to dangerous hypothermia and fluid and electrolyte imbalances. Thus it is important always to keep these patients covered as much as possible, use radiant warmers, elevate the environmental temperature, and warm inspired respiratory gases. Late complications concerning the skin include progressive scar formation, which results in movement-restricting contractures.[26]

METABOLIC EFFECTS

Many metabolic alterations follow extensive burn injury. Increased utilization of glucose, fat, and protein result in a greater oxygen demand and increased carbon dioxide production.[33,48–58] Centrally mediated or sepsis-induced hyperthermia also increases oxygen consumption and carbon dioxide production. This may persist even after complete healing of the burn wounds.

CALCIUM HOMEOSTASIS

Many acutely burned patients demonstrate an abnormally low ionized calcium level that may persist for up to seven weeks following injury.[59] A prospective study of the changes in total calcium and ionized calcium [Ca^{++}], inorganic phosphate (P$_i$), and magnesium (Mg) following major acute thermal injury compared these findings with those in patients long recovered from similar injuries (Figure 19-3).[59] This study demonstrated marked abnormalities in the indices of calcium metabolism in both acute and recovery phases. The [Ca^{++}] value could not be predicted for any patient by use of the McLean-Hastings nomogram. Hypophosphatemia and hypermagnesemia reverted toward normal during the latter phase of recovery from the acute injury. The usual reciprocal relationship between calcium and inorganic phosphate was not evident. Therefore supplemental oral or intravenous calcium is extremely important in the management of severly burned patients.

PHARMACOLOGY

Subsequent to any major thermal injury there are many changes in hepatic, renal and pulmonary functions.[27–29,32–36,57–60] Because of impaired organ perfusion during the hypovolemic phase, uptake and clearance of many drugs may be decreased. Subsequently, during the hypermetabolic phase, because of increased blood flow and enzyme induction, the activity of the clearing organs may be enhanced.[28,29,33] The massive edema present in the burned and nonburned areas, and the loss of drug through burn wound, can result in an apparent increase in the central or total volume of distribution of drugs.[60,61]

Many drugs are highly bound by plasma proteins. The activity of such drugs is likely to depend more on the unbound than total drug concentrations. The two major binding pro-

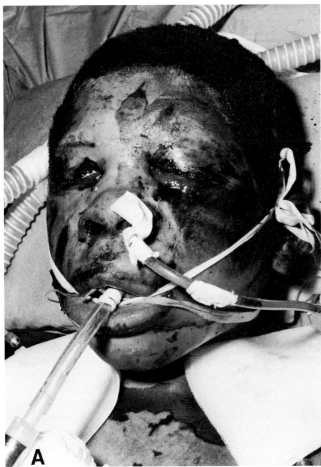
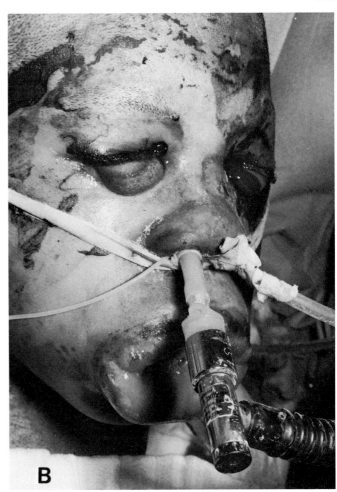

Figure 19-4. A young child who had just sustained a facial burn in a closed space (A). Note the early onset of facial edema. The same patient several hours later (B) shows massive edema formation that extends into the oropharynx, larynx, and trachea. Early prophylactic intubation is mandatory in any facial burn, or in any patient where there is potential for inhalation injury. Note that the endotracheal tube was changed from oral to nasal position, and that it is secured with cloth tape rather than adhesive tape.

teins, alpha$_1$-acid glycoprotein and albumin, increase and decrease respectively following thermal injury, resulting in either decreased and increased free fractions of those drugs with which they bind.[62,63] In addition, there is indirect evidence to suggest that burn injury, with its complications and hormonal responses, may cause changes in receptor numbers at nerve endings.[64–66] It is therefore not surprising that aberrant responses to drugs acting on adrenergic and cholinergic receptors have been reported.[64,65,67,68] Other examples of drugs affected by burn-induced kinetic and dynamic changes include aminoglycoside antibiotics, diazepam, muscle relaxants, and cimetidine.[28,29,35,61,65,69–71] Thus burn-induced alterations in kinetics and dynamics make the clinical response to any medication unpredictable. Therefore clinical effects should always be closely monitored, and plasma concentrations, protein binding, and clearance documented whenever possible.

RESUSCITATION AND INITIAL EVALUATION

The resuscitation of the burned patient must give priority to the establishment of a clear airway, maintenance of adequate oxygenation and circulating blood volume. Diagnosis and evaluation for associated injuries must also be considered.

AIRWAY AND OXYGENATION

All burned patients, especially those with inhalation injuries, must be considered hypoxemic; many will suffer from carbon monoxide poisoning (see below). Therefore on admission, administration of a high-inspired oxygen concentration is mandatory. Direct injury to the airway and alveoli occurs in patients who have sustained pulmonary inhalation injury due to the inhalation of smoke, flames, noxious gases, heated air, or steam.[4,15–25]

When a patient is burned in an enclosed space, or if thermal burns or carbonaceous material are evident about the mouth and nose, respiratory involvement is probable.[21] Upper airway obstruction caused by edema of the lips, nose, tongue, pharynx, or glottis is very common, and can be compared to the combined effects of acute epiglottitis and laryngotracheobronchitis. The decreasing patency of the airway by rapidly increasing edema, beginning in the first hours after the injury and lasting several days, make late intubation hazardous, if not impossible (Figure 19-4). Prophylactic intubation should be performed in any case of severe facial burns, or when pulmonary burn and upper airway inhalation injury is suspected. Control of the airway in the pediatric patient is usually accomplished under general anesthesia. In the case of pure

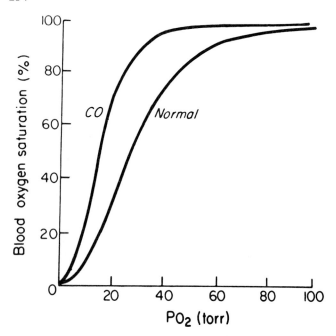

Figure 19-5. This figure presents the changes in the oxygen-hemoglobin dissociation curve which occur with carbon monoxide poisoning. The oxygen–hemoglobin dissociation curve is altered in shape as well as shifted to the left. Therefore less oxygen is available for delivery to tissues, and the oxygen carried by hemoglobin is more tightly bound. (Reproduced with permission Fein et al: *Crit Care Med* 8:94–98, 1980.)

inhalational injury without facial or upper airway burn the need for intubation should be considered individually. Clinical experience shows that endotracheal tubes can be left in place in these patients for weeks with fewer risks than the alternative tracheostomy. Tracheostomy in burned patients is associated with high mortality rates, and in some pediatric series the death rate approaches 100 percent.[72] Tracheostomy should be considered only in extreme situations where intubation is technically impossible. Although the mortality due to tracheostomy has been reduced considerably by the increased use of endotracheal tubes, morbidity due to prolonged endotracheal intubation still exists.[73] The use of soft uncuffed silastic tubes may reduce the incidence of complications, such as tracheal stenosis, tracheal erosion, and tracheomalacia. However, the narrower internal diameter of the endotracheal tube lumen may increase the work of breathing during spontaneous ventilation even with continuous positive end expiratory pressure.[74]

CARBON MONOXIDE POISONING

Carboxyhemoglobin is produced by the combination of carbon monoxide (CO) with the iron of the heme radical, the oxygen-binding site. CO combines more slowly with hemoglobin than does oxygen, but is bound more than 200 times more firmly.[75–76] The toxic effects of CO poisoning are due to tissue hypoxia from decreased oxygen delivery. Decreased delivery occurs not only because CO renders the hemoglobin unavailable to bind to oxygen, but also because carboxyhemoglobin, even in small amounts, shifts the oxygen-dissociation curve to

the left (Figure 19-5).[16,76] The majority of smoke inhalation victims have CO poisoning. Direct measurement of carboxyhemoglobin is very important to guide treatment. Estimates of its concentration may be derived by *measuring* (not calculating) oxygen saturation or arterial oxygen content. The half-life of carboxyhemoglobin is approximately four hours when breathing room air, but decreases to 30 minutes when 100 percent oxygen is administered with mechanical ventilation.[15] Immediate administration of oxygen is therefore essential to achieve the highest level of oxygen in the blood; positive pressure ventilation may be indicated.

ADEQUACY OF CIRCULATION

The various formulas for determining fluid replacement are estimates, and often need modification, depending on clinical and laboratory findings.[2,77–86]

The most widely accepted and effective fluid protocols in current use are the Parkland (Baxter) and Brooke formulas.[2] It is important to remember that all formulas are only guides to fluid therapy; they should be modified for the individual patient, depending upon the response. The Parkland formula calls for four milliliters of lactated Ringer's solution for each percent of body surface area (BSA) burned, times body weight in kilograms. The Brooke formula recommends 0.5 milliliter colloid + 1.5 milliliters crystalloid for each percent BSA burned times kilograms of body weight. Either formula gives the calculated volume, in addition to the calculated normal body maintenance fluid requirement for each day. Half of the calculated amount of both replacement volume and maintenance fluid volume is given in the first eight hours, and a fourth more is given in each of the two subsequent eight-hour periods of the first day following the burn.

The syndrome of hyperosmolar, hyperglycemic non-ketotic coma (consisting of severe dehydration, marked hyperglycemia, serum hyperosmolality, and coma in the absence of ketoacidosis) may be associated with burns, and has a high mortality.[2] This emphasizes the need to limit the use of glucose-containing solutions during the intial volume resuscitation, and the need for frequent serum glucose measurement.

The general appearance of the patient and the state of his or her sensorium provide an important guide to the effectiveness of the resuscitative therapy. In addition, urinary output is usually a helpful indicator of the need for fluid replacement, bearing in mind the possible increase of antidiuretic hormone secretion and occasional tubular dysfunction.[5,30] Every effort must be made to protect the kidneys by providing adequate fluid replacement. Renal failure, in the presence of major burns, is virtually tantamount to death. However, overly vigorous fluid therapy may result in pulmonary edema. Therefore, this situation necessitates careful titration of all fluids to replete circulating blood volume. Commonly used endpoints of satisfactory fluid resuscitation include heart rate, systemic arterial blood pressure, urinary output, central venous pressure, and arterial oxygenation and pH. In more severely ill patients, cardiac performance is appraised by pulmonary artery flow-directed catheters, and measurement of cardiac output.[9] Multiple factors, including ventricular compliance and airway pressure, distort measured atrial filling pressures. Using the thermodilution principle, mean pulmonary artery pressure, pulmonary capillary wedge pressure, central venous pressure, ventricular volume, and ejection fraction have been measured in burned young adults and

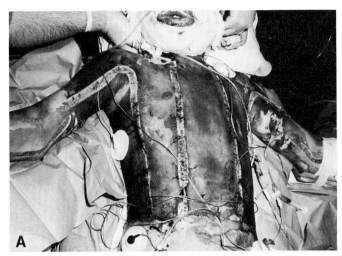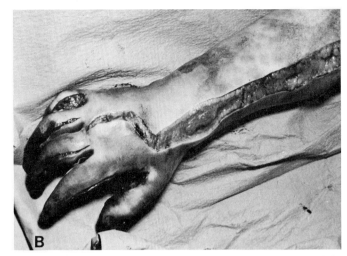

Figure 19-6. Circumferential chest burns result (A) in severe impairment of respiration secondary to the tourniquet effect of the shrinking eschar and subcutaneous edema. The widely separated escharotomy lines indicate the severity of the constriction. Similar effects occur in the circumferentially burned extremities (B). Early escharotomy may help to preserve function and prevent amputation.

teenagers to be used as a guide to the adequacy of fluid therapy.[8,10] End-diastolic ventricular volume was superior to the conventional measures in predicting the adequacy of circulating blood volume. The technique of ventricular volume and ejection fraction measurement may have applications to younger children in the future. More recently, cardiovascular function estimated by echocardiography and ^{99}Tc ventriculography have been used in the critically ill.[87]

In the child, the evaporated fluid losses exceed 4,000 milliliters for each square meter of burn surface each day, compared to only 2,500 milliliters in the adult.[85] Concomitantly, for each square meter of burn surface, 2,500 kilocalories of heat are lost each day. Minimizing caloric expenditure and providing caloric supplementation simultaneously are the only ways to prevent catabolism of body tissues. The tendency for children to be poikilothermic, particularly in the absence of protective skin as a result of the burn injury, causes profound temperature derangements. Efforts to maintain normal body temperature involve active warming (warming blanket, ambient room temperature of 22–25° C or warmed intravenous fluids), as well as prevention of heat loss by keeping the patient covered. This is especially important during this initial volume resuscitation, and in the operating room when dressings are taken down for examination and excision procedures.

ASSOCIATED INJURY

Associated injuries such as a tension pneumothorax, a ruptured spleen, liver, long bone fractures, or head injury are easy to overlook. Thus during the initial resuscitation a very careful history and physical examination is mandatory. Such injuries may compound the need for increased volume resuscitation fluids.

CIRCUMFERENTIAL BURNS

There are definite immediate cardiovascular and respiratory responses to circumferential burns of the chest, abdomen, and extremities.[11,26,86] Circumferential burns of the thorax

can contribute to respiratory failure from decreased chest-wall compliance. Functional residual capacity is reduced with airway closure and atelectasis, resulting in profound hypoxemia.[16,19–21] Deep circumferential burns of the abdomen may generate excessive intra-abdominal pressure, which may reduce the already low cardiac output by impairing venous return, in addition to restricting diaphragmatic movement (Figure 19-6).[11] When this occurs, both extra- and intrapulmonary factors can contribute to arterial desaturation.[27] Damaged tissues can also generate severe compressive forces restricting or occluding the blood flow to burned extremities; this results in ischemia, which, if left untreated, may necessitate partial or total amputation. Escharotomies of circumferential burns of the chest, abdomen, and extremities must be performed urgently, since impaired hemodynamics and respiratory mechanics can cause irreversible damage within hours following the burn injury.

ELECTRICAL BURNS

This type of injury can be associated with loss of limbs and other injuries which are not immediately obvious. The extent of the injury is unpredictable—often the surface injury is small but the extent of underlying tissue damage and necrosis is massive. Such an injury is a combination of electrical and thermal damage.[88] Very often, victims have concurrent injuries, such as fractures of vertebrae or long bones, ruptured organs, myocardial injury, or numerous contusions. These patients are often admitted in a coma with seizures. Muscle tissue surrounding bone is usually more affected than superficial muscles. Early fasciotomy is needed to preserve the blood flow to extremities. Massive myonecrosis and hemolysis may result in hyperkalemia, as well as myoglobinuria and hemoglobinuria. Follow-up of patients with electrical injuries often reveals unpredictable sequelae occurring three months to three years after injury, and may occur in organs or areas that do not necessarily appear abnormal during the acute course of illness. The latent interval between injury and the

Table 19-1

Systemic Effects of Burn Injury

System	Early	Late
Cardiovascular	↓ C.O. 2° (secondary) to decreased circulating blood volume, myocardial depressant factor	↑ C.O. 2° to sepsis ↑ C.O. 2–3 times > baseline for months (hypermetabolism) Hypertension
Pulmonary	Upper airway obstruction 2° to edema Lower airway obstruction 2° to edema, bronchospasm, particulate matter ↓ FRC ↓ Pulmonary compliance ↓ Chestwall compliance	Bronchopneumonia Tracheal stenosis ↓ Chestwall compliance
Renal	↓ GFR a) secondary to circulating blood volume b) myoglobinuria c) hemoglobinuria Tubular dysfunction	↑ GFR 2° to C.O. Tubular dysfunction
Hepatic	↓ Function 2° to circulating blood volume, hypoxia, hepatotoxins	Hepatitis ↑ Function 2° to hypermetabolism, enzyme induction ↓ Function 2° to sepsis drug interaction
Hematopoietic	↓ Platelets ↑ Fibrin split products, consumptive coagulopathy, anemia	↑ Platelets ↑ clotting factors possible AIDS, Hepatitis
Neurologic	Encephalopathy Seizures ICP	Encephalopathy Seizures ICU psychosis
Skin	↑ Heat, fluid, electrolyte loss	Contractures, scar formation
Metabolic	↓ Ionized calcium	↑ O_2 consumption ↑ CO_2 production ↓ Ionized calcium
Pharmacokinetics	Altered volume of distribution Altered protein binding	↑ Tolerance to narcotics, sedatives Enzyme induction, altered receptors Drug interaction

↓ = decrease in
↑ = increase in
C.O. = cardiac output
FRC = functional residual capacity
GFR = glomerular filtration rate
ICP = intra cranialpressure

appearance of chronic tissue damage is comparable in its time relationship to the effects of irradiation. These late complications most frequently include neurologic dysfunction, ocular damage, damage to the gastrointestinal tract, changes in the ECG, and delayed hemorrhage from large vessels.[88,89]

GUIDELINES TO ANESTHETIC MANAGEMENT

The anesthetic management of the burned pediatric patient begins with the initial resuscitation, and may continue for many years through reconstructive surgery. Knowledge and understanding of the pathophysiology of burn injury will enable the anesthesiologist to recognize and treat complications arising as a result of burn injury or its therapy (Table 19-1).

GENERAL PRINCIPLES

The patient coming to the operating room for burn wound excision and grafting must be properly prepared physiologically and psychologically. This preparation includes:

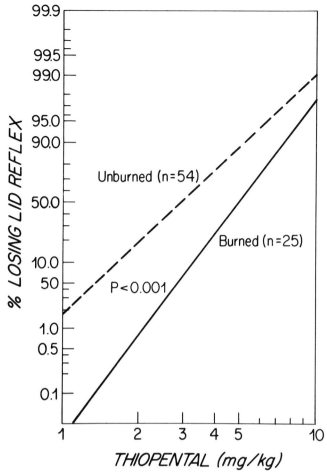

Figure 19-7. This figure compares the percent of children (burned and unburned) who lost the lid reflex versus the intravenous bolus dose of thiopental. Note the marked shift in the dose response curve. (Reproduced with permission of Coté, et al: *Anesthesiology* 55:S338, 1981.

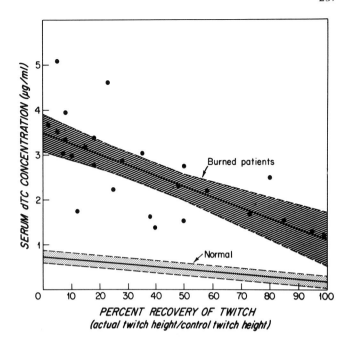

Figure 19-8. This figure correlates serum concentration of d-tubocurarine versus the percentage of recovery of the response to electrical twitch stimulation. Shaded areas represent 95 percent confidence limits. Note the marked increase in requirements for burned patients; they may have complete recovery from neuromuscular blockade despite serum concentrations which would result in complete paralysis in unburned patients. (Reproduced with permission from Martyn JAJ, et al: *Anesthesiology* 52:353–355, 1980.)

- *Psychological support* from nurses, parents, physicians and trained psychologists.
- Care to *adequately sedate* the patient prior to movement to the OR, which can be quite painful, both physically and emotionally. Intravenous narcotics, such as fentanyl and meperidine, which have minimal histamine release, are particularly helpful for this purpose. It should be noted that burned patients develop tolerance to most narcotics and sedatives, thus eventually requiring higher dosages to achieve a satisfactory clinical response.
- Correction of *intravascular volume* prior to induction of anesthesia.
- Attention to minimize patient's *heat loss* during transport.
- Adequate monitoring for major blood loss including an intra-arterial cannula, urinary catheter, ECG, and esophageal stethoscope. In the more critically ill, catheters to measure cardiac filling pressures may be useful.
- Good intravenous route for volume infusion.
- Use of specific anesthetic equipment, including a variety of sterilized laryngoscope blades, endotracheal tubes, airways and blood pressure cuffs. A ventilator is helpful to free the anesthesiologist's hands.
- Special equipment to maintain body temperature, includ-

ing a warming blanket, radiant warmer, blood warmer, a heated humidifier and a heated operating room (22–25°C).

Essential invasive monitoring (arterial line) may be established after induction of anesthesia in most patients. Thiopental in incremental doses is usually well tolerated, provided there is an adequate intravascular volume. Studies in children long recovered from acute injury found a 40 percent increase in thiopental dose needed to ablate the lid reflex, compared to unburned children; acutely burned children appear to have a similarly increased need (Figure 19-7).[90] Ketamine may on occasion be preferred if the adequacy of intravascular volume is in question; tolerance to ketamine with repeated administration has been reported.[91] High-dose fentanyl for those patients who will be ventilated postoperatively is also acceptable. However, one must be observant for chest-wall rigidity. Other methods of induction include rectal methohexital or thiopental for infants and children. An inhalation induction is preferable for patients with a compromised airway.

Succinylcholine is contraindicated in burned patients because of potentially lethal efflux of potassium ions from muscle.[64] The cause of this abnormal response is probably due to the fact that the entire muscle membrane, rather than just the myoneural junction, becomes a chemoreceptor. Such tissue can thus be resistant to non-depolarizing muscle relaxants, and sensitive to depolarizing muscle relaxants.[64,65,70,71] The duration of this dangerous response to succinylcholine is unknown. However, a recent case of a child showing marked

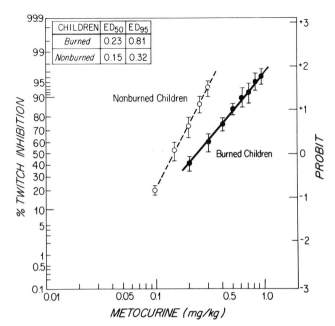

CHILDREN	ED$_{50}$	ED$_{95}$
Burned	0.23	0.81
Nonburned	0.15	0.32

Figure 19-9. This figure plots percent twitch inhibition versus metocurine dose (mg/kg) in burned children. Note the marked shift of the dose response curve. (Reproduced with permission from Martyn JAJ, et al: *Br J Anaesth* 55:263–268, 1983.)

resistance to non-depolarizing relaxants 463 days after burn injury indirectly suggests that sensitivity to succinylcholine may persist long after the acute injury phase.[92] The non-depolarizing muscle relaxants (d-tubocurarine, pancuronium bromide, metocurine) are therefore the relaxants of choice in burned patients. In this regard, it has been found that following burns of more than 25 percent BSA, both the total dose of d-tubocurarine administered and the serum concentration necessary to attain a given degree of muscle twitch depression, are increased three to five times compared to unburned subjects (Figures 19-8 and 19-9).[65,70] Recovery from neuromuscular blockade was seen at serum concentrations that would give 100 percent twitch depression in unburned patients. More recent studies with pancuronium and metocurine indicate that the hyposensitivity is highly correlated to the magnitude of burn (r = 0.88).[71,93] Protein binding and pharmacokinetic studies with d-tubocurarine indicate that these two factors contribute little to the enhanced muscle relaxant requirements.[60,62] Changes of particular tissues (namely, an increase in the number of acetylcholine receptors at the neuromuscular junction, or an altered affinity for the relaxant by those receptors) may be responsible for the elevated demand for non-depolarizing muscle relaxants.[65,71] Pharmacologic reversal of neuromuscular blockade, however, poses no special problem in burned patients.[65,71]

Maintainence of anesthesia is usually accomplished with nitrous oxide, oxygen, relaxant, and a narcotic or inhalation agent. In very ill patients anesthetic doses—but not muscle relaxant requirements—are drastically reduced; in this situation high dose fentanyl–oxygen anesthesia, or neuroleptanesthesia, appears to be well tolerated. Ketamine may be the anesthetic agent of choice in specific circumstances, such as the desire to avoid airway manipulation after application of fresh facial grafts, or for very brief procedures. The experience of

Table 19-2

Approximate Expected Blood Loss for Burn Excision as a Percentage of Body Surface Area*

Procedure	Estimated Blood Loss (EBL)
Fascial Excision	1.5 ml/cm^2**
Tangential Excision	4 ml/cm^2**

* These calculations are based on the measurement of blood loss during surgical procedures at the Shriner's Burn Institute (unpublished data). These guidelines have been used for the last five years and have proven to be useful in clinical practice.
** This includes percentage of body surface area of burn excised, and area of skin harvested. For example, if a 10 kg child with BSA of 0.45m^2 (4500 cm^2) has a 10% harvest and a 10% excision, for a total of 20%, we get 0.2 × 4500 = 900 cm^2. Therefore, tangential procedures would result in 900 × 4 = 3600 ml EBL, and fascial procedures would result in 900 × 1.5 = 1350 ml EBL.

other burn centers with ketamine as the sole anesthetic has not been unsatisfactory.

The inspired oxygen concentration is regulated according to the arterial blood gases. Because of the increased metabolic rate and carbon dioxide production, increased alveolar ventilation may be required. Blood gas analysis must therefore be assessed early, frequently, and throughout the anesthetic procedure. Constant monitoring of expired carbon dioxide is also very helpful during intraoperative management. The endotracheal tube must be secured with tracheostomy tape, since standard adhesive tape will not stick to burned tissue and wet dressings. ECG leads also will not adhere, and for this reason are placed under dependent portions of the body, or sutured onto the skin after the patient is anesthetized. The standard measures for protecting the cornea from drying, and positioning of the limbs to prevent nerve compression, must also be observed.

The most important feature of the intraoperative course is the monitoring and replacement of the patient's blood loss. For this reason invasive intravascular monitoring is essential. The Seldinger approach has proven particularly valuable for central venous cannulation,[94] and may also be of value should there be need for use of the femoral artery for monitoring.[95] It is not uncommon for the patient to loose one to three blood volumes during each burn excision. One must therefore be familiar with the surgical approach to burn excision; during a tangential excision a patient might lose three to five times more blood than during excisions down to fascia (Table 19-2). Blood loss is also quite dependent upon the expertise of the surgical team. It is difficult to estimate blood loss despite accurate weighing of surgical sponges because of significant losses in the surgical drapes. Other indicators of circulating blood volume, such as urine output, central venous pressure, arterial pressure, and wave form, must be closely monitored.

Chronic ionized hypocalcemia in association with major thermal injury was discussed earlier in this chapter. Because of these experiences, prophylactic intermittent administration of calcium is strongly recommended. To patients weighing less than ten kilograms, 10 milligrams are administered every 15–30 minutes (100–150 mg of CaCl$_2$ for every unit of plasma or albumin). The importance of this therapy is clinically demonstrated by the fact that acute reductions in ionized calcium secondary to citrate binding are avoided during rapid infusion of fresh frozen plasma or citrated whole blood (see Chapter 11).[96-98] Clinically the rapid administration of fresh frozen plasma or citrated whole blood through a central line without additional calcium may be more likely to induce severe hypotension, bradycardia, and electrical mechanical dissociation. Rapid administration of citrated blood products has been much safer in our experience through peripheral lines. Rapid administration of washed packed cells does not cause ionized hypocalcemia.

SPECIAL CONSIDERATIONS

As a general rule, burned patients require larger than normal doses of all medications, including antibiotics, cimetidine, muscle relaxants, and anesthetic drugs.[28,29,61,65,67-71,90-92] Pharmacokinetic studies in acutely burned patients indicate that the increased requirement for antibiotics and cimetidine was due in part to leakage through burn wound, rapid urinary excretion, and altered volume of distribution.[28,29] Pharmacokinetic studies of d-tubocurarine demonstrate an increased central volume of distribution, normal total volume of distribution, and increased urinary excretion, as well as increased plasma binding. It did not, however, show losses through the burn wound.[60-62] In addition, there appears to be increased tolerance to sedatives and narcotics. A pharmacokinetic study of diazepam (Valium) in adult burn patients demonstrated a significantly higher free fraction (pharmacologically active component), while the clearance of free diazepam was reduced. An increased tolerance to diazepam despite a higher fraction of pharmacologically active drug and decreased clearance suggests resistance at tissue receptors similar to that seen at the neuromuscular junction.[35] The persistence of such changes in requirements both for muscle relaxants and anesthetic drugs long after recovery from burn injury must be kept in mind and doses titrated according to needs.[90,92]

The pharmacokinetics of many medications commonly used in burned patients remains to be investigated.[34] In general one must be aware of the alterations in distribution volume and protein binding, increased or decreased metabolism, and excretion. Furthermore, these patients are frequently on multiple medications and therefore drug interactions, potentiations, and incompatibilities must be considered. Of particular importance in this context is cimetidine, which is known to inhibit the clearance of many other drugs (see Chapter 6).[35]

A less common but important source of cyanosis and hypoxemia is the development of methemoglobinemia. In burns treated with silver nitrate dressings, the presence of some strains of gram-negative bacteria, which are capable of reducing nitrates to nitrites, creates a situation in which the nitrites diffuse into the bloodstream, converting hemoglobin into methemoglobin.[2] The methemoglobin not only decreases the available oxygen-carrying capacity, but also increases the affinity of the unaltered hemoglobin for oxygen, thereby further impairing the delivery of oxygen; as a result the P_{50} curve is shifted to the left. Methemoglobinemia should, therefore, be considered in the differential diagnosis of cyanosis. Approximately five grams of deoxyhemoglobin for each deciliter of blood are necessary to produce visible cyanosis, but a comparable skin color is produced by 1.5–2 grams methemoglobin for each deciliter of blood. Blood that contains more than approximately ten percent methemoglobin usually appears dark red or even brown, despite a high oxygen tension, and does not change color even with vigorous agitation in room air. Measured oxygen saturation or content will be low. Treatment consists of removing the toxic agent, administration of methylene blue (2 mg/kg), oxygen inhalation and, possibly, hemodialysis.

Because these patients frequently undergo multiple anesthetic procedures, special considerations must be given to endotracheal tube type and size. When appropriate, uncuffed endotracheal tubes should be utilized and a record kept of the size tube and pressure at which leakage occurs for each anesthetic procedure. It is not uncommon to note the use of smaller endotracheal tubes as weeks go by, which heralds the development of a subglottic lesion (stenosis, granuloma, polyps), and should be investigated with bronchoscopy. If cuffed tubes must be used then a high volume low pressure or the silastic variety is recommended.

Hyperalimentation is frequently carried out preoperatively and intraoperatively. These fluids should be continued intraoperatively, preferably with the use of a constant infusion pump to avoid accidental over-infusion. If the hyperalimentation fluids must be terminated, (to permit blood transfusion, etc.) then frequent monitoring of blood glucose levels is mandatory. Dangerous rebound hypoglycemia may occur if infusion of these solutions is interrupted.

AWAKENING

Upon awakening from anesthesia special consideration must be given to the likelihood of severe pain. Therefore analgesic drugs should be administered, in increasingly liberal doses because of increased tolerance. Adequacy of air exchange and patency of the airway, however, must be given first priority.

SPECIAL TECHNIQUES

One decade ago controlled hypotension for burn surgery proved helpful;[99] harvesting of skin from the scalp and repeat harvesting of skin from other areas are situations which lend themselves particularly well to this technique. With better surgical techniques, we no longer use controlled hypotension, since the risks outweigh the benefits.

SUMMARY

In summary the care of the burned patient involves detailed knowledge of the early and late effects of burn injury on the respiratory, cardiac, renal, hepatic, hematopoietic, and metabolic systems. An awareness of altered pharmacokinetics and pharmacodynamics to anesthetic agents, combined with an understanding of the problems of massive blood transfusion, will also contribute to safe anesthetic care. Finally, the importance of adequate analgesia, sedation, and concern for the psychological well being of this devastatingly injured child cannot be over emphasized. All of these factors combine to produce a successful outcome.

REFERENCES

1. Lloyd JR: Thermal trauma: Therapeutic achievements and investigative horizons. *Surg Clin North Am* 57:121–138, 1977
2. Moncrief JA: Burns. *N Engl J Med* 288:444–454, 1973
3. Arturson G: Pathophysiological aspects of the burn syndrome with special reference to liver injury and alterations of capillary permeability. *Acta Chir Scand* [Suppl] 274:1–135, 1961
4. Demling RH, Smith M, Bodai B, et al: Comparison of postburn capillary permeability in soft tissue and lung. *J Burn Care Res* 1:86–92, 1981
5. Morgan RJ, Martyn JAJ, Philbin DM, et al: Water metabolism and antidiuretic hormone (ADH) response following thermal injury. *J Trauma* 20:468–472, 1980
6. Wilmore DW, Long JM, Mason AD, Jr, et al: Catecholamines: Mediator of the hypermetabolic response to thermal injury. *Ann Surg* 180:653–669, 1974
7. Martyn JAJ, Burke JF: Is there a selective increase in pulmonary capillary permeability following cutaneous burns? *Chest* 76:374–375, 1979
8. Martyn JAJ, Snider MT, Szyfelbein SK, et al: Right ventricular dysfunction in acute thermal injury. *Ann Surg* 191:330–335, 1980
9. Aikawa N, Martyn JAJ, Burke JF: Pulmonary artery catheterization and thermodilution cardiac output determination in the management of critically burned patients. *Am J Surg* 135:811–817, 1978
10. Martyn JAJ, Snider MT, Farago LF, et al: Thermodilution right ventricular volume: A novel and better predictor of volume resuscitation in burns. *J Trauma* 21:619–626, 1981
11. Turbow ME: Abdominal compression following circumferential burn: Cardiovascular response. *J Trauma* 13:535–541, 1973
12. Parks DH, Carvajal HF, Larson DL: Management of Burns. *Surg Clin North Am* 57:875–894, 1977
13. Moati F, Sepulchre C, Miskulin M, et al: Biochemical and pharmacological properties of a cardiotoxic factor isolated from the blood serum of burned patients. *J Pathol* 127:147–156, 1979
14. Kremer B, Allgower M, Graf M, et al: The present status of research in burns. *Int Care Med* 7:77–87, 1981
15. Trunkey DD: Inhalation injury. *Surg Clin North Am* 58:1133–1140, 1978
16. Fein A, Leff A, Hopewell PC: Pathophysiology and management of the complications resulting from fire and the inhaled products of combustion: Review of the literature. *Crit Care Med* 8:94–98, 1980
17. Sherwin RP, Richters V: Lung capillary permeability: Nitrogen dioxide exposure and leakage of tritiated serum. *Arch Intern Med* 128:61–68, 1971
18. Green GM, Jakab GJ, Low RB, et al: Defense mechanisms of the respiratory membrane. *Am Rev Respir Dis* 115:479–514, 1977
19. Nieman GF, Clark WR, Wax SD, et al: The effect of smoke inhalation on pulmonary surfactant. *Ann Surg* 191:171–181, 1980
20. Pruitt BA, Jr, Erickson DR, Morris A: Progressive pulmonary insufficiency and other pulmonary complications of thermal injury. *J Trauma* 15:369–379, 1975
21. Wroblewski DA, Bower GG: The significance of facial burns in acute smoke inhalation. *Crit Care Med* 7:335–338, 1979
22. Stone HH: Pulmonary burns in children. *J Pediatr Surg* 14:48–52, 1979
23. Zawacki BE, Jung RC, Joyce J, et al: Smoke, burns, and the natural history of inhalation injury in fire victims. *Ann Surg* 185:100–110, 1977
24. Stephenson SF, Esrig BC, Polk HC, Jr: The pathophysiology of smoke inhalation injury. *Ann Surg* 182:652–660, 1975
25. Powers SK (moderator): Supportive therapy in burn care. Smoke inhalation. *J Trauma* [Suppl] 19:912–922, 1979
26. Quinby WC, Jr: Restrictive effects of thoracic burns in children. *J Trauma* 12:646–655, 1972
27. Martyn JAJ, Aikawa N, Wilson RS, et al: Extrapulmonary factor influencing the ratio of arterial oxygen tension to inspired oxygen concentration in burn patients. *Crit Care Med* 7:492–496, 1980
28. Loirat P, Rohan J, Baillet A, et al: Increased glomerular filtration rate in patients with major burns and its effect on the pharmacokinetics of tobramycin. *N Engl J Med* 299:915–919, 1978
29. Martyn JAJ, Greenblatt DJ, Abernethy DR: Increased cimetidine clearance in burned patients. *Clin Pharmacol Ther* 35:258, 1984
30. Eklund J, Granberg PO, Liljedahl SO: Studies on renal function in burns. *Acta Chir Scand* 136:627–640, 1970
31. Falkner B, Roven S, DeClement FA, et al: Hypertension in children with burns. *J Trauma* 18:213–217, 1978
32. Ciaccio EI, Fruncillo RJ: Urinary excretion of D-glucaric acid by severely burned patients. *Clin Pharm Ther* 25:340–344, 1979
33. Wilmore DW, Goodwin CW, Aulick LH, et al: Effect of injury and infection on visceral metabolism and circulation. *Ann Surg* 192:491–504, 1980
34. Sawchuk RJ, Rector TS: Drug kinetics in burn patients. *Clin Pharmacokinet* 5:548–556, 1980
35. Martyn JAJ, Greenblatt DJ, Quinby WC: Diazepam kinetics in patients with severe burns. *Anesth Analg* 62:293–297, 1983
36. Czaja AJ, Rizzo TA, Smith WR, Jr, et al: Acute liver disease after cutaneous thermal injury. *J Trauma* 15:887–894, 1975
37. Sepulchre C, Moati F, Miskulin M, et al: Biochemical and pharmacological properties of a neurotoxic protein isolated from the blood serum of heavily burned patients. *J Pathol* 127:137–145, 1979
38. Antoon AY, Volpe JJ, Crawford JD: Burn encephalopathy in children. *Pediatrics* 50:609–616, 1972
39. Curreri PW, Hicks JE, Aronoff RJ, et al: Inhibition of active sodium transport in erythrocytes from burned patients. *Surg Gynecol Obstet* 139:538–540, 1974
40. Heideman M: The effect of thermal injury on hemodynamic, respiratory and hematologic variables in relation to complement activation. *J Trauma* 19:239–243, 1979
41. Simon TL, Curreri PW, Harker LA: Kinetic characterization of hemostasis in thermal injury. *J Lab Clin Med* 89:702–711, 1977
42. Munster AW: The early management of thermal burns. *Surgery* 87.29–40, 1980
43. Blackburn GL, Maini BS, Pierce EC: Nutrition in the critically ill patient. *Anesthesiology* 47:181–194, 1977
44. Czaja AJ, McAlhany JC, Andes WA, et al: Acute gastric disease after cutaneous thermal injury. *Arch Surg* 110:600–605, 1975
45. Martyn JAJ: Chemoprophylaxis of increased gastric acidity and bleeding in burned pediatric patients. *Crit Care Med* 13:1–3, 1985
46. Priebe HJ, Skillman JJ, Bushnell LS et al: Antacid versus cimetidine in preventing acute gastrointestinal bleeding. *N Engl J Med* 302:426–430, 1980
47. Goudsouzian NG, Coté CJ, Liu LMP, et al: The dose response effects of oral cimetidine on gastric pH and volume in children. *Anesthesiology* 55:533–536, 1981
48. Burke JF, Wolfe RR, Mullany CJ: Glucose requirements following burn injury. Parameters of optimal glucose infusion and possible hepatic and respiratory abnormalities following excessive glucose intake. *Ann Surg* 190:274–285, 1979
49. Baxter CR: Problems and complications of burn shock resuscitation. *Surg Clin North Am* 58:1313–1322, 1978
50. Wilmore DW, Aulick LH: Metabolic changes in burned patients. *Surg Clin North Am* 58:1173–1187, 1978
51. Kien CL, Rohrbaugh DK, Burke JF, et al: Whole body protein synthesis in relation to basal energy expenditures in healthy children and in children recovering from burn injury. *Pediatr Res* 12:211–216, 1978
52. Scholmerich J, Kremer B, Richter IE, et al: Effect of cutaneous

human or mouse burn toxin on the metabolic function of isolated liver cells. *Scand J Plast Reconstr Surg* 13:223–230, 1979

53. Aulick LH, Wilmore DW: Increased peripheral amino acid release following burn injury. *Surgery* 85:560–565, 1979

54. Turinsky J, Saba TM, Scoville WA, et al: Dynamics of insulin secretion and resistance after burns. *J Trauma* 17:344–350, 1977

55. Hessman Y, Thoren L: Glycogen storage in rat liver and skeletal muscle in thermal trauma. *Acta Chir Scand* 141:385–392, 1975

56. Hessman Y: Glycogen storage in rat liver and skeletal muscle in thermal trauma. III. Effect on adrenal demedulation. *Acta Chir Scand* 141:473–479, 1975

57. Aprille JR, Hom JA, Rulfs J: Liver and skeletal muscle mitochondrial function following burn injury. *J Trauma* 17:279–288, 1977

58. Brown WL, Bowler EG, Mason AD, Jr, et al: Protein metabolism in burned rats. *Am J Physiol* 231:476–482, 1976

59. Szyfelbein SK, Drop LJ, Martyn JAJ: Persistent ionized hypocalcemia during resuscitation and recovery phases of body burns. *Crit Care Med* 9:454–458, 1981

60. Martyn JAJ, Matteo RS, Greenblatt DJ, et al: Comparative pharmacokinetics of d-tubocurarine in burned and non-burned man. *Anesth Analg* 61:241–246, 1982

61. Flandrois JP, Marichy J, Ceyrat J: Pharmacokocinetique del'amikacine chez le brule (resultats preliminaires) *Nouv Presse Med* 8:3501–3502, 1979

62. Leibel WS, Martyn JAJ, Szyfelbein SK, et al: Elevated plasma binding cannot account for the burn related d-tubocurarine hyposensitivity. *Anesthesiology* 54:378–382, 1981

63. Martyn JAJ, Abernethy DR, Greenblatt DJ: Plasma protein binding of drugs after severe burn injury. *Clin Pharmacol Ther* 35:535–539, 1984

64. Gronert GA, Theye RA: Pathophysiology of hyperkalemia induced by succinylcholine. *Anesthesiology* 43:89–99, 1975

65. Martyn JAJ, Szyfelbein SK, Ali HH, et al: Increased d-tubocurarine requirement following major thermal injury. *Anesthesiology* 52:352–355, 1980

66. Aprille JR, Aikawa N, Bell TC, et al: Adenylate cyclase after burn injury: Resistance to desensitization by catecholamines. *J Trauma* 19:812–818, 1979

67. Cone JB, Ransom JM, Tucker WE et al: Dopamine effects on post burn myocardial depression. *J Trauma* 22:1019–1020, 1982

68. Martyn JAJ, Farago LF, Burke JF: Pulmonary hemodynamics of low dose dopamine in nonseptic burned patients. *Bull Rev Burn Inj* 1:53–54, 1984

69. Glew RH, Moellering RC, Burke JF: Gentamicin dosage in children with extensive burns. *J Trauma* 16:819–823, 1976

70. Martyn JAJ, Goudsouzian NG, Matteo RS, et al: Metocurine requirements in burned pediatric patients: The relation of plasma concentration to neuromuscular blockade. *Br J Anaesth* 55:263–268, 1983

71. Martyn JAJ, Liu LMP, Szyfelbein SK, et al: Pancuronium requirements in burned children. *Anesthesiology* 59:561–564, 1983

72. Eckhauser FE, Billote J, Burke JF, et al: Tracheostomy complicating massive burn injury—a plea for conservatism *Am J Surg* 127:418–422, 1974

73. Katlic MR, Burke JF: Severe low-pressure cuff tracheal injury in burn patients. *Int Care Med* 7:82–92, 1981

74. Macintosh R, Mushin WW, Epstein HG: *Physics for the Anaesthetist* (ed 3). Oxford, Blackwell Scientific Publications, 1972, pp 247–269

75. Haldane J, Loraine Smith J: The absorption of oxygen by the lungs. *J Physiol* 22:231–258, 1897

76. Douglas CG, Haldane JS, Haldane JBS: The laws of combination of hemoglobin with carbon monoxide and oxygen. *J Physiol* 44:275–304, 1912

77. Pruitt BA, Jr.: Fluid and electrolyte replacement in the burned patient. *Surg Clin North Am* 58:1291–1312, 1978

78. Baxter CR: Problems and complications of burn shock resuscitation. *Surg Clin North Am* 58:1313–1322, 1978

79. Shires GT: Supportive therapy in burn care. Fluid resuscitation. *J Trauma* [Suppl 11] 19:864–877, 1979

80. Baxter CR: Fluid volume and electrolyte changes of the early postburn period. *Clin Plast Surg* 1:693–703, 1974

81. Caldwell FT, Bowser BH: Critical evaluation of hypertonic and hypotonic solutions to resuscitate severely burned children: A prospective study. *Ann Surg* 189:546–552, 1979

82. Moylan JA, Jr., Reckler JM, Mason AD, Jr: Resuscitation with hypertonic lactate saline in thermal injury. *Am J Surg* 125:580–584, 1973

83. Jelenko C, Williams JB, Wheeler ML, et al: Studies in shock and resuscitation. I. Use of a hypertonic, albumin-containing, fluid demand regimen (HALFD) in resuscitation. *Crit Care Med* 7:157–167, 1979

84. Monafo WW, Chuntrasakul C, Ayvazian VH: Hypertonic sodium solutions in the treatment of burn shock. *Am J Surg* 126:778–783, 1973

85. Wilson RD: Anesthesia and the burned child in the anesthesiologist's role in pediatric acute care. *Int Anesthesiol Clin* 13:203–217, 1975

86. Boswick JA, Thompson JD, Kershner CJ: Critical care of the burned patient. *Anesthesiology* 47:164–170, 1977

87. Hoffman MJ, Breenfield LJ, Sugerman HJ et al: Unsuspected right ventricular dysfunction in shock and sepsis. *Ann Surg* 198:307–319, 1983

88. Solem L, Fischer RP, Strate RG: The natural history of electrical injury. *J Trauma* 17:487–492, 1977

89. Hiebert JM, Thacker JG, Edlich RF: Early management of commercial electronic current injuries. *Curr Concepts Trauma Care* 2:7–14, 1979

90. Coté CJ, Petkau AJ: Thiopental requirements may be increased in children reanesthetized at least one year after recovery from extensive thermal injury. Anesth Analg 64:in press

91. White PF, Way WL, Trevor AJ: Ketamine: Its pharmacology and therapeutic uses. *Anesthesiology* 56:119–136, 1982

92. Martyn JAJ, Matteo RS, Szyfelbein SK, et al: Unprecedented resistance to neuromuscular blocking effects of metocurine with persistence after complete recovery in a burned patient. *Anesth Analg* 61:614–617, 1982

93. Satwicz PR, Martyn JAJ, Szyfelbein S, et al: Potentiation of neuromuscular blockade using a combination of pancuronium and dimethyltubocurarine. *Br J Anaesth* 56:479–484, 1984

94. Coté CJ, Jobes DR, Schwartz AJ, et al: Two approaches to cannulation of a child's internal jugular vein. *Anesthesiology* 50:371–373, 1979

95. Seldinger SI: Catheter replacement of the needle in percutaneous arteriography. *Acta Radiologica* 39:368–376, 1953

96. Kahn RC, Jascott D, Carlon GC, et al: Massive blood replacement. Correlation of ionized calcium, citrate, and hydrogen ion concentration. *Anesth Analg* 58:274–278, 1979

97. Stulz PM, Scheidegger D, Drop LJ, et al: Ventricular pump performance during hypocalcemia. Clinical and experimental studies. *J Thorac Cardiovasc Surg* 78:185–194, 1979

98. Denlinger JK, Nahrwold ML, Gibbs PS, et al: Hypocalcemia during rapid blood transfusion in anaesthetized man. *Br J Anaesth* 48:995–1000, 1976

99. Szyfelbein SK, Ryan JF: Use of controlled hypotension for primary surgical excision in an extensively burned child. *Anesthesiology* 41:501–503, 1974

20

Malignant Hyperthermia

John F. Ryan

INCIDENCE

Malignant hyperthermia (malignant hyperpyrexia, MH) is an acute, potentially fatal disorder in which skeletal muscles unexpectedly increase their oxygen consumption and lactate production, resulting in greater heat production, respiratory and metabolic acidosis, muscle rigidity, sympathetic stimulation, and increased cellular permeability. It is a relatively rare disorder which is estimated to occur in one in every 50,000–100,000 adult patients undergoing general anesthesia; in children its incidence is reported to be one in every 3,000–15,000.[1,2] The difference is more likely due to the retrospective nature of the studies and the age at which most surgery is performed. MH occurs almost exclusively during or following an anesthetic procedure, and is more frequently reported with halothane anesthesia, especially when succinylcholine has been utilized.[3] However, it can occur with other halogenated agents, and even in their absence.[4–6]

Although deaths from high fever were a known complication of anesthesia, the initial descriptions of MH were not recognized as a separate entity until the syndrome was accurately characterized by Denborough and Lowell in 1960.[7] At that time the mortality rate approached 90 percent. With more awareness of the syndrome and symptomatic management, the mortality rate dropped to 60 percent. However, the real breakthrough in the management of this metabolic derangement occurred in 1979 when the specific effectiveness of dantrolene sodium was recognized in the prevention, as well as the treatment, of this syndrome.[8,9]

MH is an inherited metabolic defect best described as autosomal dominant, with reduced penetrance and variable expressivity.[10–13] Reduced penetrance implies that fewer offspring are affected than would be predicted by a totally dominant pattern. Variable expressivity implies differing susceptibility between families, with little variation within the same family. However, not all patterns of inheritance fit the above description, and consequently it is proposed that malignant hyperthermia is transmitted by more than one gene and more than one allele.[11–13]

PATHOPHYSIOLOGY

Most of the investigative work on the pathophysiology of this disease has been performed on the pig. Swine breeders and veterinarians have long known that certain strains of pig, when exposed to stresses related to slaughter, accelerated their metabolism; it was also found that the muscle in these pigs deteriorated into pale, soft, exudative pork.[14] Further observations led to the conclusion that porcine stress syndrome and malignant hyperthermia are practically the same genetic disease.[15] Episodes of both syndromes demonstrate the same biochemical changes; fever, acidosis, cyanosis, mottling, rigidity of muscles and rhabdomyolysis, cardiac arrhythmias, and eventually shock. Consequently, some porcine pedigrees particularly susceptible to MH have been identified (e.g., Landrace, Pietrain, Poland China); these strains provide a model for the study of the human syndrome.[16] Much of our knowledge of the pathophysiology of this disease and the eventual identification of the specific treatment of MH has been based on studies of this animal model.[17,18]

The target organ in malignant hyperthermia is skeletal muscle[12–14] and the disturbance of calcium flux from the sarcoplasmic reticulum membrane.[19–24] In order to understand the pathophysiological changes that occur in skeletal muscles during an episode of MH, it is important to understand the basic physiological changes that occur during normal contraction of skeletal muscle.[25]

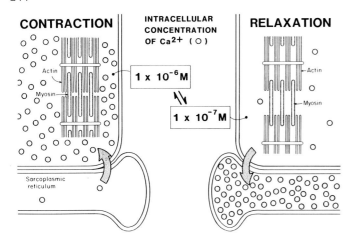

Figure 20-1. This figure depicts the actin myosin movement during calcium-stimulated muscle contraction. Biochemically the relaxation phase is the energy utilizing process of calcium transport, and contraction is a more passive event. It is the failure of lowering myoplasmic calcium, which occurs normally during the relaxation phase, that leads to the development of MH in a patient.

The nerve impulse, through its action on the neuromuscular junction, creates a chain of events that leads to depolarization of the muscle. The muscle action potential spreads on the surface of the muscle membrane from its center to its periphery. The action potential is transmitted to the interior of the muscle fiber by way of the T tubule system (Figure 20-1). When it reaches the terminal sac of the sarcoplasmic reticulum, it causes a release of the calcium ion in the cytoplasm. Ionized calcium can also be released from the sarcolemma and mitochondria. Ionized calcium bound to calmodulin initiates contraction by removing tropomyosin–troponin inhibition, which allows the actin filaments to slide across the myosin filaments, contracting the muscle fiber.[26]

During relaxation the calcium that was released during contraction is pumped back into the sarcoplasmic reticulum, sarcolemma, and the mitochondria. This restores the tropomyosin–troponin inhibition, allowing the actin and myosin filaments to separate, lengthening the muscle fiber. This is an energy requiring process provided through the generation of adenosine triphosphate (ATP) in the mitochondria.

The pathogenesis of malignant hyperthermia involves the uptake and storage of intracellular calcium. The main defect lies in the inability of the sarcoplasmic reticulum to store calcium. This is evidenced by an increase in myoplasmic free calcium.[27] At resting levels the ionized calcium [Ca^{++}] levels are three or four times normal.[24] Upon triggering of MH, the intracellular [Ca^{++}] increases up to 17 times.[27]

The elevated myoplasmic calcium level (1) activates ATPase, thus accelerating the hydrolysis of ATP or ADP, (2) inhibits troponin, thus permitting a biochemical contraction to occur, and (3) activates phosphorylase kinase and glycogenolysis, with resulting production of ATP and heat. As the calcium levels further increase, calcium diffuses into a secondary storage site, the mitochondria. This [Ca^{++}] infusion stimulates aerobic activity within this organelle, as well as the sarcolemma. The ATP will be diminished by this furious enzymatic activity; therefore, the supply of high energy bonds will diminish and the hypermetabolic muscles will be unable to cope completely with the energy demands by means of aerobic

metabolism, and consequently the muscle will resort to anaerobic metabolism, and lactic acid will start to accumulate.

As a consequence of this, the metabolic rate is accelerated, causing a high rate of oxygen consumption, as well as heat and carbon dioxide production. The circulation may allow heat dissipation early in this sequence, but soon, in an effort to supply the increased demands for oxygen to the muscles, peripheral vasoconstriction can occur, blood is shunted away from the skin, and body temperature may rise dramatically.[28]

Because of the marked increase in the oxygen uptake of muscle cells, the venous blood will therefore be markedly desaturated of oxygen, and will have a high CO_2 concentration (respiratory acidosis) due to the enhanced intracellular processes; lactic acidosis (metabolic acidosis) results when oxygen demands outstrip oxygen delivery. These factors have clinical importance since the earliest change in the fulminant hypermetabolic state will be mirrored on the venous side of the circulation as a respiratory acidosis. It is therefore very helpful to obtain a venous blood sample when seeking a diagnosis of malignant hyperthermia. End-tidal CO_2 monitoring will serve a similar purpose. Continuous measurement has enabled our pediatric anesthesia group to diagnose MH in two children.[29]

The continued uncontrolled contraction of a large group of muscles can lead to the clinically observed rigidity.[30-32] This most often occurs early after administration of succinylcholine, but it may also be seen later. In the late stages of a full-blown MH episode, development of rigidity is attributable to the temperature rise within the muscle cell.[33]

The actomyosin ATPase enzyme system ends muscle contraction. If there is an enzyme malfunction, then continued contraction leads to rigidity. Our laboratory has noted a relationship between the clinical rigid form and markedly lowered function of actomyosin ATPase.[34] This might explain the high incidence of positive results of this test with muscle from patients who presented with masseter spasm.[35,36]

Muscles are the main tissues involved in this syndrome; with a full-blown episode there may be massive swelling of the muscles, rhabdomyolysis, and a massive leak of potassium and calcium outside the cells. Both hyperkalemia and hypercalcemia thus result. Hyperkalemia is the major source of mortality; calcium channel blockers have produced fatal, evanescent rises in serum potassium in swine, and thus are contraindicated in the therapy of MH.[37] With adequate treatment, these electrolyte abnormalities reverse spontaneously.

The cardiac arrhythmias observed in this syndrome are nonspecific. Several factors contribute to their occurrence; hyperkalemia, fever, acidosis, hypoxia, and autonomic hyperactivity. There is also the possibility that the syndrome directly affects cardiac muscle.

If the patient survives, other complications may occur, including consumption coagulopathy, hemolysis, myoglobinemia, and myoglobinuria; the latter may lead to renal failure.

The cause of death in this syndrome is variable and related somewhat to the particular time that death occurs. In the initial few hours it is most probably from ventricular fibrillation. If death occurs several hours later, after a prolonged attempt at resuscitation, it may be due to pulmonary edema, coagulopathy, acid–base imbalance, or electrolyte imbalance. If it occurs days later, death is more likely to be from multiple organ failure, brain damage, or renal decompensation.[20]

It is interesting, that the height of the fever has no specific

Table 20-1

Signs and Symptoms of
Malignant Hyperthermia

- Tachycardia
- Tachypnea
- Respiratory Acidosis
- Metabolic Acidosis
- Fever
- Hyperkalemia
- Cyanosis
- Prolonged Coagulopathy

Table 20-2

Presentation of Malignant
Hyperthermia

- Masseter rigidity
- Succinylcholine induced muscle rigidity
- Full blown in operating room
- Full blown in recovery room
- Intraoperative fever alone
- Neurolept Malignant syndrome
- Heat stroke
- Episodic fever
- Sudden Infant Death syndrome

predictive effect on the outcome.[38] The author's first patient had a temperature elevation of greater than 43.8°C (110.8°F) with cardiac arrest and a plasma potassium level of 14.9 mmol/l, all occurring within an 18 minute period.[26] Approximately two hours later this patient was trying to vocalize her desire to be extubated.[39] She eventually made a complete recovery. In spite of this markedly elevated temperature, no brain damage ensued. This contrasts with the widely held view that brain damage inevitably occurs at these temperatures.

DIAGNOSIS

Since the first systemic effect of this syndrome is increased metabolism (oxygen consumption), the cardiovascular and respiratory system respond to this increased demand by increasing their output. Therefore, *the first signs of this syndrome are tachycardia and tachypnea (Table 20-1).*

Although light anesthesia is often the cause of tachycardia, in a healthy child of seven an increase from 120 to 180 beats/min (or an increase from 70 to 120 beats/min in an adult) is usually a sign of pathology. Not all tachycardia or tachypnea is attributable to "light" anesthesia. (Table 20-2). It is reasonable to deepen the depth of anesthesia, but it is also vital immediately to rule in or out other mechanical factors (endobronchial intubation, hypoventilation, circuit problem, etc.). If these prove normal and a brief trial of deepened anesthesia fails to slow the heart rate, then a simultaneous central venous and arterial blood sample should determine the presence or absence of a hypermetabolic state. In this respect *the expired CO_2 monitor is invaluable. In hypermetabolic states, the expired CO_2 will be high, especially during MH.* In this condition it becomes extremely difficult to bring the end-expired CO_2 level within the normal range, even with vigorous hyperventilation. In situations of airway obstruction the recorded CO_2 levels will be elevated; however, once the defect has been corrected, end-tidal CO_2 will return rapidly to its normal value with mild to moderate hyperventilation.

MASSETER SPASM

An early manifestation of malignant hyperthermia is masseter spasm. It usually appears as an isolated manifestation following succinylcholine. This tightness is an active spasm, completely different from inadequate relaxation, and it does not relax with further succinylcholine administration. It may last from a few minutes up to half an hour. All patients can be ventilated with a face mask despite the rigidity and the inability to open the mouth because the chest wall is relaxed. Simple

bag and mask ventilation will therefore sustain oxygenation until the masseter muscles relax.

Not all patients who have the MH syndrome develop masseter spasm, and conversely a fair number of the patients who develop masseter spasm do not have MH. However, there is a very strong correlation; 65–80 percent of patients who have succinylcholine-induced masseter spasm are susceptible to malignant hyperthermia.[35,36,40] Masseter spasm following succinylcholine is common in myotonia congenita, and may occasionally occur in patients with Duchenne muscular dystrophy.[30,32] In some patients, however, no cause can be found, even after extensive investigations.[41]

The initial response of the anesthesiologist to masseter spasm during anesthesia should be to terminate the potent inhalation agents, give oxygen, and monitor the patient for symptoms and/or signs of MH. If this is an elective case, the procedure should be postponed and the patient evaluated more closely for possible MH susceptibility. If the surgical procedure is not elective, after obtaining proper monitoring, dantrolene, and adequate help, the anesthetic process is continued by using a balanced technique. There are no controlled studies on the value of dantrolene in these "untriggered" cases. The author, at present, would not treat rigidity after succinylcholine alone, but would have dantrolene sodium available and would closely monitor the patient for signs and symptoms of a hypermetabolic state. These would be increased CO_2 production (end-tidal CO_2), development of tachypnea, tachycardia, venous oxygen desaturation, and an increased venous CO_2 level, even in the presence of minor initial arterial blood gas changes.

MUSCLE TESTING

The diagnosis of MH is primarily determined by the clinical responses. Once even a weak set of symptoms have been diagnosed as MH, the patient and his or her family usually are considered positive by all physicians thereafter. This may seem unjustified in some circumstances, and perhaps not medically correct, but it is the reality of present day medicine. It is interesting to note that in a population referred to us, 50 percent of family members of known MH-susceptible patients may themselves be susceptible to MH, which is consistent with the autosomal mode of inheritance. This supports the need for caution in administering anesthesia to members of a family in which one person is susceptible.

Muscle biopsy specimens have been utilized to determine

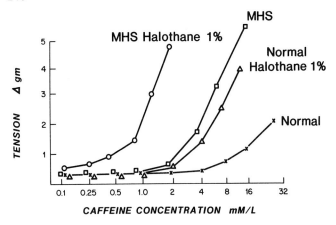

Figure 20-2. This idealized graph demonstrates response of various classifications of patients to muscle testing by caffeine contracture. Clinically there may be an overlap which clouds the diagnosis in an individual case.

the presence or absence of a consistent marker in muscle function associated with MH. One test that has gained acceptance by several laboratories is quantitation of the forces of muscle contracture following exposure of the biopsy sample to halothane, caffeine, or both. Excised muscle is placed on stretch in a bath at 37°C. After optimal length tension has been determined, halothane and/or caffeine are added, the muscle is stimulated supramaximally and the contracture amplitude is measured.[41,42]

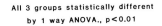

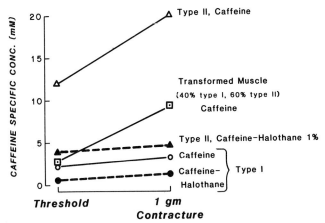

Figure 20-3. This figure presents the effect of fiber type upon caffeine contracture studies. Pure type I and II fiber samples differ in their contracture response to caffeine and halothane–caffeine. Prolonged electrical stimulation causes Type II fibers to become Type I. After three months of low-grade stimulation, the transformed fiber content is 60/40%, as shown above. The quantification of the muscle fiber type of each individual biopsy specimen is an important determinant in evaluating susceptibility to MH. (Britt BA, et al: Malignant hyperthermia: An investigation of five patients. Can Anesth Soc J 20:431–467, 1973. Reproduced with permission.)

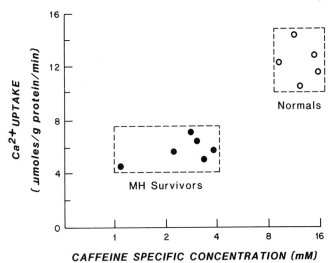

Figure 20-4. This graph relates the calcium uptake in thin cryostat section specimens to caffeine contracture in two groups of patients. The first group are MH survivors who had tachycardia, tachypnea, fever of about 103°F, metabolic acidosis, respiratory acidosis, rigidity and hyperkalemia. The "normal" muscle specimens were taken from healthy patients.

A vigorous in vitro contracture of a skeletal muscle specimen to halothane, and a reduced contracture threshold to caffeine, can identify the donor as susceptible to MH (Figure 20-2). The response to 2mM caffeine and to less than two percent halothane were the only tests that unequivocally discriminated between susceptible and normal control subjects.[43] However, simultaneous exposure to both halothane and caffeine produces considerable overlap between normal and known MH-susceptible patients, indicating that the combined test is too sensitive (Figure 20-3).

In our laboratory we have relied upon determination of calcium uptake into the sarcoplasmic reticulum. This method was first accomplished at the height of an acute episode of MH, and initially utilized the isolation of fragmented sarcoplasmic reticulum grana; now a more simplified method uses quick-frozen cryostat muscle sections.[43–45] The correlation with the previous method, reproductivity of uptake results, ease of transport, small muscle biopsy needed, and ability to perform histology of the contiguous cryostat section are advantages of this method.

However, this test has not been extensively compared to the halothane–caffeine contracture test. We have studied both methods in 16 patients and the preliminary results are encouraging (Figure 20-4).

Any widely sensitive test to confirm an unequivocal diagnosis either positive or negative will have a gray zone. In MH the problem is the clinically positive patient who tests unequivocally negative. This wide spectrum of MH susceptibility has been observed in both humans and pigs.[43] Therefore, most laboratories tend to take the conservative approach, favoring the diagnosis on the positive side (false positive) because the consequences of a false negative result are much more serious than for a false positive. It is better to treat the patient as if he or she has MH and avoid all triggering agents, than to assume the patient is negative and end with catastrophic complications.

THE PATIENT WITH SUSPECTED MH

Most of the time MH occurs in situations where it is least suspected. With a careful history, however, information can be obtained indicating that one of the patient's relatives has had a complicated anesthetic history. There are also some disorders that have an inconstant association with MH.[46] These diseases include muscular dystrophies, and of these, the Duchenne type, is the most severe and rapidly progressive, and seems to be the one most commonly associated with MH.[47–49] Other associated diseases may include central core disease, sudden infant death syndrome (SIDS), and neurolept malignant syndrome.[50–52] Other diagnoses that have an association with MH are peripheral muscle disorders such as ptosis and squint, or skeletal deformities such as scoliosis or kyphosis. The presence of muscle cramps, or increase in muscle size with weakness, may also be suggestive signs. In adults, intolerance to caffeine is one of the distinctive symptoms.

Several noninvasive tests can be performed to evaluate susceptibility, but none of them is conclusive. The most common is serum creatinine phosphokinase (CPK). It is elevated even at rest in 60–70 percent of susceptible patients.[53] The usefulness of CPK in MH diagnosis is predicated on lack of other muscle disease that would explain the elevation, as well as the peak of the elevated enzyme. We have set an arbitrary level of a ten-fold increase in CPK as being diagnostic of MH in otherwise unexplainable situations. Although a useful measure if markedly elevated, a lack of CPK elevation does not exclude the diagnosis of MH.

Another blood test that has been advocated for the detection of MH is the halothane-induced platelet ATP depletion test. It seems to be satisfactory in the hands of the original authors but does not seem to be reproducible by other researchers.[54,55]

Amplitude of thumb adduction in response to percutaneous stimulation of the ulnar nerve during and following occlusive tourniquet application to the upper extremity has been studied in MH patients.[56,57] Evoked thumb adduction was transduced and measured using a Grass FT-10 force transducer and Grass polygraph. Supramaximal square-wave pulses of 0.2 millisecond duration were applied to the ulnar nerve at the wrist through two surface electrodes at a frequency of 0.1 Hz by a Grass S-88 stimulator via a SIU-5 stimulus isolation unit. A tourniquet was applied to the upper arm with pressure set at 250 mm Hg for ten minutes. Twitch height was recorded before, during, and after tourniquet application. In normal patients, the post-ischemic neuromuscular response after ten minutes of arterial occlusion was below control at one minute, then slowly returned to normal.

MH susceptible patients can have marked post-ischemic twitch increases. This observation, termed the tourniquet test, has been of value when the post-ischemic rise is greater than 80 percent of the baseline value. It has not been a reliable predictor when normal responses (twitch depression) are measured. A promising offshoot of this investigation is the observation of a significantly lowered oxygen content in the ischemic arm of MH susceptible patients.[57]

Malignant hyperthermia can also present initially as ventricular ectopy in otherwise healthy patients; this is especially common during induction of anesthesia. If there is no airway instrumentation, hypercarbia, hypoxia, or some other stimulus to explain the arrhythmia, MH becomes suspect.

Table 20-3

Standard Treatment Regimen

- Stop anesthesia and surgery immediately
- Hyperventilate patient with 100% oxygen
- Administer dantrolene (Dantrium®) 2.5 mg/kg IV and procainamide (up to 15 mg/kg IV slowly if required for arrhythmias) as soon as possible
- Initiate cooling
- Correct acidosis
- Secure monitoring lines: EKG, temperture, Foley catheter, arterial pressure, central venous pressure
- Maintain urine output
- Monitor patient until danger of subsequent episodes is past (48–72 hr)
- Administer oral or IV, dantrolene for 48–72 hr

Electrocardiographic investigation must also be carried out, as well as myoglobin and CPK levels. If the EKG is normal and the CPK and myoglobin are elevated, one can make a tentative diagnosis of MH.

MANAGEMENT OF AN MH EPISODE

When a full-blown episode of MH is diagnosed, *immediate aggressive therapy* is indicated. Table 20-3 outlines the standard treatment regimen. The keystone of this approach is dantrolene sodium (Dantrium*). This drug has been shown to be effective at a dose of 2.5 mg/kg IV without any major adverse effect. If administered early during the episode, it reverses the biochemical changes of MH and decreases cellular metabolism.[9] If its administration is delayed for more than 24 hours, it still reverses some of the clinical signs, but does not affect the mortality rate.

Although dantrolene is the key to successful outcome, the other ancillary measures are also very important (Table 20-3). Active cooling, treating the associated acidosis, and correcting the electrolyte imbalance can make the difference between a borderline or completely adequate recovery.

Dantrolene has probably been responsible for the dramatic decrease in the mortality from MH since its intravenous use was introduced in the United States in 1979. The drug instructions recommend an initial dose of 1 mg/kg IV. However, a small number of patients do not respond to this dosage level. Since no major side effects occur after a large dose, we strongly suggest an initial bolus dose of 2.5–3.0 mg/kg IV, followed in 45 minutes by a bolus dose of 10 mg/kg if all signs and symptoms of the syndrome have not resolved. The complete cessation of (1) tachycardia, (2) tachypnea, (3) all rigidity, (4) decreased urinary output, (5) altered consciousness, (6) blood gas abnormalities, and (7) electrolyte disturbances should be attained. If this does not occur with initial therapy, a repeated higher dose of dantrolene should be administered, or an alternate diagnosis for the problem should be sought.

Two recent experiences exemplify the reasons for this recommendation. A 19-year old child who developed MH was treated with dantrolene at a dosage of 1 mg/kg IV. Twelve hours postoperatively all signs of MH were absent, except

* Norwich, NY

Table 20-4

Signs and Symptoms of
Continuing Malignant
Hyperthermia Episode

- Continued hyperkalemia
- Residual rigidity still present
- Massive fluid requirements
- Oliguria proceeding to anuria

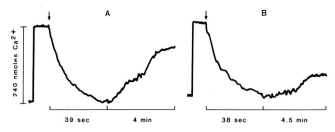

Figure 20-5. The dual spectrophotometric tracing pictured above captures the uptake and release of calcium into and from the sarcoplasmic reticulum. The tracing on the left was taken before the addition of dantrolene. The effect of dantrolene (tracing on the right) is to inhibit calcium release from the sarcoplasmic reticulum. (Van Winkle WB: Calcium release from skeletal muscle sarcoplasmic reticulum: Site of action of dantrolene sodium. Science 193:1130–1131, 1976. Reproduced with permission)

tachycardia (180 beats/min) and marked hypertension (240/150 mmmHg) despite vigorous doses of nitroprusside, nitroglycerin and hydralazine. After IV dantrolene in a dose of 3 mg/kg, a brief improvement of the cardiovascular aberrations followed. Subsequent to 10 mg/kg of dantrolene IV, dramatic return of all parameters to normal values occurred.

The second patient developed a full-blown picture of MH, and 20 hours later was still unconscious, with marked left gastrocnemius muscle spasm. He was receiving 1 mg/kg of dantrolene IV every eight hours as a maintenance dose to prevent recurrence of MH; 30 minutes following IV dantrolene in a dose of 10 mg/kg the patient was awake and the muscle spasm gone.

In our experience, the response to dantrolene takes 6–20 minutes. End-expired PCO₂ will begin to decrease in about six minutes, and monitored arterial blood gas analysis will show significant restoration toward normal in 20 minutes. The important factor is that by 45 minutes the patient should be completely normal. If not, intensive therapy should be pursued. Ten percent of MH patients following a full-blown episode redevelop the syndrome, so-called recrudescence. This usually occurs four to eight hours after the initial episode, and has been noted up to 36 hours after initial therapy. Characteristically, patients "smolder" along with modified symptoms until a triggering event ignites a renewed full-blown episode.[58] Table 20-4 outlines the signs and symptoms of a continuing subclinical episode of MH.

Patients with recrudescence have expired due to a change in muscle cellular permeability. Such patients require enormous volume infusions to maintain intravascular volume. Muscles immediately take up this volume and swell dramatically. The two patients that developed MH in our institution in 1979 gained 24 kilograms in 18 hours, and 15 kilograms in 36 hours, respectively.[59,60]

Once the initial episode has been successfully treated, patients traditionally have been given 1 mg/kg of dantrolene IV q6h for 24 hours, or by mouth for an additional 48–72 hours.

ACTIONS OF DANTROLENE

Dantrolene's action has been identified as being specific for skeletal muscles.[61] It does not affect neuromuscular transmission, or have measurable effects on the electrically excitable surface membrane. It does, however, produce muscle weakness and may potentiate non-depolarizing neuromuscular blocking agents. Indirect evidence indicates that the site of action of dantrolene sodium is within the muscle itself, and is related to the caffeine-sensitive calcium stores. It is suggested that dantrolene sodium prevents the release of calcium from the sarcoplasmic reticulum, or antagonizes calcium effects at the actin-myosin-troponin-tyopomyosin level, or both (Figure

20-5).[62,63] Such actions are proposed as explanations for the skeletal muscle relaxant activity of the drug observed clinically.

Some unique properties of the drug include:

1. At doses from 5 to 15 mg/kg/IV it produces a significant degree of muscle relaxation
2. In intravenous doses up to 15 mg/kg it has no significant action on the cardiovascular system
3. At intravenous doses up to 30 mg/kg it does not depress respiration
4. There is no indication of toxicity when the drug is administered intravenously on an acute basis.

By reducing rigidity and restoring muscle function, dantrolene normalizes all functions associated with muscle hypermetabolism in MH. One important example is the rapid reduction in serum potassium, since potassium is restored to muscle cells. This ultimately normalizes cardiac function. As cellular metabolism returns to aerobic processes and respiration normalizes, acid–base disorders are corrected. Thus, while dantrolene acts primarily on skeletal muscles, its beneficial effects are far reaching.

SUBSEQUENT ANESTHETICS

When a surgical procedure is planned in a known MH-susceptible patient, pretreatment with dantrolene sodium will help prevent triggering the syndrome.[64,65] Previously, dantrolene was recommended at a dose of 4.8 mg/kg by mouth q.i.d. for 48 hours before anesthesia.[45] Despite these precautions, however, a patient has been reported to have developed MH.[6,66] Recently, IV dantrolene has been suggested as a more effective method to achieve satisfactory blood levels. A dose of 2.5 mg/kg IV given at an interval of two hours achieves a steady state of 3.6 μg/ml for five and a half hours, then the blood level declines slowly.[61] Such a dose does not produce any adverse cardiovascular effects and does not affect respiratory variables such as peak expiratory flow rate, vital capacity, end-tidal CO₂ and respiratory rate. It is interesting that dantrolene at such doses causes peripheral muscle weakness as evidenced by marked diminution of both twitch response (75%) and grip strength (42%).[67] Fatigue is also a common problem for 24–48 hours. Consequently, common sense dictates that patients receiving dantrolene preoperatively or intraoperatively will require a smaller dose of muscle relaxant, and ambulation is preferably avoided in the first 24 hours, and then performed cautiously for at least 48 hours. Also, such doses of dantrolene in awake patients cause dizziness, light-headedness, and occasionally nausea. Difficulty in swallowing may also occur in the first 24 hours of its administration.

Other measures useful in avoiding triggering MH are (1) moderate to heavy premedication with tranquilizers (no phenothiazines, but barbiturates and opiates may be used, and in children rectal methohexital is a good choice), (2) a balanced anesthetic technique (nitrous oxide–oxygen, barbiturate, opioid tranquilizer, pancuronium) is most frequently used; droperidol may be advantageous due to its effect on MH-susceptible muscle in vitro;[68] halogenated agents are completely avoided; if there is no machine without vaporizers, it is advisable to flush the circuits with oxygen for one to three hours before the start of the anesthetic procedure; (3) careful monitoring (the most important aspect of management; all changes in heart rate should be carefully followed, and the use of end-expired CO_2 analyzers, and obviously a temperature monitor should be employed); (4) supplementary local anesthesia of the ester type, such as procaine, 2-chloroprocaine and tetracaine; and (5) availability of dantrolene.

Although caffeine induces contracture responses in vitro, it seems that these effects do not apply to related compounds, such as theophylline or aminophylline.[69]

THE FAMILY

In the time after an episode of MH, dealing with the family of the patient becomes a major challenge for the anesthesiologist. Most importantly, the family needs information and support. Frequently the stunning effect of this complication will deter the anesthesiologist from close contact with the family; yet the psychological and legal consequences for both the family and physician of such inaction, even with a good outcome of the MH episode, can be catastrophic.

At the present time, it seems reasonable to document the episode by muscle biopsy at an appropriate interval. It will then be necessary to determine which branch of the family is susceptible. Once these two goals have been accomplished, further testing within the family can be performed, if they are willing. A biopsy on these other family members should be attempted only after informing them that, the test is not a medical necessity—all anesthesiologists will treat the entire family as positive regardless of test results—but that this is a personal choice based on the need for peace of mind. Muscle biopsy during incidental surgery in family members makes eminent sense. The only restriction is the withholding of dantrolene sodium and droperidol prior to excision of the muscle specimen. These two drugs have been shown to "normalize" abnormal responses of the muscle specimens in MH-susceptible individuals.[47,68]

A common practice in planning anesthesia for family members of a known MH family is to request muscle testing separately prior to the procedure. In most instances, since a balanced technique will be utilized whether the results are normal or positive, it seems easier, and less expensive, for the patient to have a muscle biopsy taken at the time of the planned elective operation. Obviously the dantrolene will be available in the OR, and the level of vigilance and awareness of the anesthesiologist will be at a peak for this patient, based on the family history.

The long-term relationship of the anesthesiologist with the family of an MH survivor, continued education, and availability of the anesthesiologist, are important factors. The family needs literature; they need their questions answered. They need to know of the support group, the Malignant Hyperthermia Association of the United States. This organization, founded by Suellen Gallamore, has a hotline number (209-634-4917, ask for Index Zero) which is available 24 hours to physicians, and acts as a clearinghouse for information for MH families.

In summary, MH is a hypermetabolic event that can be triggered in genetically susceptible individuals by anesthesia. It has occurred in newborns and in the elderly.[70-71] With constant vigilance, it can be treated adequately with a successful outcome. If neglected, however, undiagnosed, or mistreated, it can lead to disasterous consequences.

REFERENCES

1. Britt BA: Recent advances in malignant hyperthermia. *Anesth Analg* 51:841–49, 1972
2. Relton JES, Britt BA, Stewart DJ: Malignant hyperpyrexia. *Br J Anaesth* 45:269–275, 1973
3. Britt BA, Kalow W: Malignant hyperthermia, a statistical review. *Can Anaesth Soc J* 17:293–315, 1970
4. Pan TH, Wollack AR, DeMarco JA: Malignant hyperthermia associated with enflurane anesthesia. *Anesth Analg* 54:47–49, 1975
5. Boheler J, Eger EI, II: Isoflurane and malignant hyperthermia. *Anesth Analg* 61:712–13, 1982
6. Fitzgibbons DC: Malignant hyperthermia following preoperative oral administration of dantrolene. *Anesthesiology* 54:73–75, 1981
7. Denborough MA, Lovell RRH: Anaesthetic deaths in a family (letter). *Lancet* 2:45, 1960
8. Harrison GG: Control of the malignant hyperpyrexic syndrome in MHS swine by dantrolene sodium. *Br J Anaesth* 47:62–65, 1975
9. Kolb ME, Horne ML, Martz R: Dantrolene in human malignant hyperthermia: A multicenter study. *Anesthesiology* 56:254–262, 1982
10. Britt BA, Locher WG, Kalow W: Hereditary aspects of malignant hyperthermia. *Can Anaesth Soc J* 16:89–98, 1969
11. Kalstrup J, Keske-Nielson E, Haase J, et al: Malignant hyperthermia in a family: A clinical and serological investigation of 139 members. *Acta Anaesth Scan* 18:58–64, 1974
12. Kalow W, Britt BA: Inheritance of malignant hyperthermia, in RA Gordon, BA Britt, W Kalow (eds): *International Symposium on Malignant Hyperthermia.* Springfield, IL, Charles C. Thomas, 1973, pp 67–76
13. Ellis FR, Cain PA, Harriman DGF: Multifactorial inheritance of malignant hyperthermia susceptibility, in JA Aldrete, BA Britt (eds): *Second International Symposium on Malignant Hyperthermia.* New York, Grune & Stratton, 1978, pp 329–338
14. Eikelenboom G, Minkema D: Prediction of pale, soft exudative muscle with a non-lethal test for the halothane-induced porcine malignant hyperthermia syndrome. *Neth J Vet Sci* 99:421–426, 1974
15. Rutberg H, Henrikson KG, Jorfeldt K, et al: Metabolic changes in a case of malignant hyperthermia. *Br J Anaesth* 55:461–467, 1983

16. Berman MC, Kench JE: Biochemical features of malignant hyperthermia in Landrace pigs, in RA Gordon, BA Britt, E Kalow (eds): *International Symposium on Malignant Hyperthermia.* Springfield, IL, Charles C. Thomas, 1973, pp 287–297

17. Gronert GA, Milde JH, Theye RA: Dantrolene in porcine malignant hyperthermia. *Anesthesiology* 44:488–495, 1976

18. Gronert GA, Theye RA: Halothane-induced porcine malignant hyperthermia: Metabolic and hemodynamic changes. *Anesthesiology* 44:36–43, 1976

19. Gronert GA: Malignant hyperthermia. *Anesthesiology* 53:395–423, 1980

20. Britt BA: Etiology and pathophysiology of malignant hyperthermia. *Fed Proc* 38:44–48, 1979

21. Jardon OM: Physiologic stress, heat stroke, malignant hyperthermia: A perspective. *Milit Med* 147:8–14, 1982

22. Britt BA, Kwong FHF, Endreyni L: The clinical and laboratory features of malignant hyperthermia management–A review, in EO Henschel (ed): Malignant Hyperthermia, Current Concepts edited by E.O. New York: Appleton-Century-Crofts, 1977, pp 63–77

23. Ohnishi ST, Taylor SR, Gronert G: Calcium-induced Ca^{2+} release from sarcoplasmic reticulum of pigs susceptible to malignant hyperthermia. *FEBS Let* 161:103–107, 1983

24. Lopez JR, Alamo L, Caputo C, et al: Intracellular ionized calcium concentration in muscles from humans with malignant hyperthermia. *Muscle Nerve* (in press)

25. Karamanian A: Muscle physiology, in N Goudsouzian, A Karamanian (eds): *Physiology for the Anesthesiologist.* Norwalk, CT, Appleton-Century-Crofts, 1984, pp 287–299

26. Tregear RT, Marston SB: The crossbridge theory. *Ann Rev Physiol* 41:723–736, 1979

27. Kim DH, Sreter FA, Ohnishi ST: Kinetic studies of Ca^{++} release from sarcoplasmic reticulum of normal and malignant hyperthermia susceptible pig muscles. *Biochem Biophy Res Commun* 775:320–327, 1984

28. Muhrer ME, Williams CH, Payne CG, et al: Vasoconstriction and porcine hyperpyrexia. *Science* 39:993, 1974

29. Baudendistal L, Goudsouzian NG, Coté CJ, et al: End-tidal CO$_2$ monitoring: Its use in the diagnosis and management of malignant hyperthermia. *Anaesthesia* 39:1000–1003, 1984

30. Cody JR: Muscle rigidity following administration of succinylcholine. *Anesthesiology* 29:159–162, 1968

31. Paterson IS: Generalzed myotonia following suxamethonium. *Br J Anaesth* 34:340–42, 1962

32. Inoue R, Kawamata M, Yamamura Y, et al: Generalized muscular rigidity associated with increased serum enyzmes and postoperative muscular weakness induced by general anesthesia without hyperthermia. *Hiroshima J Anesth* 13:232–235, 1977

33. Fuchs F: Thermal skeletal muscle actomyosin: A possible contributing factor in the rigidty of malignant hyperthermia. *Anesthesiology* 42:584–589, 1975

34. Allen PD, Ryan JF, Sreter FA, et al: Rigid versus nonrigid MH, studies of Ca^{2+} uptake and actomyosin ATPase. *Anesthesiology* 53:S251, 1980

35. Donlon JV, Newfield P, Sreter F, et al: Implications of masseter spasm after succinylcholine. *Anesthesiology* 49:298–301, 1978

36. Schwartz L, Rockoff MA, Koka BV: Masseter spasm with anesthesia: Incidence and implications. *Anesthesiology* 61:772–775, 1984

37. Saltzman LS, Kates RA, Corke BC, et al: Hyperkalemia and cardiovascular collapse after verapmil and dantrolene administration in swine. *Anesth Analg* 63:473–478, 1984

38. Cabral E, Muskowitz PR, Richter A, et al: Reversible profound depression of cerebral electrical activity in hyperthermia. *Electroencephalogr Clin Neurophysiol* 42:687–701, 1977

39. Ryan JF, Papper EM: Malignant fever during and following anesthesia. *Anesthesiology* 32:196–201, 1970

40. Ellis FR, Halsall PJ: Suxamethonium spasm. A differential diagnostic conundrum. *Br J Anaesth* 56:381–384, 1984

41. Rosenberg H, Reed S: In vitro contracture test for susceptibility to malignant hyperthermia. *Anesth Analg* 62:415–420, 1983

42. Britt BA, Kalow W, Gordon A, et al: Malignant hyperthermia: An investigation of five patients. *Can Anaesth Soc J* 20:431–467, 1973

43. Nelson TE, Flewellen EH, Gloyna DF: Spectrum of susceptibility to malignant hyperthermia—a diagnostic dilemma. *Anesth Analg* 62:545–552, 1983

44. Ryan JF, Donlon JV, Malt RA, et al: Cardiopulmonary bypass in the treatment of malignant hyperthermia. *N Engl J Med* 290:1121–1122, 1974

45. Mabuchi K, Sreter FA: The use of cryostat sectioning for measurement of calcium uptake by sarcoplasmic reticulum. *Anal Biochem* 86:733–742, 1978

46. Gronert GA: Controversies in malignant hyperthermia. *Anesthesiology* 59:273–274, 1983

47. Brownell AK, Paasuke RT, Elash A, et al: Malignant hyperthermia in Duchenne muscular dystrophy. *Anesthesiology* 58:180–182, 1983

48. Miller ED, Jr, Sander DB, Rowlingson JC, et al: Anesthesia-induced rhabdomyolysis in a patient with Duchenne's muscular dystrophy. *Anesthesiology* 48:146–148, 1978

49. Gronert GA: Malignant Hyperthermia. *Anesthesiology* 53:395–423, 1980

50. Frank JP, Harati Y, Butler IJ, et al: Central core disease and malignant hyperthermia syndrome. *Ann Neurol* 7:11–17, 1980

51. Denborough MA, Galloway GJ, Hopkinson KC: Malignant hyperpyrexia and sudden infant death. *Lancet* 2:1068–1069, 1982

52. Dallman JH: Neuroleptic Malignant Syndrome: A Review. *Milit Med,* 149:471–473, 1984

53. Isaacs H, Barlows MB: Malignant hyperpyrexia. Further muscle studies in asymptomatic carriers identified by creatinine phosphokinase screening. *J Neurol Neurosurg Psychiatry* 36:228–243, 1973

54. Solomon CC, Masson N: Malignant hyperthermia platelet bioassay. *Anesthesiology* 60:265, 1984

55. Giger U, Kaplan RF: Halothane-induced ATP depletion in platelets from patients susceptible to malignant hyperthermia and from controls. *Anesthesiology* 58:347–352, 1983

56. Roberts JT, Ali HH, Ryan JF: A tourniquet test for malignant hyperthermia. Presented at 53rd Congress, IARS, March, 1979

57. Roberts JT, Ryan JF, Ali HH, Allen PD: Abnormally high regional oxygen consumption in malignant hyperthermia patients induced by a non-anesthetic stress (10 minute tourniquet ischemia to the upper extremity). *Anesthesiology* 57:A229, 1982

58. Mathieu A, Bogosian AJ, Ryan JF, et al: Recrudescence after survival of an initial episode of malignant hyperthermia. *Anesthesiology* 51:454–455, 1979

59. Murphy A, Conlay A, Ryan JF, et al: Malignant hyperthermia during a prolonged anesthetic for reattachment of a limb. *Anesthesiology* 60:149–150, 1984

60. Norwich Eaton Pharmaceuticals (Division of Norwich Eaton, Ltd). Dantrium Intravenous (Dantrolene Sodium Intravenous). Product Monograph, 1979

61. Dykes MHM: Evaluation of a muscle relaxant. Dantrolene sodium (Dantrium). *JAMA* 231:862–864, 1975

62. Van Winkle WB: Calcium release from skeletal muscle sarcoplasmic reticulum: Site of action of dantrolene sodium. *Science* 193:1130–1131, 1976

63. Flewellen EH, Nelson TE, Jones WP, et al: Dantrolene dose response in awake man. Implications for management of malignant hyperthermia. *Anesthesiology* 59:275–280, 1983

64. Flewellen, EH, Nelson TE: Dantrolene dose response in malignant hyperthermia susceptible (MHS) swine: Method to obtain prophylaxis and therapeutics. *Anesthesiology* 52:303–308, 1980

65. Ruhland G, Hinkle AJ: Malignant hyperthermia after oral and intravenous pretreatment with dantrolene in a patient susceptible to malignant hyperthermia. *Anesthesiology* 60:159–160, 1984

66. Monster AW, Herman R, Meeks S, McHenry J: Cooperative study for assessing the effects of a pharmacological agent on spasticity. *Am J Phy Med* 52:163–188, 1973

67. Gratz DO, Reed S, Strobel GE: Chloropromazine potentiation of halothane contractures in skeletal muscle of frog, normal and malignant hyperthermic man: Comparison with droperidol. *ASA Annual Meeting Abstracts* 317, 1975

68. Flewellen EH, Nelson TE: Is theophylline, aminophylline, or caffeine (methylaxnthines) contraindicated in malignant hyper

thermia susceptible patients? *Anesth Analg* 52:115–118, 1983

69. Gronert GA: Puzzles in malignant hyperthermia. *Anesthesiology* 54:1–2, 1981

70. Sewall K, Flowerdo RM, Bromberger P: Severe muscular rigidity at birth: Malignant Hyperthermia. *Can Anesth Soc J* 27:279–282, 1980

71. Mayhew JF, Rudolph J, Tobey RE: Malignant hyperthermia in a six-month old infant. A case report. *Anesth Analg* 57:262–264, 1978

21

Regional Anesthesia

Charles J. Coté

Regional anesthetic techniques are underutilized in pediatric patients of the United States for three major reasons: lack of experience, fear of adverse effects, and lack of patient cooperation.[1] In this section we will discuss guidelines for selecting a suitable patient, the properties of local anesthetics, and specific blocks. It is hoped that by making anesthesiologists who care for children more aware of these blocks that they will be used more frequently for surgical procedures, and specifically for postoperative analgesia.

PATIENT SELECTION

In the selection of a patient for regional anesthesia, several factors must be considered. While nearly all pediatric patients are candidates for some form of intraoperative block placed for postoperative analgesia, there are a limited number of pediatric patients who will accept a regional technique for the entire procedure. The latter individual tends to be very mature for age and can express an understanding of the procedures. The anesthesiologist must give a sensitive, reassuring, yet honest and clear explanation of the whole experience. The most important aspect of any regional technique in the awake pediatric patient is strong psychological support, especially the dialogue which distracts the child from events in the operating room.

When a regional anesthetic technique is performed, it is mandatory that the anesthesiologist have readily available equipment and drugs for the treatment of local anesthetic overdosage. It is important that an intravenous route be established *prior* to any regional procedure to allow for appropriate sedation, hydration, and treatment of accidental overdosage.

We have found regional blocks applied intraoperatively to be particularly effective in reducing intraoperative anesthetic requirements, and to significantly reduce postoperative excitement and analgesic needs. Local blocks are a very valuable adjunct to outpatient procedures such as circumcision, urethral dilatation, and inguinal hernia.[2-4] They allow time for parents to administer analgesics such as acetaminophen *before* the block wears off; frequently this results in a nearly pain-free postsurgical recovery. In our practice, therefore, postoperative pain relief is the major indication for the use of regional anesthesia.

LOCAL ANESTHETICS

There are excellent detailed reviews of the pharmacology and mechanism of action of local anesthetics.[5-7] It should be emphasized that the type of block produced by any given local anesthetic is dependent on site of injection, concentration of the drug, and local changes in tissue pH. In addition, because of the structure of peripheral nerves, it is possible to have nearly complete block of pain receptors but minimal motor blockade; it is this latter effect that is most important for postoperative analgesia. The rapidity of onset is not significantly affected by concentration, while the depth of anesthetic block is. Thus, for analgesia one would use a low anesthetic concentration, whereas for both analgesia and motor block the use of a higher concentration is required.[5] The pH of the tissue into which the local anesthetic is injected is also important; local anesthetics are less effective in an acidic medium, such as infected tissues.

Table 21-1

Recommended Maximal Safe Dose and Duration of Action of Commonly Used Local Anesthetic Drugs

Local Anesthetic	Maximal mg/kg Dose	Duration of Action
2-Chloroprocaine	20.0	short
Procaine	10.0	intermediate
Lidocaine	7.0	intermediate
Mepivacaine	7.0	intermediate
Tetracaine	1.5	long
Bupivacaine	3.0	long

Table 21-2

Epinephrine Dilution and Its Conversion to μgm/ml

Epinephrine Dilution	Concentration μgm/ml
1:100,000	10.0
1:200,000	5.0
1:400,000	2.5
1:800,000	1.25

TOXICITY OF LOCAL ANESTHETICS

The major toxic effects are central nervous system (CNS) excitation or depression, and cardiovascular depression. CNS excitation is the most common major toxic effect, manifesting itself as agitation, confusion, or seizures, and at times heralded by a metallic taste or tinnitus. This is frequently followed by CNS depression, which may lead to respiratory arrest.

Local anesthetics produce relaxation of smooth muscle in peripheral arterioles, which may result in a fall in systemic pressure.[6,7] The combination of direct myocardial depression and peripheral vasodilation may lead to cardiac arrest.

PREVENTION OF TOXICITY

There is little data correlating anesthetic block, blood level, and dosage for pediatric patients. Most procedures in children have been carried out using data extrapolated from adult studies. Table 21-1 lists the recommended maximum dose and duration of action.

The prevention of toxic reactions is a function of (1) total drug dosage, (2) the site of injection, (3) the rate of uptake, (4) any pharmacologic alteration of toxic threshold, (5) technique, and (6) the rate of degradation, metabolism, excretion, and acid–base status of the patient.

Total Drug Dosage

Until more detailed studies are available, one must be careful to stay within the guidelines presented in Table 21-1. In addition, the markedly obese child must not be given a higher dose simply because of the increased weight; lean or normal body weight for size must guide all drug dosage.

Site of Injection

Injection of local anesthetics into vascular areas will result in higher blood levels than the same dose injected into a less vascular area. For example, the blood levels following intercostal block are significantly greater than those following brachial plexus or femoral–sciatic nerve block.[8–11]

Rate of Uptake

The rate of local anesthetic uptake is dependent on the vascularity of the site of injection; increased perfusion will result in increased rate of uptake, whereas decreased perfusion will result in decreased uptake.[12] There is some evidence to suggest that children will absorb local anesthetic agents more rapidly than adults, and that blockade will be of shorter duration.[13] The use of a vasoconstrictor will reduce the rate of uptake of local anesthetics and prolong the duration of block. Because of the risk of arrhythmias, however, the dose of epinephrine must be strictly limited when used in conjunction with potent inhalational agents, especially halothane. In a pediatric patient anesthetized with halothane, a dose of 1.0–1.5 μgm/kg epinephrine used to be the maximal recommended dosage; however, recent communications suggest that higher doses of epinephrine may be safe in children.[14–16] If enflurane or isoflurane is used, a larger dose of epinephrine may safely be administered (3–5 μgm/kg).[17] If no potent inhalational anesthetic is to be used then, up to 10 μgm/kg, with a maximum of 250 μgm, may safely be utilized. A concentration of 1:100,000 should not be exceeded. A quick reference for converting local anesthetic concentrations and epinephrine to easily calculated figures is presented in Tables 21-2 and 21-3. Epinephrine is contraindicated in blocks where vasoconstriction could lead to tissue necrosis, as in digital and penile blocks.

Alteration of Toxic Threshold

Pharmacologic alteration of the toxic threshold is a valuable adjunct to regional techniques. Diazepam, a potent amnesic and sedative, also raises the seizure threshold. Thus, premedication of a patient with diazepam will aid in alleviating the anxiety of the anesthetic procedure in addition to offering some protection to the patient from toxic side effects.[18]

Technique

The rate of injection may also be an important factor in the development of drug toxicity. If the injection will be partially or completely intravascular, a slow injection of a low dose might not exceed toxic levels, whereas a rapid injection could. Similarly, the duration of a toxic reaction would be shorter from a single small injection compared to toxicity secondary to a large injection.[19] In addition, repeated injections exceeding the recommended maximum dose could result in prolonged toxic reactions compared to a single injection.

Metabolism, Excretion, Acid–Base Factors

Local anesthetics are divided into ester and amide groups. The ester group (procaine, tetracaine, and 2-chloroprocaine) is metabolized chiefly by means of hydrolysis by plasma pseudocholinesterase. 2-Chloroprocaine, with its short plasma half-life, is particularly advantageous because it is less likely to produce toxic reactions. Prolonged toxic effects are possible, however, in those patients with atypical pseudocholinesterase.[7] Patients with liver disease, and neonates, may have prolonged toxicity due to the greater half-lives of ester types of local anesthetics in the presence of diminished production of pseudocholinesterase.[20] Hypoproteinemia may also result in less protein binding, and thus higher free plasma levels of all local anesthetics; this also may contribute to developing toxicity. The amide group (lidocaine, mepivacaine, and bupivacaine) is metabolized primarily by the liver; thus patients with severe liver dysfunction may be prone to systemic toxic reactions.[21] Renal excretion plays a small role in the elimination of both amide and ester local anesthetics; its major role is excretion of the breakdown products. Patients with congestive heart failure are also at risk for increased toxicity due to altered volume of distribution and poor drug clearance both by the liver and the kidneys.[22] In addition, both metabolic and respiratory acidosis increase the likelihood of toxicity.[23,24]

PEDIATRIC CONSIDERATIONS

It is often stated that if a patient cannot tolerate a general anesthetic he or she will tolerate a local anesthetic. *This is a potentially dangerous approach for infants and children.* As outlined above, the potential for significant toxicity is increased in the presence of congestive heart failure, liver disease (or immature neonatal liver), decreased protein binding (well documented in the neonate for most medications), decreased renal function (or immature kidneys in the neonate), and acidosis. All of these problems, combined with the very small doses of local anesthetic which can be safely used in infants, make this alternative a potentially disasterous situation. For example, a child weighing two kilograms may receive 5 mg/kg of lidocaine, which equals ten milligrams, which is equivalent to one milliliter of a one percent solution. Thus it is very easy to exceed toxic levels. In addition, it is difficult to determine if a block is successful. For example, if a child is restless, the anesthesiologist could easily misinterpret this as indicating a need for additional local anesthetic when hypoxia may be the cause of the restlessness; hence the ease of achieving toxic levels. Another consideration is the technical difficulties of securing the airway once a small patient has been prepped, draped, and is undergoing the surgical procedure. It is our feeling that *the sick child or infant is not a good candidate for performing an entire procedure under local anesthesia.* A well placed local block with minimal doses may, however, reduce the anesthetic requirements for selected surgical procedures, but the dose chosen must be drastically reduced for the previously stated reasons.[2–4]

TREATMENT OF TOXIC REACTIONS

The most common toxic reaction to local anesthetics is central excitation with seizures; it is only with massive overdose that myocardial depression occurs. The key to treatment is recognition of impending reaction and urgent management following the procedures outlined below.

1. Clear the airway to assure adequate oxygen delivery and ventilation.
2. Administer medications which specifically antagonize the central excitatory effects, such as diazepam (0.1–0.3 mg/kg IV) or thiopental (1–3 mg/kg IV).
3. Supply cardiovascular support with intravenous fluids and, if necessary, a vasopressor and/or vasoconstrictor.
4. Induce rapid excretion, i.e., hydration and alkalinization, of the urine if appropriate.[6,7]

Table 21-3

Local Anesthetic Concentration and Its Conversion to Mg/ml

Local Anesthetic Concentration	
Percent	mg/ml
3.0	30.0
2.0	20.0
1.0	10.0
0.5	5.0
0.25	2.5

ALLERGY TO LOCAL ANESTHETICS

An allergic reaction to a local anesthetic drug is rare. When it does occur, it is more common with the ester types.[7] Many of the allergic reactions reported are secondary to the preservative methylparaben, rather than the anesthetic agent itself.[25] True anaphylaxis is possible, however, and if there is any question of local anesthetic allergy, this must be ruled out. It is important that all the facilities for treating anaphylaxis be readily available and that the patient be observed for a minimum of one hour following injection of the local anesthetic. A more detailed protocol is described elsewhere.[26]

SPECIFIC PROCEDURES

INGUINAL FIELD BLOCK

The use of a field block for inguinal hernia repair is often indicated in the sick, debilitated, adult patient. However, there is minimal experience utilizing this technique in modern pediatric anesthesia. Blockade of the ilioinguinal and ileohypogastric nerves, however, is very effective for postoperative analgesia.[4]

Technique. This block may be inserted either at the commencement of surgery or shortly prior to the termination of general anesthesia. Locating a point 1.0–1.5 cm cephalad and 1.0–1.5 cm toward the midline from the anterior superior iliac spine, a blunted 22 gauge needle is inserted through the external and internal oblique muscles (Figure 21-1)—two popping sensations are useful indicators of proper needle placement. At this point 1–5 ml of *0.25 percent* bupivacaine, with or without epinephrine diluted 1:100,000, is injected in fan-like fashion cephalad toward the umbilicus, caudad toward the groin, and medially. Just prior to removal from the skin another 0.5–1.0 ml of local anesthetic is injected subcutaneously to block the ileohypogastric nerve. Care must be taken to avoid entering the peritoneal cavity. The maximum allowable dose of bupivacaine is estimated to be 3 mg/kg.

PENILE BLOCK

The single injection penile block is a very valuable adjunct to postoperative analgesia following circumcision, urethral dilatation, and hypospadias repair.[2,27] The agent most useful

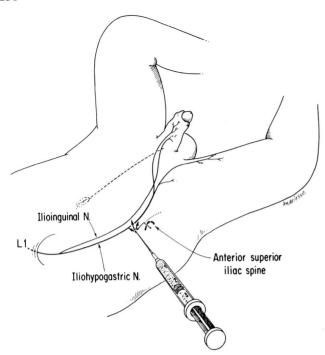

Figure 21-1. Ilioinguinal nerve block. The anterior superior iliac spine is palpated, and a point 1–1.5 cm cephalad and toward the midline is located. A 22 gauge needle is passed through the external and internal oblique muscles, and 1–5 ml of local anesthetic deposited in a fan-like fashion cephalad toward the umbilicus, medially, and caudad toward the groin. Just prior to removal from the skin another 0.5–1.0 ml of local anesthetic is injected subcutaneously to block the iliohypogastric nerve.

is 0.25 percent bupivacaine; *epinephrine must not be used because of the danger of inducing penile necrosis.*

Technique. After cleansing the skin, a 23–25 gauge needle is inserted in the midline one centimeter above the symphysis pubis at an angle of 30 degrees to the skin, and directed slightly caudad and toward the midline (Figure 21-2). At a distance of about half a centimeter after piercing the penile fascia, and following a negative aspiration for blood, 1–4 ml of local anesthetic (preferably 0.25% bupivacaine) is injected.[2]

INTERCOSTAL BLOCKS

Intercostal blocks inserted by the surgeon or anesthesiologist during or immediately following thoracotomy may be very helpful in reducing narcotic requirements, optimizing respiratory mechanics, and encouraging early ambulation.[28–30] The drug of choice is 0.5 percent bupivacaine, with epinephrine diluted 1:100,000, in a dose of 1–5 ml for each block, depending on the size of the patient. A recent report has found a more rapid rise in local anesthetic concentrations in the blood of children receiving intercostal blocks compared to adults.[13]

Technique. The site of injection may be either

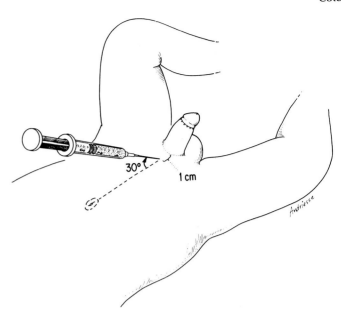

Figure 21-2. Penile block. After preparing the skin, a 23–25 gauge needle is inserted in the midline one cm above the symphysis pubis at an angle of 30° and directed caudad. After piercing the penile fascia (0.5–1.0 cm) and negative aspiration for lack of blood, 1–4 ml of local anesthetic *without epinephrine* is injected.

paravertebral or on the mid-axillary line. The lower rib margin is located, and a skin wheal inserted (Figure 21-3A). The skin is then retracted so that the skin wheal is now located over the rib, and the injecting needle is passed until contact is made with the rib (Figure 21-3B). The skin is then released and the needle carefully "walked" off the edge of the rib (Figure 21-3C). An appropriate volume of drug is deposited. This is determined by the number of ribs to be blocked, drug concentration, and total drug dosage. To minimize the possibility of a pneumothorax, the physician should make contact with the rib using a small needle, and carefully position the needle while stabilizing the hand on the chest wall.

BRACHIAL PLEXUS BLOCK

Brachial plexus block at the axilla is probably one of the most useful blocks for the pediatric anesthesiologist.[31,32] Its advantages include ease of insertion, low incidence of serious morbidity, and suitability for orthopedic or plastic surgical repairs on hand or forearm injuries in the child with a full stomach. There are many variations in the technique; however, any procedure that requires paresthesia as an indicator of a successful needle location is a disadvantage in the pediatric patient.[1]

Technique. In children, where the artery is so easily palpable, it is relatively simple to deposit a volume of local anesthetic on both sides of the artery or to traverse the artery and inject both posterior and anterior to the artery. Either technique will usually result in adequate infiltration of the neurovascular sheath and a satisfactory block. The need for cutaneous infiltration to block the musculocutaneous nerve

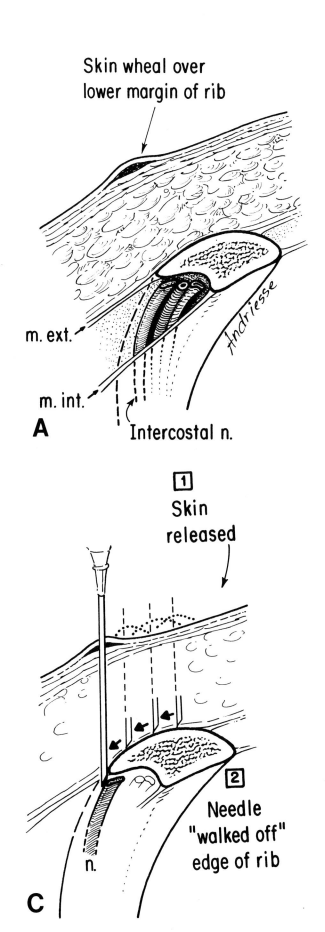

Skin wheal over
lower margin of rib

m. ext.

m. int.

A

Intercostal n.

Andriesse

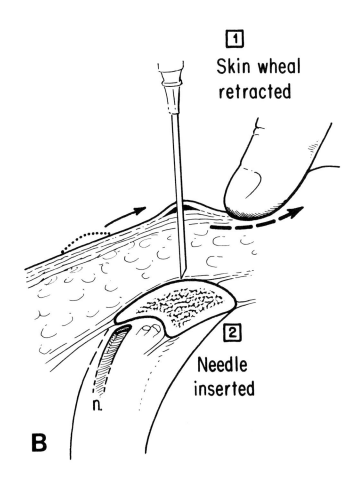

1
Skin wheal
retracted

2
Needle
inserted

n.

B

1
Skin
released

2
Needle
"walked off"
edge of rib

n.

C

Figure 21-3. Intercostal nerve block. A skin wheal is inserted on the lower rib margin (A). The skin wheal is retracted over the body of the rib and a needle inserted until contact is made with the rib (B). The skin is released and the needle carefully "walked" off the edge of the rib margin (C). After negative aspiration for blood, the appropriate volume of drug is injected.

257

and intercostal brachial nerve is variable. If the paravascular technique of Winnie is utilized there is often no need to block the musculocutaneous nerve.[33] A valuable adjunct to this technique, which aids in stabilizing the needle, is to use either a Butterfly (Abbott) and a local anesthetic syringe, or an intravenous extension tubing between the needle and syringe.[34] Another useful adjunct in the anesthetized pediatric patient is the use of a nerve stimulator to aid in localization of the neurovascular bundle.[35] We have not found the need for this with axillary blocks, but have found it useful for femoral–sciatic blocks.

The volume and concentration of local anesthetic chosen must be modified according to patient size and depth of block required. A volume of 0.5–1.0 ml/kg is generally satisfactory, provided the total dose is adjusted for weight. If postoperative analgesia is desired, 0.25 percent bupivacaine would be most appropriate. If deep anesthesia with motor paralysis is necessary, however, 0.5 percent bupivacaine or a combination of one percent lidocaine (maximum of 7 mg/kg) and tetracaine (maximum 1–2 mg/kg) may be utilized. This latter combination would provide a rapid onset with a prolonged block.[36] The use of bupivacaine for analgesia in children has greatly diminished the need for postoperative narcotics.[37]

Example: A 20 kg child with wrist fracture, using a 0.5% solution.

Bupivacaine maximal dose = 3 mg/kg
3 × 20 = 60 mg,
0.5% = 5 mg/ml
60 mg÷5 mg = 12 ml maximum volume

INTRAVENOUS REGIONAL ANESTHESIA

Intravenous regional anesthesia was first described in 1908, and is frequently referred to as a Bier block.[38] This has proved to be a particularly valuable technique, with rapid onset of anesthesia for procedures of brief duration, such as suturing of a large laceration or a closed reduction of a fracture.[39,41] Disadvantages include the possibility of toxic reactions in the presence of tourniquet failure. Strict attention to detail, i.e., elevation or exanguination of the extremity to be blocked, proper application of a double pneumatic cuff, and careful calculation of total anesthetic dose, is important in order to avoid serious complications and provide a successful block.[1] A low dose of neuromuscular blocking agent, such as curare (0.03 mg/kg) or pancuronium (0.005 mg/kg), may also improve the quality of motor blockade.

Example: A 20 kg child with a wrist fracture.

Lidocaine 3-5 mg/kg maximum safe dose using a 0.5% solution (5 mg/ml)

5 × 20 = 100 mg

0.5% = 5 mg/ml

100 mg ÷ 5 mg = 20 ml

SPINAL ANESTHESIA

Successful subarachnoid blocks have been performed in patients of all ages, including neonates.[42–47] Medicolegal issues and parental concern over permanent paresis, however, have resulted in diminishing pediatric application. Our experience has been limited to adolescents undergoing lower abdominal, urologic, or orthopedic procedures. One publication reported

less effect on blood pressure in children under five years of age, but widely varying effects in children six years of age or older. The reasons for the apparent stability of the cardiovascular system in the younger patients are not clear, but lower proportional blood volume of the lower extremities and an incompletely developed sympathetic nervous system have been postulated. There was also a very strong inverse relationship of duration of block with age.[47]

The dangers of spinal anesthesia in children are similar to those in the adult population. It is therefore important to hydrate the patient prior to administration of the block, as well as to have available appropriate vasopressors and the means for airway management.

The anatomy of the spinal cord is the same as the adult by one year of age (i.e., terminating at L-1; in the newborn it extends to L-3). When positioning a small child for spinal puncture, the anesthesiologist must carefully check for adequate air exchange. Recommended doses to achieve lower abdominal block are a 1 percent solution of tetracaine in dosages of 0.2–0.3 mg/kg.[42]

Adhesive arachnoiditis has been reported in adults with 2-chloroprocaine; until further studies are carried out this drug should not be used for spinal or epidural anesthesia.[48]

EPIDURAL/CAUDAL BLOCK

The use of epidural anesthesia has become less popular in children for the same reasons as spinal anesthesia.[49] Most recent pediatric reports describe the use of caudal anesthesia for lower abdominal surgery or postoperative pain relief.[50–59] The dose requirements for epidural blockade rise rapidly until the age of 18. There are several formulae that may be consulted to calculate the appropriate dose.[56,57,59,60,61] If only analgesia is desired, a much lower drug concentration will suffice; if motor blockade is necessary, a higher drug concentration will be required. It is important to remain within the safe guidelines presented in Table 21-1 to minimize toxic reactions from injecting into a relatively vascular area. In addition, it must be noted that in the neonate the sacral sac of the spinal cord may extend to the fourth sacral vertebra, thus making accidental total spinal blockade more likely.

SUMMARY

While regional blocks are extremely useful for postoperative analgesia in many common procedures, they are also valuable as the sole anesthetic in selected patients. Often, if a mild analgesic (e.g., acetaminophen) is administered prior to the block dissipating, the patient will be nearly pain free when the block does wear off. The anesthesiologist must be familiar with these techniques and must have a working knowledge of pediatric anatomy, the appropriate sedation, the various local anesthetics, and, perhaps most important, should be able to calm the child through sensitive preoperative explanation and constant intraoperative attention. Any block performed in adult patients may be performed in pediatric patients, provided the circumstances are carefully chosen.

REFERENCES

1. Eather KF: Regional anesthesia for infants and children. *Int Anesth Clin* 13:19–48, 1975

2. Soliman MG, Tremblay NA: Nerve block of the penis for

postoperative pain relief in children. *Anesth Analg* 57:495–498, 1978

3. Lunn JN: Postoperative analgesia after circumcision: A randomized comparison between caudal analgesia and intramuscular morphine in boys. *Aneasthesia* 34:552–554, 1979

4. Shandling B, Steward DJ: Regional analgesia for postoperative pain in pediatric outpatient surgery. *J Pediatr Surg* 15:477–480, 1980

5. deJong RH: Local anesthetic mechanisms. *Anesth Rev* 3:18–23, 1974

6. Covino BG: Local anesthesia (part 1). *N Engl J Med* 286:975–983, 1972

7. Covino BG: Local anesthesia (part 2). *N Engl J Med* 286:1035–1042, 1972

8. Tucker GT, Moore DC, Bridenbaugh PO, et al: Systemic absorption of mepivacaine in commonly used regional block procedures. *Anesthesiology* 37:277–287, 1972

9. Braid DP, Scott DB: The systemic absorption of local analgesic drugs. *Br J Anaesth* 37:394–404, 1965

10. Ritchie JM, Greene NM: Local anesthetics, in Gilman AG, Goodman LS, Gilman A (eds): *The Pharmacological Basis of Therepeutics* (ed 6). New York, Macmillan, 1980, pp 300–320

11. Mather LE, Cousins MJ: Local anesthetics and their current clinical use. *Drugs* 18:185–205, 1979

12. Morikawa KI, Bonica JJ, Tucker GT, et al: Effect of acute hypovolemia on lignocaine absorption and cardiovascular response following epidural block in dogs. *Br J Anaesth* 46:631–635, 1974

13. Rothstein P, Arthur GR, Felman H, et al: Pharmacokinetics of bupivacaine in children following intercostal block. *Anesthesiology* 57:A426, 1982

14. Melgrave AP: The use of epinephrine in the presence of halothane in children. *Can Anaesth Soc J* 17:256–260, 1970

15. Karl HW, Swedlow DB, Lee KW, et al: Epinephrine–halothane interactions in children. *Anesthesiology* 58:142–145, 1983

16. Ueda W, Hirakawa M, Mae O: Appraisal of epinephrine administration to patients under halothane anesthesia for closure of cleft palate. *Anesthesiology* 58:574–576, 1983

17. Johnston RR, Eger EI, II, Wilson C: A comparative interaction of epinephrine with enflurane, isoflurane, and halothane in man. *Anesth Analg* 55:709–712, 1976

18. deJong RH, Heavner JE: Local anesthetic seizure prevention: Diazepam versus pentobarbital. *Anesthesiology* 36:449–457, 1972

19. Alper MH: Toxicity of local anesthetics (editorial). *N Engl J Med* 295:1432–1433, 1976

20. Reidenberg MM, James M, Dring LG: The rate of procaine hydrolysis in serum of normal subjects and diseased patients. *Clin Pharm Ther* 13:279–284, 1972

21. Selden R, Sasahara AA: Central nervous system toxicity induced by lidocaine: Report of a case in a patient with liver disease. *JAMA* 202:908–909, 1967

22. Thompson PD, Melmon KL, Richardson JA, et al: Lidocaine pharmacokinetics in advanced heart failure, liver disease, and renal failure in humans. *Ann Int Med* 78:499–508, 1973

23. Englesson S: The influence of acid–base changes on central nervous system toxicity of local anesthetic agents. I. An experimental study in cats. *Acta Anaesthesiol Scan* 18:79–87, 1974

24. Englesson S, Grevsten S: The influence of acid–base changes on central nervous system toxicity of local anaesthetic agents. II. *Acta Anaesthesiol Scand* 18:88–103, 1974

25. Aldrete JA, Johnson DA: Allergy to local anesthetics. *JAMA* 207:356–357, 1969

26. Arora S, Aldrete JA: Investigation of possible allergy to local anesthetic drugs: Correlation of intradermal with intramuscular injections. *Anesth Rev* 5:13–16, 1976

27. Kirya C, Werthmann MW, Jr: Neonatal circumcision and penile dorsal nerve block—a painless procedure. *J Pediatr* 92:998–1000, 1978

28. Bridenbaugh PO, Bridenbaugh LD, Moore DC, et al: The role of intercostal block and three general anesthetic agents as predisposing factors to postoperative pulmonary problems. *Anesth Analg* 51:638–644, 1972

29. Fleming WH, Sarafian LB: Kindness pays dividends: the medical benefits of intercostal nerve block following thoracotomy. *J Thorac Cardiovasc Surg* 74:273–274, 1977

30. Crawford ED, Skinner DG, Capparell DB: Intercostal nerve block with thoracoabdominal incision. *J Urol* 121:290–291, 1979

31. Small GA: Brachial plexus block anesthesia in children. *JAMA* 147:1648–1651, 1951

32. Clayton ML, Turner DA: Upper arm block anesthesia in children with fractures. *JAMA* 169:327–329, 1959

33. Winnie AP: The perivascular techniques of brachial plexus anesthesia, in Hershey SG (ed): *Refresher Courses in Anesthesiology* (vol 2). Philadelphia, J.B. Lippincott, 1974, pp 149–162

34. Winnie AP: An "immobile needle" for nerve blocks. *Anesthesiology* 31:577–578, 1969

35. Montgomery SJ, Raj PP, Nettles D, et al: The use of the nerve stimulator with standard unsheathed needles in nerve blockade. *Anesth Analg* 52:827–831, 1973

36. Moore DC, Bridenbaugh LD, Bridenbaugh PO, et al: Does compounding of local anesthetic agents increase their toxicity in humans? *Anesth Analg* 51:579–585, 1972

37. Neill RS: Postoperative analgesia following brachial plexus block. *Br J Anaesth* 50:379–382, 1978

38. Bier A: Uber einen neuen Weg Localanasthesie an den Gliedmassen zu erzeugen. *Arch Klin Chir* 96:1007–1016, 1908

39. Carrel ED, Eyring EJ: Intravenous regional anesthesia for childhood fractures. *J Trauma* 11:301–305, 1971

40. FitzGerald B: Intravenous regional anaesthesia in children. *Br J Anaesth* 48:485–486, 1976

41. Gingrich TF: Intravenous regional anesthesia of the upper extremity in children. *JAMA* 200:405, 1967

42. Calvert DG: Direct spinal anaesthesia for repair of myelomeningocoele. *Br Med J* 2:86–87, 1966

43. Berkowitz S, Greene BA: Spinal anesthesia in children: Report based on 350 patients under 13 years of age. *Anesthesiology* 12:376–387, 1951

44. Slater HM, Stephen CR: Hypobaric pontocaine spinal anesthesia in children. *Anesthesiology* 11:709–715, 1950

45. Junkin CI: Spinal anaesthesia in children. *Can Med Assoc J* 28:51–53, 1933

46. Abajian JC, Mellish P, Browne AF, et al: Spinal anesthesia for surgery in the high-risk infant. *Anesth Anal* 63:359–362, 1984

47. Dohi S, Naito H, Takahashi T: Age-related changes in blood pressure and duration of motor block in spinal anesthesia. *Anesthesiology* 50:319–323, 1979

48. Reisner LS, Hochman BN, Plumer MH: Persistant neurologic deficit and adhesive arachnoiditis following intrathecal 2-chloroprocaine injection. *Anesth Analg* 59:452–454, 1980

49. Dawkins CJM: An analysis of the complications of extradural and caudal block. *Anaesthesia* 24:554–563, 1969

50. Ruston FG: Epidural anesthesia in pediatric surgery. *Anesth Analg* 36:76–82, 1957

51. Jensen BH: Caudal block for post-operative pain relief in children after genital operations. A comparison between bupivacaine and morphine. *Acta Anaesth Scand* 25:373–375, 1981

52. Lourey CJ, McDonald IH: Caudal anaesthesia in infants and children. *Anaesth Intens Care* 1:547–548, 1973

53. Kay B: Caudal block for postoperative pain relief in children. *Anaesthesia* 29:610–611, 1974

54. Bramwell RGB, Bullen C, Radford P: Caudal block for postoperative analgesia in children. *Anaesthesia* 37:1024–1028, 1982

55. McGown RG: Caudal analgesia in children: Five hundred cases for procedures below the diaphragm. *Anaesthesia* 37:806–818, 1982

56. Hassan SZ: Caudal anesthesia in infants. *Anesth Analg* 56:686–689, 1977

57. Schulte-Steinberg O, Rahlfs, VW: Spread of extradural anal-
     gesia following caudal injection in children. *Br J Anaesth*
     49:1027–1034, 1977
58. Takasaki M, Dohi S, Kawabata Y, et al: Dosage of lidocaine for
     caudal anesthesia in infants and children. *Anesthesiology*
     47:527–529, 1977
59. Soliman MG, Ansara S, Laberge R: Caudal anaesthesia in pae-
     diatric patients. *Can Anaesth Soc J* 25:226–229, 1978
60. Spiegel P: Caudal anesthesia in pediatric surgery: A preliminary
     report. *Anesth Analg* 41:218–221, 1962
61. Bromage PR: Physiology and pharmacology of epidural analge-
     sia. *Anesthesiology* 28:592–622, 1967

22

Recovery from Anesthesia and the Postoperative Recovery Room

Charles B. Berde
I. David Todres

In contrast to many other forms of central nervous system depression, a striking feature of general anesthesia is its relatively rapid reversibility. It is not surprising that recovery of normal consciousness is not instantaneous; indeed it is remarkable that recovery is so rapid. Recovery rooms became widespread following the realization that the period of emergence from anesthesia has several common and potentially catastrophic problems that can generally be obviated by an environment which facilitates close observation and rapid institution of therapy. This chapter will outline general principles governing recovery from anesthesia, procedural and organizational issues in pediatric recovery room care, and common clinical problems that arise in the care of children in the recovery room.

RECOVERY FROM ANESTHESIA

Contemporary anesthetic practice frequently employs combinations of inhalation anesthetics, muscle relaxants, and intravenous hypnotics and narcotics. We will discuss each class separately, realizing that the effects of these agents in clinical practice can be synergistic, and that the effects of such synergy on recovery have been poorly characterized.

INDICATORS OF WAKEFULNESS

While complete recovery of mental acuity following an inhalation anesthetic may take one to four days, much of our concern in recovery rooms focuses on the more rapid process of return of protective reflexes necessary for cardiorespiratory stability. These include the ability to prevent airway obstruction from posterior displacement of the tongue or secretions, the ability to remove tracheobronchial secretions by coughing, baroreceptor reflexes to support perfusion, and chemorecep-

tor reflexes to support respiration in response to hypercarbia and hypoxemia. The principles governing recovery from inhalation anesthesia are well summarized by Eger.[1] MAC-awake, the alveolar concentration at which 50 percent of patients respond to a simple command such as "open your eyes." has been shown to be roughly 60 percent of MAC for four inhalation anesthetics.[2] A general clinical impression is that adults at MAC-awake levels of anesthesia (if unimpeded by other factors) are able to maintain and protect their airways without assistance. A recent study confirms the clinical impression that spontaneous eye opening predicts safe airway maintenance in children recovering from anesthesia.[3]

PHYSICOCHEMICAL FACTORS GOVERNING RECOVERY FROM INHALATION ANESTHESIA

On discontinuation of inhalation anesthesia, the rate of fall of alveolar concentration of the gas is a function of alveolar ventilation, anesthetic solubility (blood/gas solubility coefficient or λ), cardiac output, and the venous-to-alveolar partial pressure difference. Increased ventilation results in a more rapid fall in alveolar concentration, which will result in more rapid recovery, provided the $PaCO_2$ is not so low as to diminish cerebral blood flow and anesthetic removal from the brain. The blood/gas solubility coefficient is a major determinant of recovery time. MAC-awake is generally reached within two minutes for nitrous oxide; it may take several hours for a highly soluble agent such as ether. The potent inhalation agents in current use are intermediate between nitrous oxide and ether. Effects of cardiac output on recovery are complex.[1] Maintenance of high anesthetic concentrations will also result in greater accumulation in tissues and will prolong recovery time. A frequent rationale for the use of nitrous oxide and muscle relaxants is that they permit use of smaller concentrations of more soluble agents and result in more rapid recovery.

The duration of anesthesia affects recovery, and these effects are more pronounced the more soluble an agent is. For example, a halothane anesthetic procedure maintained at 1.1 MAC for 15 minutes results in recovery to MAC-awake in aproximately four minutes, whereas it may take 15 minutes to reach MAC-awake for a two-hour anesthetic procedure at 1.1 MAC. A practical question for current-day outpatient anesthesia is whether the use of isoflurane ($\lambda = 1.48$) or enflurane ($\lambda = 1.90$) results in clinically significantly shorter recovery times than halothane ($\lambda = 2.3$). Although isoflurane should theoretically result in the fastest induction-to-recovery time, two pediatric outpatient studies involving brief cases have not found any significant advantage.[4,5] Several hypotheses are suggested for this lack of a difference:

1. The cases may have been too short to allow sufficient equilibration.[6]
2. The studies did not maintain patients at comparable multiples of MAC.
3. Clinicians in these studies may have been less familiar with clinical signs of depth for isoflurane and may have maintained patients at relatively higher anesthetic concentrations.

RECOVERY OF RESPIRATORY REFLEXES

Response to Carbon Dioxide

While patients at MAC-awake levels of inhalation anesthesia may in general maintain airway patency, they have variable depression of other reflexes. There is a dose-related reduction in the ventilatory response to carbon dioxide; however, even at levels between 0.6–1.0 MAC, patients with patent airways and normal lungs do not generally become dangerously hypercarbic. Patients with obstructive lung disease or other causes of increased work of breathing may become increasingly hypercarbic. The level of ventilation is also a function of the degree of painful stimulation; patients with a surgical stimulus will breathe more vigorously than less stimulated patients. However, if the act of breathing increases incisional pain, as is common for thoracic and upper abdominal surgery, they may have diminished tidal volumes.

Response to Oxygen

Of potentially greater significance to recovery room care than responses to carbon dioxide are the effects of residual volatile anesthetic agents on the ventilatory response to hypoxemia.[7] The responsiveness of the peripheral chemoreceptors, which govern hypoxic drive in man, is blunted by alveolar halothane concentrations as low as 0.1 percent, and abolished entirely at 1.1 percent halothane. Patients in recovery rooms are frequently predisposed to hypoxemia; causes include airway obstruction, central hypoventilation (inhalation anesthetics, narcotics), atelectasis with ventilation–perfusion imbalance, and diminished tidal volume secondary to pain, tight dressings, casts, etc. With residual anesthesia, they may not struggle or hyperventilate, and may lapse into unconsciousness. A major rationale for the routine administration of supplemental oxygen in the recovery room is to prevent episodic hypoxemia, which may occur even after uneventful surgical procedures. In newborns, the ventilatory response to hypoxemia is attenuated even in the absence of anesthetic agents.[8–12] Use of oxygen in this population must be judicious and must involve a consideration of the risks of retrolental fibroplasia.[13–15]

RECOVERY FROM NEUROMUSCULAR BLOCKADE

Recovery in this situation may be monitored by peripheral nerve stimulation and clinical indices, such as an inspiratory force greater than -20 cm H_2O, vital capacity greater than 15–20 ml/kg, ability to protrude the tongue and head lift for longer than five seconds.[16] In small infants, who may not lift their heads well, brisk flexion of hips and knees to lift the feet off the table is associated with return of adequate muscular recovery.[17] Incomplete reversal may result in loss of airway patency and diminished ventilation, and may be especially dangerous in combination with residual anesthetics and narcotics. Reversal by cholinesterase inhibitors has been well studied in infants and children; train-of-four monitoring can be performed in all age groups.[18–20] (See Chapter 9.)

RECOVERY FROM INTRAVENOUS NARCOTICS AND HYPNOTICS

Recovery in this situation may be more variable and difficult to quantify than recovery from the inhalational and neuromuscular blocking agents. Clearance of these agents is characterized by rapid phase due to redistribution, and a slower phase due to elimination via the liver and kidneys. Kinetic parameters may be misleading if one fails to consider biologic activity of metabolites (e.g., the prolonged action of diazepam's metabolites). In the case of other agents such as scopolamine and ketamine, biologic effects on memory and other cognitive functions are not easily accounted for by plasma disappearance curves. The depressant effects of narcotics and hypnotics on the ventilatory response to carbon dioxide are well known; it is worth noting that they may depress the hypoxic drive as well. Further studies should address the effects of varying doses of narcotics on MAC-awake for inhalation agents, as well as the effect of painful stimulation on MAC-awake.

Intravenous narcotics and hypnotics are frequently given in combination with each other and with inhalation agents; a general impression is that combinations of such agents are commonly synergistic in their depression of respiratory and circulatory reflexes; this is well described for combinations of narcotics with benzodiazepines.[21] Although narcotic-induced depression is antagonized by naloxone, we would encourage its use only for specific indications, (e.g., severe hypoventilation), routine use at the termination of an anesthetic can produce acute pain, anxiety, and vomiting. Large or repeated doses of ketamine and droperidol are especially associated with prolongation of recovery time.

PROCEDURAL ASPECTS OF RECOVERY ROOM CARE

Recovery from anesthesia is a process of consecutive steps. As noted by Smith[22]

Recovery begins as soon as the anesthesiologist stops active administration of anesthetic agents. It follows a definite progression, first in the operating room, where respiration is reestablished and tracheal extubation is accomplished, then in the recovery room, where the patient regains full consciousness and cardiopulmonary stability (or in the intensive care unit for prolonged support), and finally in the nursing division or ward, where he recovers his strength and becomes ambulatory and ready for discharge.[22]

In addition to this excellent summary, we would include the time of transport from the operating room to the recovery room as an essential step in the anesthesiologist's care.

ENDOTRACHEAL EXTUBATION

Criteria for Extubation

In most cases extubation may be safely performed in the operating room. However, the child's condition may necessitate leaving the endotracheal tube in place and planning extubation at an appropriate time in the recovery room or intensive care unit.

For certain circumstances, there is widespread agreement that the child or infant should be awake prior to extubation; these include children who have been anesthetized with a full stomach, children with a risk of airway obstruction (including those with jaws wired shut and those with Pierre Robin, Treacher-Collins, hemifacial microsomia, and other syndromes associated with a difficult airway), and premature and other infants predisposed to apnea. Beyond this, the timing of extubation is a matter of dispute. For example, the practice at some institutions is to extubate when the patient is awake and demonstrating eye-opening and other purposeful movement; at others the practice is to extubate under deep inhalation anesthesia; clinicians at both institutions report very rare problems with either approach. Most clinicians would agree that either of these approaches is preferable to extubation in a very light plane of anethesia when laryngospasm is a high probability and vomiting may occur without protective reflexes intact. Our approach is to extubate most children awake with protective airway reflexes intact; exceptions include severe asthmatics, global eye injuries and cases in which severe coughing would jeopardize the surgical outcome.

Procedure for Extubation

The stomach is routinely emptied prior to discontinuation of anesthesia; indeed it is our general practice to empty the stomach immediately following induction. When anesthesia is administered by mask, it is important that this and other manipulations occur at a sufficient depth of anesthesia so that laryngospasm or vomiting does not occur. Extubation is preceded by pharyngeal suctioning, and occurs with a full inspiration. Immediately following extubation, oxygen should be administered and the child observed for adequate ventilation, color of the mucous membranes, and the presence of laryngospasm or vomiting. *Transport of the patient should not be undertaken until the patency of the airway and adequacy of respiration are confirmed.*

TRANSPORT TO THE RECOVERY ROOM

A brief clean up of the patient follows, and a check of the security and patency of the intravenous line, etc. The child should be kept warm throughout the transport to avoid the dangers of cooling or overheating. Unless the patient is wide awake (i.e., with protective airway reflexes intact), or unless there is a specific contraindication, it is sensible to transport

extubated patients in the lateral position, so that the tongue, secretions and possible vomitus are less likely to cause airway obstruction. A hand holding the chin up will help maintain the patient's airway as well as provide a breath monitor; one can feel the exhaled breath on the hand. For sleepy children, continued use of the precordial stethoscope serves as a monitor of respiration and circulation; in screaming, crying, or otherwise highly active children, this may be more of a nuisance. For potentially unstable patients, we recommend transport with an ECG, and monitoring of blood pressure with a cuff and anaeroid manometer, or with a transduced arterial line. These patients should have their monitoring lines, intravenous drips, and other paraphernalia clearly sorted out and simplified prior to transport. For sick patients, intubated patients, and patients with potential airway difficulties, appropriate resuscitation bags, face masks, oral airways, oxygen tanks (check levels!), functioning laryngoscopes, endotracheal tubes, portable suction, and medications (including atropine and succinylcholine) should be carried enroute to the recovery room or intensive care unit. Patients receiving vasopressors or vasodilators require battery powered infusion pumps.

Transport to the recovery room or intensive care unit is a time of potential danger. Often a patient appears awake following the stimulation of extubation and transfer to the stretcher, but may subsequently become more obtunded, and obstruction of the airway may occur while in transit. Equally as common is a child who becomes restless in transit. Guardrails may be helpful, but most important is the constant observation of the patient by the anesthesiologist. A gentle hand on the head may prevent bumping against guardrails. As always, *the cause of restlessness must be sought* (see below).

ARRIVAL IN THE RECOVERY ROOM

Attention is first directed to airway patency, the color of lips and mucous membranes, adequacy of ventilation, perfusion, and central nervous system function. Pulse, blood pressure, respiratory rate and temperature are recorded. Oxygen is administered. In rare cases (preterm infants, late-stage cystic fibrosis) it may be necessary to regulate the inspired concentration of oxygen more precisely. Many children oppose placement of an oxygen mask, and a funnel type mask or open hose with high flow rates may be less objectionable (although less optimal). Thereafter, report should be given to the nurses and physicians in attendance. This report should include at least a description of the patient's current problem, past medical history, medications and allergies, operative procedure, premedication, anesthetic agents and techniques, blood loss, fluid replacement, intraoperative medications, and problems with either surgery or anesthesia and possible anticipated problems in the recovery unit.

ORGANIZATION OF THE RECOVERY ROOM

This will vary with the particular need of each hospital and its surgical practice. In general, it is recommended that the recovery room be located adjacent to the operating room, in order to permit rapid transport of patients to and from the operating room, and to allow ready access to surgeons and anesthesiologists. On one hand recovery rooms may function almost as intensive care units, with critically ill patients, and on the other hand, recovery rooms for ambulatory surgery areas may see only relatively healthy patients. Even in the latter case,

Table 22-1

Recovery Room Supplies

Essential Bedside Equipment

1. Oxygen supply with regulated flows.
2. Oxygen face masks and face tents for spontaneous ventilation (various sizes).
3. Resuscitation Bags: Self-inflating (Ambu) and Mapleson type
4. Anesthesia face masks for positive pressure ventilation (pediatric sizes 0, 1, 2, 3, e.g. Rendell-Baker Soucek; adult sizes, small, medium, large)
5. Oral airways (sizes 00, 0, 1–5)
6. Suction and appropriate suction catheters (sizes 6 1/2– 10 French); Tonsil-type (Yankauer) attachment
7. Needles, syringes, alcohol wipes, betadine solution, gauze pads.
8. Arterial blood gas kit.

Emergency Supplies for "Crash Cart" or Central Location

1. Laryngoscopes with blades: Miller 0, 1, 2, 3, Macintosh 3, 4
   Extra-laryngoscope bulbs
2. Endotracheal tubes
   Sizes 2.5mm ID (internal diameter) through 8mm ID (Cuffed tubes for sizes > 5.5mm ID.)
   Stylette appropriate for each tube size
   Syringe for cuff inflation
   Tape and benzoin for tube fixation
3. 14 gauge catheter over needle, e.g. Medicut® or Jelco®) with 3.0mm ID endotracheal tube adaptor for emergency cricothyroidotomy
4. Back-up resuscitation bags and masks, oral airways, as described above for each bedside.
5. Nasogastric tubes
6. Intravenous infusion solutions, tubing, drip chambers.
7. Supplies for intravenous cannulation catheter over needle sets sizes 24 to 14 gauge.
8. Cut-down tray, tracheostomy, and suture sets.
9. Central venous catheter insertion set.
10. Tube thoracostomy set and system for suction and underwater seal.
11. Defibrillator
12. Electrocardiogram
13. Pressure transducer system and oscilloscope monitor
14. Sterile gowns, gloves, masks, towels, drapes
15. Foley catheter
16. Bed-board for C.P.R.

Table 22-2

Recovery Room Medications

Emergency Medications on "Crash Cart"

Atropine
Epinephrine
Sodium bicarbonate
Dextrose
Calcium chloride and Calcium Gluconate
Lidocaine (intravenous and topical)
Succinylcholine
Thiopental or methohexital
Diphenhydramine
Hydrocortisone, Dexamethasone, methyl-prednisolone
Neostigmine, Edrophonium
Physostigmine
Naloxone
Aminophylline
Furosemide
Dopamine
Isoproterenol
Norepinephrine
Sodium Nitroprusside
Heparin
Verapamil
Quinidine
Bretylium
Propranolol
Diphenylhydantoin
Mannitol
Racemic epinephrine (for inhalation)

Medications to be Kept Under Lock

Morphine
Meperidine
Diazepam
Phenobarbital
Cocaine (for nasal intubation)

Other Medications for Central Location

Antibiotics (e.g. ampicillin, gentamicin, keflin, etc)
Acetaminophen
Dantrolene
Digoxin
Pancuronium, or other non-depolarizing relaxants
Antiemetics-droperidol, promethazine, prochlorperazine
Protamine
Insulin
Potassium chloride (KC1)

it is essential that full facilities be available for resuscitation, and that there be a regular protocol for transfer to an acute care environment.

The number of beds required is largely a function of the surgical volume and acuity. Recommendations commonly indicate two recovery room beds for each operating room; each bedspace should include oxygen, suction, blood pressure cuffs, and the equipment listed in Table 22-1. Depending on the case mix, there should be a variable number of ECG monitors and pressure transducers for arterial and venous catheters, etc. We recommend the use of portable "crash carts," which can be moved to the bedside for acute airway management, resuscitation, defibrillation, and so on. Medications should be readily

accessible; a representative listing of necessary medications is included in Table 22-2.

The physical layout of a recovery room is generally made to support optimum visibility of patients, so that events can be observed and treated rapidly; usually, large open rooms are used. While such visibility is essential, large noisy rooms can be frightening to children. When appropriate, drawing curtains to give a child some privacy should be allowed; this is particularly true if acute interventions are occurring with other patients. In all cases, but especially for adolescents, it is important to appreciate their modesty and wish not to be unnecessarily exposed.

Patients awakening from anesthesia often complain of strange or loud noises, and increased noise may even be

Table 22-3

Discharge Criteria (In-patients)

1. Recovery of airway and respiratory reflexes adequate to support gas exchange and to protect against aspiration of secretions, vomitus or blood.
2. Stability of circulation and control of any surgical bleeding.
3. Absence of anticipated instability in categories 1 & 2.
4. Reasonable control of pain and vomiting.
5. Appropriate duration of observation following narcotic administration (a minimum of 30 minutes following an intravenous dose).

Table 22-4

Discharge Criteria (Out-patients)

1. All criteria in Table 22-3.
2. Recovery of consciousness to near base-line levels.
3. For older children: return to stable gait. For smaller children it may be permissible for parents to carry their children without full recovery of gait. For this circumstance, parents must be advised that the child is at risk of injury if improperly supervised.
4. Control of pain to permit adequate analgesia via the oral route thereafter.
5. Control of nausea and vomiting to allow for oral hydration (see text under "Discharge Criteria").

associated with increased patient discomfort.[23] Noise levels in recovery rooms commonly average between 50–70 dB; these levels produce measurable autonomic changes suggestive of a stress reaction.[24] Every effort should be made to diminish unnecessary noise and commotion in recovery rooms.

Staffing is also a function of the particular needs of the hospital. For non-acute patients, a nurse-to-patient ratio of one to three is generally deemed sufficient; for acutely ill patients, the ratio may be one to one or even two to one. Ideally, nurses caring for pediatric patients should have specific training in topics including pediatric airway and circulatory problems, the pharmacology of anesthetics, narcotics and other common medications in children, and the emotional and behavioral responses of children at various ages. A description of nursing considerations in pediatric recovery room care is given in other texts.[25] Physician coverage also varies widely. In many hospitals, the anesthesiologist who administered an anesthetic remains responsible throughout the recovery, while many busy hospitals, including many teaching hospitals, have a separate physician responsible for the recovery room. Regardless of the system used, anesthesia personnel should be readily available for acute evaluation and intervention. Following the guidelines of the Joint Committee on Accreditation of Hospitals (JCAH), we advise that an anesthesiologist supervise care in the recovery rooms.

DISCHARGE CRITERIA

A variety of criteria for discharge from recovery rooms have been given; these considerations are summarized elsewhere.[26] Attempts have been made to use formal criteria to assess readiness for discharge, but readiness is also a function of the situation to which the patient is being discharged. As an extreme example, a patient having a slight degree of postintubation croup might be discharged to a ward or pediatric intensive care unit with nurses and physicians skilled at assessment of pediatric airways, while a patient with an identical problem might not be appropriate for discharge following outpatient surgery with parents of questionable reliability who anticipate driving seventy miles to their home through a snow storm. For inpatients not going to an intensive care unit, the general features of readiness for discharge are summarized in Table 22-3. Outpatients are generally required to satisfy these criteria, as well as the additional criteria in Table 22-4. The issue of ability to keep down oral fluids in outpatients must be tailored to the individual case. Pediatric outpatients are frequently quite deficient in

fluids at the time of induction of anesthesia; this applies most to small children and infants who are scheduled for later cases and have been kept NPO for prolonged periods. We attempt to replace a greater fraction of their deficits intravenously in the operating and the recovery rooms, so that even if they take very little fluid thereafter, it will be less likely for them to become dehydrated. Attempts to force fluids often result in vomiting in the recovery room or during a journey home. In many cases, where the parents are reliable, the deficit is small, and the likelihood of vomiting is small, it may be more sensible to let the child go home and try to take fluids again in a more comfortable environment.

RECOVERY ROOM PROBLEMS

Major problems encountered in the postoperative recovery room phase are discussed below, with an emphasis on pathophysiological changes. This approach allows one to deal with the problem irrespective of the nature of the surgical or anesthetic procedure.

PAIN

Besides being a problem in its own right, pain may bring on several of the other signs discussed here, including tachycardia, hypertension, nausea, vomiting and anxiety.[27] Untreated pain appears to exacerbate emergence delirium.

Although we believe in the prompt and vigorous treatment of patients in pain, it should be recalled that a patient's pain must be assessed, and that the presence of pain which is inappropriate to the patient's condition may be of diagnostic significance. For example, severe limb pain following a limb procedure requires ruling out compartment syndromes; shoulder pain following cystoscopy may suggest bladder perforation and peritoneal irritation.

Several generalizations about treatment of pain in pediatric postoperative patients apply.

1. As with adults, preoperative encouragement and instruction of patients who are old enough to understand, diminishes the experience of pain. Pain is exacerbated by anxiety and a feeling of helplessness and of uncertainty regarding what will happen.[28]
2. Where possible, use long-acting local anesthetics, such as bupivacaine, to diminish pain. Infiltration of the sper-

matic cord and incision can make hernia repair much less painful; intercostal nerve blocks can diminish pain of thoractomy.

3. Distraction and the company of parents or other familiar individuals is helpful; teddy bears and other favorite personal objects which make the child feel more secure should be brought to the recovery room when appropriate.

4. Rectal administration of acetaminophen is effective for mild pain, aids in the alleviation of more severe pain by narcotics, and has a very high therapeutic ratio.

5. For moderate and severe pain, intravenous narcotics are the mainstay of treatment. Incremental doses of morphine (0.05–0.2 mg/kg) or meperidine (0.5–2 mg/kg) should be *titrated to effect*, recognizing the following qualifiers: doses should be greatly diminished or preferably omitted in the patient who has a compromised airway or is hemodynamically unstable; the biological effects of an intravenous dose of morphine may not be maximal for ten minutes, therefore observation for an overdose must not end two minutes after a dose is given but continue through the appropriate observation period; respiratory rate is a reasonable guide to effect, and it is usually unlikely that a tachypneic patient has received too much narcotic, despite what may seem to be a high dose; the intravenous route for narcotics is preferred to the intramuscular route in the recovery room because onset of action is more rapid (pain is more easily controlled before it becomes severe), and because peak effects are more readily seen. The reaction to an intramuscular dose may not peak until the patient has left the recovery room, when observation may be less than optimal. Most recovery rooms require that a patient who has received narcotics remain there for 20–30 minutes following a last dose; when there is any doubt, it is prudent to watch patients for longer periods.

In most cases, it is not possible or prudent to remove pain entirely, but it should be possible to attenuate the pain enough to make it tolerable. It is probable that there are more errors in undertreatment than in overtreatment, because of preconceptions about the diminished experience or memory of pain in infants and children, and because of inordinate fears of respiratory depression by narcotics. With step-by-step administration of narcotics, titration to desired effect, and observation, respiratory depression should be rare. Should respiratory depression occur, however, the child must receive assisted ventilation until narcotic antagonists (e.g., naloxone) take effect.

ANXIETY AND AGITATION

Frequently, infants and children in recovery rooms may be restless and agitated, or may cry uncontrollably. While these may be "normal" responses to emergence from anesthesia in a strange and unfriendly environment, it is imperative that physicians and nurses first investigate whether these are serious signs of physiologic distress. Causes include:

- Hypoxemia and/or hypercarbia secondary to upper airway obstruction (tongue, secretions, blood, vomitus), lower airway obstruction (bronchospasm, mucus plugs), or ventilation–perfusion imbalance (atelectasis, poor inspiratory effort due to casts, bandages or pain, pulmonary edema, pneumothorax).
- Hypotension and inadequate perfusion (hypovolemia, cardiac failure).
- Metabolic disturbance, including hypoglycemia and hyponatremia.
- Increased intracranial pressure (ICP) or other primary CNS pathology.
- Excitatory effects of drugs (scopolamine, ketamine).
- "Pure" emergence delirium from inhalation anesthesia.
- Untreated or undertreated pain (watch especially for unanticipated causes of pain, such as metal instruments left under patients, traction on nasogastric tubes, Foley catheters, chest tubes, tight casts and occlusive taping of IV boards).
- Behavioral reaction of an awake child to threatening circumstances.

In many cases, consideration of the circumstances of the surgery and a brief examination, with attention to the adequacy of ventilation, should suffice for ruling out the first four causes above when there is doubt, measure arterial blood gases, electrolytes, and blood sugar as needed. Oxygen should be administered in most cases. Since a tight mask may increase agitation, it may be necessary to use a funnel mask or open hose. If one is confident that these factors are not causing the problem, then use narcotics, physostigmine, and reassurance and cuddling as indicated by the particular circumstances. We believe that emergence delirium is exacerbated by emergence from inhalation anesthesia with untreated pain, and we encourage the use of narcotics intraoperatively or before emergence when appropriate. Emergence delirium appears less common in children and adolescents when a predominantly nitrous oxide–narcotic technique is used. Among the inhalation agents, there may be a higher incidence of stormy emergence when enflurane is employed.[4,29]

NAUSEA AND VOMITING

Although rarely life threatening (except when vomiting occurs in patients unable to protect themselves from aspiration), nausea and vomiting are major causes of unpleasant experience and recollection in anesthetized children. A review of the literature and our own experience suggests to us that (1) although reported incidences vary from less than 1 percent to over 80 percent, it is clear to us that nausea and vomiting are very common problems; we suggest that the lower figures represent either under-reporting or too strict inclusion criteria; (2) although the variation in incidence may be related to the individual patient, the operative procedure, and the anesthetic agents used, there is little basis for choosing one current anesthetic regimen over another in this regard; (3) stomach emptying before emergence should be encouraged, thereby diminishing the quantity of potential vomitus, relieving stomach distension, which may trigger vomiting, and possibly removing blood clots following oral or pharyngeal surgery, which can be a chemical irritant stimulus for vomiting; and (4) patients who report a serious tendency towards motion sickness are more likely to vomit. The use of antiemetics both prophylactically and after vomiting has begun is a controversial subject. A number of studies in adults and children have shown considerable efficacy for phenothiazines and butyrophenones, most notably droperidol, in diminishing the incidence and especially the severity of postoperative vomiting. Many studies include patients who have had several different types of operations and anesthetics, and effects may be obscured by the uncontrolled variables. Two recent studies with commendable designs are those of Abramowitz et al. in which patients undergoing strabismus surgery under halothane–nitrous oxide anesthesia were given either saline or varying doses of droperidol.[30,31] Several points are noteworthy. First, in their experience, higher doses (75–100 μg/kg) had greater efficacy than moderate doses (50 μg/kg), which had greater efficacy than a placebo. Second, no extrapyramidal reactions were seen. Third, despite a widespread impression that droperidol can prolong recovery time, they noted that ambulatory patients who received prophylactic droperidol were ready for discharge sooner than those who did not, because of a higher incidence of delayed discharge due to vomiting in the latter group.

Other groups reported efficacy of lower doses of droperidol (10–30 μg/kg) and find higher incidences of extrapyramidal reactions with higher doses.[32,33] Suffice it to say that the matter requires further study, and that at present there is no guaranteed effective treatment for postoperative nausea and vomiting, although droperidol and other agents significantly reduce the incidence and severity of these problems.

Especially for small children and infants, specific intravenous fluid and electrolyte replacement of losses due to vomiting (in addition to maintenance fluids) should be given in the recovery room and in the postoperative ward.

UNRESPONSIVENESS

Following a surgical procedure, there may be concern because of a child's slow awakening. Frequent causes include:

- Hypoxemia
- Hypercarbia (CO_2 narcosis)
- Hypovolemia (inadequate cerebral perfusion)
- Hypoglycemia
- Residual anesthetic, narcotic, or hypnotic effect
- Residual neuromuscular blockade
- Increased intracranial pressure or other intracranial pathology (hemorrhage, tumor, etc)
- Water and electrolyte imbalance (hyponatremia)
- Postictal state

The approach to such a patient begins with a brief examination and review of the pertinent history, including preexisting conditions and the anesthetic record. In many cases, it is easy to rule in or out conditions from the history and examination alone. For example, not all somnolent patients need a blood gas to rule out ventilatory disturbance, or serum electrolyte values to rule out metabolic derangements. Pupillary signs, patterns and frequency of respiration, and the smell of volatile agent on a patient's breath may give clues to the presence of excessive narcotic effect or of residual anesthetic effect. If there is any doubt, the burden of proof lies on the physician to perform tests (blood gases, Dextrostix, etc.) to rule out life-threatening causes of unresponsiveness, most of which can be readily treated.

RESPIRATORY INSUFFICIENCY

We emphasize again that respiratory insufficiency in the recovery room may present with obvious stigmata of difficult breathing, but it may also present as anxiety, unresponsiveness, tachycardia, bradycardia, hypertension, arrhythmia, seizures or cardiac arrest. When any of these other conditions are present, adequacy of respiration must be assured and ruled in or out as a cause.

Airway Difficulties

Initially, the patency of the airway is checked and, when necessary, stimulation of the patient, positioning, mandibular displacement, placement of oral and nasal airways, and suctioning of secretions may be needed to open and clear the upper airway. In many cases, respiration will improve with these measures alone. If they fail, however, one must consider the patency of the laryngeal inlet and the lower airway, i.e., whether laryngospasm, subglottic narrowing secondary to edema, bronchospasm, or tracheal secretions are compromising airflow. Laryngospasm may require administration of oxygen under positive pressure by mask, or in rare cases, succinlycholine. Postintubation croup or subglottic edema has been associated with a number of factors, including traumatic intubation, tight-fitting endotracheal tubes, coughing on the tube, a change in the patient's position during surgery, prolonged duration of intubation, and surgery on the head and neck.[34] For reasons that have not been adequately explained, postintubation croup is less common in infants under three months of age than it is in older infants and toddlers. Treatment initially consists of inhalation of cool mist. If the symptoms are sufficiently severe, racemic epinephrine by inhalation is generally effective, although its effects are temporary, and rebound edema may follow its use. In general, a decision to use racemic epinephrine implies that there will be prolonged observation of the patient thereafter. For outpatients, this implies that the child will be admitted to the hospital overnight.

Respiratory Effort

If the airway is patent, attention turns to the adequacy of respiratory effort. Residual neuromuscular blockade can be diagnosed using peripheral nerve stimulation. Depending on the severity and the clinical situation, it may be treated with either further doses of reversal agents or ventilatory assistance. If the signs of narcotic overdosage are present, naloxone will have immediate effect. Administration of naloxone (standard dose is 0.01 mg/kg) in small incremental doses (0.002 mg/kg), if the situation permits, may prevent precipitation of acute anxiety or pain.

Patients may have an adequate airway and the potential for adequate ventilatory effort, but have difficulty breathing due to pain, restriction from bandages or casts, abdominal distension, pneumothorax, atelectasis, aspiration or pneumonitis, or cardiogenic pulmonary edema. In most cases, history and examination will narrow the differential, and when necessary, chest radiographs and invasive hemodynamic monitoring will further guide diagnosis and treatment.

Recent studies have disclosed an alarming tendency towards postoperative apnea in preterm infants.[35,36] We recommend apnea and ECG monitoring overnight in small preterm infants and in any infant with a previous history of apnea; outpatient surgery in these patients should be discouraged. The immediate availability of pediatric intensive care should exist for facilities undertaking elective surgery in this population. In many cases, spells of periodic breathing or apnea can be terminated merely by stimulation; in others assisted ventilation with a bag and mask is required.

HYPOTENSION

In assessing hypotension the anesthesiologist should be familiar with the normal blood pressure ranges in infants and children (see Chapter 2).

The measurement should be obtained with appropriate sized blood pressure cuffs (two thirds the length of the upper arm). Inappropriately sized cuffs will give spurious readings. The proper placement of the cuff is essential to avoid errors in interpretation.

The most common cause of hypotension in children is hypovolemia. This may result from inadequate replacement of blood and fluid loss (third space loss) during the surgical procedure, or from continuing losses.

Drugs, large doses of inhalational and local anesthetic agents, and narcotics may produce hypotension through vasodilation (relative hypovolemia) and direct myocardial depression; these are rarely contibutory in the recovery room care of children.

Increased temperature will cause vasodilation and a relative hypovolemia. In addition, the increased metabolic demands of the fever may compromise an already-stressed myocardium, with resultant heart failure and hypotension. Any factor which interferes with venous return will result in hypotension; for example, tension pneumothrorax, pericardial tamponade, and compression of the inferior vena cava.

HYPERTENSION

Postoperative hypertension is less common than hypotension. Too small a cuff may give a spuriously high blood pressure reading.

Other factors include hypervolemia, pain, distended bladder, hypercarbia, and drugs (e.g., ketamine, epinephrine). Pheochromocytoma will occasionally cause hypertension, but this is rare.

TACHYCARDIA

Tachycardia is an important postoperative sign signifying an attempt of the body's compensatory mechanism to maintain an adequate cardiac output, or a response of the body to reflex stimuli (pain) or drugs (epinephrine, atropine). In addition, tachycardia may be due to hypoxemia, hypercarbia, hypovolemia, sepsis (fever), overtransfusion, or heart failure.

BRADYCARDIA

Bradycardia in the recovery room most commonly reflects hypoxemia. It may also reflect a vagal response to a number of stimuli (e.g., passage of a nasogastric tube). Drugs (such as prostigmine and fentanyl) may also induce bradycardia. In neurosurgical cases it may accompany increased intracranial pressure.

HYPOTHERMIA

Hypothermia is a serious postoperative problem in the infant. The response to hypothermia is to increase body temperature by shivering; this response is not well developed in the first few weeks of life. When shivering occurs, oxygen consumption increases and imposes a possible life-threatening stress, i.e., oxygen demand may outstrip oxygen delivery. In addition, the vasoconstrictor response to diminish heat loss results in metabolic acidosis from intense peripheral vasoconstriction and resultant inadequate perfusion. Acidosis in turn causes respiratory and cardiac depression and possibly cardiopulmonary arrest.

HYPERTHERMIA

Elevation of temperature may be due to simple causes, such as overheating, but may be of serious import when its origin is the malignant hyperthermia syndrome (see Chapter 20). Other causes are bacterial sepsis, dehydration, pyrogenic reaction to infusion of fluids and blood. Suspicion of sepsis necessitates a complete examination to localize the source.

OLIGURIA

Oliguria is defined as a urine output of less than 1 ml/kg/hour. The cause may simply be a blocked catheter. If a catheter is not in place it may be advisable to insert one when a diagnosis is needed. A significant cause of oliguria is hypovolemia. Urine output is also a valuable indication of adequacy of cardiac output. Another cause of oliguria is acute tubular necrosis, which usually has its origin in intraoperative or preoperative ischemia. Oliguria may occur with intraoperative manipulation of the kidney, or the aorta (even when the aorta is cross-clamped infrarenally).

The approach to oliguric patients begins with assessment of the clinical signs of adequate perfusion and with appropriate treatment of circulatory insufficiency by expanding the intravascular volume with fluids and blood and administrating inotropic agents as needed. Diuretics should be administered only when there is clinical and/or physiologic evidence of intravascular volume overload, and not merely to treat a urine output number. Conversely, it should be realized that in pediatric patients who have had an adequate blood pressure preoperatively and intraperatively without the support of alpha-adrenergic agents it is extraordinarily rare to develop renal failure in the postoperative period, and one can err in too strict adherence to numerical guidelines for urine output in otherwise physiologically stable patients.

SEIZURES

Seizures may occur in the recovery room, and may be due to hypoxemia or metabolic imbalance (hypoglycemia, hyponatremia). On occasion patients receiving anticonvulsant drugs may have missed a necessary dose. Every effort should be made to maintain therapeutic levels either by oral administration on the day of surgery, or intravenous administration at the time of surgery. Treatment consists of attention to the establishment of a clear airway, adequate oxygenation and ventilation, and seeking the underlying cause.

PARENTS IN THE RECOVERY ROOM

In recent years there has been a healthy trend towards accommodating the presence of parents in the recovery room. Having the parents at the bedside of the child is a judgement that will depend upon the child's clinical status. There is a significant emotional benefit for the child awakening in strange surroundings to the presence of its parents. This emotional benefit is shared, too, by the parents who feel quite helpless when cut off from their child at this stage. The presence of parents may be especially invaluable in dealing with the mentally handicapped child. However, it should be appreciated that flexibility in this arrangement is necessary, and that allowing parents in the recovery room has to be evaluated on an individual basis.

REFERENCES

1. Eger EI, II: *Anesthetic Uptake and Action.* Baltimore, Williams & Wilkins, 1974, pp 228–248

2. Stoelting RK, Longnecker DE, Eger EI: Minimum alveolar concentrations in man on awakening from methoxyflurane, halothane, ether and fluroxene anesthesia: MAC awake. *Anesthesiology* 33:5–9, 1970

3. Lee KWT, Dougal RM, Downes JJ: Criteria for tracheal extubation in children following anesthesia. Abstract 30, American Academy of Pediatrics, Spring Meeting 1984, p 33

4. Horne JA, Ahlgren EW: Halothane, Enflurane and Isoflurane for outpatient surgery. A pediatric case series. Abstract, American Society of Anesthesiology, 1973, pp 269–270

5. Pandit UA, Leach AB, Steude GM: Induction and recovery characteristics of halothane and isoflurane anesthesia in children. *Anesthesiology* 59:A445, 1983

6. Stoelting RK, Eger EI, II: The effects of ventilation and anesthetic solubility on recovery from anesthesia: An in vivo and analog analysis before and after equilibrium. *Anesthesiology* 30:290–296, 1969

7. Knill RL, Gelb AW: Ventilatory responses to hypoxia and hypercapnia during halothane sedation and anesthesia in man. *Anesthesiology* 49:244–251, 1978

8. Cross KW, Oppé TE: The effect of inhalation of high and low concentrations of oxygen on the respiration of the premature infant. *J Physiol* 117:38–55, 1952

9. Rigatto H, Brady JP, Torre Verrolusco R: Chemoreceptor reflexes in preterm infants. I. The effect of gestational and postnatal age on the ventilatory response to inhalation of 100% and 15% oxygen. *Pediatrics* 55:604–613, 1975

10. Rigatto H, Torre Verduzio R, Cortes DB: Effects on O_2 on the ventilatory response to CO_2 in preterm infants. *J Appl Physiol* 39:896–899, 1975

11. Gerhardt T, Bancalari E: Apnea of prematurity. I. Lung function and regulation of breathing. *Pediatrics* 74:58–62, 1984

12. Gerhardt T, Bancalari E: Apnea of prematurity. II Respiratory reflexes. *Pediatrics* 74:63–66, 1984

13. Flynn JT, O'Grady GE, Herrem J, et al: Retrolental fibroplasia. I. Clinical observations. *Arch Ophthalmol* 95:217–223, 1977

14. Kinsey VE, Arnold HJ, Kalina RE, et al: PaO₂ levels and retrolental fibroplasia. A report of the cooperative study. *Pediatrics* 60:655–668, 1977

15. Betts EK, Downes JJ: Retrolental fibroplasia and oxygen administration during anesthesia. *Anesthesiology* 47:518–520, 1977

16. Ali HH, Savarese JJ: Monitoring of neuromuscular function. *Anesthesiology* 45:216–249, 1976

17. Mason EJ, Betts EK: Leg lift and maximum inspiratory force. *Anesthesiology* 52:441–442, 1980

18. Meakin G, Sweet P, Bevan JC, et al: Neostigmine and edrophonium as antagonists of pancuronium in infants and children. *Anesthesiology* 59:316–321, 1983

19. Fisher DM, Cronelly R, Miller RD, et al: The neuromuscular pharmacology of neostigmine in infants and children. *Anesthesiology* 59:220–225, 1983

20. Fisher DM, Cronelly R, Sharma M, et al: Clinical pharmacology of edrophonium in infants and children. *Anesthesiology* 61:428–433, 1984

21. Stanley TH, Webster LR: Anesthetic requirements and cardiovascular effects of fentanyl–oxygen and fentanyl–diazepam-oxygen anesthesia in man. *Anesth Analg* 57:411–416, 1978

22. Smith RM: *Anesthesia for Infants and Children* (ed 4). St. Louis, C.V. Mosby, 1980

23. Minckley BB: A study of noise and its relationship to patient discomfort in the recovery room. *Nurs Res* 17:247–250, 1968

24. Falk SA, Woods NS: Hospital noise levels and potential health hazards. *N Engl J Med* 289:774–780, 1973

25. Luczun ME: *Postanesthesia Nursing.* Rockville, MD, Aspen Publications, 1984, pp 169–185

26. Hartwell PN: Recovery room care. *Int Anesthiol Clin* 21:107–114, 1983

27. Andersen R, Krogh K: Pain as a major cause of postoperative nausea. *Can Anaesth Soc J* 24:366–369, 1976

28. Egbert LD, Battit GE, Welch CE, et al: Reduction of postoperative pain by encouragement and instruction of patients. *N Engl J Med* 270:825–827, 1964

29. Steward DJ: A trial of enflurane for paediatric outpatient anaesthesia. *Can Anaesth Soc J* 24:603–608, 1977

30. Abramowitz MD, Elder PT, Friendly DS, et al: Antiemetic effectiveness of intraoperatively administered droperidol in pediatric strabismic outpatient surgery. Preliminary report of a controlled study *J. Pediatr Opthalmol Strabismus* 18:22–27, 1981

31. Abramowitz MD, Oh TH, Epstein BS, et al: The antiemetic effect of droperidol following strabismus surgery in children. *Anesthesiology* 59:579–583, 1983

32. Patton CM: Rapid induction of acute dyskinesia by droperidol. *Anesthesiology* 43:126–127, 1975

33. Dupre LJ, Stieglitz P: Extrapyramidal syndromes after premedication with dropendol in children. *Br J Anaesth* 52:831–833, 1980

34. Koka BV, Jeon LS, Andre JM, et al: Postintubation croup in children. *Anesth Analg* 56:501–505, 1977

35. Steward DJ: Preterm infants are more prone to complications following minor surgery than are term infants. *Anesthesiology* 56:304–306, 1982

36. Liu LMP, Coté CJ, Goudsouzian NG, et al: Life threatening apnea in infants recovering from anesthesia. *Anesthesiology* 59:506–510, 1983

23

Pediatric Equipment

Daniel F. Dedrick
Charles J. Coté

BASIC EQUIPMENT FOR ANESTHESIA AND LIFE SUPPORT

OPERATING ROOM AIR CONDITIONING SYSTEMS

Although few think of the operating room as an item of equipment, it does provide the physical environment for the conduct of anesthesia, and may be compared to a huge infant incubator.[1] Either the warmth provided by the air conditioning in the winter or the cooling provided during the summer may be crucial for thermal stability. Temperature regulation is a more significant problem in the small child than in the adult due to the higher ratio of body-surface-area-to-body-mass. If the patient is a neonate or small infant, the room temperature should be warmer (24–27°C) than for an adult patient; this may be reduced somewhat once the patient is prepped and draped. Older children may have the room temperature progressively lowered toward 21–22°C as they reach the adult size. *Exposure* during anesthetic induction and surgical preparation *prior to draping* causes a significant thermal stress.[2–4]

SUCTION APPARATUS

As in the adult population, the presence of *functioning suction* apparatus *is mandatory prior to beginning any anesthetic* procedure. The device should be capable of regulated pressures. Suctioning the oropharynx may require a higher vacuum level than that necessary for endotracheal suction. Special circumstances may require the availability of an additional suction line; a child with esophageal atresia may need a separate suction dedicated solely to continuous drainage of the proximal pouch. We use 6.5 French suction catheters with a thumb-control side port for neonates, and 8 or 14 French "Oxygen Catheters" for older children. It is helpful to have

several sizes of suction catheters available because of the wide size range of pediatric patients. We routinely suction the stomach contents after induction of anesthesia; in larger patients, vented catheters may be more efficacious than unvented catheters. Tracheal suction should be gently performed with blunt tipped, well lubricated catheters. Additional suction equipment must also provide the capability of venting ("scavenging") waste anesthetic agents (see section below).

OPERATING TABLE

While not generally thought of as such, the operating table is a vital piece of *anesthesia* equipment. The table should provide readily available Trendelenberg controls, in case of either regurgitation or the need to increase venous return from the lower extremities. The table should allow for the full range of positioning for all anticipated surgical procedures. Several manufacturers offer special narrow tables for infant and neonatal surgery; these offer the advantage to the surgeon of proximity to the patient. The operating room table must also have appropriate padding to prevent patient contact with any metal support structures. Ability both to remove the head support and to lower the foot section can provide a smaller table for infants. For extremely long operative procedures, an alternating pressure air mattress placed between the patient and the operating table may help to guard against decubitus injuries. Periodically changing the position of the patient's head may be important in preventing bald spots as a result of prolonged contact pressure in one position.[5]

WARMING DEVICES

A hypothermic baby may become acidotic and apneic, may have slowed induction or awakening following anesthesia, and may have problems with reversal of neuromuscular block-

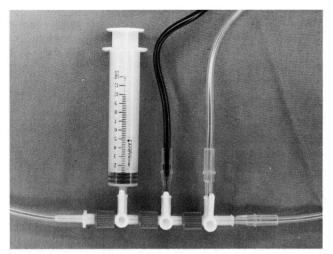

Figure 23-1. Multiple 3-way stopcocks allow syringe to be used to precisely administer blood, plasma, albumin, or other fluids.

ing drugs.[6–9] It cannot be emphasized enough that the operating room itself, via its air conditioning system, is an important factor in temperature regulation for all patients.[10] Other methods for reducing cold stress are presented below.

Radiant Warmers

Overhead radiant heating units with servo-temperature control are very useful. Because of the risk of skin burn, however, the servo-control sensor must be applied to the warmed skin and *should not measure body core temperature*.[11,12] A maximum skin temperature of 37°C should preclude surface burns from the radiant warmer. Not only must the radiant warmer be employed during the anesthetic setup time and surgical preparation, but also it should be brought back over the patient immediately as the drapes are removed at the end of the operative procedure. In the rush to move the patient to the recovery room or intensive care unit, one must not forget that exposure *at the end of the case* is as much of a thermal stress as exposure at the beginning. If infrared light bulbs are used, rather than direct infrared radiators, their red cast may make accurate evaluation of the patient's color difficult.

Warming Blankets

Circulating water mattresses have been shown to be useful in maintaining normothermia in patients with body surface area of less than a half square meter; in the normally developing child this is about ten kilograms body weight.[13] Above this weight limit, the decreasing ratio of body-surface-area-to-body-mass generally makes heat transfer at safe temperatures inefficient enough to minimize the benefit of this device. To avoid surface burns, the fluid temperature should never exceed 39°C, and must be monitored.[14] In addition, several layers of sheet should be interposed between the patient and the warming blanket to avoid direct contact.

Other Means for Minimizing Thermal Stress

Fluid Warmers. Most anesthesiologists accept the importance of warming intravenous fluids and blood products,

particularly during rapid infusion. The effectiveness of fluid warmers is dependent on the time IV fluids or blood products are in contact with the warmer.[15] There may also be a significant thermal stress from cystoscopy, wound irrigation, or antibiotic irrigation solutions.[16] All of these solutions should be warmed to body temperature, particularly prior to use in infants and neonates.

Heated Humidifiers. Heated humidifiers in the anesthetic circuit also may be a significant aid to maintaining thermal stability. Airstream warming and humidification may have its greatest value in cases with continuing thermal loss during the operation, as happens with exposed peritoneum or pleura.[17–22] The effects of these devices on the efficiency of the breathing circuit are considered in more detail below.

Wrapping. Any form of wrapping can reduce radiant and convective heat losses, thus reducing thermal stress.[23] Cotton wadding wrapped around extremities and plastic self-adhesive drapes have both been very effective for this purpose. Covering of an infant's head may be of particular value since the head represents such a large proportion of the body surface area. As with the other warming devices described above, there are hazards, particularly with plastic drapes.[24] The adhesive plastic drapes not only reduce conductive losses but also eliminate sweating as a mechanism of thermal regulation; hyperthermia may result.

EQUIPMENT FOR INTRAVENOUS THERAPY

It is necessary to have available the appropriate range of intravenous (IV) equipment for the patient population being anesthetized. It is our practice to establish IV access in all anesthestized patients. The only exception to this practice is the very short case where it will take longer to start the IV than to complete the surgery. In this situation an IV is set up ready for use should it be needed.

The size of the infusion bottle should not exceed the patient's estimated fluid deficit, unless a volume limiting device is interposed between the IV container and the patient. We generally employ an intravenous set with a micro drop outlet (50–60 drops/ml) until the adolescent size range is reached. The IV setup should also include easily accessible injection ports; often IV extension tubings are required when IV's are started in the foot. Air bubbles should be purged from all infusion sets prior to patient use.[25] In children with known intracardiac defects or arteriovenous malformation, the potential for paradoxical air emboli is always present, and in these circumstances intravenous air traps should be employed.[26] In the smallest patients, we terminate the intravenous line with a T-connector. This places a self-sealing port directly over the hub of the IV catheter, allowing the direct injection of drugs with minimal fluid dead space.

When carefully metered transfusion of colloid and/or blood is necessary, a multiple-stopcock manifold incorporated into the infusion line allows the main line to continue infusing maintenance fluid except during the actual administration of either blood or colloid (Figure 23-1). This manifold has an outlet to attach the blood administration set, another outlet to connect the colloid administration set, and a third outlet for a metering syringe. (Formulae employed to estimate fluid requirements and colloid and blood replacement needs are given in Chapters 10 and 11.)

Careful control of infusion rates may be facilitated by the use of infusion pumps or intravenous rate controllers. The infusion pump chosen for use in the pediatric patient must suit the circumstances. In most situations a device with precise volume limits, and air bubble and pressure alarms is the safest.

There are few well documented data concerning both the mechanical elements of intravenous infusion systems and the characteristics of the various fluids which are employed clinically. It has been clearly demonstrated that flow of crystalloid is not a simple linear function of perfusion pressure when using currently available types of infusion sets; the relationship is highly non-linear, best described as the quadratic model.[27]

$$P = R_L F + R_T F^2$$

where P = pressure, F = flow, R_L = resistance for laminar flow, and R_T = resistance for turbulent flow. Both the parameters R_L and R_T show a linear increase with the length of the tubing set, but certain elements of the IV systems have been shown to have isolated effects on one term or the other. A five micron filter will alter R_L; a check valve will significantly alter R_T.[27] The same investigators have subsequently shown that a similar quadratic function describes the pressure/flow relationship of intravenous cannulae.[28] They further found that the effects of the tubing set *add* to the effects of the cannula itself to determine the total flow resistance character of the complete administration set. These studies were done strictly with crystalloid, and show steep rises in resistance with increasing pressure in a very non-linear manner as smaller size cannulae are used (Figure 23-2, Table 23-1). The Abbot T-connector does not alter crystalloid flow up to driving pressures of 300 torr.[28]

The method of accelerating flow through an IV line is also a concern in emergency situations. Dula and his associates have shown that the pressure infusion cuff is the best method for increasing flow rates for bags of crystalloid, colloid, or blood components.[29] Next in order of efficacy were both the Abbott blood pump and a stop-cock and syringe arrangement. Gravity was the slowest method of infusion. Since we often use the syringe technique in pediatrics (primarily for metering), it is worth noting that it is similar in efficiency to the blood pump IV set. However, the pressure infusion cuff remains the fastest way to administer large volumes quickly in the resuscitation of the hypovolemic shock state.

The choice of fluid itself can make a major difference in the rate of infusion, primarily because of differences in viscosity. Crystalloid will pass most readily, followed by colloid, whole blood, and packed red blood cells. The present recommendation is for dilution of packed erythrocytes with normal saline.[30] Dilutions will not only increase the flow rate but also can decrease hemolysis of the red cells during rapid infusion. Questions remain about the clinical significance of this hemolysis, however; Eurenius and Smith have shown that even through a 26-gauge needle with a driving pressure of 300 torr, the plasma hemoglobin will increase only from the normal baseline of 22.3 mg/100 ml to 32.1 mg/100 ml in seven day old blood stored in citrate-phosphate-dextrose, CPD.[31] Their study showed a greater degree of hemolysis with larger-size IV cannulae.

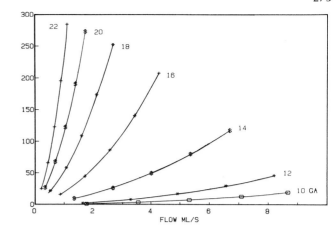

Figure 23-2. The pressure–flow relationship of intravenous catheters. Note that the pressure–flow relationship is non-linear. (Reproduced with permission BK Philip, JH Philip)

AIRWAY APPARATUS

Masks

The smaller the patient, the more important is the elimination of mechanical dead space. Rendell-Baker-Soucek masks were developed from molds of the facial contours of many children. They are designed to minimize mechanical dead space without the inflatable cuff or high dome usually seen in adult masks. The transparent plastic model is preferable to the classic black conductive rubber, since it allows observation of the patient's color and condensate from exhaled humidity with respiration. Vomiting may be seen under the mask.

Airways

Oral. A complete variety of oral airways must always be readily available. The infant has a relatively large tongue which easily obstructs the airway once consciousness is lost. If too large an airway is inserted, damage to laryngeal structures (traumatic epiglottis, uvular swelling) may result in postoperative airway obstruction.[32–34] Improperly inserted airways, by obstructing venous and lymphatic drainage, may also result in airway obstruction secondary to swelling of the tongue.[35–36] In general, a tongue blade is useful to help insert the airway without kinking the tongue or catching the tongue or lips between the airway and the teeth. The proper size airway may be estimated by comparing the artificial airway to the external anatomy of the patient (See Fig. 5-12).

Nasopharyngeal. Nasopharyngeal airways are not as frequently employed in pediatric patients because the internal diameter is often small, resulting in significantly increased work of breathing. In addition, adenoidal hypertrophy, so common in children, makes the child liable to bleeding following nasopharyngeal airway insertion. If such an airway is desired, a well lubricated endotracheal tube cut off at the appropriate length may be used.

Endotracheal Tubes

For the pediatric patient population, endotracheal tube sizes 2.5–6.0 mm internal diameter (ID), must be available, with appropriate sizes of stylettes. There are several methods for selecting the proper size endotracheal tube. (see Chapter 5). There may be considerable variability from one manufac-

Table 23-1

Flow Parameters of Isolated Devices

	IV Tubing	Catheter						
Gauge		10	12	14	16	18	20	22
Length (cm)		7.6	7.6	5.1	5.1	5.1	3.2	2.5
R_L	11.57	0.20	0.26	4.58	11.16	27.98	57.51	76.77
R_T	2.34	0.22	0.65	1.93	8.74	24.99	57.42	162.10

Unpublished data. (Reproduced with permission from BK Philip and JH Philip.)

turer to another in wall thickness, external diameter, kink resistance, direction and angle of bevel, as well as variation in endotracheal tube cuff length and thickness.[37] Despite these differences in endotracheal tube wall thickness, a first approximation for the correct endotracheal tube size for an *average* child older than two years is 4.5 mm ID + the patient's age/4.[38] A *full-term neonate* usually accepts a 3.0 or 3.5 mm ID tube, a normal one-year-old accepts a 3.5–4.0 ID tube, and a two-year-old accepts a 4.5–5.0 mm ID tube. One should always have at hand endotracheal tubes *at least* one half size larger *and* smaller than estimated in order to accomodate airway size variability. The only true test for appropriate size selection is a leak between 20 and 30 cm H_2O peak inflation pressure. The leak may easily be assessed by closing the circuit pop-off valve and slowly increasing the pressure by gently squeezing the anesthesia bag while listening over the larynx with a stethoscope.

It is important to remember that in the smaller child the cricoid ring is *narrower* than the glottic opening. A snug fitting tube may therefore result in edema formation and postoperative airway obstruction (post-intubation croup). We employ *uncuffed tubes* on elective cases until a 6 mm ID size is reached. Traditional teaching suggests that this is appropriate practice. However, this has not been confirmed on a scientific basis. Because the external diameter of a cuffed tube is larger, one must use a smaller ID tube for a given tracheal size, therefore resulting in a narrower airway and increased work of breathing. Cuffed endotracheal tubes are available down to 3.0 mm ID and may be appropriate for use in cases where the patient has very non-compliant lungs, a full stomach, or hiatus hernia with reflux. One must also realize that the endotracheal tube cuff pressure will increase during a nitrous-oxide-supplemented anesthetic due to diffusion of nitrous oxide into the cuff.[39] This may present a special additional hazard to children, where the cricoid ring is the narrowest portion of the larynx and unanticipated cuff pressure may result in mucosal swelling. Standard endotracheal tubes are implant-tested, Z-79 certified, disposable plastic.[40]

Molded preformed tubes are especially useful for head and neck surgery because they remove the anesthesia circuit connections from the surgical field.[41,42] Although the newer plastic tubes are fairly incompressible, when the possibility of excessive external pressure applied to the airway is anticipated, a tube with Tovell spiral wire reinforcement may be used. Its kink resistance is well known, but its additional wall thickness limits its applicability in smaller patients. This spiral spring-like construction has resulted in it "popping" out of the airway; in addition, repeated improper sterilization may lead to bubble formation within the rubber, which can lead to airway obstruction when used with nitrous oxide.[43] The use of

Cole tubes should be abandoned; because of the tapered configuration, they tend to serve as a laryngeal wedge. Significant damage to the larynx and cricoid cartilage has been observed following their use.[44] The difference in flow resistance from non-tapered tubes, said to be their principal advantage, is not clinically significant, especially with assisted or controlled ventilation. There is, however, a significant increase in resistance with Cole tubes of 2.5 mm ID or smaller.[45,46]

The recent use of the carbon dioxide laser beam for the treatment of laryngeal polyposis has introduced the problem of ignition of the endotracheal tube. Protection of the endotracheal tube surface with aluminum foil or wet sponges, as well as the use of red rubber endotracheal tubes which have a much lower ignition potential, will decrease this hazard. Avoidance of high levels (75%) of oxygen and nitrous oxide, which both support combustion, will also diminish the risks of fire.[47]

INTUBATION EQUIPMENT

Routine Equipment

Intubation equipment must also suit all sizes of pediatric patients. Magill forceps are available in two pediatric sizes. Laryngoscopes are available with lightweight small handles and a full range of blades. Generally a straight blade design is better in smaller children, infants, and neonates because of the higher position of the larynx within the neck. (See Chapter 5) A straight blade may be used in children as one would use a curved blade in an adult, i.e., displacing the epiglottis by lifting the base of the tongue at the vallecula, rather than by directly picking up the epiglottis with the tip of the blade. A special laryngoscope called the Oxyscope,* which incorporates a small-bore oxygen delivery tube, has been demonstrated to reduce significantly the incidence of cyanosis and bradycardia in neonates should laryngoscopy be prolonged (Fig. 5-14).[48]

Special Equipment

There are occasional difficult airways that may require special intubation equipment. Both flexible and rigid fiberoptic laryngoscopes are available for the pediatric population. They may be employed essentially as "optical stylets" over which an endotracheal tube may be passed.[49–51] The rigid device demands a straight-line approach to the airway. The external diameter of most presently available fiberoptic equip-

---

* Puritan-Bennett Corp., Foregger Medical Division, Langhorne, PA

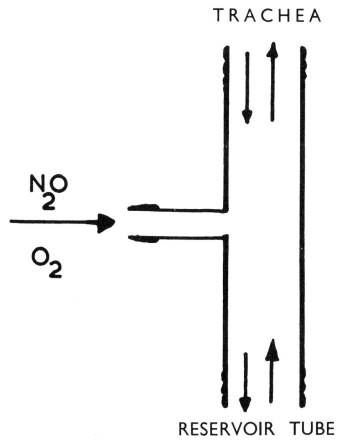

TRACHEA

N₂O

O₂

RESERVOIR TUBE

Figure 23-3. The T-piece as described by Ayre. (Reproduced with permission from Ayre P: The T-piece technique. *Br J Anaesth* 28:520–523, 1956.)

ment is quite large, and therefore such devices will only pass through larger endotracheal tubes. The marketplace may soon provide smaller diameter units. In addition, such equipment should only be used by an experienced individual, especially when approaching a difficult airway problem.

THE ANESTHESIA MACHINE AND ITS APPENDAGES

Anesthesia Machine

While many pediatric patients may be anesthetized with standard adult machinery, anesthesia machines customized for pediatric use are of great value. In addition to the usual flow meters and vaporizers, they incorporate a cylinder yoke and a flow meter for air. Premature infants are at risk for retrolental fibroplasia, and hyperoxia *may* be a contributing risk factor.[52] Furthermore, expansion of the bowel caused by diffusion of nitrous oxide into gas-containing loops *may* present the surgeon with a proportionately more difficult problem in small children than in adults.[53] In cases where there are contraindications to the use of nitrous oxide, air can be blended into the circuit to titrate the inspired oxygen concentration. An in-line oxygen analyzer is indicated in order to use an air–oxygen blend safely.

Scavenger

The waste anesthetic gas scavenging system used for the pediatric machine must be carefully designed to eliminate the application of either negative or positive pressure to the patient. Unless the system is able to open to the atmosphere by either a "tube within a tube" or a negative pressure relief valve design, the wall suction may vent vital oxygen and anesthetic gases from the circuit and patient.[54–56]

Circuits

A full spectrum of anesthetic circuits, varying with the size of the patient, must be available. Adolescents and older children may be anesthetized with a standard adult semiclosed circle absorber system, perhaps with the substitution of a smaller rebreathing bag. Younger children may be anesthetized with the circuit modified by replacement of the hoses with small-sized "pediatric" tubing, and by substituting a smaller rebreathing bag.[57] Infants and neonates (10 kg or less) may be anesthetized with non-rebreathing systems, such as the Mapleson D variety. Mapleson D systems do not have directional valves or a carbon dioxide absorber; this eliminates the resistance intrinsic to the opening pressure of circuit valves and to turbulent flow through soda lime.[58]

The work of breathing is particularly important for infants and children, and thus most pediatric circuits and masks are designed to eliminate both dead space and resistance. The classic example of such as a system is the Ayre's T-piece; with this circuit there are no valves or reservoir bags (Figure 23-3).[59] Later modifications include changes of the T-piece and expiratory limb.[60] The Jackson-Rees modification involves the addition of a respiratory reservoir (bag) to the expiratory limb.[61] The most popular pediatric system is the Magill and its various modifications, Mapleson A–E (Figure 23-4).[62] These systems each consist of fresh gas flow into the circuit, a reservoir bag, a pressure-relief (pop-off) valve, tubing of varying lengths connecting all of the above, and an adaptor for the mask or endotracheal tube. Each of these has advantages and disadvantages which are well reviewed elsewhere.[63] The Mapleson D variety is the most commonly used today because of its safety and versatility with controlled or spontaneous ventilation.[58] The pop-off valve is at the end of the expiratory limb, just prior to the reservoir bag; thus fresh gas washes alveolar gas out of the expiratory limb during expiration. The efficiency of this wash out (to prevent rebreathing) is dependent on the volume of the expiratory limb, the fresh gas flow, and the size of the tidal volume.[63] Larger patients (heavier than 15 kg) require high fresh gas flow rates to prevent rebreathing; up to 20 l/min may be required in adults.[64,65] The advantages of minimal dead space and low resistance to flow are counter-balanced by the disadvantages of heat and humidity lost to the anesthetic gases and significant waste of anesthetic agents because of the high flows required.[63]

Humidifiers

A heated humidifier is necessary in order to maintain body temperature and to prevent drying of secretions whenever a non-rebreathing circuit is used.[66,67] This, in turn, may lead to other problems, such as additional connections that may leak or become disconnected, "rainout" from humidified gas (resulting in water collection within the circuit), resistance to gas flow, and bubbling noises which distract from the ability to auscultate heart tones and breath sounds. Inhalation of hot anesthetic gases may result in "hot pot tracheitis;" this can be

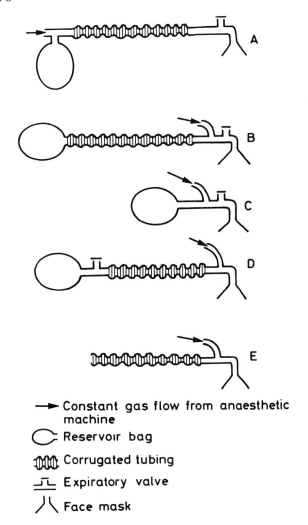

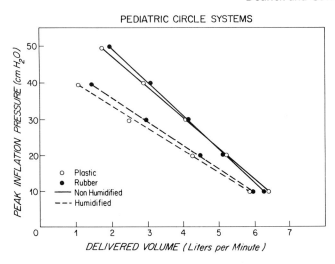

Figure 23-5. When a humidifier is added to the circuit, a significant reduction in delivered minute ventilation occurs secondary to increased compression volume (broken lines v. solid lines). This must be compensated with increased minute ventilation. (Reproduced with permission from Coté CJ et al: Wasted ventilation measured in vitro with eight anesthetic circuits used on children with and without inline humidification. *Anesthesiology* 59:442–446, 1983.)

Figure 23-4. The Mapleson categories of breathing circuits. The most commonly used circuit for infants is the Mapleson D configuration. (Reproduced with permission from Mapleson WW: The elimination of rebreathing in various semi-closed anaesthetic systems. *Br J Anaesth* 26:323–332, 1954.)

avoided by monitoring inspired gas temperature just proximal to the mask or endotracheal tube.[68]

A heated humidifier helps to maintain body temperature with adult pediatric circle systems as well as with non-rebreathing systems.[17–20] Whenever a heated humidifier is added, the extra gas-containing volume of the tubing and humidifier increase the total volume of the anesthetic circuit.[69] This in turn increases both the volume of gas that can be compressed and the length of compliant tubing that can stretch during controlled positive-pressure ventilation. This may result in clinically important reductions in delivered minute ventilation, particularly if the humidifier is added after the anesthesia ventilator has been adjusted and no further compensation has been made for the increased compression volume and compliance losses. The addition of a heated humidifier decreases the efficiency of all anesthetic circuits to which they are applied (Figure 23-5). The degree to which anesthetic circuit efficiency is affected depends upon the gas-containing volume of the humidifier and the distensibility of the tubing used. Thus, highly compliant adult rubber tubing

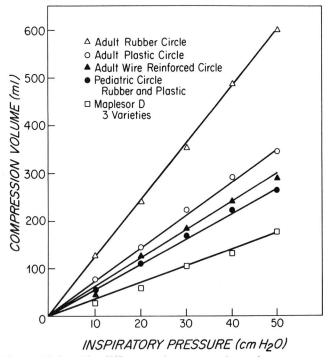

Figure 23-6. The differences in compression volumes among five anesthetic circuits. The Mapleson D systems are the most efficient with the lowest compression volume, whereas the adult rubber circle system has the highest compression volume and is the least efficient circuit. (Reproduced with permission from Coté CJ et al: Wasted ventilation measured in vitro with eight anesthetic circuits used on children with and without inline humidification. *Anesthesiology* 59:442–446, 1983.)

will have greater adverse effects than wire-reinforced, small-diameter tubing (Figure 23-6).[69]

Our practice at present is to use plastic disposable Mapleson D circuits with a humidifier for children weighing ten kilograms or less, pediatric wire-reinforced circle systems with a humidifier for children weighing 10–30 kilograms, and adult wire-reinforced circle systems for children heavier than 30 kilograms.

ANESTHESIA VENTILATORS

Nearly any adult volume ventilator may be used in pediatric patients by making appropriate adjustments in the respiratory rate, fresh gas flow, tidal volume, and inspiratory-to-expiratory time ratio. However, ventilators designed specifically for pediatric use are preferable. Our practice emphasizes the value of manual bag ventilation for teaching purposes; this provides immediate feedback regarding patient lung compliance or problems with the circuit (e.g., kinked tube, disconnections). However, under specific circumstances the use of a ventilator provides valuable assistance by freeing the anesthesiologist's hands for other tasks. *Whenever the immediate hand-bag feedback is given up for the convenience of a mechanical ventilator, a disconnect/apnea alarm system should be used as an aid to vigilance.*

Whenever a ventilator is used, one must understand what effects alterations in fresh gas flow may have on delivered ventilation. *For most ventilators used in the operating room, fresh gas flow into the circuit is added to the ventilator output during the inspiratory time*; this augmentation effect may result in potentially serious errors in calculating delivered minute ventilation ($\dot{V}E$), especially during use on infants and small children. This is exemplified by the following examples.

An *adult* patient with $\dot{V}E$ of 7 l/min, I:E ratio of 1:2, and fresh gas flow of 6 l/min. If there were no compliance or compression volume losses, the patient would receive 7 l/min + (1/3 × 6 l/min) = 9 l/min. If the fresh gas flow were reduced to 3 l/min, the patient would receive 7 l/min + (1/3 × 3 l/min) = 8 l/min. This is a change of about *11%*.

A *pediatric* patient with $\dot{V}E$ of 2 L/min, I:E ratio of 1:2, and fresh gas flow of 6 l/min. Again, assuming no compression or compliance volume losses, the patient would receive 2 l/min + (1/3 × 6 l/min) = 4 l/min. If the fresh gas flow was now reduced to 3 l/min the patient would receive 2 l/min + (1/3 × 3 l/min) = 3 l/min. This is a *25%* change in delivered minute ventilation (Figure 23-7).

Thus, whenever a change is made in fresh gas flow for *any* circuit used in children, the adequacy of chest expansion, breath sounds, and peak inspiratory pressure must each be reevaluated. If this is not done, serious, potentially life-threatening alterations in delivered ventilation may result.

EQUIPMENT CART

Because of the wide range of sizes of so many different items necessary to care for the full spectrum of pediatric patients, we find it advantageous to use mobile, multi-drawer carts. The various drawers should be organized for ease of use: *separate* airway equipment, drugs, intravenous supplies, monitoring equipment, and so forth, each in an appropriately labeled drawer. Since pediatric anesthesia in our hospital is often administered outside of the main operating room suite (e.g., radiology, radiation therapy, cardiac catheterization laboratory), these mobile carts simplify the safe practice of anesthesia for children and guarantee the availability of all the

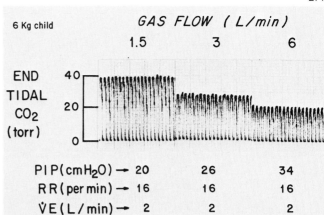

Figure 23-7. Changes in delivered minute ventilation using a pediatric circle system, as reflected by end-tidal carbon dioxide measurement, in a 6 kg child on a pediatric, electronically controlled ventilator. The only change made was in fresh gas flow. Note the near halving of end-expired CO_2 when fresh gas flow was increased from 1.5 l/min to 6 l/min. Whenever a change is made in fresh gas flow during controlled ventilation new ventilatory settings must be determined.

necessary equipment even outside of the operating room. A list of the equipment and drugs which we stock in our carts is provided in Table 23-2.

DEFIBRILLATOR

Every anesthetizing location should be equipped with a D-C defibrillator. It is not necessary to have a unit specifically for pediatrics, as long as the energy range may be adjusted to the appropriate levels (2 watt sec/kg) and a set of pediatric paddles is kept with the device. Ideally, the design should incorporate all controls in the paddles, facilitating use without leaving the patient. Another desirable feature is a sensing circuit, providing the capacity for synchronous defibrillation, should that be needed.

MONITORING EQUIPMENT

ROUTINE MONITORING FOR THE HEALTHY CHILD

Chart

Besides its obvious role as a medical–legal document, the anesthetic record can be a very important monitor. Proper recording of the patient's status upon arrival in the operating room encourages evaluation of the effects of any premedication, confirmation of NPO status, weight, and fluid balance. Careful logging of intraoperative fluid administration and losses allows assessment of the patient's replacement needs. *Concurrent* charting of the patient's vital signs and anesthetic drug administration allows correlations to be made, and encourages trend analysis. Many changes that are too subtle to interpret on a moment-to-moment basis become obvious when plotted out over time. In addition, a numbering system correlating events with time on the anesthesia record documents the sequence of anesthetic management and may prove very useful should a medicolegal case arise (Figure 23-8).

Table 23-2

Pediatric Equipment Cart Inventory

Drawer 1
Laryngoscope handles (functioning)
Laryngoscope blades (functioning)

Miller	Macintosh	Wis-Hipple
0 (1)	1 (2)	1½ (2)
1 (2)	2 (2)	
2 (2)	3 (1)	
3 (1)		

Magill Forceps, 1 pediatric, 1 adult, Tape 1″ (4), ½″ water proof tape (4), Penrose Drains 4 each ¾″ & ¼″ (for tourniquets), Scissors, Flashlight.

Drawer 2
Masks: #3 (3), #2 (4), #1 (3), #0 (3)
Airways: #3 (5), #2 (5), #1 (5), #000 (5)

Drawer 3
Gauze Sponges (sterile and non-sterile), Double-stick discs, rubber bands, bandaids, alcohol swabs, antibiotic ointment, water soluble surgical lubricant, Lidocaine ointment 5%, Bulldog clips, safety pins, corneal lubricant, pedi blood tubes (blue, red, purple, and green), neuro eye patches.

Drawer 4
Adult sodium bicarbonate (2), pediatric sodium bicarbonate 8.4% (2), infant sodium bicarbonate 4.2% (2), cardiac lidocaine 100 mg (2), dextrose 50% (1), mannitol 25% (1), diphenhydramine 50 mg (2), potassium chloride 20 mEq (1), hydrocortisone 100 mg (2), calcium chloride 10% (4), sterile water, methohexital sodium 500 mg (8), lidocaine 1.0% (5), phenylephrine (5), prostigmine:1:2000 (10), ephedrine (5), atropine (10), isoproteronol (2), furosemide (3), epinephrine 1:1000 (10), succinylcholine (1), curare (1), dexamethasone 4 mg/ml (2), dopamine (2).

Drawer 5
Pediatric uncuffed endotracheal tubes: #2.5 (6), #3.0 (6), #3.5 (5), #4.0 (6), #4.5 (6), #5.0 (6), #5.5 (6), #6.0 (6), Adult cuffed endotracheal tubes: 2 each of #6.0, #6.5, #7.0, stylettes in a variety of appropriate sizes.

Drawer 6
Pediatric esophageal stethoscope (6), adult ECG pads (10), pediatric ECG pads (10), #6.5 suction catheters (6), oxygen catheters (20) 10 of each size 8F & 14F.

Drawer 7
Syringes: 12cc (10), 6cc (10), 3cc 22GA (20), 3cc 25GA (20), 1cc 27GA (20), 1cc insulin (10).
Needles: 15GA 1½″, 19GA 1½″, 20GA 1½″, 25GA ⅜.
Butterfly: 23GA, 25GA (10).

Drawer 8
Medicut 22GA, 20GA, 18GA, Angiocath 22GA 1″, 20GA 1½″, 18GA, 24G Cathalon
Pedi IV Boards—2 sizes (4), T-connectors, 3 way stopcocks.

Drawer 9
Pedi IV Sets (6), pediatric metriset (2), IV extension sets (10), 250 ml D_5LR (4), lactated ringer's solution 250 ml (6), air trap filters, head strap, blood pressure cuffs (2 each size), 1 adult size with stethoscope, oximeter sensors.

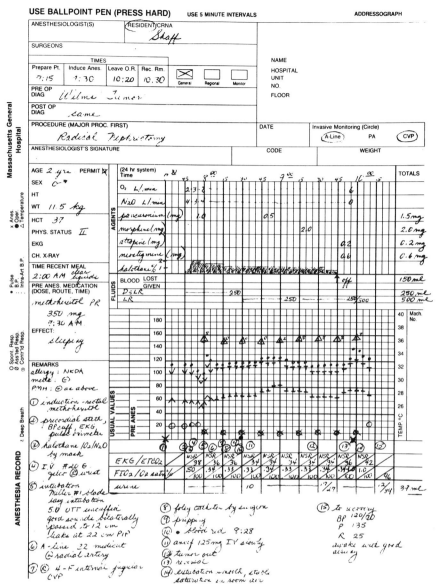

Figure 23-8. Typical anesthetic record with numbering system to correlate events with time.

Precordial/Esophageal Stethoscope

If one were only allowed a single monitoring device, a stethoscope would be it. In the infant, neonate and small child, the experienced ear can easily diagnose many arrhythmias, assess cardiac output, and estimate blood pressure, all without interference from electrocautery or other electrical artifacts that can confound elaborate electronic monitors. In addition, one can also auscultate for pulmonary gas entry. The precordial stethoscope we use is generally a weighted metal bell device, with its location stabilized by a double adhesive disc. For certain specialized needs, such as bronchography or angiography, a plastic stethoscope which is not radiopaque may be used. Before the adhesive disc is applied, we generally listen to find the optimal site where both heart tones and breath sounds can be heard. Usually this is at the apex of the heart, but occasionally the suprasternal notch provides better listening conditions. The latter position may be better during induction and emergence, since airway information may more readily be obtained.

Whenever a patient has been intubated, the precordial stethoscope may be exchanged for an esophageal. These are available in both pediatric and adult sizes; the pediatric size may be introduced atraumatically even in newborns. The less expensive adult variety is often usable in children age six or older. Commercially available disposable esophageal stethoscopes are now marketed which incorporate a thermistor, allowing the introduction of two monitors at once. One possible relative contraindication to esophageal stethoscopes is use during a pediatric tracheostomy. Misidentification of the esophageal stethoscope as an endotracheal tube has resulted in the surgeon opening the esophagus. In this circumstance, *either* the stethoscope should not be used, *or* the surgeon must be clearly informed that *two* stiff tubes pass through the neck structures, since this complication has occurred even in the hands of very experienced surgeons.[70]

The only major defect of a stethoscope as a monitor is that it provides information only when it is connected to the anesthesiologist. Custom-molded ear pieces, which better exclude room noises, are much more effective and more comfortable to wear than the conventional binaural stethoscope. These special ear pieces have the added advantage of leaving the other ear open for communication with the surgeon and ancillary personnel.

Blood Pressure Devices

Blood pressure measurement is as useful in children as in adults, and must be followed in every patient. Hypovolemia and anesthetic depth may be assessed just as in adults. An appropriate size of blood pressure cuff should be applied to the arm or thigh, covering approximately two-thirds of the length of the upper arm or thigh. The bladder should rest over the artery chosen for monitoring. In adolescents and older children, a stethoscope may be secured over the artery to listen for Korotkoff's sounds. In smaller children, one may use the flicker of the needle in an aneroid sphygmomanometer dial as an indicator of systolic pressure; with experience, one may estimate diastolic pressure as well.[71] When this flicker is not clearly readable, a distal pulse sensor is needed. This can be either a photoelectric plethysmograph over a digit, looking for return of the signal as the cuff is deflated, or a Doppler flow detector positioned over a distal artery.[72] The Infrasonde device and several electronic oscillometer units (Dinamap, Century, and others) offer convenient alternatives. These monitors are available with automatic time cycling. Remember that the cuff chosen must be of the appropriate size and properly located if one is to obtain accurate data from any of these instruments.[73–75] If one of these automatic devices is utilized, it is mandatory that proper application, function and adequate deflation time be assured; venous stasis, petechiae, and nerve compression damage are possible.[76] In addition, a factiously low blood pressure and heart rate may result from malfunctioning automated devices that have microprocessors which reset to "atmospheric" when residual pressure is left in the cuff; the residual pressure in the cuff is interpreted as atmospheric pressure and also interferes with pulse amplitude. Therefore heart rate and blood pressure determination are lower than they should be.[77] The oscillotonometer may also be useful in children. Care to apply an appropriate size of cuff, and to use proper technique, will result in accurate blood pressure determination.[78]

Electrocardiograph

Although many arrhythmias may be diagnosed by careful attention to the heart sounds conducted via the precordial or esophageal stethoscope, the electrocardiogram is still a mandatory monitor. In the healthy child, lead placement may differ from that selected for adults, since the principal need is for diagnosis and resolution of arrhythmias, rather than the detection of ischemia; this may not be true in cardiac surgery. With the greater right heart predominance in the younger ages, a cross chest lead generally provides the optimal combination of atrial and ventricular voltage signals. A QRS detector with beeper is a useful accessory, particularly when vagal stresses are applied to the patient. Most newer monitors incorporate either a cardiotachygraph based on the QRS detector, or a triggered sweep on the oscilloscope face for readout of the heart rate with a calibrated scale. A built-in lead fault detector is also useful to check the cables and patient leads themselves when a poor signal is obtained. We employ standard adult disposable electrodes on older children, reserving the much more expensive pediatric size for infants and neonates. Cleaning, gently abrading, and defatting the skin

with an alcohol wipe can improve the contact. Tincture of benzoin may also help to maintain good adhesion in areas near surgical prep solutions. Care must be taken to isolate the leads from the electrocautery dispersive electrode to avoid electrical burns.[79,80]

Oxygen Monitor

Monitoring of the inspired oxygen concentration is now mandated medicolegally in some states.[81] In neonates, especially the premature, one must be alert to the possible ocular toxicity of high arterial oxygen tensions resulting from high inspired-oxygen concentrations.[82] In all patients, oxygen monitoring can help prevent hypoxemia. Remember that the standard, so-called "fail safe" device built into most anesthesia machines is keyed only to *pressure* in the oxygen line; should the oxygen *flow* be turned off, the patient may receive an hypoxic mixture without warning from the alarm. An oxygen monitor on the inspiratory limb would show the oxygen decline, and provide an accurate alarm. With the more frequent use of closed-circuit anesthesia and air–oxygen blends, oxygen monitoring assumes even greater importance.[81] Since prolonged exposure to greater than 50 percent inspired oxygen can cause pulmonary damage, beginning with impaired mucociliary function, a high as well as a low level alarm on the monitor is desirable.[83] This equipment should be calibrated prior to each use and alarm limits set for each case; by setting a narrow band of alarm limits, early detection of changes in gas flow is possible.

Temperature Monitor

Although there is medicolegal pressure in some jurisdictions to monitor temperature in every patient because of the danger of malignant hyperthermia (MH), we feel that temperature monitoring is mandated by other patient care needs. *Hypothermia* is much more common in the operating room than hyperthermia, and may be associated with acidosis, myocardial irritability, respiratory depression, greater absorption of inhalation agents, and delayed emergence from anesthesia.[2,3,6–9]

The choice of monitoring site depends on the nature of the anesthetic course and associated surgical procedure. Most of our mask anesthetics are monitored either with rectal, tympanic, or axillary probes. The rectal probe is less accurate and subject to cooling during urologic or major peritoneal surgical procedures. The tympanic probe accurately reflects core temperature, but if improperly inserted may injure the tympanic membrane.[84,85] The axillary temperature monitor is only a trend monitor and not a core measurement. A well placed axillary thermistor (positioned high in the axilla with the arm adducted, preferably an arm without an IV) will generally track the body temperature well, except in severe shock states, when it trails by about 1–1.5°C below true core temperature.[86]

When patients have been intubated, we usually employ either tympanic or esophageal thermistors. Occasionally we will use a nasopharyngeal probe. An esophageal probe may be influenced by the gas stream in the trachea, so for accuracy it must be placed near the great vessels or the heart (two thirds the length of the esophagus). A nasopharyngeal probe very nearly reflects core temperature, but may induce epistaxis when inserted. A newer device, based on liquid crystal displays, called the TempAStrip, is intended for placement over the forehead, using its own adhesive backing.[87] This is only a crude trend monitor and may in fact be inadequate for

Table 23-3

Temperature Probes

Temperature Probe Location	How to Insert	Advantages	Disadvantages
Axillary	High in axilla with arm closely adducted	Ease of insertion Noninvasive	Easy to dislodge Trend monitor only (not true core temperture) May be influenced by IV fluid therapy in ipsilateral arm
Rectal	Insert with disposable cover sleeve (well lubricated past rectal sphincter)	Ease of insertion	May cause bleeding May be influenced by peritoneal cooling or bladder cooling May cause bacteremia
Nasopharyngeal	Insert to the depth equal to the distance between the nose and external auditory canal (well lubricated)	Ease of insertion Accurate core temperature monitor	May cause epistaxis May cause bacteremia
Esophageal	Insert to a depth $\frac{2}{3}$ the length of the esophagus	Ease of insertion Accurate core temperature	May be influenced by tracheal temperature Esophageal perforation
Tympanic	Gently insert probe into external auditory meatus	Most accurate core monitor	Expensive Contraindicated with external otitis or otitis media May cause damage to tympanic membranes if improperly inserted
Skin	Place liquid crystal strip on forehead	Ease of placement	Inaccurate monitor Expensive

intraoperative monitoring.[88] The advantages and disadvantages of most temperature monitoring devices are presented in Table 23-3.

Blood Loss Monitoring

While *close observation of the surgical field* is the best single monitor, two ancillary devices may help. We place a small volume trap on the suction line prior to the major evacuation trap. This mini-trap is arranged so that the outlet leading to the large suction bottle is at the top allowing emptying into the main container by inverting the mini-trap (Figure 23-9). This is particularly useful for cases involving a fluid-filled organ, such as the bladder, since it can be "re-zeroed" by dumping the mini-trap; it is also helpful when caring for infants or small children. We routinely weigh surgical sponges on a dietary scale, making the approximation that one gram is equivalent to one milliliter of blood. Greatest accuracy is obtained by immediate weighing as the sponges come off the surgical field, thus minimizing evaporative losses. However, the ultimate determinant of blood loss is the patient's physiological response.

Neuromuscular Transmission Monitoring

Measuring the indirectly elicited twitch response is indicated when neuromuscular blocking agents are employed. The most helpful clinical monitor during the use of non-depolarizing competitive blockers is the train-of-four instrument; this is available from several manufacturers. The train-of-four does not require any recording capability or baseline, since it works strictly by comparison with its own internal standard, the first twitch.[89,90] The unit may also be used with depolarizing relaxants, looking instead only at first twitch amplitude. If there is a significant decrement (greater than 50%) between the first and fourth twitch in this context, it suggests phase two blockade (this is discussed further in Chapter 9).[91]

We do not employ needle electrodes, since they are more hazardous to the patient. They may cause bleeding, infection, burns, or nerve injury. Current density may be very high due to the limited contact surface and due to resistance of surrounding skin. Self-adhesive electrodes designed specifically for twitch monitors are available, but they are unnecessary, expensive, and tend to be too large for infants and small children. In these small patients, our usual alternative is a pair of infant-size EKG electrodes.

The choice of monitoring location depends upon the nature of the surgery. One may choose any site where a motor nerve is close to the body surface and its associated muscle group is available for observation. The most common stimulation site in our practice is the ulnar nerve in the forearm, observing the thumb (adductor pollicis brevis). This is the

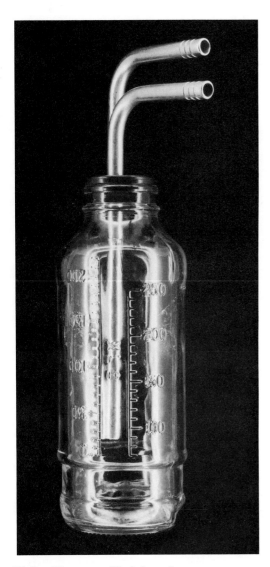

Figure 23-9.   The type of "mini trap" we use more accurately to quantitate suctioned blood losses. It consists of an empty IV bottle with inlet and outlet connections. One goes to larger wall suction bottles, the other to patient suction. With frequent emptying one can separate irrigation fluid from actual blood losses.

standard site for most research reports. Using the facial nerve may result in *false positive* responses, since the muscles may easily be stimulated directly. We switch the power off between readings to avoid possible injury secondary to prolonged, repetitive exposure to electrical current.

ADVANCED MONITORING TECHNIQUES

Invasive Blood Pressure

When clinically indicated, even in healthy patients, one should insert the proper cannulae for arterial, right atrial, or pulmonary arterial pressure monitoring. Properly inserted by percutaneous or open approaches, these lines are all of relatively low risk to the patient.

Percutaneous arterial cannulation is performed with a

22–24-gauge catheter-over-needle device in infants, neonates, and small children, with a 20-gauge device in older children (see Chapter 24).[92] Central venous and pulmonary artery cannulation are usually achieved using the Seldinger technique.[93,94] The proper reference location for all pressure transducers is usually the level of the patient's right atrium. If intracranial pressure monitoring is also employed, many practitioners prefer to use a reference zero position at some easily reproducible *cranial* site (e.g., the external ear canal) to facilitate the estimation of cerebral perfusion pressure. In cases with moderate blood loss or small circulatory alterations, an oscilloscopic display is adequate. In more difficult cases, however, the addition of a multi-channel recording polygraph capable of slow paper speed assists in trend analysis. Because of the limitations inherent in monitor electronics, *digital* display systems may occasionally give erroneous pressure readings.

Placement of any of these invasive monitors provides additional benefits other than direct hemodynamic monitoring. Serial pH and arterial blood gas tension measurements from an arterial line, or serial chemistries, glucose, hematocrits, and osmolalities, through either an arterial, venous or pulmonary artery line, allow continual assessment of the complex patient. "Mixed venous" sampling from the pulmonary arterial catheter yields a measure of oxygen extraction. Cardiac output may be determined by Fick, thermodilution, or dye dilution techniques with appropriate catheters. Furthermore, in cases performed in the sitting position, a right atrial catheter provides an approach to therapy for air embolism (see Chapter 17).

Disconnect/Apnea Alarms

Whenever a ventilator is employed during anesthesia, the tactile feedback from the rebreathing bag is lost. We feel that a disconnect alarm is then mandatory. Most newer anesthesia ventilators incorporate such a monitor, but it may be bought as a separate add-on item for older designs. These monitors generally sense time cycling of pressure events. *Most of these alarms will detect complete ventilator disconnects but may not be sensitive enough to detect extubations with small endotracheal tubes or partial circuit disconnects because of the continued presence of flow resistance.* Other types of alarms, such as heat-sensing devices or capnographs, can provide more reliable means of detecting both inadequate ventilation and accidental extubation.

Besides the sensing of pressure *cycles*, many newer monitors include detection ability to alarm on very *high pressure*, *continuous* positive pressure, and *negative* pressure. Some products include automatic switch-on when shifting from hand ventilation to machine, thereby avoiding failure to monitor. While these devices are not perfect substitutes for the educated hand, they do provide much of the information given up by the use of ventilators.

Apnea monitors, whether based on transthoracic impedance, motion, or other patient parameters, are mandatory in both the perioperative and recovery room phases for any prematurely born infant under 50 weeks conceptual age with a *history* of apnea spells, or any child with *ongoing* spells. Even if the patient has had a period of some months with a normal respiratory pattern at home, the anesthetic state may bring about a temporary return of apnea spells.[95,96]

Volume Meter/Spirometer

In some instances, it may be desirable to follow a patient's respiratory gas exchange. Either a Wright turbine respirometer or Drager positive displacement spirometer may be employed. In addition, newer designs based on either the pneumotachygraph operating principle, vortex detectors, or thermistor flow meters, are available. Our practice ordinarily is only to use spirometers as a secondary check on controlled ventilation. Most of these devices are fairly inaccurate at the very low flows an infant might be able to generate.[97]

Inspiratory Pressure Gauge

In patients with the need for ventilatory assistance, a precise pressure gauge applied *at the airway* can help to minimize barotrauma. When using the adult circle absorber system or a ventilator, the gauges built into these devices are remote from the airway and may therefore be inaccurate. Airway pressure should ideally be measured as close to the endotracheal tube as possible. Clearly, infants requiring PEEP or CPAP are more accurately managed with pressure monitoring close to the airway.

Urinary Catheter

Aseptically inserted, a catheter in the bladder connected to a closed drainage system is of little risk to the patient. Urine output is as useful in the operating room as in the intensive care unit as an indicator of volume and perfusion status. Also, the presence of hematuria or hemoglobinuria can aid in the diagnosis of surgical trauma to the urinary system, bleeding dyscrasia, or major transfusion reaction.

Some of the indications for a urinary catheter include massive fluid shifts, prolonged radiologic procedures with large doses of contrast material, prolonged surgical procedures, neurosurgical procedures with osmotic diuretic therapy, and urinary reconstructive procedures. In most children the urinary catheter is inserted after the induction of anesthesia. In infants the usual urinary catheter might be difficult to insert; a feeding tube works well. Since the urine output is small in these infants, connecting a feeding tube to a syringe will provide an adequate system for measurement. Obviously the urinary catheter should be in an area near the anesthesiologist so the output can be closely followed. As a general rule, the minimum acceptable urinary output in a child is 0.5–1.0 ml/kg/hr. This is especially important in the infant where the concentrating ability of the kidney is limited to about 700 mosmol/l compared to 1,200 mosmol/l in the older child and adult.

Carbon Dioxide Analyzers

The most commonly used gas analyzer in our anesthetic practice is the quantitative expired carbon dioxide analyzer. It is particularly useful in teaching ventilation and airway management to resident physicians and student nurse-anesthetists, provided the response time of the instrument is rapid enough to accurately reflect *end-expired* carbon dioxide tension.[98] These monitors are generally made in either of two configurations, one where the expired gas is suctioned from the anesthesia circuit (side stream sampler), and the other a mainstream airway cuvette optical sensor; both types are infrared analyzers. Measurement of expired carbon dioxide tensions can be an essential monitoring tool in patients operated upon in any position where air embolism may occur. Clinically significant air embolism will cause a transient change

in carbon dioxide excretion because the lung tissue is ventilated but not perfused. In addition, with quantitative measurement any change in circuit flows, disconnections, tube kinks, or extubations may be detected. The early diagnosis of malignant hyperpyrexia and the adequacy of its therapy may also be made.[99] In critically ill neonates or hypermetabolic burned children, ventilatory requirements may be as high as 4.3 times normal, and therefore a rapid means of assessing adequacy of ventilation is extremely helpful.[100] Peak carbon dioxide sensors are especially useful when narrow limits to carbon dioxide (low or high) are set. A capnograph with recorder is even more useful, since the carbon dioxide wave form may help in diagnosing events other than those directly related to the airway.

Anesthetic Gas Analyzers

Anesthetic gas analyzers range from the simple to the complex. The most basic design is the Drager Narkotest elastomeric sensor; this is no longer on the market. This analyzer employs the change in length of a silocone elastomer, which occurs with the adsorption of halothane or other agents, to alter the position of a needle on a dial. Its response time is quite slow (minutes), thus it is inadequate for end-tidal determinations, but it is useful for time-weighted averages, such as in closed-system anesthetic techniques. A device of intermediate cost, the Engstrom EMMA, also depends upon adsorption of halothane or another agent. In this device, such adsorption changes the effective mass of a quartz crystal oscillator and thus its frequency response. Internal circuitry then converts this information to a volume percentage, on a time scale fast enough to resolve breath-to-breath values when the optional recorder is attached. This device, however, has a serious problem with artifacts caused by sensing water vapor exhaled from the patient, and is therefore more useful on the inspired gas portion of the anesthesia circuit far from the patient's airway.[101,102]

Much more expensive devices based either on ultraviolet or infrared absorption, or on mass spectrometry, can also provide a rapid time response.[103] Careful assessment of the end-expired gas or vapor tensions may give some indication of the patient's anesthetic depth, but each patient must be assessed on an individual basis. In addition, some of these devices may be used to advantage in monitoring efficacy of antipollution measures, checking scavenging valves, anesthesia machine leaks, and high pressure piping system leaks, as may soon be mandated by National Institute of Occupational Safety and Health (NIOSH) under the Occupational Safety and Health Act (OSHA).

Acute Care Laboratory

When critically ill patients are in the operating room, serial measurements of blood chemistries, arterial blood gas tensions, pH, and other parameters may be needed on a time scale faster than that provided by the main laboratory facilities of the hospital. Our anesthesia department coordinates a laboratory serving primarily the operating rooms and associated intensive care units. This Acute Care Laboratory performs measurements of blood gas tensions, pH, hematocrit, osmolarity, total protein, sodium, potassium, glucose, and ionized calcium, all on small heparinized samples. These measurements must be available on a short turnaround time. Our laboratory usually works on a standard of 10–15 minutes, but can provide nearly instantaneous answers for emergency situations. Since the laboratory works with heparinized samples, dry heparin may eliminate volume artifacts from liquid solutions of heparin when performing studies on small patients.

Transcutaneous Oxygen–Carbon Dioxide Monitor

Serial sampling of arterial blood gas tensions through an indwelling cannula is unfortunately an episodic monitor. Continuous monitoring of oxygen and carbon dioxide tensions is possible through electrodes mounted on the skin. The area underlying the electrode is warmed, "arterializing" the region. Response time depends upon the thickness of the skin and the temperature of the electrode, and is faster in small infants and neonates.[104] Correlation with arterial levels in the clinical range is generally good, but *variations in perfusion can alter the readings,* particularly for oxygen.[105] With certain combinations of membrane material and polarization current, the Clark oxygen electrode may reduce halothane, yielding erroneous data for transcutaneous oxygen ($TCpO_2$). This problem may be minimized by changing to a Teflon membrane and altering polarization voltage.[106] These devices are not without hazard, for the heater will provide a first degree burn if the electrode remains in place for any length of time.

This technology has been of limited utility in operating rooms, but is very helpful in the ICU, where changes in perfusion are slower and are not altered by anesthetic gases or anesthetic depth, electrocautery, or continued bumping of the electrode by surgical staff.[107,108]

Pulse Oximetry

A new monitor is the pulse oximeter. This monitor determines the oxygen saturation of hemoglobin by spectrophotoelectric oximetric techniques; the detection of the amount of light transmitted through tissue between a two-wavelength light source and a detector allows continuous calculation of arterial saturation.[109] Use of two frequencies helps to eliminate interfering absorption by other molecules. This monitor is easy to use, noninvasive, and our experience has found it to be reasonably accurate. While it is useful in most patients, its greatest utility is as a noninvasive monitor in individuals with anatomic or physiologic shunts, since the effects of anesthetics and positive pressure ventilation are difficult to predict. This monitor is part of the next generation of on-line, real-time event detectors; it may prevent many significant anesthetic mishaps by providing immediate diagnosis of hypoxic events. *If one used both a pulse oximeter and end-tidal carbon dioxide monitoring it would be extremely difficult to miss significant gas-exchange problems. This monitor is now part of our routine standard of care.*

Intracranial Pressure Monitoring

In the patient with the likelihood of increased intracranial pressure (ICP), whether associated with trauma, tumor, metabolic disorder, or other cause, there is no substitute for direct monitoring of ICP. Measurement may be accomplished by transduced pressures through either a ventricular cannula placed through a burr hole, or by a Becker bolt or equivalent. Measurement can be performed noninvasively by aplanation if the fontanelles remain open. See Chapter 17 for further discussion.

TRANSPORT APPARATUS

Because transport environments (particularly outside the hospital in ambulances, helicopters, and fixed-wing aircraft) are exceedingly noisy, we depend upon electronic monitoring more than we would in the operating theater. When heart sounds are audible, a precordial or esophageal stethoscope is very useful. However, we generally must rely upon the electronic signal of a portable EKG. This must have battery-mode capability, and if possible also aircraft and ambulance power, as well as routine line current. If the monitor incorporates a QRS beeper, it should be capable of high volume to compete with the noisy transport environment. If there is an oscilloscopic display, the phosphors must be fairly bright, to be visible under all conditions. For transport within the hospital, these constraints may be loosened, the only strong need being battery operation.

PURCHASE OF ANESTHESIA EQUIPMENT

With the increasing sophistication of monitoring and life support equipment, purchasing decisions can no longer be intuitive. A proper grounding in the underlying engineering concepts would probably require four years at the Massachusetts Institute of Technology, but a good working knowledge of the operating principles, advantages, and special hazards of the various types of apparatus may be simply obtained. While your vendors are happy to provide the manufacturer's literature about their products, there is an advantage to obtaining information from an unbiased source. In our outside lives many of us refer to *Consumer Reports* for the evaluation of household appliances. There is an equivalent periodical, *Health Devices,* published by ECRI (formerly the Emergency Care Research Institute) of Plymouth Meeting, Pennsylvania. The safety office of your hospital probably subscribes to this periodical. ECRI will send a second copy of the journal to another individual at the same address for a small added price.

Another useful source of information is the specialty pediatric hospital. Whether through inquiry at medical meetings or by direct solicitation, practitioners at these unique resource institutions are often willing to share their special expertise. Remember that while many of the tools described in this chapter are specific to the younger patients, some items are useful for adults as well.

Finally, there are seven general principles to keep in mind for any equipment purchase.

1. *New purchases should work with what you already own.*
2. *The sales person is inherently biased.* He or she may be able to provide accurate mechanical specifications, but clearly has a vested interest in convincing you that the *company's view* of the capabilities and advantage of *its* product is correct.
3. Always *try out* samples of proposed purchases. You should test equipment *in the environment in which it will be used, with the people who will be using it.* What looks attractive in a display may not work well in your hands or in your special circumstances.
4. *Do not* use equipment for any purpose other than that for which it has been designed.
5. Have your hospital safety office check for electrical leakage and other safety features.
6. Spend as much on *maintenance* as on the product. Consider a maintenance contract, if available. Ask that the

company assure the future availability of parts, and the compatibility of subsequent modifications or design evolutions with your equipment.

7. If two products are comparable, but one has *local service facilities*, it may be the better choice.

If there are areas of special needs, try to be as detailed in your specifications as you can when dealing with your suppliers. For example, if a monitor is to be used *strictly* in the operating room, it may be a reasonable decision to operate it from the electrical lines. Conversely, if the monitor is to serve *not only* in the operating room, *but also* in transport between the operating theatre and the recovery room or intensive care unit, it must obviously have its own internal battery backup. The more precisely you can define your needs, the more accurate will be the comparisons that you can make between the bids of rival vendors. Remember that any given piece of equipment will occasionally be out of service, whether for regular preventive maintenance or for some unanticipated repair; although it is difficult in this era of cost containment to convince the hospital administration, this fact dictates an *absolute need* for additional units as spares.

REFERENCES

1. Roizen MF, Sohn YJ, L'Hommedieu CS, et al: Operating room temperature prior to surgical draping: Effect on patient temperature in recovery room. *Anesth Analg* 59:852–855, 1980

2. Bennett EJ, Patel KP, Grundy EM: Neonatal temperature and surgery. *Anesthesiology* 46:303–304, 1977

3. Farman JV: Heat loss in infants undergoing surgery in air-conditioned theatres. *Br J Anaesth* 34:543–557, 1962

4. Harrison GG, Bull AB, Schmidt HT: Temperature changes in children during general anesthesia. *Br J Anaesth* 32:60–68, 1960

5. Patel KD, Henschel EO: Postoperative alopecia. *Anesth Analg* 59:311–313, 1980

6. Munson ES, Eger EI, II: The effects of hyperthermia and hypothermia on the rate of induction of anesthesia: Calculations using a mathematical model. *Anesthesiology* 33:515–519, 1970

7. Brewin EG: Physiology of hypothermia. *Int Anesthesiol Clin* 2:803–827, 1964

8. Nishet HIA: Acid–base disturbance in hypothermia. *Int Anesthesiol Clin* 2:829–855, 1964

9. Dundee JW, Clarke RSJ: Pharmacology of hypothermia. *Int Anesthesiol Clin* 2:857–872, 1964

10. Bennett EJ, Patel KP, Grundy EM: Neonatal temperature and surgery. *Anesthesiology* 46:303–304, 1977

11. Levison H, Linsao L, Swyer PR: A comparison of infrared and convective heating for newborn infants. *Lancet* 2:1346–1348, 1966

12. Price HV, Whelpton D, McCarthy J: Newborn-infant heater. *Lancet* 2:1294, 1971

13. Goudsouzian NG, Morris RH, Ryan JF: The effects of a warming blanket on the maintenance of body temperature in anesthetized infants and children. *Anesthesiology* 39:351–353, 1973

14. Crino MH, Nagel EL: Thermal burns caused by warming blankets in the operating room. *Anesthesiology* 29:149–150, 1968

15. Russell WJ: A review of blood warmers for massive transfusion. *Anaesth Int Care* 2:109–130, 1974

16. Meyers MB, Oh TH: Prevention of hypothermia during cystoscopy in neonates. *Anesth Analg* 55:592–593, 1976

17. Hall GM: Body temperature and anesthesia. *Br J Anaesth* 50:39–44, 1978

18. Stone DR, Downs JB, Paul WL, et al: Adult body temperature and heated humidification of anesthetic gases during general anesthesia. *Anesth Analg* 60:736–741, 1981

19. Chalon J, Patel C, Ramanathan S, et al: Humidification of the circle absorber system. *Anesthesiology* 48:142–146, 1978

20. Tausk HC, Miller R, Roberts RB: Maintenance of body temperature by heated humidification. *Anesth Analg* 55:719–723, 1976

21. Berry FA, Jr, Hughes-Davies DI: Methods of increasing the humidity and temperature of the inspired gases in the infant circle system. *Anesthesiology* 37:456–462, 1972

22. Rashad KF, Benson DW: Role of humidity in prevention of hypothermia in infants and children. *Anesth Analg* 46:712–718, 1967

23. Baum JD, Scopes JW: The silver swaddler. *Lancet* 1:672–673, 1968

24. Bacon C, Scott D, Jones P: Heat stroke in well wrapped infants. *Lancet* 1:422–425, 1979

25. Petty C: Needle venting of air from intravenous tubing. *Anesth Analg* 53:1016–107, 1974

26. Gronert GA, Messick JM, Jr, Cucchiara RF, et al: Paradoxical air embolism from a patent foramen ovale. *Anesthesiology* 50:548–549, 1979

27. Philip BK, Philip JH: Characterization of flow in intravenous infusion systems. IEEE Transactions on Biomedical Engineering. *BME* 30:702–707, 1983

28. Philip BK, Philip JH, Joseph D: Personal communications.

29. Dula DJ, Muller HA, Donovan JW: Flow rate variance of commonly used IV infusion techniques. *J Trauma* 21:480–482, 1981

30. Calkins JM, Vaughan RW, Cork RC, et al: Effects of dilution, pressure, and apparatus on hemolysis and flow rate in transfusion of packed erythrocytes. *Anesth Analg* 61:776–780, 1982

31. Eurenius S, Smith RM: Hemolysis in blood infused under pressure. *Anesthesiology* 39:650–651, 1973

32. Shulman MS: Uvular edema without endotracheal intubation. *Anesthesiology* 55:82–83, 1981

33. Sesgne TP, Felske A: Uvular edema. *Anesthesiology* 49:375–376, 1979

34. Haselby KA, McNiece WL: Respiratory obstruction from uvular edema in a pediatric patient. *Anesth Analg* 62:117–118, 1983

35. Bennett RL, Lee TS, Wright BD: Airway obstructing supraglottic edema following anesthesia with the head positioned in forced flexion. *Anesthesiology* 54:78–80, 1981

36. Moore MW, Rauscher LA: A complication of oropharyngeal airway placement. *Anesthesiology* 47:526, 1977

37. Bernhard WN, Yost L, Turndorf H, et al: Cuffed tracheal tubes—physical and behavioral charateristics. *Anesth Analg* 61:36–41, 1982

38. Corfield HMC: Orotracheal tubes and the metric system. *Br J Anaesth* 35:34, 1963

39. Munson ES, Stevens DS, Redfern RE: Endotracheal tube obstruction by nitrous oxide. *Anesthesiology* 52:275–276, 1980

40. American National Standares Institute, Inc., Committee on Anesthetic and Ventilatory Equipment, 1430 Broadway, New York, New York, 10018.

41. Ring WH, Adair JC, Elwyn RA: A new pediatric endotracheal tube. *Anesth Analg* 54:273–274, 1975

42. Morgan GAR, Steward DJ: A pre-formed paediatric orotracheal tube design based on anatomical measurements. *Can Anaesth Soc J* 29:9–11, 1982

43. Ohn KC, Wu WH: Another complication of armored endotracheal tubes. *Anesth Analg* 59:215–216, 1980

44. Brandstater B: Dilatation of the laryx with Cole tubes. *Anesthesiology* 31:378–379, 1969

45. Hatch DJ: Tracheal tubes and connectors used in neonates—dimensions and resistance to breathing. *Br J Anaesth* 50:959–964, 1978

46. Glauser EM, Cook CD, Bougas JP: Pressure-flow characteristics

and dead spaces of endotracheal tubes used in infants. *Anesthesiology* 22:339–341, 1961

47. Patel KF, Hicks JN: Prevention of five hazards associated with the use of carbon dioxide lasers. *Anesth Analg* 60:885–888, 1981

48. Todres ID, Crone RK: Experience with a modified laryngoscope in sick infants. *Crit Care Med* 9:544–545, 1981

49. Nussbaum E: Flexible fiberoptic bronchoscopy and laryngoscopy in children under 2 years of age: Diagnostic and therapeutic applications of a new pediatric flexible fiberoptic bronchoscope. *Crit Care Med* 10:770–772, 1982

50. Taylor PA, Towey RM: The broncho-fiberscope as an aid to endotracheal intubation. *Br J Anaesth* 44:611–612, 1972

51. Davis NJ: A new fiberoptic laryngoscope for nasal intubation. *Anesth Analg* 52:807–808, 1973

52. James CS, Lanman JT: History of oxygen therapy and retrolental fibroplasia. *Pediatrics* [suppl] 57:591–642, 1976

53. Eger EI, II, Saidman LJ: Hazards of nitrous oxide anesthesia in bowel obstruction and pneumothorax. *Anesthesiology* 26:61–66, 1965

54. Lecky JH: Anesthetic pollution in the operating room: A notice to operating room personnel. *Anesthesiology* 52:157–159, 1980

55. Mazze RI: Waste anesthetic gases and the regulatory agencies. *Anesthesiology* 52:248–256, 1980

56. Patel KD, Dalal FY: A potential hazard of the Drager scavenging interface for wall suction. *Anesth Analg* 58:327–328, 1979

57. Rackow H, Salanitre E: Modern concepts in pediatric anesthesiology. *Anesthesiology* 30:208–234, 1969

58. Bain JA, Spoerel WE: A streamlined anaesthetic system. *Can Anaesth Soc J* 19:426–435, 1972

59. Ayre P: The T-piece technique. *Br J Anaesth* 28:520–523, 1956

60. Harrison GA: Ayre's T-piece: A review of its modifications. *Br J Anaesth* 36:115–120, 1964

61. Jackson-Rees G: Anaesthesia in the newborn. *Br Med J* 2:1419–1422, 1950

62. Mapleson WW: The elimination of rebreathing in various semi-closed anaesthetic systems. *Br J Anaesth* 26:323–332, 1954

63. Dorsch JA, Dorsch SE: *Understanding Anesthesia Equipment. Construction, Care, and Complications.* Baltimore, Williams & Wilkins, 1975.

64. Sykes MK: Rebreathing circuits. *Br J Anaesth* 40:666–674, 1968

65. Bain JA, Spoerel WE: Carbon dioxide output in anesthesia. *Can Anaesth Soc J* 23:153–162, 1976

66. Chalon J, Loew DAY, Malbranche J: Effects of dry anesthetic gases on tracheobronchial ciliated epithelium. *Anesthesiology* 37:338–343, 1972

67. Weeks DB: Provision of endogenous and exogenous humidity for the Bain breathing circuit. *Can Anaesth Soc J* 23:185–190, 1976

68. Klein FF, Graves SA: Hot pot tracheitis. *Chest* 65:225–226, 1974

69. Coté CJ, Petkan AJ, Ryan JF, et al: Wasted ventilation measured in vitro with eight anesthetic circuits used on children with and without inline humidification. *Anesthesiology* 59:442–446, 1983

70. Schwartz AJ, Downes JJ: Hazards of a simple monitoring device, the esophageal stethoscope. *Anesthesiology* 47:64–65, 1977

71. Van Bergen FH, Weatherhead DS, Treloar AE, et al: Comparison of indirect and direct methods of measuring arterial blood pressure. *Circulation* 10:481–490, 1954

72. Poppers PJ: Controlled evaluation of ultrasonic measurement of systolic and diastolic blood pressures in pediatric patients. *Anesthesiology* 38:187–191, 1973

73. Yelderman M, Ream AK: Indirect measurement of mean blood pressure in the anesthetized patient. *Anesthesiology* 50:253–256, 1979

74. Friesen RH, Lichter JL: Indirect mesurement of blood pressure in neonates and infants utilizing an automatic non-invasive oscillometric monitor. *Anesth Analg* 60:742–745, 1981

75. Kimble KJ, Darnall RA, Jr, Yelderman M, et al: An automated oscillometric technique for estimating mean arterial pressure in critically ill newborns. *Anesthesiology* 54:423–425, 1981

76. Sy WP: Ulnar nerve palsy possibly related to use of automatically cycled blood pressure cuff. *Anesth Analg* 60:87-88, 1981

77. Roy RC, Morgan L, Beamer D: Factitiously low blood pressure from the Dinamap. *Anesthesiology* 59:258–259, 1983

78. Hutton P, Prys-Roberts C: The oscillotonometer in theory and practice. *Br J Anaesth* 54:581–591, 1982

79. Aronow S, Bruner JM: Electrosurgery. *Anesthesiology* 42:525–526, 1979

80. Chandra P: Severe skin damage from EKG electrodes. *Anesthesiology* 56:157–158, 1982

81. Westenskow DR, Jordan WS, Jordan R, et al: Evaluation of oxygen monitors for use during anesthesia. *Anesth Analg* 60:53–56, 1981

82. Merritt JC, Sprague DH, Merritt WE, et al: Retrolental fibroplasia: A multifactorial disease. *Anesth Analg* 60:109–111, 1981

83. Winter PM, Smith G: The toxicity of oxygen. *Anesthesiology* 37:210–241, 1972

84. Benzinger M: Tympanic thermometry in surgery and anesthesia. *JAMA* 209:1207–1211, 1969

85. Wallace CT, Marks WE, Adkins WY, Mahaffey JE: Perforation of the tympanic membrane, a complication of tympanic thermometry during anesthesia. *Anesthesiology* 41:290–291, 1974

86. Kuzucu EY: Measurement of temperature. *Int Anesthesiol Clin* 3:435–449, 1965

87. Lees DE, Schuette W, Bull JM, et al: An evaluation of liquid-crystal thermometry as a screening device for intraoperative hyperthermia. *Anesth Analg* 57:669–674, 1978

88. Vaughan MS, Cork RC, Vaugham RW: Inaccuracy of liquid crystal thermometry to identify core temperature trends in postoperative adults. *Anesth Analg* 61:284–287, 1982

89. Ali HH, Savarese JJ: Monitoring the neuromuscular junction. *Anesthesiology* 57:215–249, 1976

90. Goudsouzian NG, Liu LMP, Coté CJ: Comparison of equipotent doses of non-depolarizing muscle relaxants in children. *Anesth Analg* 60:862–866, 1981

91. Churchill-Davidson HC, Katz RL: Dual, Phase II, or desensitization block. *Anesthesiology* 27:536–538, 1966

92. Todres ID, Rogers MC, Shannon DC, et al: Percutaneous catheterization of the radial artery in the critically ill neonate. *J Pediatr* 87:273–275, 1975

93. Todres ID, Crone RK, Rogers MC, et al: Swan-Ganz catheterization in the critically ill newborn. *Crit Care Med* 7:330–334, 1979

94. Coté CJ, Jobes DR, Schwartz AJ, et al: Two approaches to cannulation of a child's internal jugular vein. *Anesthesiology* 50:371–373, 1979

95. Steward DJ: Preterm infants are more prone to complications following minor surgery than are term infants. *Anesthesiology* 56:305–306, 1982

96. Liu LMP, Coté CJ, Goudsouzian NG, et al: Life threatening apnea in infants during recovery from anesthesia. *Anesthesiology* 59:506–510, 1983

97. Mushin WW, Rendell-Baker L, Thompson PW, et al: *Automatic Ventilation of the Lungs* (ed 3). Oxford, Blackwell Scientific Publications, 1980, p 46

98. Evan JM, Hogg MIJ, Rosen M: Correlation of alveolar PCO_2 estimated by infra-red analysis and arterial PCO_2 in the human neonate and the rabbit. *Br J Anaesth* 49:761–764, 1977

99. Baudendistel L, Goudsouzian NG, Coté CJ, Strafford M: End-tidal CO_2 monitoring: Its use in the diagnosis and management of malignant hyperthermia. *Anaesthesia* 39:1000–1003, 1985

100. Epstein RA, Hyman AI: Ventilatory requirements of critically ill neonates. *Anesthesiology* 53:379–384, 1980

101. Hayes JK, Westenskow DR, Jordan WS: Monitoring anesthetic vapor concentrations using a piezoelectric detector: Evaluation of the Engstrom EMMA. *Anesthesiology* 59:435–439, 1983

102. Linstromberg JW, Muir JJ: Cross-sensitivity in water vapor in the Engstom EMMA. *Anesth Analg* 63:75–88, 1984

103. Gillbe CE, Heneghan CPH, Branthwaite MA: Respiratory mass spectrometry during general anaesthesia. *Br J Anaesth* 53:103–109, 1981

104. Huch R, Lucey JF, Huch A: Oxygen: Noninvasive monitoring. *Perinatal Care* 2:18–25, 1978

105. Gothgen I, Jacobsen E: Transcutaneous Oxygen tension measurement. II. The influence of halothane and hypotension. *Acta Anaesth Scan* [suppl] 67:71–75, 1978

106. Sugioka K, Woodley C: The use of transcutaneous oxygen electrodes in the presence of anaesthetic agents. *Can Anaeth Soc J* 28:498–505, 1981

107. Dennhardt R, Fricke M, Mahal S, et al: Transcutaneous PO_2 monitoring in anaesthesia. *Eur J Intensive Care Med* 2:29–33, 1976

108. Rafferty ID, Marrero O, Nardi D, et al: Transcutaneous PO_2 as a trend indicator of arterial PO_2 in normal anesthetized adults. *Anesth Analg* 61:252–255, 1982

109. Yelderman M, New W, Jr: Evaluation of pulse oximetry. *Anesthesiology* 59:349–352, 1983

24

Procedures

I. David Todres
Charles J. Coté

VASCULAR CANNULATION

Vascular cannulation is vital to the anesthetic and intensive care management of all children. It covers the spectrum from a simple intravenous (IV) line to the more sophisticated pulmonary artery catheterization. The indications for the insertion of these devices in children are the same as for the adult, e.g., to provide a route for fluid and drug administration and to monitor cardiopulmonary function. However, the materials employed, insertion techniques, and complications are often specific to children. While the technique of insertion may be extremely difficult in the young infant, inability to perform the procedure must not preclude its use. No child should be denied an indicated procedure because of operator inexperience; appropriate consultation should be employed.

VENOUS CANNULATION

Peripheral Intravenous Cannulation:
Percutaneous

Indications: ideally in all anesthetized patients.

Rationale:

1. To prevent hypovolemia during induction, maintenance, and recovery from anesthesia.
2. To provide access for drugs, fluid and electrolytes, glucose, and blood products.
3. To have access to the circulation for resuscitation drugs.
4. To provide a route for immediate postoperative pain relief.

Methods:

1. If awake, establish a healthy cooperative patient/anesthesiologist interaction.
2. Secure extremity for IV site, preferably one in close proximity to the anesthesiologist.
3. "Scalp vein" (Butterfly-Abbott) for induction followed by insertion of appropriate size catheter under anesthesia, or vascular catheter inserted after injection of local anesthetic with a small gauge (27) needle.
4. T-connector (Abbot) to minimize dead space for neonates.
5. Antibiotic ointment, "bandaid," and tape appropriately applied.
6. Calibrated burette to limit total infusion.
7. Flow limiting infusion pump for neonates and infants.

Complications:

1. Hematoma—usually of no serious consequence.
2. Infection/thrombosis—may be limited by good aseptic technique and application of antibiotic ointment.[1-4]
3. Skin sloughing—usually caused by subcutaneous infiltration of calcium, potassium, or hypertonic solutions. May be avoided by frequent inspection, such as checking IV function prior to injection of potentially sclerosing agents.[5,6]

Peripheral Intravenous Cannulation: Intravenous
Cut Down

Indications:

1. Any patient in whom percutaneous cannulation is unsuccessful.

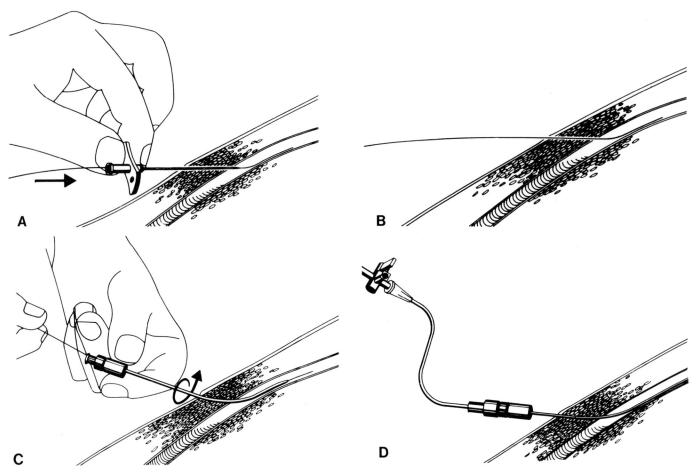

Figure 24-1. Seldinger technique for catheter placement. The needle is inserted into the target vessel and the flexible end of the guide wire is passed freely into the vessel (A). The needle is then removed leaving the guide wire in place (B). The catheter is advanced with a twisting motion into the vessel (C). Finally, the wire is removed and the catheter connected to appropriate flow or monitoring device (D). (Reproduced with permission. Scientific Exhibit. Central venous catheterization in Pediatrics. Schwartz AJ, Coté CJ, Jobes DR, Ellison N.)

2. Any patient in whom percutaneous cannulation is tenuous.
3. If the catheter in place would be too small for the planned surgical procedure.

Methods. This procedure is most commonly performed by surgeons, but may be carried out by other experienced individuals. Standard texts should be consulted.

Sites. The most common sites for insertion are the saphenous vein at the ankle (medial malleolus) and the brachiocephalic vein in the arm (antecubital fossa).

Complications:

These are the same as for percutaneous techniques; however, there is a higher incidence of infection and therefore it should be used only on a short term basis.[7]

Central Venous Cannulation

Indications:

1. To provide a secure means for rapid fluid administration where major shifts in intravascular volume are anticipated, e.g., multiple trauma, intestinal obstruction, burns.

2. To monitor cardiac filling pressures.
3. For infusion of drugs that are sclerosing to peripheral veins, e.g., antibiotics, vasopressors, and hyperalimentation fluids.
4. Measurement of mixed venous acid–base balance or estimation of cardiac output (Fick Principle).
5. Measurement of cardiac output (dye dilution).
6. Route for aspiration of air emboli.

Sites. The common sites for central venous cannulation are external and internal jugular veins, the subclavian and brachiocephalic veins, femoral veins, and the umbilical vein in the neonate. The more invasive approaches (internal jugular and subclavian) should not be used in the presence of a bleeding diathesis.

Methods and Materials. In our experience the percutaneous approach to central venous cannulation is most successful using modified Seldinger* techniques. This approach is demonstrated in Figure 24-1. The advantages of this technique include that (a) it avoids the need for a cutdown, (b) there is only one venipuncture with a thin walled small gauge needle,

---

* Cook, Inc., Bloomington, Ind.

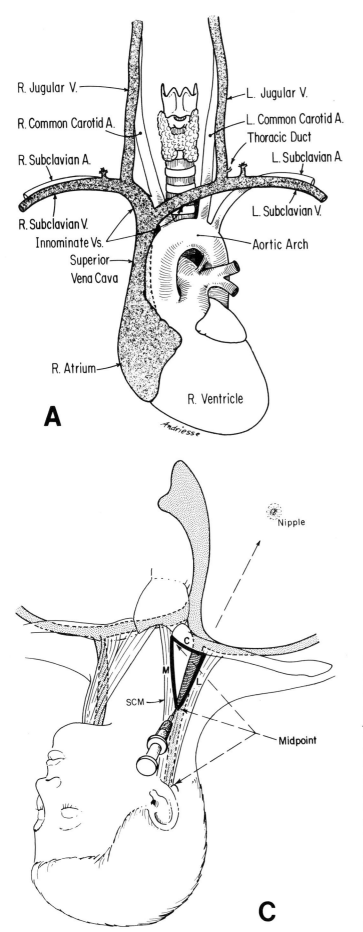

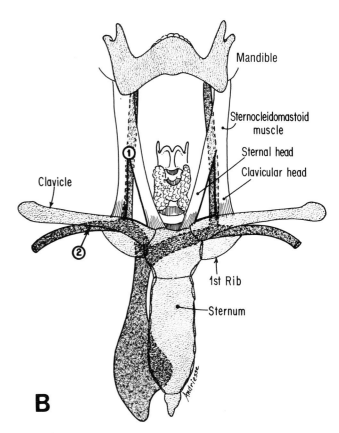

Figure 24-2. Anatomy. Figure (A) depicts the anatomical relationships of major chest and neck structures. Note how the internal jugular vein is in close proximity to the carotid artery. Also note that a nearly straight line is formed by the internal jugular vein, innominate vein, superior vena cava, and right atrium; thus it is rare for a right internal jugular catheter to migrate anywhere but the right atrium. Figure (B) demonstrates the relationship of external anatomical landmarks with the anatomy of figure (A). Note the triangle formed by the two bellies of the sternocleidomastoid muscle and the clavicle. The number one indicates the preferred point of needle insertion at the apex of this triangle for internal jugular vein puncture. The number two indicates the point of needle insertion for subclavian vein puncture. Figure (C) demonstrates the anatomical landmarks as they would appear to the anesthesiologist. Note that the needle is introduced at the apex of the triangle outlined in (B), and directed at an angle of 30° to the skin toward the ipsilateral nipple. This point of entry is half the distance between the mastoid process and the clavicle.

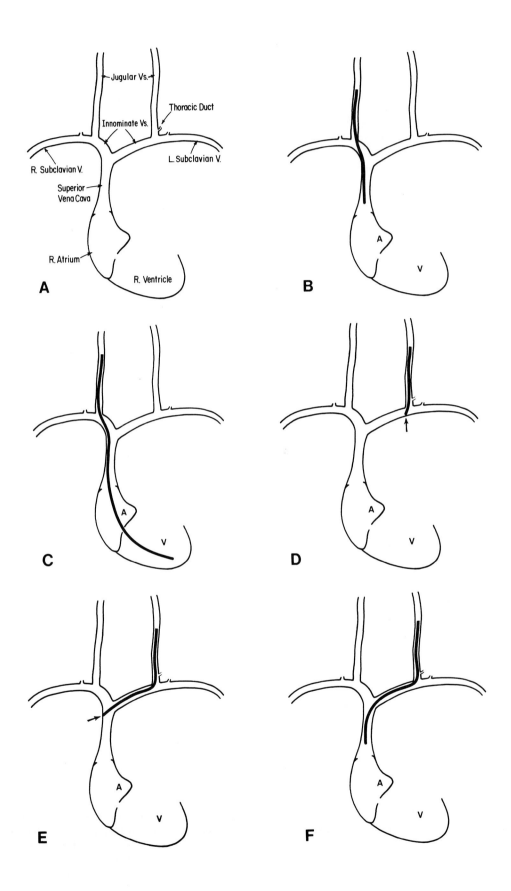

A

Jugular Vs.

Thoracic Duct

Innominate Vs.

R. Subclavian V.

L. Subclavian V.

Superior Vena Cava

R. Atrium

R. Ventricle

B

A

V

C

A

V

D

A

V

E

A

V

F

A

V

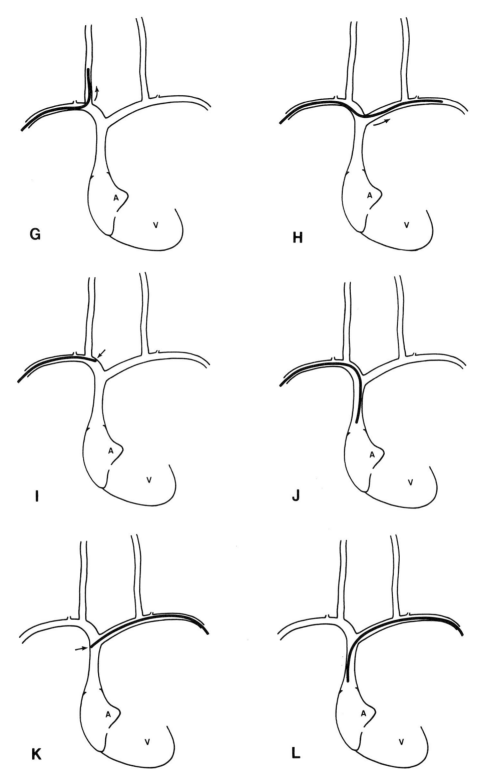

Figure 24-3. Proper and improper CVP placement. (A) Normal vascular anatomy. (B) Proper location for right internal jugular catheter, i.e., right atrium or superior vena cava. (C) Ventricular location of any catheter is dangerous and contraindicated. (D) A short left-sided internal jugular catheter may erode through the innominate vein. (E) A left-sided internal jugular catheter striking the lateral wall of the superior vena cava may erode through and must be partially withdrawn or advanced further. (F) Proper location for left internal jugular catheter. (G) A right subclavian catheter may pass into the internal jugular vein; the catheter should be withdrawn and repositioned. (H) A right subclavian catheter may pass to the opposite subclavian vein; this catheter should be withdrawn and repositioned. (I) A short right subclavian catheter may strike the lateral wall of the innominate vein and erode through; this catheter should be advanced or withdrawn. (J) Proper location for right subclavian line. (K) Short left subclavian line may erode through the superior vena cava; this catheter should be advanced or withdrawn. (L) Proper location for left subclavian vein catheter.

(c) a guide wire directs the catheter within the blood vessel, (d) the introduction of a large catheter through the small venipuncture site minimizes the chances of significant hematoma formation even after systemic heparinization, and (e) this procedure can often be accomplished in an emergency situation in less than one minute.

Alternative techniques involve locating the vein with a small gauge needle following by venipuncture with a large needle (Intracath)** through which the catheter is threaded. This technique is successful in the hands of the experienced individual, but has the disadvantage of requiring several venipunctures, and the larger needle may cause damage to surrounding tissues or result in hematoma formation.[10]

External Jugular Vein Catheterization: Technique:

1. The patient is placed in Trendelenberg position with the head turned 45 degrees away from the side of cannulation.
2. A pillow or rolled sheet is placed under the shoulders to extend the head and allow complete access to the neck.
3. Under proper aseptic conditions venipuncture and catheter insertion is completed according to the techniques shown in Figure 24-1. (Usually a J-wire is more useful to circumvent the plexus of veins at the clavicle.)[11,12]
4. Antibiotic ointment, occlusive dressing (Op-Site[†]), suture or tape appropriately.

A significant number of catheters will not pass beyond the clavicle or will pass into the axillary vein.[13] The right side is generally more successful than the left.[14] If a shorter catheter is used (Angiocath, Jelco, Medicut) infusion and pressure monitoring is very dependent on position.[15]

Internal Jugular Vein Catheterization. There are many approaches and techniques for internal jugular vein cannulation.[16–24] We have had the most success with a high approach using as landmarks for insertion, the apex of a triangle formed by the two bellies of the sternocleidomastoid muscle and the clavicle (Figure 24-2). Using the Seldinger technique our success rate even in neonates approaches 75 percent on first attempt, and 90–95 percent on second attempt.[9] Cannulation of the right side virtually assures a central location, since the internal jugular vein, the superior vena cava, and the right atrium are in a straight line (Figure 24-2). Left-sided cannulation risks injury to the thoracic duct and possible pneumothorax, since the apex of the lung is higher on the left. In addition, if a catheter inserted on the left is too short it is not unusual for the tip to rest against the wall of the superior vena cava, be position dependent, and possibly erode through the wall of the vessel (Figure 24-3). The principal advantage to the high approach is that the most common complication (arterial puncture approximately 10%) is easily recognized and usually treated uneventfully. A lower approach risks unrecognized life-threatening complications (pneumothorax, hemothorax).[9,21]

Technique:

1. The patient is positioned as for external jugular vein cannulation.

_____
** Deseret, Sandy, Utah.
† Acme United Corporation, Bridgeport, CT

2. The apex of a triangle formed by the two bellies of the sternocleidomastoid muscle is located. This point is usually where the external jugular vein crosses the sternocleidomastoid muscle or the midpoint between the mastoid process and the sternal notch.
3. The carotid artery is palpated and the needle is introduced just lateral to it at an angle of 30° to the skin surface. In some children the internal jugular vein is quite superficial, thus even a less acute angle may be indicated. While continuously aspirating, the needle is advanced toward the ipsilateral nipple a distance of no more than 2.5 cm. If no blood is freely obtained the needle is slowly withdrawn while maintaining aspiration. Often the needle kinks the vessel upon entry, and it unkinks during withdrawal allowing free aspiration of blood.
4. Once venipuncture is accomplished the syringe is carefully removed and the end of the needle occluded (to prevent air embolism) until a flexible guide wire is inserted (Figure 24-1).[8] The wire should advance with almost no resistance. However, if the wire cannot be advanced, the needle has passed out of the vessel lumen or its tip rests against the vessel wall. In this situation the wire and needle should be withdrawn simultaneously so as not to sheer the wire. If the wire passes easily, then cannulation proceeds as demonstrated in Figure 24-1. Catheter tip location should be confirmed radiologically and repositioned as indicated (Figure 24-3).
5. Generally the catheter site is covered with antibiotic ointment, sutured, and protected with an occlusive dressing which is changed daily.

Contraindications:

1. Bleeding diathesis
2. Contralateral pneumothorax
3. Raised intracranial pressure (Trendelenberg position as well as venous occlusion by the catheter may increase intracranial pressure)
4. Aberrant vessels (e.g., cervical aortic arch)
5. Emphysematous bleb

Subclavian Vein Catheterization. The subclavian vein is also a popular site for central vein cannulation.[25–31] The advantages include fixed landmarks, ease of securing the line to the patient for long term management, and patient comfort. Disadvantages include potential life-threatening complications, e.g., pneumothorax, hemothorax.[28,31] If this site is chosen preoperatively we routinely obtain a chest roentgenogram after the catheter is inserted and before surgery commences to circumvent the danger of an unrecognized intraoperative tension pneumothorax. The use of the Seldinger technique (our preference) may reduce the incidence of damage to intrathoracic structures compared to other techniques. As with left-sided internal jugular vein cannulation if a left subclavian catheter tip rests against the wall of the superior vena cava it is possible to erode through, resulting in hemothorax or hydrothorax (Figure 24-3).

Technique:

1. The patient is prepped and positioned as previously described for internal jugular puncture.
2. A needle is inserted immediately inferior to the clavicle at

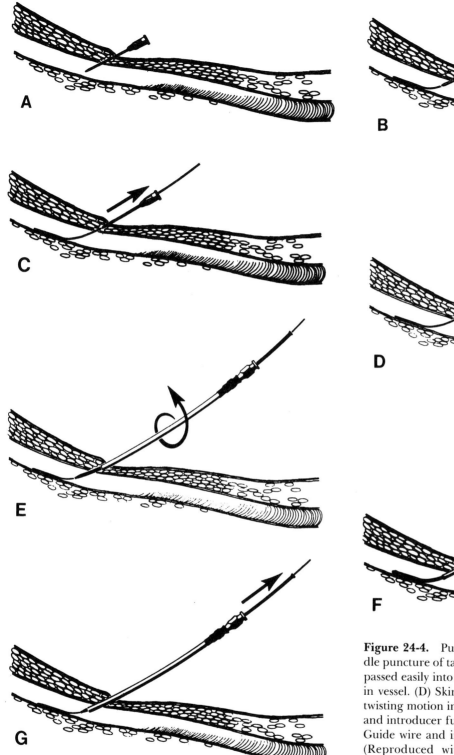

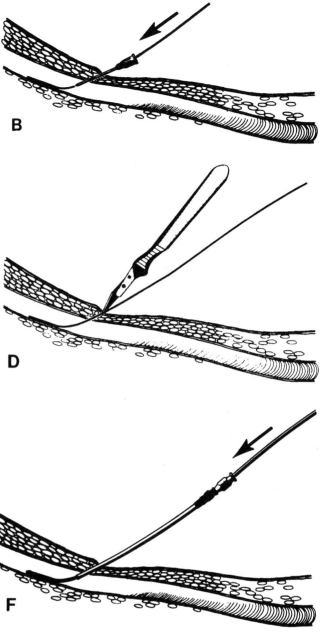

Figure 24-4. Pulmonary artery catheter insertion. (A) Needle puncture of target vessel is made. (B) Flexible guide wire is passed easily into vessel. (C) Needle is withdrawn leaving wire in vessel. (D) Skin incision made with scalpel blade. (E) With twisting motion introducer follows wire into vessel. (F) Sheath and introducer further advanced as a unit into the vessel. (G) Guide wire and introducer removed leaving sheath in place. (Reproduced with permission, Conahan TJ, III, *JAMA* 237:447, 1977.)

a point 1/2 to 2/3 its length from the sternal end; while hugging the under surface of the clavicle the needle is directed toward the suprasternal notch maintaining continuous aspiration.

3. As soon as free blood flow is obtained proceed as in Figure 24–1. If the Seldinger technique is not used, then first locating the subclavian vein with a small gauge needle is recommended.

4. The catheter insertion site is covered with antibiotic ointment, sutured in place, and an occlusive dressing applied.

Contraindications. The same as for internal jugular cannulation.

Brachiocephalic Vein Catheterization. This vein offers the advantage of being far removed from vital intrathoracic struc-

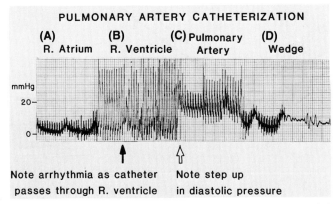

Figure 24-5. Pulmonary artery catheterization. Right atrial tracing (A) Right ventricular tracing (B); note arrhythmia when catheter tip strikes ventricular tissue (solid arrow). Pulmonary artery tracing (C); note the step up in diastolic pressure that is hallmark of the catheter in the pulmonary artery (open arrow). Wedge location (D); note the loss of pulmonary artery tracing, and that pattern tracing is very similar to right atrial.

tures.[32–34] The main disadvantage is that a significant number of these catheters will not pass centrally, i.e., they are caught in the axilla, or pass up the jugular vein (internal or external).[35–37] Other disadvantages include significant catheter migration with movement of the arm, and possibly an increased incidence of infection.[7]

Technique:

1. The patient is aseptically prepped and draped.
2. The brachiocephalic vein is cannulated using either the modified Seldinger technique (special long catheters and wires for this purpose), or by standard catheter through needle equipment (Intracath). If one is unable to thread the catheter once the vein is entered, initiating rapid IV fluid administration, cephalad positioning of the arm, and anterior displacement of the shoulder may assist advancement. If percutaneous techniques are not possible, direct venous cutdown is indicated.[38]

Femoral Vein Catheterization. The femoral vein may also be used for access to the central circulation. However, the catheter must pass into the thorax to provide accurate pressure measurements. Advantages include a large vein with easy access distant from vital intrathoracic structures. Disadvantages include difficulty in securing the catheter to the patient, kinking of the catheter with leg flexion, and keeping the site of insertion sterile.[39]

Technique:

1. The patient is prepped and draped with aseptic technique.
2. The femoral artery is palpated at a point midway between the pubic tubercle and the anterior superior iliac spine.
3. Using the Seldinger technique the vein is entered at a point just medial to the femoral artery and 1–2 cm below the inguinal ligament. A catheter is inserted as in Figure 24-1. Again, as for the brachiocephalic vein, special long

catheters and wires are needed in order to achieve a central location.
4. The catheter insertion site is protected as previously described (see internal jugular vein catheterization).

If an alternative technique is utilized (e.g., catheter through the needle), compression of the cannulation site should be maintained until hemostasis is assured. The saphenous vein may be cannulated by direct venous cutdown at its junction with the femoral vein if percutaneous techniques are unsuccessful.

Pulmonary Artery Cannulation

Measurement of pulmonary artery occlusion pressure (PAOP) has become increasingly important for operative and intensive care management of selected pediatric patients.[40–45] These catheters come in a variety of sizes ((2–7 French) with varying capabilities, including pressure monitoring, thermodilution of cardiac output, and cardiac pacing. We have used these catheters in children of all ages, including newborns. The internal jugular route is the most successful approach.[43]

Indications:

1. Measurement of left- and right-sided filling pressures (hypovolemia versus congestive heart failure).
2. Pulmonary artery hypertension.
3. Measurement of cardiac output.
4. Measurement of mixed venous oxygen tension and saturation.
5. Cardiac pacing.
6. A means of diagnosing and treating air emboli.

Technique:

1. The patient is prepped, draped, and positioned as for central venous catheterization.
2. The Seldinger technique is used to gain access to a large vein (internal jugular, subclavian, femoral, or brachiocephalic).
3. Instead of a catheter introduced over a wire, a dilator and sheath of appropriate size is inserted (Figure 24-4).
4. All air is flushed from the pulmonary artery catheter and it is attached to a pressure transducer.
5. The catheter is slowly advanced until a central venous (right atrial) tracing is obtained (Figure 24-5A). The balloon tip is then inflated with a measured amount of air (carbon dioxide for children with possible intracardiac shunts).
6. The catheter is further advanced until a right ventricular tracing appears (Figure 24-5B). Once this is obtained further advance of 2–3 cm usually results in successful pulmonary artery cannulation. Note: there mut be a step-up in diatolic pressure signalling the cross-over from right ventricle to pulmonary artery (Figure 24-5C).
7. The catheter is further advanced until a wedge tracing is obtained (Figure 24-5D). A return of the pulmonary artery tracing should occur with deflation of the balloon. Wedge pressure should return with *gentle* reinflation of the balloon. Confirmation of wedge position should be

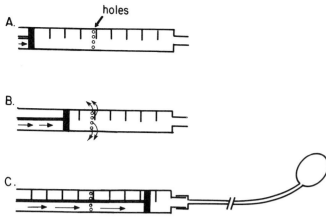

holes

A.

B.

C.

Figure 24-6. In order to prevent accidental overinflation of a pulmonary artery catheter balloon, the inflation syringe is punctured several times at the appropriate volume (A). As the plunger is depressed, air will vent out the puncture holes (B). Only the volume distal to the puncture holes will be transmitted to the balloon (C). (Reproduced with permission, Coté' CJ: A simple technique to avoid over distension of flow directed catheters. *Anesthesiology* 49:154, 1978.)

made by roentgenogram, pressure wave form, and by obtaining blood gas analysis both with and without the balloon inflated. With the balloon inflated arterialized blood should be obtained; if not, then either the catheter is against the wall of the vessel, the balloon has herniated over the tip of the catheter giving a false impression of occlusion position, or the catheter is wedged into the wall of the heart chamber, usually the right ventricle.

8. The introducer sheath is withdrawn so that only the distal portion of it remains in the SVC. The sheath site is then covered with antibiotic ointment, the catheter sutured in place, and covered with an occlusive dressing, which is changed daily.

Complications. The complications associated with pulmonary artery cannulation are similar to central venous cannulation, i.e., hematoma, arterial puncture, pneumothorax, hemothorax, arrhythmias, and air emboli. Pulmonary infarction, rupture of the pulmonary artery, thrombocytopenia, and altered pulmonary blood flow are additional significant risks.[46-53] These latter complications may be minimized by avoiding prolonged measurement of PAOP and by not over-inflating the balloon. One method of achieving this is to continuously transduce the PA tracing in order to immediately diagnose catheter migration. Another is to determine how much air results in successful occlusion. Once the latter is achieved, holes punctured in the air syringe at the desired volume may prevent accidental over-inflation (Figure 24-6).[54]

Umbilical Vein Catheterization

Indications. The umbilical vein provides easy access to the central circulation of the newborn infant for the restoration of blood volume, administration of glucose, and drugs.[55,56] It is also an important site for the procedure of exchange transfusion. In the critically ill neonate, it provides a means for measuring central venous pressure.

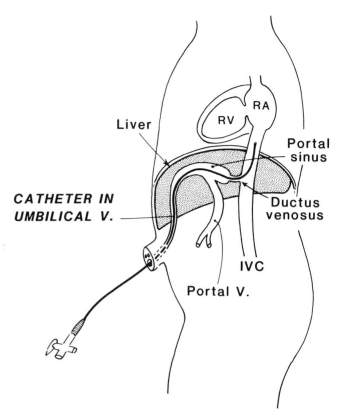

Figure 24-7. Umbilical vein catheterization. Umbilical vein is thin walled and patulous, while umbilical arteries are thicker walled and smaller diameter. Caudal traction on umbilical stump may facilitate catheter advancement. Catheter should be advanced through liver into the central circulation prior to administration of any medications.

Materials:

- Umbilical artery catheter sizes 3 1/2 and 5 French (Argyle[‡])
- Scalpel and blade
- Fine curved forceps
- Mosquito hemostats
- Umbilical tape
- Scissors
- Sutures with needle (3.0 silk)
- Antiseptic solutions (betadine and alcohol)
- 3-way stopcocks
- 10 ml syringe
- Infusion solution of 10% dextrose in water, with 2 units of heparin/ml

Procedure. After prepping and draping, cut the umbilical cord approximately one centimeter above the umbilicus. The umbilical vein orifice is more patulous and thin walled (Figure 24-7). The blood clot at the entrance to the vein is removed. Holding the catheter filled with heparinized solution, two centimeters from the tip, it is gently introduced into the vein. In some situations, forceps will aid in directing the catheter. Traction of the umbilical stump caudally may facilitate the catheter's advance (Figure 24-7). The catheter is

‡ Sherwood Medical Industries, St. Louis, MO.

passed a distance that approximates the length between the umbilical stump and the right atrium. Blood should freely aspirate into a syringe. Inability to withdraw blood may be due to the tip of the catheter resting against a vessel wall or a clot within the catheter lumen. *It is important that the tip of the catheter be placed in the proper position, i.e. at the junction of the inferior vena cava and right atrium.* An x-ray will confirm proper catheter position. At times, the catheter may fail to traverse the ductus venosus and may become wedged in the liver. This position is potentially dangerous should hyperosmolar or sclerosing solutions be injected (calcium chloride, sodium bicarbonate, 50% glucose) as this may lead to portal necrosis and subsequent cirrhosis. The catheter is sutured in place, its insertion site covered with antibiotic ointment, and taped to the abdominal wall. The catheter is then connected to a constant infusion system and should be removed as soon as the indications for its insertion have passed.

Complications:

1. Thrombosis of portal or mesenteric veins.
2. Infection—septicemia.
3. Endocarditis.
4. Pulmonary infarction—misplacement of catheter into pulmonary vein via patent foramen ovale.
5. Portal cirrhosis and esophageal varices.[57-62]

ARTERIAL CANNULATION

Umbilical Artery Catheterization

Indications. The umbilical artery in the neonate is a convenient site for monitoring arterial blood pressure, blood gases, and pH. In addition, it provides emergency access to the infant's circulation for restoration of blood volume, and administration of glucose and drugs.[63-67]

Materials. The materials employed for cannulation are identical to those described for umbilical venous catheterization. In addition, equipment is required for continuous monitoring of blood pressure (transducer, oscilloscope with pressure alarms, and constant infusion pumps).

Procedure. After prepping and draping, cut the umbilical cord approximately one centimeter above the umbilicus. The two umbilical arteries are identified (see Figure 24-8). The cut vessel ends are thicker-walled and smaller than the vein, and are usually in spasm. The artery is entered in the manner described for umbilical vein catheterization, except that cephad traction is applied to the umbilical stump (Figure 24-8A). The catheter courses through the umbilical artery into the iliohypogastric artery and then into the descending aorta. Proper position of the catheter tip is crucial. If the catheter is advanced too far up the aorta it may pass through the ductus arteriosus into the pulmonary artery. If this is not recognized, blood pressure and blood gas measurements may be misleading. Care should also be taken to ensure the placement of the catheter in the descending aorta distal to the origin of the renal arteries (lumbar vertebra 1) and inferior mesenteric artery. The catheter should be ideally just above the bifurcation of the descending aorta, that is, at lumbar vertebrae 3–4 (Figure 24-8A). This position can be difficult to maintain, and if the catheter tip slips into one of the iliac arteries it could lead to ischemia (Fig. 24-8B). The alternative accepted placement, at the level of the diaphragm, is easier to maintain, but predisposes the infant to the increased risk of embolization to renal or mesenteric vessels.[68-78] Correct positioning is confirmed radiologically. Once the catheter is properly positioned, the system is connected to a constant infusion pump, and heparinized fluids (10% dextrose in water, or normal saline) are infused. The catheter is sutured, taped, and antibiotic ointment applied as for umbilical vein catheters.

Complications:

1. Disconnection of stop-cocks and catheters can lead to potentially dangerous exsanguination.
2. Embolization of blood clot or air. Blood clots may embolize retrograde or, more likely, distally, leading to ischemia or infarction of the infant's gut, kidneys, or the lower limbs.
3. Vascular spasm, usually transitory, which may be resolved by withdrawal of the catheter.
4. Sepsis. The infant is always at risk for sepsis and, therefore, clear indications for the insertion of this catheter are mandatory with removal at the earliest possible time.
5. Hypertension as a result of renal artery emboli causing ischemia and infarction of the kidney.
6. Complications may be minimized by using the umbilical artery as a source for blood pressure monitoring and blood gas analysis only and reserving alternative sites for glucose and drug administration.

Radial Artery Cannulation

Radial artery cannulation has been developed as an alternative to umbilical artery cannulation in the neonate and is the primary site of arterial cannulation in infants and children in our institution. Percutaneous radial artery cannulation has become widely practiced with minimal morbidity.[79-82] Failure to cannulate the artery percutaneously may be followed successfully by direct arterial cut down.

Indications. Monitoring of arterial blood gases and pH and monitoring of arterial blood pressure. The right radial artery is preferred in the neonate as it is representative of pre-ductal blood flow.

Materials:

1. Betadine and alcohol.
2. Number 22 or 24 "intravenous" cannula. (Medicut[§], Jelco[‖]).
3. Number 19–20-gauge needle for skin puncture.
4. T-connector.
5. Infusion system and pump with heparinized isotonic saline (1–2 units/ml).
6. Tape and armboard.

Procedure. Adequacy of ulnar artery collateral flow is confirmed by the modified Allen test (Figure 24-9).[83] The color of the hand is noted. The hand is passively clenched and the radial and ulnar arteries are simultaneously compressed at the wrist. The ulnar artery is then released and flushing

§ Argyle-Sherwood Medical Industries, St. Louis, MO.
‖ Critikon Inc., Tampa, FL.

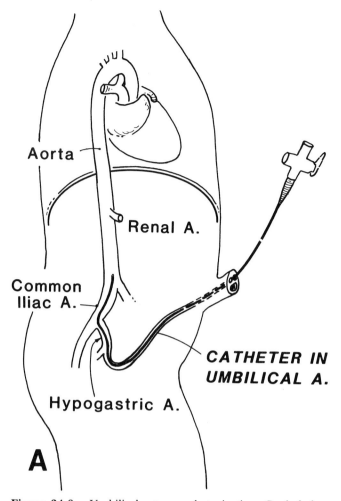

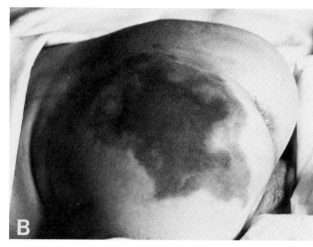

Figure 24-8. Umbilical artery catheterization. Cephalad traction on umbilical stump (A) may facilitate catheter advancement. Catheter tip at lumbar 3–4 vertebrae just above aortic bifurcation is ideal position. An alternative accepted location is at the level of the diaphragm. Figure (B) illustrates an area of necrosis resulting from a catheter migrating into the internal iliac vessel occluding one of its branches.

(reperfusion) of the blanched hand is noted. If the entire hand is well perfused while the radial artery remains occluded, indicating adequate collateral flow, catheterization of the radial artery is performed. The hand is secured on an armboard with slight extension of the wrist to avoid excessive median nerve stretching. The fingertips should be left exposed when the hand is taped down so that any peripheral ischemic changes due to spasm, clot, or air can be observed.

The course of the radial may be "visualized" in the neonate with the aid of a fiberoptic light source directed towards the lateral side or dorsal aspect of the wrist. Use of a doppler may also be of some value.[84–86] A number 20-gauge needle is used to make a small skin puncture over the point of maximal pulsation of the radial artery, usually at the second proximal wrist crease. This will ease passage of the cannula by reducing resistance offered by the skin. Cannulation is accomplished either on direct entry of the artery at an angle of 15–20°, or on withdrawing the cannula following transfixion of the artery (Figure 24-10A). The catheter is then firmly attached to a T connector to permit continuous infusion of heparinized isotonic saline (1–2 units/ml) at the rate of 1–2 ml/hr via a constant infusion pump (Figure 24-10B). Antibiotic ointment

and "bandaid" are applied, the surrounding skin is coated with tincture of benzoin, and the catheter securely taped in place (Figures 24-10C-D). A pressure transducer is then connected in line with this system to allow continuous arterial pressure monitoring to be recorded on an oscilloscope. In order to assure accurate blood pressure measurement it is essential that the transducer be calibrated with mercury to the patient's heart level, that all air bubbles are removed from the system, and that no more than three feet of tubing be used between the patient and the transducer.[87]

Blood samples are obtained by clamping off the distal end of the T-connector, cleaning the rubber end of the T-connector with betadine, and introducing a 22-gauge needle, and allowing 3–4 drops of blood to flow out (Fig. 20-10E). A sample of saline-free blood can be easily obtained by use of a heparinized syringe with minimal blood loss and minimal manipulation of the system (Figure 24-10F).[80,88] After sampling, the clamp is released and continuous infusion is resumed. This method of sampling avoids the use of stop-cocks, which are potential sources of infection. In addition, bolus flushes are avoided. These are associated with retrograde blood flow to the brain and may be disastrous if an air bubble

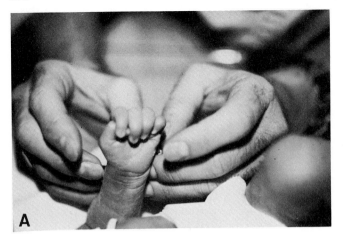

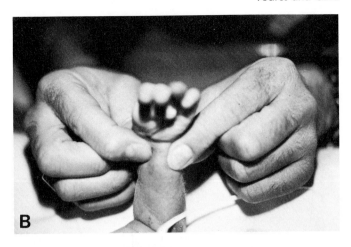

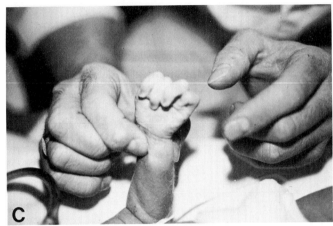

Figure 24-9. Modified Allen's test: color and perfusion of the hand is noted (A). The hand is passively clenched (B) and both radial and ulnar vessels occluded. The ulnar artery is released while the radial artery remains occluded (C). If flow through the ulnar artery is adequate, then the color and perfusion should rapidly return

or blood clot should accompany a bolus flush.[89] Only heparinized normal or half-normal saline is infused in order to avoid arterial damage and thrombosis. *All arterial lines must be clearly identified (red tape) in order to avoid accidental infusion of hypertonic solutions and sclerosing medications.*

Complications:

1. Infection at the site of the catheter, with possible septicemia.
2. Arterial thrombus formation. This is dependent on the size catheter inserted, the material of which it is constructed, and the technique of insertion.
3. Emboli. A clot or air may embolize to the digits, resulting in arteriolar spasm or more serious ischemic necrosis.
4. Disconnection of catheter from infusion system. Blood loss may be life-threatening, especially in the infant.
5. Ischemia. The radial artery cannula should be withdrawn if ischemic changes develop.

The previous method has described the traditional percutaneous radial artery cannulation at the ventral aspect of the wrist. The radial artery on the dorsal aspect of the wrist within the anatomical "snuff box" may be used as an alternative site.[81] Once an attempt at cannulation of the radial artery is made, the ulnar artery should be left untampered in order to assure adequate perfusion of the entire hand. Strict indica-

tions for the insertion of radial artery catheters are mandatory, and their removal considered at the earliest possible time.[90–100]

Temporal Artery

When the radial artery has been previously cannulated or is inaccessible, the temporal artery may be used.[101,102] Recently the serious complication of cerebral infarction has been described with this technique. The infarction appears to be related to retrograde embolization of air or blood clot.[103]

An advantage of this sampling site is that it provides preductal blood gas values. However, in our experience, the tortuous course of the artery and the resultant apposition of the distal tip of the catheter to the arterial wall have caused difficulties in freely drawing blood samples.

Technique. This artery may be cannulated either percutaneously or by direct cut down.[101,102,103]

Femoral Artery Cannulation

This site is more commonly used in adults. In situations where peripheral arterial cannulation is impossible, e.g., burned patients, the femoral artery may be utilized.[104]

Procedure. The femoral artery is located by palpation at the groin. Anatomically it is situated midway between the anterior superior iliac spine and the pubic tubercle.

After proper sterile preparation of the skin, a number 3 or 4 Cook catheter is inserted into the femoral artery using the

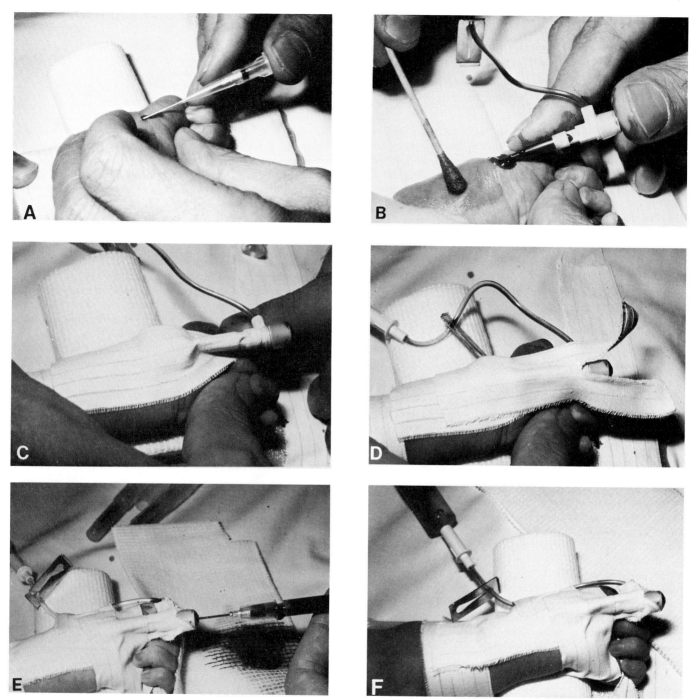

Figure 24-10. After adequate collateral circulation has been assured, the radial artery is palpated and the appropriate catheter advanced into the vessel (A). A T connector with appropriate flush solution is connected (B) and antibiotic ointment and benzoin are applied. A piece of tape is wrapped around the catheter and T connector (C). A second piece of tape torn down the center (D) is applied and wrapped around the catheter and T connector (E). Blood gas samples may be obtained by occluding the T connector, passing a small gauge needle into it, allowing a few drops of blood and flush solution to be drained, and then withdrawing the sample (F).

Seldinger technique. The artery is entered at the point of maximal pulsation, approximately one centimeter below the line joining the anterior superior iliac spine and the pubic tubercle. Following cannulation, the catheter is connected to a continuous flow system and transduced as described under the section on radial artery cannulation. The catheter is sutured in place and covered with antibiotic ointment and occlusive dressing. This is particularly important because of the likelihood of fecal and urinary contamination.

Complications:

1. Infection.
2. Emboli of clot and air leading to ischemic necrosis of the lower limb.

3. Poor arterial puncture technique has led to osteoarthritis of the hip joint. Severe trauma to the femoral artery has resulted in gangrene of the lower limb, retroperitoneal hemorrhage, and arteriovenous fistula formation.[104–105]

Dorsalis Pedis Artery Cannulation and Posterior Tibial Artery Cannulation

These are additional useful sites for arterial cannulation in children when more desirable locations are inaccessible. Collateral circulation should always be checked. Should one cannulate or attempt to cannulate one artery, the other should always be left free to ensure adequate collateral blood flow.

Procedure. The artery is cannulated in the same manner as the radial artery cannulation technique. The cannulation is attempted at a point of maximal pulsation. One should have a clear picture of the anatomy of the dorsalis pedis and posterior tibial arteries before attempting this procedure. If percutaneous cannulation is impossible, then the cut-down technique should be carried out to ensure successful cannulation.

PEDIATRIC VENTILATORS

It is always advantageous to have pediatric ventilators available. However, this is not always practical, and thus alternative techniques using adult ventilators must occasionally be adopted. Most adult ventilators used in the operating room are of the volume variety, i.e., the desired volume is delivered with each breath once this volume has been determined electronically, by adjusting the bellows, or adjusting inspiratory/expiratory (I/E) time and fresh gas flow. Setting the rate and tidal volume will determine minute ventilation. Pressure ventilators may be adjusted by altering flow and rate. Adjustment of the inspiratory-to-expiratory ratio may affect the amount of actual delivered ventilation with all ventilators, i.e., a shorter inspiratory time will usually deliver less volume to the patient, since a greater portion of the cycle is lost to compression of the circuit. An I/E ratio of 1:2 will usually be adequate for most children (with compliant lungs). Less compliant lungs will require a greater inspiratory time (I/E ratio 1:1, and occasionally 2:1). Newborns usually require a rate of 25 to 30 breaths each minute, children one to eight years old 12–15 breaths each minute, and children older than eight will usually be adequately ventilated at a rate of 8–10 breaths each minute, provided the correct inspiratory pressure and I:E ratio is selected.

GUIDELINES FOR SETTING UP A VENTILATOR

1. Open "pop-off" valve to anesthesia circuit.
2. Turn on ventilator and adjust to appropriate rate and tidal volume (10–15 ml/kg/breath to start).
3. Connect ventilator tubing to anesthesia circuit in place of anesthesia bag.
4. Gradually close pop-off valve until the peak inspiratory pressure (PIP) reaches 20–25 cm H_2O.
5. If PIP is 20–25, check breath sounds, symmetry of chest excursion, patient's color.
6. If PIP is less than 20 and pop-off is completely closed, increase tidal volume slowly so that the desired PIP and chest excursion is reached. Recheck step 5.

Note: some adult volume ventilators must be converted to pressure preset ventilators by leaving the pop-off valve partially open. For this situation frequent inspection of chest movement must be made, since accidental alteration of the pop-off, change in compliance, or airway resistance (kinked tube, mucus plug), might lead to clinically dangerous hypoventilation. Accidental closure of the pop-off in this circumstance would lead to hyperventilation, while opening of the pop-off would lead to hypoventilation. It is for these reasons that dedicated pediatric ventilators are most helpful and recommended.

If the patient has a small endotracheal tube, or poorly compliant lungs or chest wall, high inflation pressures may be required. In addition, the compression volume and compliance of each circuit is different, so that with very compliant circuits it is possible to have significant hypoventilation secondary to losses from stretching of the circuit. The addition of a heated humidifier will significantly decrease the efficiency of any anesthetic circuit (increased compression volume) and must be considered when added to the anesthesia system after the ventilator has been set. In addition, the rate of fresh gas flow into the circuit may also affect delivered minute ventilation, even with circle systems. (See Fig. 23-7)

In summary, the anesthesiologist setting a ventilator for pediatric use must consider the circuits utilized, humidification, chest wall and pulmonary compliance, airway resistance (small diameter tube), peak inspiratory pressure, chest movement, breath sounds, patient color, I/E ratio, and fresh gas flow into the circuit. Yet despite considering all of the above, the only accurate way to assess adequacy of ventilation is to measure end-tidal or arterial carbon dioxide tensions, and closely observe the patient.

REFERENCES

1. Duma RJ, Warner JF, Dalton HP: Septicemia from intravenous infusions. *N Engl J Med* 284:257–260, 1971
2. Collins RN, Braun PA, Zinner SH, et al: Risk of local and systemic infection with polyethylene intravenous catheters—a prospective study of 213 catheterizations. *N Engl J Med* 279:240–243, 1968
3. Smits H, Freedman LR: Prolonged venous catheterization as cause of sepsis. *N Engl J Med* 276:1229–1233, 1967
4. Cheney FW, Jr, Lincoln JR: Phlebitis from plastic intravenous catheters. *Anesthesiology* 25:650–652, 1964
5. Yosowitz P, Ekland DA, Shaw RL, et al: Peripheral intravenous infiltration necrosis. *Ann Surg* 182:553–556, 1975
6. Haynes RC, Jr, Murad F: Agents affecting calcification: Calcium, parathyroid hormone, calcitonin, vitamin D, and other compounds, in Gilman AG, Goodman LS, Gilman A (eds): *The Pharmacological Basis of Therapeutics.* New York, Macmillan, 1980
7. Moran JM, Atwood RP, Rowe MI: A clinical and bacteriologic study of infections associated with venous cutdowns. *N Engl J Med* 272:554–560, 1965
8. Seldinger SI: Catheter replacement of the needle in percutaneous arteriography. *Acta Radiol* 39:368–376, 1953
9. Coté CJ, Jobes DR, Schwartz AJ, et al: Two approaches to cannulation of a child's internal jugular vein. *Anesthesiology* 50:371–373, 1979
10. Prince SR, Sullivan RL, Hackel A: Percutaneous catheterization of the internal jugular vein in infants and children. *Anesthesiology* 44:170–174, 1976
11. Schwartz AJ, Jobes DR, Levy WJ, et al: Intrathoracic vascular

catheterization via the external jugular vein. *Anesthesiology* 56:400–402, 1982

12. Blitt CD, Wright WA, Petty WC, et al: Central venous catheterization via the external jugular vein—a technique employing the J-wire. *JAMA* 229:817–818, 1974

13. Belani KG, Buckley JJ, Gordon JR, et al: Percutaneous cervical central venous line placement: A comparison of the internal and external jugular vein routes. *Anesth Analg* 59:40–44, 1980

14. Blitt CD, Carlson GL, Wright WA, et al: J-wire versus straight wire for central venous system cannulation via the external jugular vein. *Anesth Analg* 61:536–537, 1982

15. Stoelting RK: Evaluation of external jugular venous pressure as a reflection of right atrial pressure. *Anesthesiology* 38:291–294, 1973

16. Brinkman AJ, Costley DO: Internal jugular venipuncture. *JAMA* 223:182–183, 1973

17. Jernigan WR, Gardner WC, Mahr MM, et al: Use of the internal jugular vein for placement of central venous catheter. *Surg Gynec Obstet* 130:520–524, 1970

18. Mostert JW, Kenny GM, Murphy GP: Safe placement of central venous catheter into internal jugular vein. *Arch Surg* 101:431–432, 1970

19. Boulanger M, Delva E, Maille, J-G, et al: Une nouvelle voie d'abord de la veine jugulaire interne. *Can Anaesth Soc J* 23:609–615, 1976

20. Civetta JM, Gabel JC, Gemer M: Internal-jugular-vein puncture with a margin of safety. *Anesthesiology* 36:622–623, 1972

21. Rao TLK, Wong AY, Salem MR: A new approach to percutaneous catheterization of the internal jugular vein. *Anesthesiology* 46:362–364, 1977

22. Tsueda K, Jean-Francois JL, Gonzales EC: Cannulation of the superior vena cava—a new approach. *Anesthesiology* 40:304–307, 1974

23. English ICW, Frew RM, Pigott JF, et al: Percutaneous catheterization of the internal jugular vein. *Anesthesiology* 24:521–531, 1969

24. Daily PO, Griepp RB, Shumway WE: Percutaneous internal jugular vein cannulation. *Arch Surg* 101:534–536, 1970

25. Borja AR: Current status of infraclavicular–subclavian vein catheterization. *Ann Thorac Surg* 13:615–624, 1972

26. Groff DB: Complications of intravenous hyperalimentation in newborns and infants. *J Pediatr Surg* 4:460–464, 1969

27. Phillips SJ: Technique of percutaneous subclavian vein catheterization. *Surg Gynecol Obstet* 127:1079–1080, 1968

28. Defalque RJ: Subclavian venipuncture: A review. *Anesth Analg* 47:677–682, 1968

29. Butts DR, Glass HG: Percutaneous subclavian vein catherization in children. *Texas Med* 66:46–48, 1970

30. Filston HC, Grant JP: A safer system for percutaneous subclavian venous catherization in newborn infants. *J Pediatr Surg* 14:564–570, 1979

31. Groff DB, Ahmed N: Subclavian vein catherization in the infant. *J Pediatr Surg* 9:171–174, 1974

32. Klein MD, Rudd M: Successful central venous catheter placement from peripheral subcutaneous veins in children. *Anesthesiology* 52:447–448, 1980

33. Richards CC, Freeman A: Intra-atrial catheter placement under electrocardiographic guidance. *Anesthesiology* 25:388–391, 1964

34. Holt MH: Central venous pressures via peripheral veins. *Anesthesiology* 28:1093–1095, 1967

35. Kuramoto T, Sakabe T: Comparison of success in jugular versus basilic vein technique for central venous pressure catheter positioning. *Anesth Analg* 54:696–697, 1975

36. Webre DR, Arens JF: Use of cephalic and basilic veins for introduction of ventral venous catheters. *Anesthesiology* 38:389–392, 1973

37. Burgess GE, III, Marino RJ, Peuler MJ: Effect of head position on the location of venous catheters inserted via basilic veins. *Anesthesiology* 46:212–213, 1977

38. Hill GJ, II: Central venous pressure technique. *Surg Clin North Am* 49:1351–1359, 1969

39. Bansmer G, Keith D, Tesluk H: Complications following use of indwelling catheters of inferior vena cava. *JAMA* 167:1606–1611, 1958

40. Forrester JS, Ganz W, Diamond G, et al: Thermodilution cardiac output determination with a single flow-directed catheter. *Am Heart J* 83:306–311, 1972

41. Swan HJC, Ganz W, Forester J, et al: Catheterization of the heart in man with use of a flow directed balloon-tipped catheter. *N Engl J Med* 283:447–451, 1970

42. Swan HJC: The role of hemodynamic monitoring in the management of the critically ill. *Crit Care Med* 3:83–89, 1975

43. Todres ID, Crone RK, Rogers MC, et al: Swan-Ganz catheterization in the critically ill newborn. *Crit Care Med* 7:330–334, 1979

44. deLange SS, Boscoe MJ, Stanley TH: Percutaneous pulmonary artery catheterization via the arm before anesthesia: Success rate, frequency of complications, and arterial pressure and heart rate response. *Br J Anaesth* 53:1167–1172, 1981

45. Marshall WK, Bedford RF: Use of a pulmonary-artery catheter for detection and treatment of venous air embolism: A prospective study in man. *Anesthesiology* 52:131–134, 1980

46. Berry AJ, Geer RT, Marshall BE: Alteration of pulmonary blood flow by pulmonary artery occluded pressure measurement. *Anesthesiology* 51:164–166, 1979

47. Chun GMH, Ellestad MH: Perforation of the pulmonary artery by Swan-Ganz catheter, *N Engl J Med* 284:1041–1042, 1972

48. Kim YL, Richman KA, Marshall BE: Thrombocytopenia associated with Swan-Ganz catheterization in patients. *Anesthesiology* 53:261–262, 1980

49. Hoar PF, Stone JG, Wicks AE, et al: Thrombogenesis associated with Swan-Ganz catheters. *Anesthesiology* 48:445–447, 1978

50. Richman KA, Kim YL, Marshall BE: Thrombocytopenia and altered platelet kinetics associated with prolonged pulmonary-artery catheterization in the dog. *Anesthesiology* 53:101–105, 1980

51. Foote GA, Schabel SI, Hodges M: Pulmonary complications of the flow-directed balloon-tipped catheter. *N Engl J Med* 290:927–931, 1974

52. Doblar DD, Hinkle JC, Fay ML, et al: Air embolism associated with pulmonary artery introducer kit. *Anesthesiology* 56:389–391, 1982

53. Conahan TJ, III: Air embolism during percutaneous Swan-Ganz catheter placement. *Anesthesiology* 50:360–361, 1979

54. Cote' CJ: A simple technique to avoid over distension of flow directed catheters. *Anesthesiology* 49:154, 1978

55. Kitterman JA, Phibbs RH, Tooley WH: Catheterization of umbilical vessels in newborn infants. *Pediatr Clin North Am* 17:895–906, 1970

56. Symansky MR, Fox HA: Umbilical vessel catheterization. Indications, management and evaluation of the technique. *J Pediatr* 80:820–826, 1972

57. Erkan V, Blankenship W, Stahlman MT: The complications of chronic umbilical vessel catheterization. *Pediatr Res* 2:317, 1968

58. Vos LJM, Potocky V, Broker FHL, et al: Splenic vein thrombosis with esophageal varices: A late complication of umbilical vein catheterization. *Ann Surg* 180:152–156, 1974

59. Brans YW, Ceballos R, Cassady G: Umbilical catheters and hepatic abscesses. *Pediatrics* 53:264–266, 1974

60. Fey D, Perrotta L: Peritoneal perforation resulting from umbilical vein catheterization: An unusual pattern. *J Pediatr* 83:501, 1973

61. Scott JM: Iatrogenic lesions in babies following umbilical vein catheterization. *Arch Dis Child* 40:426–429, 1965

62. Krauss AN, Albert RF, Kannan MM: Contamination of umbilical catheters in the newborn infant. *J Pediatr* 77:965–969, 1970

63. Cole AFD, Rolbin SH: A technique for rapid catherization of the umbilical artery. *Anesthesiology* 53:254–255, 1980

64. Sherman NJ: Umbilical artery cutdown. *J Pediatr Surg* 12:723–724, 1977

65. Tooley WH: What is the risk of an umbilical artery catheter? *Pediatrics* 50:1–2, 1972

66. Vidyasagar D, Downes JJ, Boggs TR, Jr: Respiratory distress syndrome of newborn infants. II. Technique of catheterization of umbilical artery and clinical results of treatment of 124 patients. *Clin Pediatr* 9:332–337, 1970

67. Gregory GA: Resuscitation of the newborn. *Anesthesiology* 43:225–237, 1975

68. Cochran WA, Davis HT, Smith CA: Advantages and complications of umbilical artery catheterization in the newborn. *Pediatrics* 42:769–777, 1968

69. Neal WA, Reynolds JW, Jarvis CW, et al: Umbilical artery catheterization: Demonstration of arterial thrombosis by aortography. *Pediatrics* 50:6–13, 1972

70. Bauer SB, Feldman SM, Gellis SS, et al: Neonatal hypertension, a complication of umbilical artery catheterization. *N Engl J Med* 293:1032–1033, 1975

71. Plumer LB, Kaplan GW, Mendoza SA: Hypertension in infants—a complication of umbilical arterial catheterization. *J Pediatr* 89:802–805, 1976

72. Rudolph N, Wang HH, Dragutsky D: Gangrene of the buttock: A complication of umbilical artery catheterization. *Pediatrics* 53:106–109, 1974

73. Knudsen FU, Petersen S: Neonatal septic osteo-arthritis due to umbilical artery catheterization. *Acta Paediatr* 66:225–227, 1977

74. Fort KT, Teplick SK, Clark RE: Renal artery embolism causing neonatal hypertension. *Radiol* 113:169–170, 1974

75. Andersson A, Hofer PA, Holmlund DEW, et al: Colonic perforation secondary to thrombo-embolus from an umbilical artery catheter. *Acta Paediatr Scand* 63:155–156, 1974

76. Symchych PS, Krauss AN, Winchester P: Endocarditis following intracardiac placement of umbilical venous catheters in neonates. *J Pediatr* 90:287–289, 1977

77. Goetzman BW, Stadalnik RC, Bogren HG, et al: Thrombotic complications of umbilical artery catheters: A clinical and radiographic study. *Pediatrics* 56:374–379, 1975

78. Powers WF, Swyer PR: Limb blood flow following umbilical arterial catheterization. *Pediatrics* 55:248–256, 1975

79. Todres ID, Rogers MC, Shannon DC, et al: Percutaneous catheterization of the radial artery in the critically ill neonate. *J Pediatr* 87:273–275, 1975

80. Cole FS, Todres ID, Shannon DC: Technique for percutaneous cannulation of the radial artery in the newborn infant. *J Pediatr* 92:105–107, 1978

81. Amato JJ, Solod E, Cleveland RJ: A "second" radial artery for monitoring the perioperative pediatric cardiac patient. *J Pediatr Surg* 12:715–717, 1977

82. Ryan JF, Raines J, Dalton BC, et al: Arterial dynamics of radial artery cannulation. *Anesth Analg* 52:1017–1023, 1973

83. Allen EV: Thromboangiitis obliterans: Methods of diagnosis of chronic occlusive arterial lesions distal to the wrist with illustrative cases. *Am J Med Sci* 178:237–244, 1929

84. Brodsky JB, Wong AL, Meyer JA: Percutaneous cannulation of weakly palpable arteries. *Anesth Analg* 56:448, 1977

85. Buakham C, Kim JM: Cannulation of a nonpalpable artery with aid of a doppler monitor. *Anesth Analg* 56:125–126, 1977

86. Morray J-P, Brandford HG, Barnes LF, et al. Doppler-assisted radial artery cannulation in infants and children. *Anesth-Analg.* 63(3):346–348, 1984.

87. Shinozaki T, Deane RS, Mazuzan JE: The dynamic responses ofliquid-filled cathter systems for direct measurement of blood pressure. *Anesthesiology* 53:498–504, 1980

88. Galvis AG, Donahoo JS, White JJ: An improved technique for prolonged arterial catheterization in infants and children. *Crit Care Med* 4:166–169, 1976

89. Lowenstein E, Little JW, III, Hing HL: Prevention of cerebral embolization from flushing radial artery cannulas. *N Engl J Med* 285:1414–1415, 1971

90. Miyasaka K, Edmonds JF, Conn AW: Complications of radial artery lines in the paediatric patient. *Can Anaesth Soc J* 23:9–14, 1976

91. Hager DL, Wilson JN: Gangrene of the hand following intra-arterial injection. *Arch Surg* 94:86–89, 1967

92. Knill RL, Evans D: Pathogenesis of gangrene following intra-arterial injection of drugs: A new hypothesis. *Can Anaesth Soc J* 22:637–646, 1975

93. Katz AM, Birnbaum M, Moylan J, et al: Gangrene of the hand and forearm: A complication of radial-artery cannulation. *Crit Care Med* 2:270–272, 1974

94. Downs JB, Rackstein AD, Klein EF Jr, et al: Hazards of radial-artery catheterization. *Anesthesiology* 38:283–286, 1973

95. Johnson RW: A complication of radial-artery cannulation. *Anesthesiology* 40:598–600, 1974

96. Bedford RF, Wollman H: Complications of percutaneous radial-artery cannulation: An objective prospective study in man. *Anesthesiology* 38:228–236, 1973

97. Bedford RF: Percutaneous radial-artery cannulation—increased safety using Teflon catheters. *Anesthesiology* 42:219–222, 1975

98. Bedford RF: Radial arterial function following percutaneous cannulation with 18- and 20-gauge catheters. *Anesthesiology* 47:37–39, 1977

99. Jones RM, Hill AB, Nahrwald ML, et al: The effect of the method of radial artery cannulation on post cannulation blood flow and thrombus formation. *Anesthesiology* 55:76–78, 1981

100. Davis FM: Radial artery cannulation: Influence of catheter size and material on arterial occlusion. *Anaesth Intensive Care* 6:49–53, 1978

101. Gauderer M, Holfersen LO: Peripheral arterial line insertion in neonates and infants: A simplified method of temporal artery cannulation. *J Pediatr Surg* 9:875–877, 1974

102. McGovern B, Baker AR: Temporal artery catheterization for the monitoring of blood gases in infants. *Surg Gynecol Obstet* 127:600–602, 1968

103. Prian GW, Wright GB, Rumack CM, et al: Apparent cerebral embolization after temporal artery catheterization. *J Pediatr* 93:115–118, 1978

104. Park MK, Guntheroth WG: Direct blood pressure measurements in brachial and femoral arteries in children. *Circulation* 41:231–237, 1970

105. McKay RK, Jr: Thrombosis of the femoral artery following femoral venipuncture. *Pediatrics* 40:319, 1967

Index

RESUSCITATION DRUGS

	Dilution	Dose
Epinephrine	1 mg + 9 ml saline = 1:10,000	10 μg/kg (0.1 ml)
Sodium bicarbonate	1 mEq/ml	1-2 mEq (1-2 ml)/kg
Atropine	1.0 mg/ml	0.02 mg/kg
Calcium Chloride	100 mg/ml (10%)	5 mg (0.05 ml)/kg
Calcium Gluconate	100 mg/ml (10%)	15 mg (0.15 ml)/kg
Lidocaine	20 mg/ml (2%)	1 mg (0.05 ml)/kg

VASOPRESSORS

	Dilution	
Epinephrine	1 mg (1 ml)/100 ml = 10 μg/ml	
	start 0.1 μg/kg/min	
	0.01 ml/kg/min	
	0.6 ml/kg/hr	
Isoproterenol	1 mg (5 ml)/100 ml = 10 μg/ml	
	start 0.1 μg/kg/min	
	0.01 ml/kg/min	
	0.6 ml/kg/hr	
Neosynephrine	1 mg (1 ml)/100 ml = 10 μg/ml	
	start 0.1 μg/kg/min	
	0.01 ml/kg/min	
	0.6 ml/kg/hr	
Dopamine	30 mg (0.75 ml)/100 ml = 300 μg/ml	
	start 5 μg/kg/min	
	0.017 ml/kg/min	
	1.0 ml/kg/hr	

DEFIBRILLATION

start at two watt-seconds/kg. Increase until effective (double-dosing).
(check acid/base status and correct before increasing dose to high levels to optimize defibrillation.)

ANESTHETIC DRUGS

Drug	Dose/kg	Intravenous	Intramuscular	Rectal
VAGOLYTIC				
Atropine	mg	0.01–0.02	0.02	
Scopolamine	mg	0.005–0.01	0.01 up to 0.6 mg	
Glycopyrrolate	mg	0.005–0.01	0.01	
NARCOTICS				
Morphine	mg	0.1–0.2	0.1–0.2	
Meperidine	mg	1–2	1–2	
Fentanyl	μg	1–2	1–2	
MUSCLE RELAXANTS				
Succinylcholine	mg	1–2	4–5	
Curare	mg	0.3–0.6		
Metacurine	mg	0.2–0.4		
Pancuronium	mg	0.05–0.10		
Atracurium	mg	0.3–0.6		
Vecuronium	mg	0.05–0.10		
SEDATIVES/ANESTHETICS				
Thiopental	mg	4–6		20–30
Methohexital	mg	1–3		20–30
Diazepam	mg	0.1–0.3		0.1–0.3
Ketamine	mg	0.5–2.0	5–8	